MEDICAL MICROBIOLOGY

VOLUME 1

FOUNDATIONS OF INFECTION, IMMUNITY, AND DIAGNOSTICS

Ankur Mittal

ALLIED HEALTH PRESS

Medical Microbiology

Volume 1: Foundations of Infection, Immunity, and Diagnostics

Author: **Ankur Mittal**

Allied Health Press
4164 Lakeshore Road
Burlington ON L7L 1A4
Canada
www.alliedhealthpress.com
Email: orders@arclereducation.com

ISBN: 978-1-77956-780-2

ABOUT THE AUTHOR

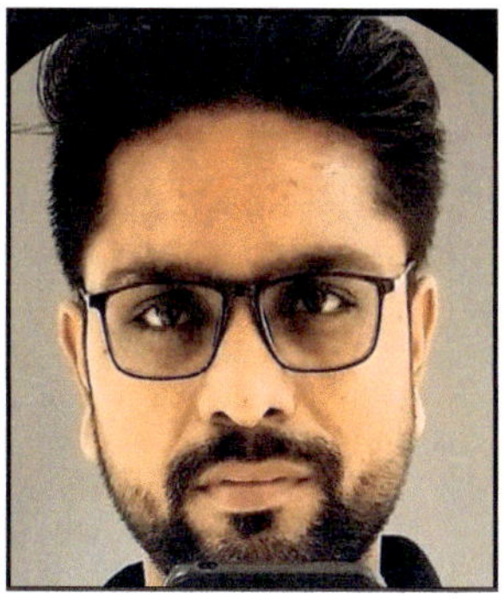

Ankur Mittal is a dedicated biomedical researcher specializing in molecular biology, microbiology, and clinical biochemistry, currently engaged in basic research on infectious and metabolic diseases. His work focuses on developing rapid molecular diagnostic platforms for Fungal Endophthalmitis and employing metagenomic sequencing for advanced microbial characterization. His research aims to integrate molecular diagnostics with clinical applications to enhance early disease detection and therapeutic outcomes.

He previously contributed to significant projects exploring Diabetic Retinopathy (DR) and Age-Related Macular Degeneration (AMD), particularly investigating the role and balance of VEGF165 and VEGF165b proteins in pathological angiogenesis. His work elucidated mechanisms underlying impaired protein expression in retinal disorders, contributing to a deeper understanding of molecular processes in ocular pathology.

Mr. Mittal completed his Master of Science (M.Sc.) in Biochemistry from the Postgraduate Institute of Medical Education and Research (PGIMER), Chandigarh (2014–2016), where he specialized in cell and molecular biology, immunogenetics, bioinformatics, and gene-based diagnostics. He earned his Bachelor of Science (B.Sc.) in Microbiology from Delhi University (2010–2013), graduating with a strong foundation in medical, industrial, and molecular microbiology.

His research contributions are documented through publications in reputed journals, including Kidney Diseases (2018), International Journal of Drug Development & Research (2016), and Pharmacology Research (2016). Additionally, he has presented his work at several national scientific conferences, such as ACBICON 2015 and the National Conference on Frontiers in Applied Biotechnology, and has participated in numerous workshops on flow cytometry, big data science, immunology, and biotechnology at leading institutions such as INSA, ILBS, and TERI University.

Brief Table of Contents

Getting Started with This Book

Chapter Openers

A list of Chapter Outline is presented providing a brief Introduction to what will be covered in the chapter.

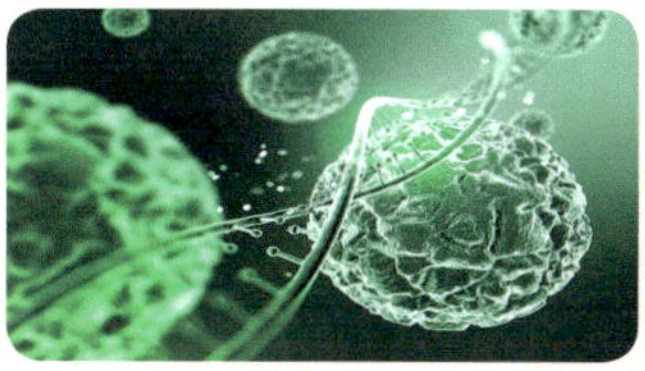

LEARNING OBJECTIVES

After studying this chapter, you will be able to:

1. Discuss the scientific method in biology;
2. Explain the cell theory;
3. Discuss the genetics and heredity;
4. Evolution and natural selection;
5. Focus on ecology and ecosystems;
6. Learn about human biology;
7. Evaluate the plant biology;
8. Explain the microbiology;
9. Focus on current trends in biology.

Introduction

Often referred to as the science of life, biology is a broad field of study aimed at comprehending the several kinds of life on Earth, from tiny creatures to sophisticated multicellular entities. Comprising several subfields, including molecular biology, ecology, and evolutionary biology, each of which advances our knowledge of living systems, this field clarifies the mechanisms controlling life events, including development, reproduction, and interaction with the surroundings, which is the central goal of biology. Moreover, biology fills in the void between the natural sciences and medicine by offering a necessary understanding of health, illness, and the interactions between organisms and their environments. Dealing with urgent global issues such as climate change, biodiversity loss, and new diseases depends on an awareness of these complex biological interactions, therefore highlighting the critical part biology plays in modern civilization. Fundamentally, biology explores and tests ideas about the living world using the scientific method. Through methodical observation and experimentation,

1.1. The Scientific Method in Biology

Learning Outcome

1. Describe the steps of the scientific method;
2. Focus on hypothesis formation;
3. Learn about experimental design.

Learning Outcomes

The beginning of each section of every chapter contains a set of Learning Outcomes that inform students of concepts they should understand. These outcomes help students understand what they should be able to do if they have mastered the material in that section.

Test Your Knowledge

Throughout each chapter, Test Your Knowledge cues you to note which topics have been covered and to self-test your understanding of the material presented.

Test Your Knowledge

1. Explain why correlation does not imply causation in scientific experiments.
2. How does the scientific method help reduce the influence of personal opinions in research?

Chapter Summary

The Summary Section appear at the end of each chapter and summarize main concepts covered throughout the chapter. These points provide key concepts in an engaging and meaningful way.

Summary

The investigation of biological principles highlights the importance of a comprehensive view of life by reflecting the intricate interactions that occur within living systems. The complexity of biology goes beyond individual species or systems, as this essay highlights; it also includes the interactions that mold ecosystems and affect biodiversity. Researchers can conduct in-depth analyses of metabolomic data using sophisticated technologies like MetaboAnalyst, which offer insights into the molecular mechanisms underlying these interactions. As demonstrated by the developments in MetaboAnalyst, for example, the integration of diverse omics data promotes a thorough understanding of metabolic pathways and helps identify important biological markers necessary for research on development and disease (Chong et al., 2018). Additionally, the phenomenon of ecological invasions is a key component of biological research and a vital field of study. The introduction of non-native species into unfamiliar habitats has significant ramifications and calls for multidisciplinary management strategies. Examining the origins and effects of these biological incursions, invasion science has become a crucial field that highlights the need to comprehend ecological dynamics and community interactions. As interest in biological invasions increases, new findings are emerging that put conventional ecological theories and practices to the test. The importance of incorporating various scientific viewpoints is shown by this developing discipline, which also highlights how invasive species shape ecosystems and advances our knowledge of ecological resilience (David et al., 2013). When taken as a whole, these discoveries from invasion science and metabolomics highlight the value of multidisciplinary biology research. Fostering cross-disciplinary collaboration and utilizing technological breakthroughs to improve our comprehension of intricate biological interactions are crucial as we look to the future of biological research. In addition to deepening our understanding of the complexities of life, this method lays the groundwork for tackling urgent environmental issues. Future studies can ensure the continued relevance of biology in a world that is constantly changing by acknowledging the interconnection of biological systems and opening the door to creative solutions that support sustainability and biodiversity conservation. We might imagine a thorough comprehension of life that serves both academia and society at large through ongoing investigation and integration of scientific knowledge.

Knowledge Assessment

The chapter includes material designed to review and reinforce each content. It includes Critical Thinking Questions to help test of your understanding of information presented in the chapter and Short answer Questions to review your understanding of the key concepts presented in the chapter.

Critical Thinking Questions

1. **Who is known as the "Father of Modern Biology"?**
   a. Aristotle
   b. Charles Darwin
   c. Gregor Mendel
   d. Louis Pasteur
2. **What is the basic unit of life?**
   a. Atom
   b. Molecule
   c. Cell
   d. Organism
3. **Which branch of biology studies the interaction of organisms with their environment?**
   a. Genetics
   b. Ecology
   c. Physiology
   d. Botany
4. **Which macromolecule is the main source of energy for living organisms?**
   a. Proteins
   b. Lipids
   c. Carbohydrates
   d. Nucleic acids
5. **DNA is primarily responsible for which function in living organisms?**
   a. Energy production
   b. Protein synthesis
   c. Storing genetic information
   d. Regulating body temperature

Short Answer Questions

1. What is biology, and why is it important to study biology?
2. What are the three main domains of life, and how are they different from one another?
3. Define homeostasis and give an example of how it works in living organisms.
4. What is the cell theory, and why is it fundamental to biology?
5. How do autotrophs and heterotrophs differ in the way they obtain energy?
6. What is the scientific method, and how is it applied in biological research?
7. Discuss how biology helps address global challenges such as climate change, disease, and food security.
8. Explain the levels of biological organization from the smallest unit to the largest. Provide examples at each level.
9. Describe the relationship between structure and function in biology, giving specific examples from cells or organs.
10. How has the discovery of genetics shaped our understanding of inheritance and variation among organisms?

Supplementary Materials

Key Terms: A list of key terms is given for quick reference

KEY TERMS FROM THIS CHAPTER

Annotation enrichment analysis	Biological structure	Cell
Cell theory	Cellular structure	Ecology
Ecosystems	Genetics	Human biology
Microbiology	Natural selection	Organism
Plant biology		

Further Resources: Recommendations for additional readings, websites, and multimedia resources.

References

1. Argelaguet, R., Velten, B., Arnol, D., Dietrich, S., Zenz, T., Marioni, J. C., Buettner, F., et al. (2018). Multi-omics factor analysis—A framework for unsupervised integration of multi-omics data sets. *Molecular Systems Biology, 14*. https://doi.org/10.15252/msb.20178124.
2. Bacher, S., Blackburn, T. M., Essl, F., & Genovesi, P. (2017). *Socio-Economic Impact Classification of Alien Taxa (SEICAT)*. https://core.ac.uk/download/286567949.pdf (accessed on 8th March 2025).
3. Barnett, R., Brace, S., Cucchi, T., & Dobney, K. (2013). *Divergent Evolutionary Processes Associated with Colonization of Offshore Islands*. https://core.ac.uk/download/20664364.pdf (accessed on 8th March 2025).

Detailed Table of Contents

CHAPTER 5

Bacterial Structure and Genetics 143

CHAPTER 6

Gram-positive Cocci 179

CHAPTER 7

Gram-Negative Cocci 215

CHAPTER 8

Gram-positive Bacilli 247

CHAPTER 9

Gram-Negative Bacilli 277

CHAPTER 12

Cells and Organs of the Immune System 383

CHAPTER 13

Hypersensitivity and Autoimmunity 419

Index 455

LIST OF FIGURES

PREFACE

Clinical microbiology is a core discipline in the explanation of the clinical and biological nature of infectious diseases. It is the scientific foundation on which identification of the pathogenic microorganisms, their patterns of spread, and studies on how they interact with the human host are based. Medical microbiology supports a range of clinical activities that include diagnosis and treatment, prevention, and planning for public health. As infectious diseases continue to pose a serious worldwide threat, especially with the threat of antibiotic resistance and new pathogens arising, the role of medical microbiology continues only to grow stronger. Clinical clinicians rely on reliable microbiological information to be able to make accurate and timely decisions that protect patient health and limit outbreaks at the community level.

Medical microbiology extends beyond the classroom and laboratory; it is practiced in hospitals, clinics, and research centers where microbial threats are met daily. To be familiar with pathogens in and out, how they are built, how they invade and affect the human host, and how the immune system responds to them, is fundamental to medicine today. From detecting bacterial forms under the microscope to differentiating immune responses during infection, the field is a combination of basic science and clinical practice. Training students, scientists, and clinicians in this helps build solid healthcare systems and improve patient outcomes worldwide.

The *Medical Microbiology Volume 1* publication is intended to be an exhaustive scholarly textbook for learners and practitioners requiring a comprehensive and organized approach to the subject. The volume establishes a firm foundation in the biological concepts of microbiology with specific emphasis on microorganisms that are of medical importance. The aim is to present clear and clinically applicable information that facilitates theoretical learning and practical use. The book integrates fundamental biological concepts with an in-depth study of microbial populations and immune responses, giving useful information for the comprehension of infectious diseases and their therapy.

Chapter 1 provides a general overview of medical microbiology, the historical development, clinical relevance, and the role of healthcare in the contemporary age. It emphasizes what types of microorganisms are studied under this science, such as bacteria, viruses, fungi, and parasites, and familiarizes readers with terminology and classification systems employed throughout the book. It also addresses the importance of aseptic technique and culture methodology and biosafety practices.

Chapter 2 focuses on staining and microscopy procedures and their principles and applications. The chapter outlines the different types of microscopes used in medical microbiology, namely bright-field, phase-contrast, and fluorescence microscopy. The chapter continues with descriptions of staining procedures such as Gram staining, acid-fast staining, and special stains used to identify certain cellular constituents or microorganisms. The rationale and diagnostic significance of each technique are discussed below in order to enlighten readers as to how visual identification supports clinical microbiology.

Chapter 3 describes various methods used for microorganism identification. It elaborates on culture characteristics, biochemical tests, molecular techniques, and immunological assays. The chapter also refers to automated identification systems that are now common in the clinical laboratory. It provides examples of the identification of pathogens in real-life diagnostic settings, with emphasis on accuracy and efficiency in clinical microbiology.

Chapter 4 explains how microorganisms interact with the host and cause disease. It summarizes microbial colonization, entry into the body, mechanisms of damage, and host responses. Special emphasis is laid on virulence factors, e.g., toxins and enzymes, that play a part in pathogenicity. The chapter also deals with patterns of infection, e.g., localized and systemic infections, and outlines the general principles of disease progression and symptomatology.

Chapter 5 covers bacterial genetics and structure. This entails the detailed coverage of bacterial cell walls, membranes, cytoplasmic structures, and appendages like pili and flagella. Replication, mutation, and expression of bacterial genetic material are covered. Plasmids, transposons, and methods of genetic transfer such as conjugation, transformation, and transduction are covered in the chapter, which are beneficial in terms of antibiotic resistance and diversity of strains.

Chapter 6 explores the group of Gram-positive cocci, focusing on clinically significant genera such as *Staphylococcus* and *Streptococcus*. It includes their classification, laboratory identification features, virulence attributes, and the diseases they cause. The clinical importance of antibiotic susceptibility testing is highlighted along with current treatment options. The chapter also outlines infection control practices relevant to hospital settings, where these organisms are common culprits.

Chapter 7 extends this discussion to Gram-negative cocci, particularly the genus *Neisseria*. The focus is on organisms like *Neisseria meningitidis* and *Neisseria gonorrhoeae*, their routes of transmission, diagnostic markers, and epidemiological patterns. Vaccine strategies and antibiotic resistance issues are included to provide a current view of how these pathogens are managed in public health and clinical contexts.

Chapter 8 shifts to Gram-positive bacilli, including both spore-forming and non-spore-forming organisms. Bacteria such as *Bacillus anthracis, Clostridium* species, *Listeria monocytogenes*, and *Corynebacterium diphtheriae* are discussed in terms of morphology, pathogenesis, and laboratory identification. Particular attention is paid to the clinical conditions caused by these organisms, ranging from tetanus to listeriosis, and their public health implications.

Chapter 9 covers Gram-negative bacilli, a medically very significant group of diverse bacteria. The chapter categorizes them based on their oxygen requirement and metabolic characteristics and covers *Escherichia coli, Klebsiella, Pseudomonas, Salmonella, Shigella*, and others. Every genus is addressed in terms of its pathogenic characteristics, resistance patterns, and treatment implications. Case studies and outbreak examples help bridge theoretical understanding to practice in the clinic.

Chapter 10 enters and discusses acid-fast bacteria with special emphasis on *Mycobacterium* species such as *M. tuberculosis* and *M. leprae*. The chapter explains why acid-fastness is such a significant trait when it comes to diagnosis and how unique staining and culture methods are employed. The diseases they cause, including tuberculosis and leprosy, are discussed in detail with emphasis on global health concerns, vaccine research, and multi-drug resistance strains.

Chapter 11 warns us of the immunological foundations pertaining to microbial infections. Chapter 11 provides an initial outline of the organization of the innate and adaptive immune system and explains the generation of immune responses. The roles of antigens, antibodies, complement proteins, and cytokines are introduced, to be further explained in greater detail later in later chapters.

Chapter 12 deals with the individual cells and organs of the immune system. It goes into detail about the function of lymphocytes, macrophages, dendritic cells, and other immune components. The function of primary and secondary lymphoid organs is explained in terms of immune maturation and response. The interaction of these components in the scenario of microbial infection is addressed in relation to real examples.

Chapter 13 addresses hypersensitivity and autoimmunity. It classifies hypersensitivity reactions into four groups and describes their mechanisms by way of clinical examples such as anaphylaxis, hemolytic anemia, and serum sickness. Autoimmunity presentation addresses diseases such as rheumatoid arthritis, systemic lupus erythematosus, and type 1 diabetes, highlighting diagnostic markers and possible inducers responsible for causing immune misrecognition of self-tissues.

The book is intended for undergraduate and postgraduate students of medical, dental, and allied health sciences. It will also be suitable for microbiologists, laboratory technologists, clinicians, and medical practitioners who need a sound grounding in clinical microbiology. The book will find favour with teachers and researchers as a teaching and consultation reference, and with examination students due to the logical arrangement and easy explanations.

INTRODUCTION TO MEDICAL MICROBIOLOGY

1

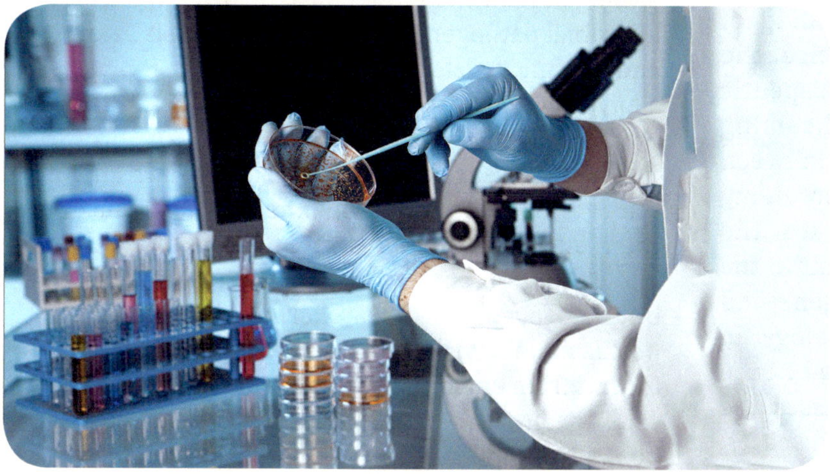

LEARNING OBJECTIVES

After studying this chapter, you will be able to:

1. Understand the types of microorganisms
2. Discuss about pathogenesis of infectious diseases
3. Describe diagnostic techniques in medical microbiology
4. Define antimicrobial agents
5. Focus on infection control and prevention
6. Explain how emerging infectious diseases pose significant challenges to global public health

Introduction

The field of medical microbiology is an important contact area between the medical sciences and microbiology, focusing on the role of microorganisms in human disease and health. Perception of the wide variety of pathogens, including bacteria, viruses, fungi, and parasites, is vital to make diagnoses and treat infectious disease. This initial exposure sets the stage for appreciation of host-pathogen interactions, which are critical for the design of effective therapeutic regimens. Understandable knowledge of medical microbiology not only helps clinicians identify and neutralize infecting hazards but also determines preventive strategies and public health policy. Increased international travel and trade cause the effects of microbial infections to extend beyond a single case, and a firm grasp of microbial pathogenesis and epidemiology is mandatory. Through this foundation, the discipline teaches students to practice in the evolving environment of infectious disease care in contemporary medicine. Within medical microbiology, the laboratory plays a central role as the front desk for diagnosis and research. Through the application of techniques such as culture, microscopy, and molecular biology, medical microbiologists can identify and determine pathogens so clinicians can make informed treatment decisions. Furthermore, recent developments in molecular diagnostics have revolutionized the science field through the ease of faster and more accurate identification of pathogens and, consequently, containment of infectious disease epidemics. Through the use of complex technologies, scientists and healthcare professionals can gain an understanding of trends in microbial resistance, hence the creation of new antibiotics and therapeutic interventions for coping with forthcoming dangers to public health. Collaboration between the clinical and academic settings is providing a stage for innovation, which makes the practice of medical microbiology vibrant in the endeavor of confronting new pathogens and emerging infections. Medical microbiology, in its fundamental nature, is not only the science of microorganisms but also encompasses the ethical and social scenario of microbial diseases. As medical decisions increasingly depend on microbiological data, the role of microbiologists also extends to informing the public about the importance of hygiene, vaccination, and antimicrobials. Writing about the beneficial as well as pathological aspects of microbial interactions further highlights the need to appreciate microbial ecology. For instance, while some microbes are very pathogenic, others are essential in maintaining us in good health, meaning an interdisciplinary model of microbial association is necessary (Ludwig et al., 2018). Not only does the model assist with infectious disease control, but it also supports the ongoing argument regarding the role of biotechnology in health care that corresponds with broader interests in the use of microbes for agriculture and industry (Wilcox, 1983). Thus, the background to medical microbiology must emphasize its interdisciplinary nature, conveying science with ethics and public engagement.

Definition and Scope of Medical Microbiology

In biological science, there is a turning point in medical microbiology that focuses on microorganisms responsible for disease in humans. It is a specialized branch of science that explores pathogenic bacteria, viruses, fungi, and protozoa and mechanisms of infection, host interaction, and susceptibility to therapy. Medical microbiology's role is greater than mere pathogen identification; it also involves work in microbial pathogenesis, antimicrobial resistance, and vaccine development, and therefore, it plays a pivotal role in public health. The discipline enables improved understanding of how infectious diseases impact populations and how interventions could be maximized to reduce their effect. Such extensive coverage not only allows for the control of current health crises but also prepares researchers and healthcare professionals with the ability to address future threats from emerging pathogens and pandemics. Additionally, medical microbiology is observed to be multidisciplinary, blending ideas from diverse fields of science such as immunology, molecular biology, and epidemiology. This holistic method enables scientists to investigate the complexity of microbial existence and its interaction with human physiology on a holistic level. Techniques such as genome sequencing, bioinformatics, and advanced imaging are now established tools used within medical microbiology to interpret the genetic makeup of pathogens and their interaction with host cells. This evolving context is underlined by the importance of identifying clinical pathways, as evidenced by research showing the interconnectedness of different hospital departments in managing infectious diseases (Boucherie et al., 2009). Medical microbiology, thus, not only enhances scientific understanding of infectious agents but also enhances practical application within healthcare systems. The scope of medical microbiology also highlights the importance of traditional remedies alongside modern medical care, particularly where aspects of culture shape health practices. For example, in most African cultures, traditional medicine holds a significant position, with a large percentage of the population relying on alternative healing activities (Diallo et al., 2013). This discipline of medical microbiology encourages the convergence of various healthcare traditions to create holistic therapeutic methodologies. Appreciation of these varied contributions allows the creation of more suitable public health practices that are culturally responsive and accommodate scientific precision. By reconciling modern medical microbiology with traditional practices, healthcare practitioners are in a position to enhance the standards of care, enhance patient safety, and ultimately establish an equitable health system capable of accommodating inclusive medical practices (Figure 1.1).

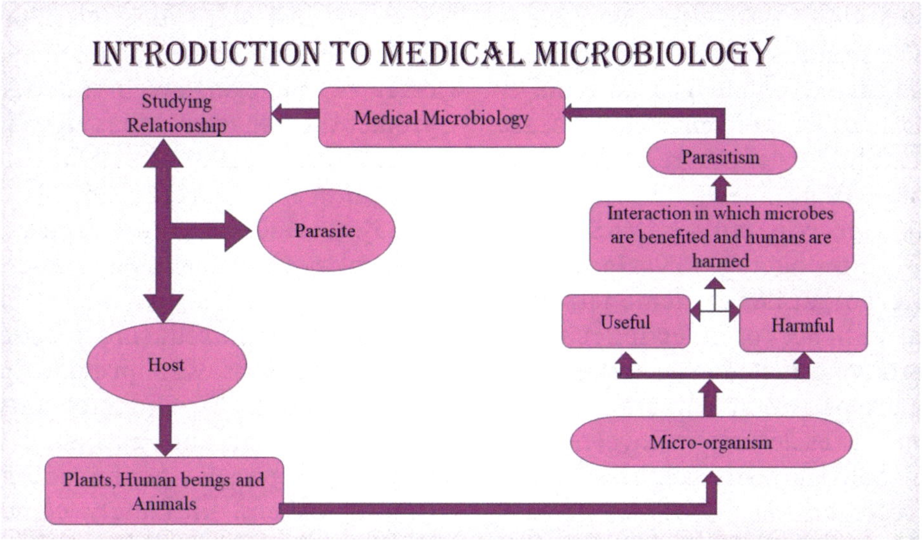

Figure 1.1. Medical microbiology.

Source: https://i.ytimg.com/vi/cvcsMeLGxf4/maxresdefault.jpg.

Historical Development of the Field

The historical development of medical microbiology has been pivotal in shaping our understanding of infectious diseases and the role of microorganisms in human health. In the late 19th century, pioneers such as Louis Pasteur and Robert Koch established the germ theory of disease, fundamentally altering the perception of pathogens. Pasteur's experiments demonstrated the function of microorganisms in spoilage and fermentation, and Koch's postulates made it possible to link certain bacteria with certain diseases. This intersection of experimentation and theory gave a boost to developments in sterilization and vaccination, which acquired a vital role in public health measures. The recognition of microorganisms as etiologic factors laid the groundwork for later research on microbial diversity, resistance, and pathogenicity, finally extending medical microbiology into an advanced, multidisciplinary science in a state of change today. Advances in technology and growing biochemical understanding of microorganisms also helped shape medical microbiology in the 20th century. The discovery of antibiotics, beginning with penicillin by Alexander Fleming in 1928, revolutionized the treatment of bacterial infections and emphasized microbial resistance. Researchers started applying newer techniques such as serology and molecular biology as the discipline expanded.

The invention of culture media and selection techniques allowed for the more accurate identification and characterization of pathogens. Additionally, the initiative to study the human microbiome, particularly through initiatives like the Human Microbiome Project, has uncovered the intricate relationships between humans and their microbial inhabitants. This revised story highlights how clinical microbiology has shifted away from its initial focus on pathogens to a broader exploration of symbiotic associations that impact disease and health. In contemporary discourse, medical microbiology is increasingly envisioned in the context of worldwide disease loads, its ancient history of progression against outbreaks and resistant infections. Methicillin-resistant *Staphylococcus aureus* (MRSA) is a case point for the ongoing struggle against resistant microorganisms, demonstrating the historical salience of infection control actions. Experts who include the well-known individuals in attendance at Witness Seminars have performed a basic role in investigating the biological behaviors of such strains and geographic forces on the prevalence of such strains. Besides, interdisciplinary research that combines genomic study and clinical utilization reflects a constant metamorphosis in the discipline where traditional microbiology comes into contact with cutting-edge genomic science. The study of the human microbiome, as it is defined in the Human Microbiome Project, is a paradigm shift toward the view of humans as superorganisms, thus increasing our knowledge of disease and health in today's globalized world (Reynolds et al., 2008; Huss et al., 2009).

Importance in Modern Medicine

The contribution of medical microbiology in contemporary medicine cannot be exaggerated because it entails the examination of the causative microorganisms responsible for inflicting disease on man. Medical microbiology plays a critical role in infection diagnosis, management, and designing proper public health measures. The understanding of microbial pathogens and the mechanism of infection has enabled healthcare providers to plan specific therapeutic measures. For instance, the emergence of antibiotic-resistant strains such as methicillin-resistant *Staphylococcus aureus* (MRSA) presents stringent challenges within a hospital setting. Infection control microbiologists have developed many assays that can effectively detect the resistant strains and facilitate better patient management with less risk of secondary outbreaks. With the evolution in microbiological research, clinicians are in a better position to predict the behavior of pathogens and thereby enhance the quality of patient care and safety in healthcare environments (Reynolds et al., 2008). Another very important role played by medical microbiology is in vaccine production and the prevention of disease. Immunization has succeeded in reducing infectious diseases' prevalence that was previously attributed to high morbidity and mortality. Based on microbiological and antigenic research, it is possible to specify the potential vaccine candidates and ultimately come up with a better and safer immunization. The process of vaccine development, such as in bacterial and viral pathogens, has relied heavily on the principles of microbiology and immunology. Moreover, constantly changing pathogens also illustrate the need for constant research and innovation. Changing patterns of resistance necessitate constant revision and updating in immunization efforts, and the importance of a strong microbiological foundation in public health initiatives is thus established. This ever-changing division not only treats current health challenges but also tries to prevent future epidemics through foresight in surveillance and research (Gillen et al., 2010).

Integration of medical microbiology into modern medical practice has enabled it to contribute significantly to personalized medicine. The ability to explore the microbiome and host interaction creates new dimensions for disease understanding and individually customized treatment development. It has been demonstrated that an individual's customized microbial community can influence how they respond to treatment, particularly in oncology and the treatment of chronic diseases. Utilizing microbiologic knowledge, practitioners can create drug regimens that provide the maximum therapeutic benefit with a low risk of inducing harmful effects. This new discipline illustrates the potential of medical microbiology to transform patient care into more efficient treatment protocols that take individual differences in microbiota into consideration. As a result, the value of medical microbiology transcends disease management, covering a wider range of medical practice focused on patient-centered health and well-being (Reynolds et al., 2008) (Figure 1.2).

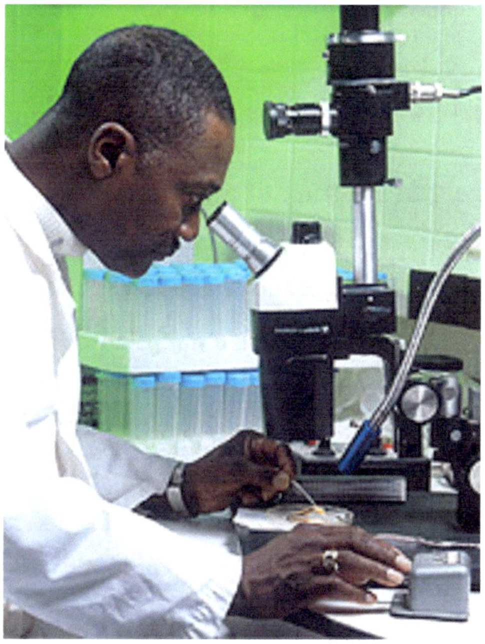

Figure 1.2. A microbiologist examining cultures under a dissecting microscope.

Source: https://upload.wikimedia.org/wikipedia/commons/b/b8/Manusingmicroscope.jpg.

1.1. Types of Microorganisms

Learning Outcome

1. Understand characteristics and classification of bacteria
2. Discuss the structure of viruses
3. Describe fungi and parasites

The classification of microorganisms is the foundation upon which medical microbiology is studied, as it entails the range of biological organisms classified on various grounds, such as morphology, physiology, and the possibility of causing disease. The basis of this classification is rooted in the separation of prokaryotic and eukaryotic microorganisms. Prokaryotes, which include bacteria and archaea, are referred to as bacteria and archaea with no membrane-bound organelles and nucleus, whereas eukaryotes, such as fungi and protozoa, consist of a complex cellular structure. This separation not only provides details about the metabolic process of the organisms but also assists in determining their function in varied ecosystems, such as human hosts. Medical microbiologists need to know such differences as they determine treatment and prophylactic measures against infection originating from pathogenic microorganisms. Bacteria constitute one of the largest, most diverse groups of microorganisms, and they can be further subdivided according to shape, conditions of growth, and metabolic function. For instance, cocci (ball-shaped), bacilli (rod), and spirilla (spiral) provide examples of the variation in form seen in bacteria. In a hospital environment, certain bacteria have been identified as being pathogenic and as playing a role in disease in humans. *Pathogenic* bacteria can cause a range of health issues from minor infection to life-threatening disease. For example, certain strains like *Escherichia coli* and *Staphylococcus aureus* are well-known for their ability to cause foodborne illness and skin infections, respectively. Use of standardized descriptors for bacterial habitats, as highlighted by the OntoBiotope ontology, can enhance precision in studies and finally lead to improved treatment outcomes through facilitation of microbiological data consistency with modern medical standards (Bossy et al., 2017). Fungi and protozoa are also other types of microorganisms that each have unique characteristics and effects on health. Fungi, comprising yeasts, mushrooms, and molds, cause opportunistic infections, primarily among immunocompromised individuals. For instance, Candida fungi are notorious for causing yeast infections and have further been implicated in systemic infection in vulnerable individuals. Conversely, protozoa, which are predominantly unicellular organisms, are responsible for diseases such as malaria and giardiasis. An understanding of these pathogens' life cycles, as well as environmental factors, is basic in the development of effective intervention strategies. From the viewpoint of food safety, it has been proven that the application of some treatments and packages inhibits the germination of psychrotrophic microorganisms, extending the shelf life of food products and making them safe (Bigeon et al., 2014). By careful analysis of various forms of microorganisms, medical microbiology is slowly evolving, stimulating innovation in clinical practice and public health programs.

1.1.1. Bacteria: Characteristics and Classification

In studying bacteria, their distinguishing features should be realized, as they are classified. Bacteria are single prokaryotic microbes that lack membrane-bound organelles and have a special structural content. Their cell walls, consisting of a general content predominantly peptidoglycan, may be of different thicknesses, rendering them susceptible or resistant to antibiotics and their classification into two wide ranges: Gram-positive and Gram-negative bacteria. This Gram staining technique is a cornerstone of microbiology because it not only serves to differentiate between bacterial species but also informs clinical treatment protocols. Bacterial shape, arrangement, and metabolic properties also contribute their share to classification, as they work to assist microbiologists in identifying their ecological niches and potential pathogenicity (Figure 1.3).

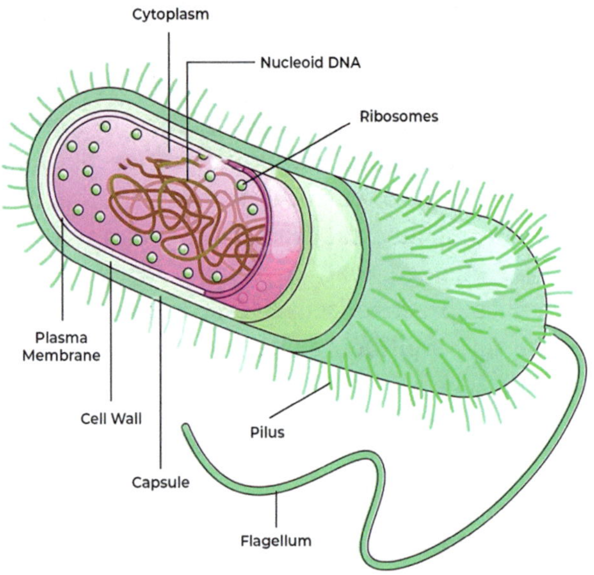

Figure 1.3. Diagram of a bacterial cell.

Source: https://media.geeksforgeeks.org/wp-content/uploads/20240226123534/Bacterial-Cell.jpg.

Bacterial classification extends to more than physical morphology to include genetic and biochemical test processes. More advanced microbial processes have given rise to the tools for developing complex systems of classification that look to utilize molecular processes such as Polymerase Chain Reaction (PCR) and multilocus sequence typing (MLST). These new methods have been key to the discovery and identification of highly genetically diverse species, broadening our information regarding their evolutionary history. For instance, *Brachyspira* species studies revealed that past culture and biochemical analyses supplemented with DNA-based techniques yield the most reliable identification procedures in such challenging pathogens (Råsbäck, 2007). Interweaving the classical and modern approaches is crucial when it comes to developing bacterial nomenclature and illuminates their ecological flexibility. In clinical practice, the importance of bacterial classification is especially highlighted when considering infections and their treatment. Different bacteria possess unique pathogenicities and resistance to antibiotics that are major factors in determining suitable treatment methods. In a study of diabetic foot ulcers caused by infection, various bacterial pathogens were cultured, including methicillin-resistant *Staphylococcus aureus* and *Escherichia coli*, and this highlights the relevance of individualized empirical antibiotic therapy in considering the most prevalent organisms in a particular case (Hayatshahi et al., 2012). Understanding the properties and classification of bacteria allows medical practitioners to make the right decision, thus promoting better patient outcomes and effective control of infectious diseases. The combination of bacteria identification and targeted treatment thus highlights the necessity of robust classification systems in medical microbiology (Figure 1.4).

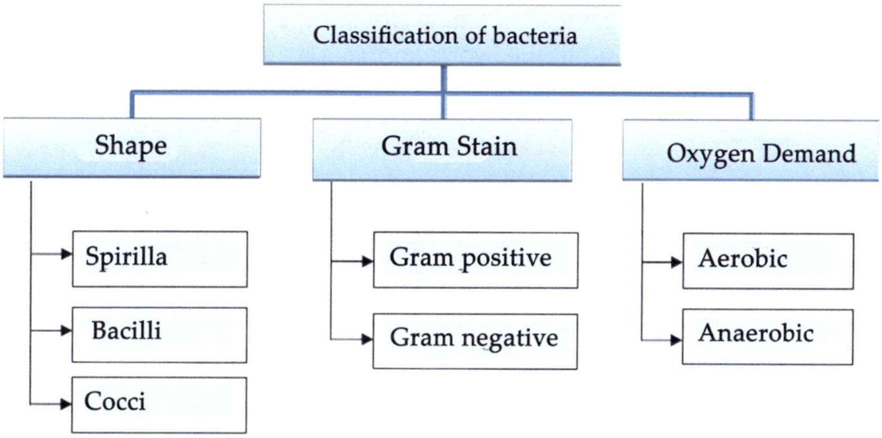

Figure 1.4. Classification of bacteria.

Source: https://www.researchgate.net/profile/Magudeaswaran-Palanisamy/publication/314141609/figure/fig1/AS:512301108088832@1499153510912/Classification-of-bacteria.png.

1.1.2. Viruses: Structure and Replication

The viral architecture is by its nature different from that of cellular life, as suited to their specialized way of life as obligate intracellular parasites. Viruses consist of a nucleic acid core, either DNA or RNA, covered with a protective protein layer known as a capsid. The capsid can be enveloped in a lipid membrane formed from the parasitized cell as well. The structural variation of viruses underlies their taxonomy; for example, enveloped viruses, such as influenza, possess a lipid bilayer to enhance their ability to fuse with host membranes. However, non-enveloped viruses, such as adenoviruses, possess structural stability that enhances resistance against external environmental forces. Understanding these structural variations not only illuminates the process by which viruses infect host cells, but also how they can be targeted to beneficial effect in therapeutic attacks in medical microbiology. Replication is a central phase in the viral lifecycle, involving hijacking of the host cellular machinery for replication. Upon entering a permissive host cell, a virus uncoats and delivers its nucleic acid into the cytoplasm or nucleus of the cell, depending on its type. The replication strategy of a virus is determined in part by its nucleic acid; DNA viruses tend to utilize the host's replication apparatus, whereas RNA viruses might encode their own polymerases. The complexity is even greater in the instance of retroviruses, such as HIV, which reverse transcribe to their RNA genome to DNA before they can integrate into the host genome. One replication cycle can result in thousands of viral particles, thereby causing spread within the host organism and to new hosts with relative ease. Knowledge of these mechanisms of replication is important in developing antiviral therapy that can break the viral life cycle. Viral interactions with the immune system of the host reiterate the significance of antiviral defense and the evolution of the host species. Research has indicated that several proteins that play a central role in innate immunity have been characterized, such as the IFIT (interferon-induced with tetratricopeptide repeats) proteins. These proteins are crucial since they recognize viruses with specific genetic features, distinguishing between pathogenic and avirulent viruses. However, differences in antiviral specificity, e.g., differences in human and murine IFIT proteins, uncover the evolutionary divergence of immune responses among species. Such understanding of host-pathogen interactions serves medical microbiology by illuminating the discovery of targeted drugs and vaccines that take advantage of these innate immune processes against viral infections, enhancing public health responses to emerging viral threats (Figure 1.5).

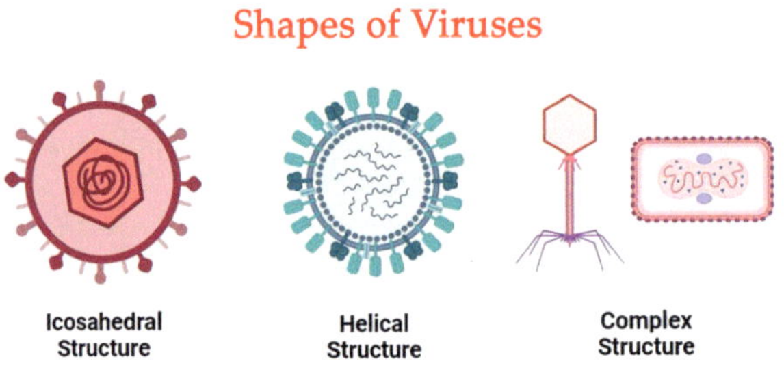

Figure 1.5. Shape of viruses.

Source: https://microbenotes.com/wp-content/uploads/2023/09/Shape-and-Size-of-Viruses.jpeg.

1.1.3. Fungi and Parasites: Overview and Significance

Fungi and parasites are significant components of medical microbiology due to their complex biological interaction with the human body and their ability to cause different diseases. Fungi such as yeasts, molds, and mushrooms are opportunistic pathogens, particularly in immunocompromised hosts. They possess specialized cellular structures, such as chitin within the cell walls, that are capable of evoking inflammatory responses and reactions in the human host. Pathogenic fungi , such as Candida and Aspergillus fumigatus have recently gained prominence for their increased prevalence in the clinical setting in concurrence with increased rates of antifungal resistance. In light of this background, there is a necessity for enhancing more efficient diagnostic and treatment methods of controlling such infections, hence placing greater value on knowledge of fungi in human disease and health in general. The significance of parasitic infections continues to be one of the central areas of research in medical microbiology due to their impact on human health. Parasites, including protozoa, helminths, and ectoparasites, have complex life cycles and routes of transmission, sometimes challenging the diagnosis and treatment. Some parasitic infections, e.g., malaria and schistosomiasis, are significant public health issues, particularly in the developing world. The World Health Organization categorizes various parasites as risk groups based on their pathogenicity and public health relevance, giving a policy platform to prevention and control strategies. Prevention and control of such parasitic infections are to be addressed from all directions in the form of public health interventions, vaccine production, and improved sanitation, which identifies the crucial role of medical microbiology in combating such serious disease hazards. New diagnostic tools, , such as metagenomic next-generation sequencing (mNGS), are transforming our understanding of parasites and fungi. Through mNGS, the entire microbial genetic material in clinical specimens can be interrogated, providing an unrivaled degree of information about the microbial cause of infection. Of special utility for recognition of recalcitrant pathogens and for the identification of resistance mechanisms, mNGS is transforming clinical practice and therapeutic strategy. Besides, it enhances our understanding of the complex interrelation between fungi, parasites, and the human microbiome. With each advancement in technology, overcoming challenges and opportunities of adopting mNGS into clinical laboratories becomes imperative to advance patient outcomes and public health, rendering its significance in combating infectious disease absolutely essential (Chiu & Miller, 2019). Additionally, complete classification systems, , such as the World Health Organization's systems, offer efficient risk assessment and containment procedures for a broad spectrum of pathogens, such as parasites and fungi, which are essential for effective disease control (Van Vaerenbergh et al., 2010) (Figure 1.6).

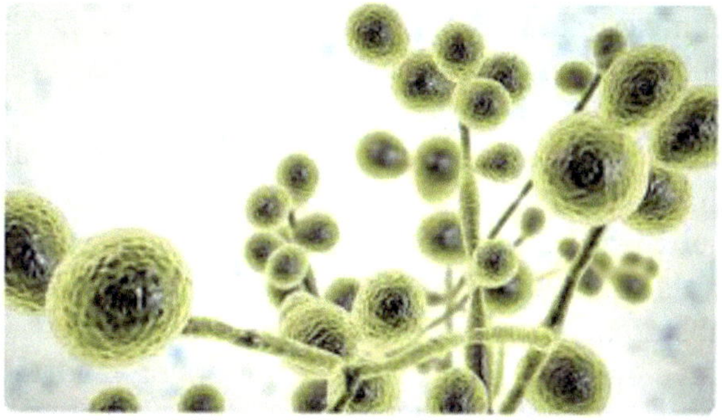

Figure 1.6. Fungi.

Source: https://encrypted-tbn0.gstatic.com/images?q=tbn:ANd9GcRHUfBzqF2yFho1H8vDS_T6JxcvErcUZQwO8Q&s.

Test Your Knowledge

1. What is the main difference between bacteria and viruses in terms of how they reproduce?
2. Which microorganism can be unicellular or multicellular: fungi, bacteria, viruses, or parasites?

1.2. Pathogenesis of Infectious Diseases

Learning Outcome

1. Understand the mechanisms of microbial infection
2. Explain the host immune response to pathogens
3. Discuss factors influencing disease severity

The pathogenesis of infectious diseases is a multifaceted process based on the complex interaction between the host and pathogens. Microorganisms , such as bacteria, viruses, and parasites employ various mechanisms to penetrate host tissues, circumvent the immune system, and disseminate within the body. For instance, enteric pathogens like *Lawsonia intracellularis* and *Brachyspira hyodysenteriae* will induce acute intestinal illness in pigs, in which pathogenicity is due to specific virulence factors enabling adhesion to epithelial cells and disrupting cellular integrity (Jacobson et al., 2003). Understanding such interactions is necessary in order to develop protective and therapeutic interventions because the nature of host-pathogen interactions can influence the course and the severity of the disease. Clinical manifestation of infectious diseases is not only pathogen dependent but also host factors like immune response and genetic susceptibility. Notably, asymptomatic long-term viral infections , such as those caused by herpesviruses, illustrate the role of the host immune environment in clinical manifestation. They can range from being entirely asymptomatic to extremely severe, depending largely on co-infections that may alter the pathogenesis of the underlying viral infection (Gentile et al., 2016). The relationship between the immune system and the pathogen calls for acuteness of knowledge on how host reactions can promote or hinder disease development. Thus, the education of medical practitioners in the uncertainty of infections gives an overall approach to patient management. Further, the development of appropriate models for infectious disease studies is important in clarifying pathogenesis mechanisms. Advanced techniques, such as polymerase chain reaction (PCR) assays, have provided access to the specific identification of pathogens in clinical specimens, as shown by studies of enteric illnesses in pigs. By employing these diagnostic tools, researchers are able to establish important associations between microbial presence and disease manifestation, ultimately casting more information about pathophysiologic mechanisms (Jacobson et al., 2003). Integration of both therapeutic and diagnostic innovations is essential in the fight against infectious diseases, bringing into focus the need for continued research in medical microbiology to help counter the existing challenges created by microbial pathogens.

1.2.1. Mechanisms of Microbial Infection

Understanding microbial mechanisms of infection is central to medical microbiology since it determines how pathogens interact with and use host systems. Microbial pathogens employ various strategies in their effort to gain entry into host organisms so that they may infect them. These involve adherence to host tissues, invading host physical barriers, and evading the host's immune response. For instance, certain bacteria possess specialized surface features, e.g., fimbriae or pili, that allow them to stick to host cells, a necessity for colonization and infection. Upon attachment, the majority of pathogens secrete toxins or enzymes that can weaken cellular function and erode the host's defense, demonstrating the complex interplay among microbial virulence factors and host response. A vintage example of microbial mechanisms of infection arrives in the guise of uropathogenic *Escherichia coli* (UPEC), and UPEC is the preeminent cause of urinary tract infections (UTIs). UPEC has a collection of virulence factors that render it adept at colonizing and establishing infection in the urinary tract. These involve adhesins that allow the bacteria to adhere to the uroepithelium, as well as toxins capable of causing damage to host tissue. The UPEC strains' genetic heterogeneity leads to pathogenicity variations, and therefore, it is imperative to appreciate such mechanisms to formulate efficacious interventions and treatments. Model organism research, , such as *Caenorhabditis elegans*, has provided valuable information concerning the virulence methods of UPECs. Through the examination of infection and survival processes in these models, researchers can identify important virulence factors and mechanisms that can be addressed therapeutically and thus increase our understanding of microbial pathogenesis (Amos et al., 2018).

Host immune response manipulation is also a critical element of microbial infection mechanisms. Pathogens have evolved numerous approaches for evading detection and clearance by the host immune response. For instance, microbial pathogens can alter their surface antigens or secrete immunosuppressive substances that interfere with the activation of immune cells. Such resistance of the host's defense is demonstrated in the behavior of various pathogens as they become engaged in infection mechanisms. A descriptive study of foodborne pathogens is used to demonstrate the effectiveness of ozone as an antimicrobial agent in lowering microbial load, exhibiting the environmental interaction between microbial survival mechanisms and external pressures (Anderson et al., 2003). Thus, this emphasizes the importance of being aware of the cell-level infection mechanisms not only for developing specific treatment protocols but also for developing effective prevention against microbial infections in a broad spectrum of cases (Figure 1.7).

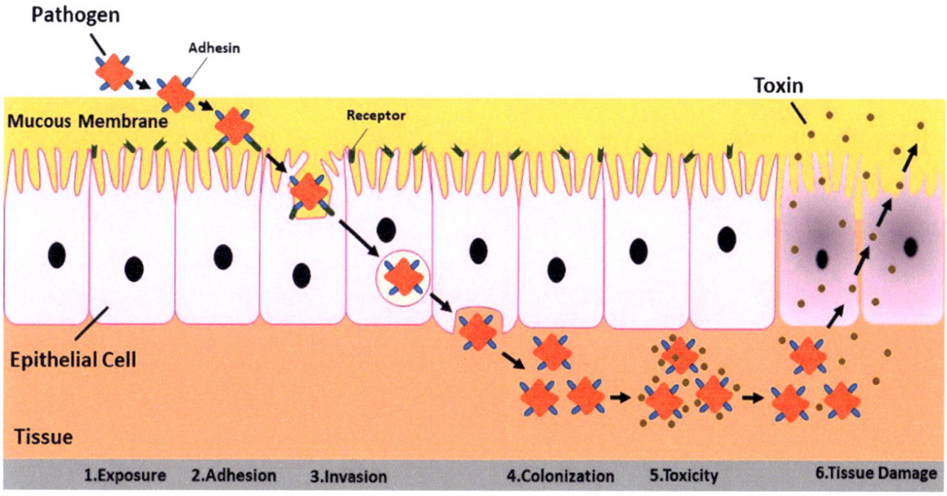

Figure 1.7. Mechanisms of microbial infections.

Source: https://www.researchgate.net/publication/366998039/figure/fig3/AS:11431281112236440@1673371521823/Mechanisms-of-microbial-infections.jpg.

1.2.2. Host Immune Response to Pathogens

Host immune response against pathogens is a complex and multifaceted process that plays a critical role in the maintenance of health. The response primarily consists of two distinct arms: innate and adaptive immunity. The innate immune system is the first line of defense, using physical barriers and cellular components to immediately recognize and eliminate pathogens. Key players, , such as macrophages and dendritic cells, recognize pathogen-associated molecular patterns (PAMPs) through pattern recognition receptors (PRRs), initiating inflammation and an immune response cascade. It not only aggressively targets the pathogens but also lays the foundation for the adaptive immune response characterized by specificity and memory. The relationship between these two systems indicates the importance of coordinated immune response in effectively combating infection and enhancing the defenses of the body against repeated exposure to pathogens. The adaptive immune response, while slower to develop, offers a very specialized means of destroying pathogens. It is lymphocyte-based, B cells and T cells, which can recognize individual antigens presented by pathogens. B cells have the role of producing antibodies that inactivate pathogens and mark them for destruction, whereas T cells can kill infected host cells directly or help in organizing the immune response. Central to this adaptive response is the process of immunological memory, such that the response upon later exposure to the same pathogen is quicker and more effective. Vaccination exploits this effect, basically preparing the immune system to combat a real threat by presenting it with non-harmful versions of the disease agent.

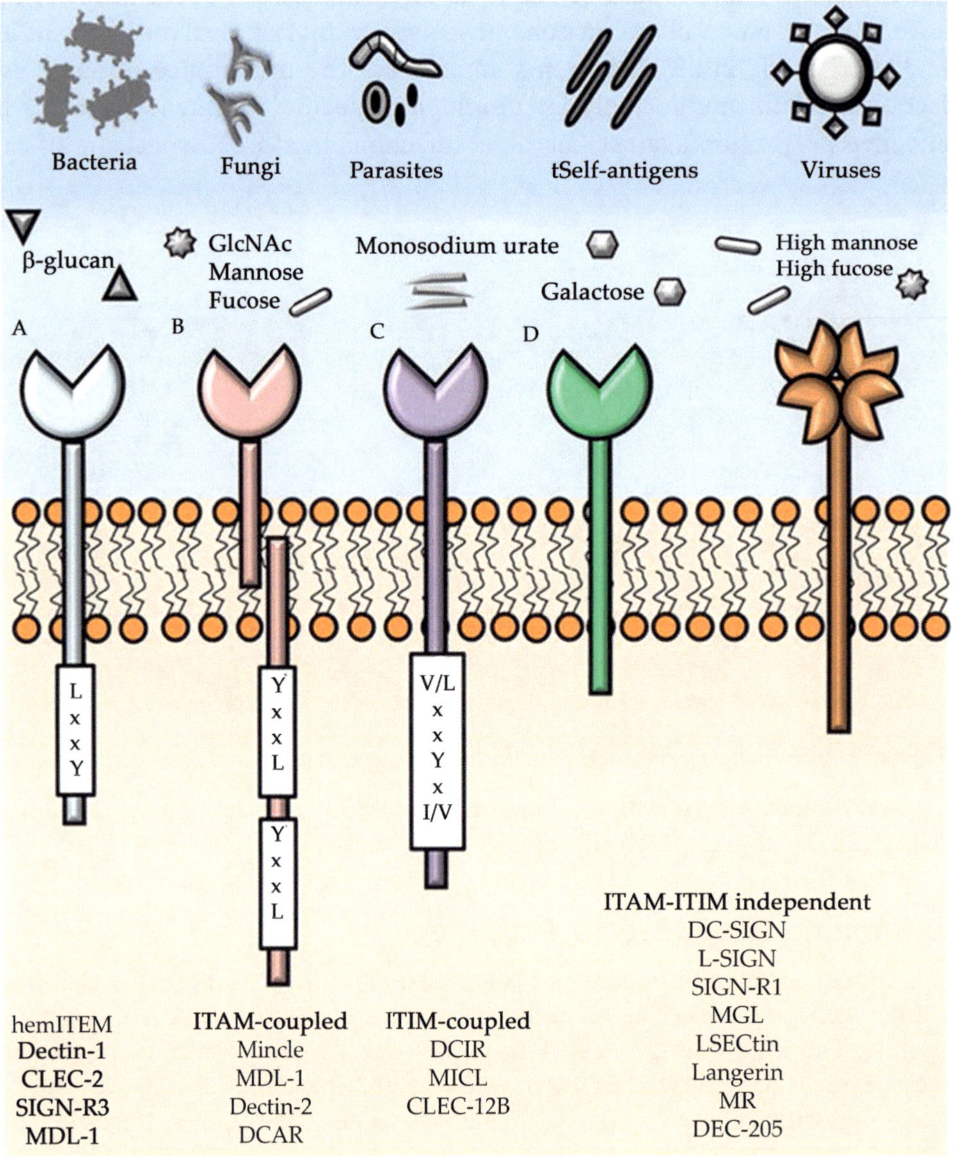

S

Figure 1.8. Recognition of pathogen-associated molecular patterns (PAMPs).

Source: https://www.researchgate.net/publication/315545987/figure/fig1/AS:11431281212090042@1702549962053/Recognition-of-pathogen-associated-molecular-patterns-PAMPs-damage-associated.tif.

Hence, understanding the mechanisms of innate and adaptive responses is essential in developing effective medical interventions against infectious illnesses. Recent studies have highlighted the role of the microbiome in determining the host immune response, illustrating the intricate relationship between microbial inhabitants and host defenses. The microbiome aids in immunological development, regulating innate and adaptive immunity. For instance, the presence of specific beneficial bacteria can trigger the generation of antimicrobial peptides and stimulate the differentiation of immune cells, resulting in a heightened protective response. Conversely, microbial imbalance or dysbiosis has been linked with increased susceptibility to infections and autoimmune disorders. The growing body of evidence suggests the necessity of a balanced microbial population to promote ideal health and underlines the therapeutic application of microbiome-based therapies in medical microbiology. As our knowledge progresses, measures like prebiotics and probiotics could further increase host resistance to pathogens, as described in Anderson et al. (2003) and Gow et al. (2017) (Figure 1.8).

1.2.3. Factors Influencing Disease Severity

The severity of disease caused by pathogenic microbes depends on a multifactorial interaction between host factors, pathogen virulence, and environmental factors. Host determinants, including age, genetic predisposition, and comorbid illnesses, may significantly affect the immune response and, therefore disease outcome. For instance, the older population mostly possesses a compromised immune function that exposes them to profound expressions of infections, for instance, invasive pneumococcal disease (IPD). Studies have established that patients over the age of 75 years record the highest mortality caused by IPD, showing how host intrinsic factors increase disease severity. In addition, individuals with compromised immune function, , such as chronic illnesses or immunosuppressive therapy, have a higher chance of developing critical disease outcomes, pointing to host vulnerabilities' contribution to infectious disease severity (Smith et al., 2011). Aside from host factors, disease severity is also significantly influenced by the virulence of the invading pathogen. Pathogens have many virulence factors that enhance their ability to invade host tissue, evade immune defense, and cause damage. For instance, some *Streptococcus pneumoniae* serogroups have been shown to have a higher association with deadly outcomes than others, which means that there are some strains that harbor determinants in the genome that are responsible for their lethality. In contrast, serogroup 1 has a reduced chance of causing death, and this signifies that not all strains present the same risk to infected humans. Understanding the relationship between these serogroups and the severity of disease will inform therapy as well as vaccine development, which will ultimately enhance public health practice in managing bacterial infections (Smith et al., 2011).

Environmental influences are also important in defining the severity of disease. Socio-economic status, climate, and geographical location can affect patterns of pathogen transmission and host exposure. For example, the environmental conditions may support the growth of some pathogens, leading to seasonal outbreaks that increase disease severity among susceptible groups. Moreover, interactions between multiple microorganisms within a host may trigger deviations along the parasitism-mutualism continuum, as is the situation with *Helicobacter pylori*. This gram-negative bacteria have the ability to be pathogenic but still confer some health advantages to the host, both aspects which highlight the precarious balance of microbial populations within the human body. Adequate knowledge of the environmental interactions is crucial to the development of successful disease control methods and dealing with public health problems caused by microbial pathogens.

Test Your Knowledge

1. What is the first step in the pathogenesis of most infectious diseases?
2. How do pathogens evade the host immune system? Give one example.
3. How does the host's immune status affect disease severity?

1.3. Diagnostic Techniques in Medical Microbiology

Learning Outcome

1. Describe culture methods and identification
2. Explain molecular techniques
3. Understand serological tests and their applications

Advances in the technology of diagnostic techniques have transformed medical microbiology practice, with the ability to quickly identify etiologic agents and enhance control of disease. The application of digital biosensors is a remarkable advancement that utilizes the ability to detect single molecules and nanoparticles to make diagnostics more sensitive than ever before. These devices not only increase the sensitivity of pathogen detection but also minimize the occurrence of false positives and false negatives, potentially making diagnostic outcomes more reliable. Improvements on techniques , such as Single-Particle Interferometric Reflectance Imaging Sensor (SP-IRIS) are the best examples of this advancement, with the capacity to accurately count biomolecules. With such developments in technologies, they promise to bring through their advances and enhancements what is critical to diagnostic findings interpretation in the clinic and ultimately their integrations into routine medical diagnostics (Avci et al., 2017).

Another emerging technique that is transforming the clinical world of medical microbiology is clinical metagenomic next-generation sequencing (mNGS). This integrative strategy analyzes microbial and host genomic material from clinical samples to provide a multi-dimensional understanding of infectious diseases. mNGS allows physicians to infer antimicrobial resistance patterns and comprehend the effect of the human microbiomes on disease. While this emerging approach has enormous diagnostic potential, operational hurdles remain immense. Translating mNGS from the laboratory to the clinic requires problem-solving around issues of protocol standardization, result interpretation, and integration into workflow streams. The promise of mNGS to transform patient management and inform public health programs is not disputable; however, with the capacity to better understand microbial populations and how they interact with the human host (Chiu & Miller, 2019). With increased medical microbiology advancements, the merging of several diagnostic technologies will define future disease detection and management policies. The combined benefits of leveraging advanced techniques like digital biosensing and mNGS enhance diagnostic sensitivity as well as drive personalized medicine concepts by tailoring therapy based on an individual's microbiome or pathogen profile. This trend towards more individualized care is a paradigm shift from traditional to new-age solutions that can address the complexity of infectious disease. In the years to come, there needs to be an interprofessional effort by clinicians, microbiologists, and researchers to enhance these diagnostic modalities. These innovations will enable healthcare systems to respond adequately to the evolving microbial world, leading to improved patient outcomes in the ever-changing war against infectious organisms.

1.3.1. Culture Methods and Identification

Culture methods are fundamental in medical microbiology for the identification and diagnosis of pathogens. The methods are founded upon culturing microbes within artificial laboratory environments in order to examine their morphology, growth, and biochemical properties. Traditional culture methods typically encompass inoculation of specific media that provide needed nutrients and environmental requirements for microbial growth. For instance, during the characterization of the genus *Brachyspira*, researchers have witnessed immense success by employing both culture and biochemical analysis, though these methods are challenging due to the species' complex biological characteristics. The adaptation of molecular techniques, particularly PCR, into the current culture routines has been vital to reinforce the accuracy of microbial identification during laboratory diagnostics, confirming clinical impressions as well as guiding treatment options effectively (Råsbäck, 2007). Apart from culture methods, molecular techniques significantly expand the identification range in medical microbiology. The introduction of DNA amplification methods, as illustrated in the research on *Mycobacterium avium* subsp. Paratuberculosis, highlights the importance of combining both culture and molecular diagnosis. These molecular methods based on DNA have been shown to be promising in detecting low bacterial loads, particularly in subclinically infected animals. Greater sensitivity in diagnosis is required in diseases like paratuberculosis, where containment can differ from full infection as the detection is made early. However, authors have cited an excess reliance on PCR that has sometimes led to misidentifications, with a focus on other methods , such as involving culture techniques to support findings and authenticate diagnostics (Englund et al., 2002). Lastly, the combination of culture techniques and molecular methods represents a paradigm change in the identification of microorganisms in medical microbiology. With growing insights into bacterial genetics, the use of sophisticated molecular typing methods , such as multilocus sequence typing (MLST) and genomic DNA studies, offers superior epidemiological data that cannot be obtained through culture. For instance, the genetic variability encountered within the *Brachyspira* genus necessitates not just culture technique but also good molecular technology to properly identify. This overlap produces a multidimensional approach to the diagnosis of infection and treatment protocol implementation, ultimately contributing to better clinical outcomes. With the intricacy of microbial interactions and newly arisen pathogens, synergistic use of culture methods and newer molecular identification will continue to be pivotal in bringing more precision to medical microbiology practice (Figure 1.9).

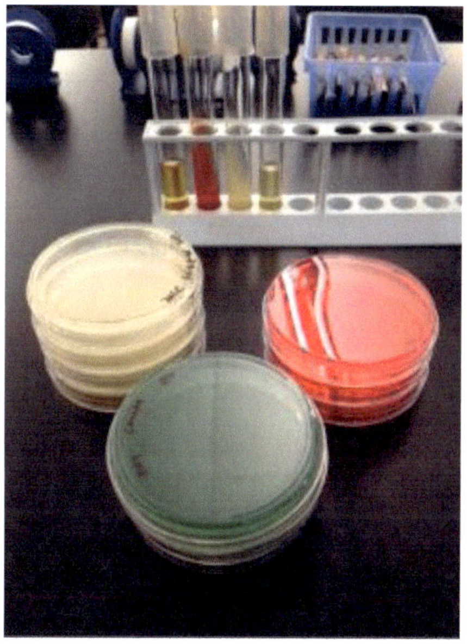

Figure 1.9. Different types of culture.

Source: https://milnepublishing.geneseo.edu/app/uploads/sites/14/2016/12/image1.jpeg.

1.3.2. Molecular Techniques: PCR and Sequencing

The invention of molecular techniques, Polymerase Chain Reaction (PCR), and DNA sequencing revolutionized the field of medical microbiology. PCR is a powerful technique that allows amplification of customized DNA sequences, which can be employed to identify pathogens in a highly sensitive and specific way for detection. This technique is invaluable for clinical diagnosis because it allows rapid identification of the causative pathogens, e.g., bacteria and viruses, from a variety of sample sources. PCR speed and accuracy have made it the laboratory gold standard for pathogen detection, especially where standard culture-based methods are too time-consuming or fail altogether, significantly improving patient care and epidemiological follow-up. New high-throughput sequencing methods complement PCR with useful data on the genetic makeup of microbes. Sequencing not only allows detection of known pathogens but also aids detection of new species and identification of their phylogenetic relationships. For instance, in a study on the *Brachyspira* genus, a blend of PCR and sequencing methods has yielded massive genetic diversity, which complicates the identification of the organisms with accuracy using DNA methods only (Råsbäck, 2007). Moreover, applying molecular typing techniques to identify bacteria , such as using Multi-Locus Sequence Typing (MLST), researchers can further understand the pathogenicity properties and epidemiology of specific strains of bacteria to assist in focused interventions. The marriage of PCR and sequencing technologies extends beyond identification; it also encompasses analysis of antimicrobial resistance and strain heterogeneity. Among the research on *Mycobacterium tuberculosis*, the application of such molecular techniques has confirmed the presence of complex patterns of DNA from ancient skeletons, which further illuminated the historical epidemiology (Donoghue et al., 2002). They emphasize the applicability of molecular techniques not only in contemporary clinical practices but also in the explanation of the long-term history of infectious diseases. With the progress of the discipline, continuous improvement of these techniques will certainly lead to ever more sophisticated techniques in medical microbiology, thus addressing the problems of emerging infectious disease control (Figure 1.10).

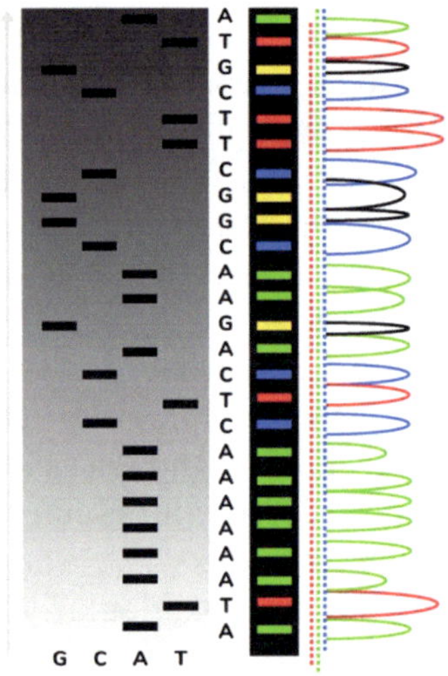

Figure 1.10. An example of the results of automated chain-termination DNA sequencing.

Source: https://upload.wikimedia.org/wikipedia/commons/3/3d/Radioactive_Fluorescent_Seq.jpg.

1.3.3. Serological Tests and Their Applications

Serological exams play a crucial role in medical microbiology since they are essential tools for diagnosing infectious diseases. Serological exams test the body's immune reaction to microorganisms by detecting the presence of antibodies or antigens in the serum. They are most valuable as they present a non-invasive means to identify current and previous infections. For example, serological tests can be applied to diagnose viral infections like

HIV or hepatitis according to the identification of specific antibodies for such pathogens. Furthermore, classical serological tests are used to determine infectious agents accurately because of the sensitivity and specificity of the tests, allowing healthcare providers to offer proper treatments according to the infectious agent detected. With the expansion in the field of human immunology, diagnostics by serological methods also continue to advance and mature in lockstep, becoming a routine component in the laboratory diagnosis of clinics. Aside from diagnostics, serological assays are also crucial in epidemiological studies, wherein they help track the transmission of infectious diseases within populations. By measuring antibody prevalence among a population, public health officials can gain data on exposure and immunity rates that will inform immunization policy and control efforts. As a case in point, when mumps or measles outbreaks occur, serology can identify unvaccinated cases and detect immunity levels among the population. In addition, serological testing is applied in surveillance programs to detect emerging pathogens, thus allowing preventive interventions against outbreaks. The application is particularly relevant in global health, where rapid detection and response to infectious diseases are essential. Its application in public health programs, thus, reflects its relevance beyond clinical diagnosis. The increasing sophistication of serological diagnostic tools, e.g., Enzyme Linked Immunosorbent Assay (ELISA), makes it more useful in all fields—space missions included. Scientists anticipate that the environment of long-duration space travel might lead to unique microbial disease manifestations, which will demand reliable diagnostic capabilities. As observed in contemporary research, membrane-supported ELISA systems were developed to meet the specific requirements of Health Maintenance Facilities in space and enable the detection of pathogens , such as Legionella pneumophila in microgravity conditions (Hejtmancik et al.). These innovations reflect the broader environment of serological tests and their possible use in diverse environments. Besides, with advancing laboratory technology, quick and dependable serological testing will continue to be an important consideration in both Earth-based and extraterrestrial public health scenarios, being a living part of medical microbiology (Generalov et al., 2014) (Figure 1.11).

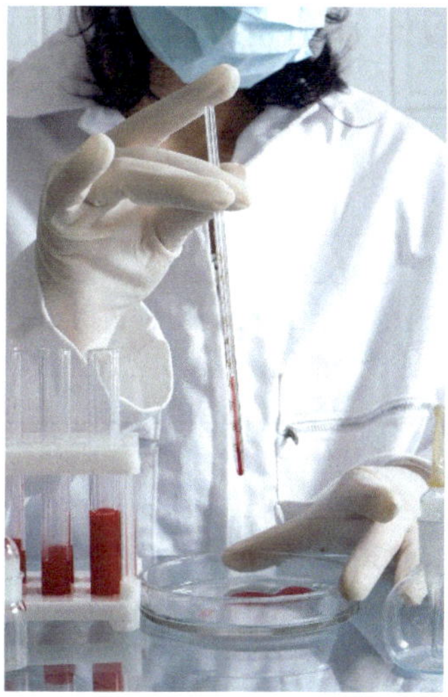

Figure 1.11. Serological testing.

Source: https://cdn.britannica.com/04/114504-050-3191864D/Blood-analysis-blood-sample-properties-diagnosis-disease.jpg.

Test Your Knowledge

1. What are the limitations of culture-based diagnostic methods?
2. How can serological tests help in diagnosing a past infection?

1.4. Antimicrobial Agents

Learning Outcome

1. Explain the classes of antibiotics and their mechanisms
2. Understand antiviral and antifungal medications
3. Discuss the challenges of antimicrobial resistance

Antimicrobial drugs are of utmost significance in the field of medical microbiology, since they play a crucial role in combating infections resulting from varied pathogens, , such as bacteria, fungi, and viruses. Antimicrobial agents can be classified into several groups, , such as antibiotics, antifungals, and antivirals, which act against specific microorganisms with different modes of action. This specificity is necessary for limiting damage to human cells while effectively killing pathogens. The understanding of microbial resistance has, nevertheless, become a significant impediment to the effectiveness of such agents. Multifaceted characteristics of pathogens like biofilm formation and genetic adaptation can render traditional antimicrobial therapies ineffective, and there is a need for ongoing research directed towards the discovery of new agents and approaches to broaden our medical protection against infection. Emerging research is showing ever-increasing prospects for novel antimicrobial agents from non-conventional resources , such as natural products and synthetic nanoparticles. For instance, yeasts like Pichia anomala have shown immense antimicrobial activity and are being put forward as potent biocontrol agents in a wide range of industries, most notably food safety and preservation (Walker et al., 2010). These yeasts possess diverse metabolic and physiological properties, and these can be employed for the design of targeted antimicrobial applications. Underpinning fundamental investigation on their cell physiology is still critical in determining how well yeasts of these types can be applied in clinical medicine and how they impact existing infection control protocols. A variety of such agents necessitates thorough studies in order to fully exploit their potential to defend against microbial attacks while within the safety and regulatory limits. Recent advances in nanotechnology have introduced a novel aspect to the synthesis of antimicrobial agents, the best case in point being magnesium oxide nanoparticles (nMgO). These nanoparticles have demonstrated highly effective antimicrobial activity against a broad spectrum of pathogens, including drug-resistant bacteria, which are more commonly encountered in clinical settings (Grelling et al., 2018). The effectiveness of nMgO lies in its ability to destabilize the microbial membrane and affect metabolic processes through several mechanisms, , such as the generation of reactive oxygen species. With inhibitory and lethal concentrations lowered, use of nMgO in medical devices is of large potential in reinforcing infection control management. Further studies are warranted to investigate potential cytotoxicity effects on host cells, with new applications in the area of medical microbiology and treatment options for infectious disease.

1.4.1. Classes of Antibiotics and Their Mechanisms

The extensive range of antibiotic classes is an integral part of the treatment of bacterial infections, with their individual mode of action against bacterial cells. Penicillins , such as amoxicillin, function by interfering with cell wall synthesis by binding to penicillin-binding proteins, thus stopping bacterial growth and multiplication. The action of cephalosporins is similar, but with enhanced spectrum activity against resistant organisms. By comparison, macrolides like erythromycin disrupt protein synthesis by binding to the 50S ribosomal subunit, ultimately inhibiting bacterial ability to synthesize essential proteins. Tetracyclines also disrupt protein synthesis but do so with the 30S ribosomal subunit, demonstrating the diversity in antibiotic mechanisms that leverage underlying differences between prokaryotic and eukaryotic cells. Understanding these mechanisms not only enhances therapeutic practice but also determines the protocols for correct antibiotic usage, critical in avoiding resistance development in frequent bacterial infections. The need for innovation along the antibiotics discovery frontier is brought out by the leveling off since the 1980s, since nearly all new antibiotics brought to market are a spin on something previously known. This emergence, coupled with the rapid emergence of antibiotic-resistant infections, is a powerful threat to global health. Green antibiotics, intended for use in animals, have been proposed as a solution to this threat, discussing the coupling between animal and human resistomes. Greening antimicrobial production aims at minimizing ecological traces while effectively breaking the flow of resistance from animals to humans. This strategy envisions that currently available classes of antibiotics would serve as a platform to create new formulations with characteristics highly suitable for veterinary administration and thus address resistance without exacerbating the environmental issue (Toutain et al., 2016).

Though the need for new antibiotics remains as pressing as before, prudent utilization of the currently available antibiotics is vital to preserve their efficacy. Overuse and misuse of antibiotics have accelerated the development of resistance, and treatment challenges and increased mortality as a result of otherwise treatable infections ensue. Public health measures aim to improve the correct prescribing of antibiotics and emphasize strict compliance with therapeutic regimens. Ongoing surveillance of bacterial resistance patterns, along with education on the risks of misuse of antibiotics, is paramount. Moreover, long-term investment in the research and development of antibiotics, particularly novel classes of antibiotics, is required to stem the looming risk of antimicrobial resistance. As the epidemiology of infectious diseases continues to evolve, proper antibiotic stewardship needs to be initiated by the medical and scientific communities together while pursuing cutting-edge efforts to combat resistance (Coukell et al., 2016) (Figure 1.12).

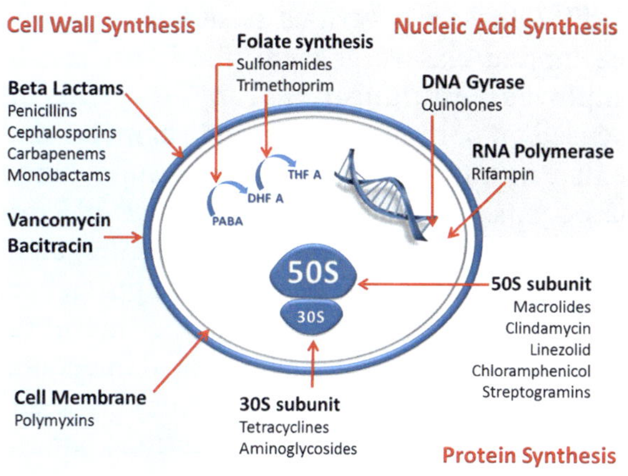

Figure 1.12. Classification of antibiotics by mechanism of action.

Source: https://www.researchgate.net/publication/272835216/figure/fig1/AS:601689551802390@1520465376371/Classification-of-antibiotics-by-mechanism-of-action-Image-by-Kendrick-Johnson.png.

1.4.2. Antiviral and Antifungal Medications

The treatment landscape for viral infections has been revolutionized with the emergence of antiviral drugs, which target various stages of viral replication. Such drugs work by inhibiting key viral enzymes and proteins, thus reducing the viral load and arresting the disease process. A few examples include nucleoside analogs that interfere with viral DNA synthesis, protease inhibitors that block crucial viral proteins, and neuraminidase inhibitors that interfere with viral release from host cells. Antiviral drugs have had wide-ranging implications in managing diseases like HIV, Hepatitis C, and Influenza, converting once devastating conditions into chronic, manageable ailments. But with the emergence of drug-resistant viral strains, there is a serious issue, and so there is a necessity for ongoing research and development of treatment methods to maintain the current antiviral drugs' activity. In contrast to antiviral drugs, the situation with antifungal medications is different, with various issues that involve the limited classes of medication that can be employed. Antifungal therapy is primarily focused on polyenes, azoles, and echinocandins with varying modes of action against fungal pathogens. The growing prevalence of drug resistance among the common pathogens , such as Candida and *Aspergillus* spp. genera complicates their treatment and increases morbidity and mortality from fungal infections. Increasing research shows a worrying trend towards increased fungal infections among immunocompromised individuals, further vindicating the need for new antifungal drugs. While most studies address the design of drugs, an understanding of antifungal mechanisms of resistance becomes imperative since it informs clinical management of the infection, as well as designing new drug molecules that can overcome resistance patterns (Vitiello et al., 2023).

The integration of nanotechnology into medical microbiology has provided new avenues for designing drug delivery systems, namely for antiviral and antifungal drugs. Nanoparticles enable targeted delivery, increased bioavailability, and can be formulated to release therapeutic agents in the targeted locations, thus enhancing the effectiveness of treatment and decreasing side effects. This new concept holds the promise to shatter new ground towards eliminating the disadvantages of traditional drug formulations, ushering in greater control over infections. But it raises new challenges regarding the safety and environmental sustainability of nanoparticles used as drugs. Therefore, extensive scrutiny of such nanomaterials is necessary the guarantee that benefits might outweigh the risks and that a balanced view of their interactions with biological systems is needed. With these advances, the fate of antiviral and antifungal therapy may be significantly determined by wise utilization of nanotechnology in medicine (Joseph et al., 2023) (Figure 1.13).

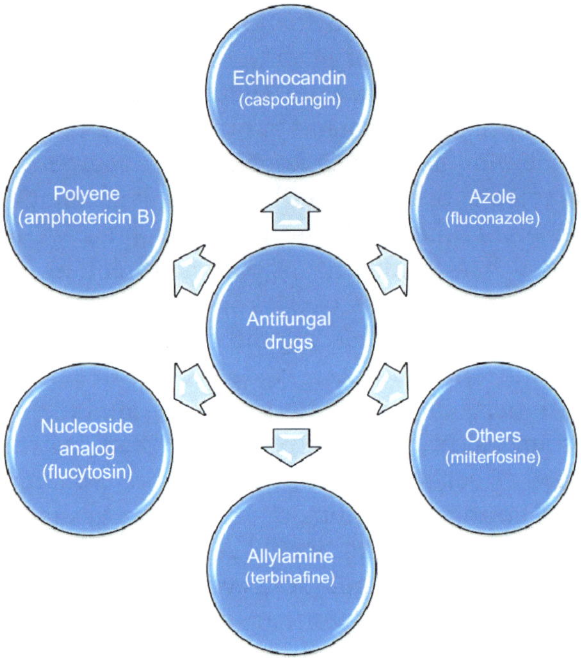

Figure 1.13. Different classes of antifungal drugs.

Source: https://www.researchgate.net/profile/Ruchi-Semwal/publication/341343991/figure/fig1/AS:890652179038209@1589359435854/Different-classes-of-antifungal-drugs.png.

1.4.3. Challenges of Antimicrobial Resistance

The growing danger of antimicrobial resistance (AMR) has emerged as one of the most critical worldwide public health issues. Antibiotics, which were recently heralded as a pillar of modern medicine, are progressively losing their effectiveness due to the rapid appearance of resistant strains of bacteria. This phenomenon is largely accounted for by the overuse and misuse of antibiotics in human medicine and agriculture. As bacteria are evolving to survive even in antibiotic presence, the efficacy of the drugs in question diminishes, with cases of treatment failure and the return of previously manageable infections. Ironically, exacerbating this issue is a sharp decline in research and development into new antibiotics, resulting in a therapeutic environment where older and weaker drugs prevail. Consequently, the compounded rate of resistance growth and antibiotic discovery plateau exacerbates the necessity to make AMR a priority as a matter of utmost public health importance (Coukell et al., 2016). The economic impact of antimicrobial resistance is vast, touching healthcare systems globally and patient outcomes.

The cost of treatment for resistant infections is significantly higher due to longer hospitalization, the administration of more expensive drugs, and other medical procedures driven by complications arising from the infections. Further, greater AMR also accounts for increased rates of morbidity and mortality infections become harder to treat or even outright untreatable. These trends put tremendous strain on healthcare resources, as well as driving a cycle of escalating healthcare expenditure. Addressing these needs through intervention in maximizing antibiotic prescription practices and improving infection prevention practices. For instance, promoting measures like hand hygiene can be a crucial step toward curbing the spread of resistant organisms and, in the long term, reducing the effects of AMR on the healthcare system (Borg, 2009). Preventing the threat of antimicrobial resistance is a multi-stakeholder response that involves stakeholders ranging from healthcare providers, policymakers to the general public. Awareness programs and educational campaigns are critical in terms of education, reinforcing a greater appreciation of AMR and its implications. Such programs can increase the awareness of health care providers and patients to guide the proper use of antibiotics. In addition, policy actions to manage the use of antibiotics in animal agriculture and livestock can further reduce the frequency of resistance in food production environments. Effective joint actions at local, national, and international levels are important in developing robust surveillance systems and research funding to support alternative treatments and new alternatives to traditional antibiotics. By embracing an interdisciplinary policy that incorporates education and strict legislation, the global community can aim at tackling antimicrobial resistance problems in a more effective way (Borg, 2009; Coukell et al., 2016) (Figure 1.14).

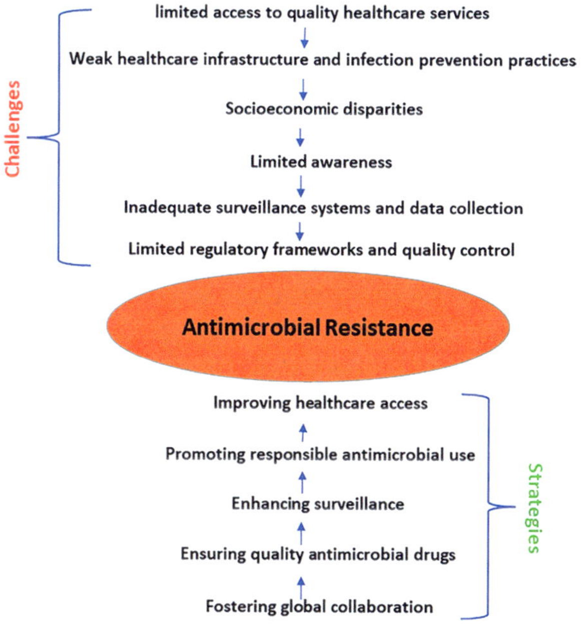

Figure 1.14. Challenges and strategies concerning antimicrobial resistance.

Source: https://www.researchgate.net/publication/373330775/figure/fig1/AS:11431281194339872@1696041505022/Challenges-and-strategies-concerning-antimicrobial-resistance.png.

Test Your Knowledge

1. Name two major causes of antimicrobial resistance in bacteria.
2. What are antifungal and antiviral drugs?

1.5. Infection Control and Prevention

Learning Outcome

1. Explain the importance of hygiene and sanitation
2. Describe vaccination strategies and public health
3. Understand the role of healthcare settings in infection control

Over the recent past, the transmission of multidrug-resistant organisms (MDROs) has posed a significant challenge to infection control and prevention in healthcare institutions. Infection control practices are central to the elimination, or at least control, of MDROs. Literature indicates that the cost of adhering to stringent infection control practices for the prevention of MDROs ranges from €285 to €57,532 per infected patient. Of special interest is that most of these costs relate to the disruption of new admissions, which can be up to 69% of the costs.

The extremely labor-intensive nature of preventing such infections makes it necessary to rethink economic models informing infection control policies, and this highlights the necessity of cost-effective measures to contain outbreaks without unproportionally weighing healthcare expenditure (Birgand et al., 2015). Moreover, infection control practices must be enhanced by the management of biofilm-related infections. Biofilm-producing bacteria are more resistant to traditional antibiotics, and thus, eradication becomes complex. Recent studies on bacteriophage therapies reveal a new approach to treating such problems. In vitro tests affirm that commercial preparation of phage can effectively prevent and treat infections caused by methicillin-resistant *Staphylococcus aureus* (MRSA), particularly in biofilm conditions. Of specific note, co-incubation with high titers of phage for extended periods resulted in positive results in biofilm eradication. In addition, these formulations increased the survival rate of *Galleria mellonella* larvae in experimental infections, which points to the potential of such formulations as an adjunct or alternative to traditional antibiotics (Luca et al., 2020).

Such integration of novel therapeutic agents into known schemes of infection control can significantly help develop the discipline of medical microbiology. By the integration of bacteriophages into the treatment and prevention regimens, hospitals would be able to strengthen their resistance against microbial resistance. The successful application of such methods does depend, however, on constant research to maximize phage delivery systems and determine their long-term effectiveness in clinical scenarios. While the paradigm in treating infectious disease is shifting, there remains an acute need for a multidisciplinary approach that combines older methods of infection control with newer treatments in order to better overall patient outcomes and mitigate the disease burden of MDRO and biofilm infections (Birgand et al., 2015; Luca et al., 2020).

1.5.1. Importance of Hygiene and Sanitation

Sanitation and hygiene are the pillars of public health and two of the most significant subjects in medical microbiology. They not only minimize microbial load but also avert the spreading of infectious disease. In the majority of developing nations, unhygienic sanitation conditions are directly responsible for health crises. Poor hygiene is mostly accountable for the prevalence of diarrheal diseases that disproportionately affect vulnerable populations , such as the elderly and young children. Addressing these underlying causes through improved sanitation facilities is central to reducing the disease burden. A targeted strategy that acknowledges the importance of hygiene among all age groups, particularly among adolescents who are often overlooked, is essential in formulating effective policies on health based on empirical evidence as revealed in the Indian villages' study (Dutta et al., 2012). Access to proper sanitation facilities also plays a critical role in schools, with implications on both health and learning achievement. Proper sanitation facilities in schools significantly enhance the hygiene behavior of students, thus reducing the incidence of infectious diseases , such as diarrhea among students. Poor maintenance of school sanitation can deter students, particularly girls, from attending school, hence exacerbating educational inequalities. The impact of this issue implies that their mere installation is not the solution, but that proper maintenance and promotion thereof are imperative for long-term success. Long-term sustainable financial models that provide room for appropriate practices of hygiene and sanitation in the learning environment are vital for the development of a healthier future population and an educated society (Dutta et al., 2012). Moreover, the broader linkages of sanitation and hygiene extend to global efforts to achieve the Millennium Development Goals (MDGs). Without a sustainable sanitation system, health improvements will be fleeting, and initiatives will fail, eroding gains in all areas. Governments and public health authorities must recognize the central role sanitation has in achieving health targets and raising living standards. Inattention to the aspect of sanitation is a failure that leads to a prolongation of preventable mortality and morbidity that can otherwise be managed. Consequently, putting a focus on hygiene and sanitation is not only essential for short-term health benefits but also is imperative in creating health-resilient populations that are capable of sustaining health benefits in the long term (Figure 1.15).

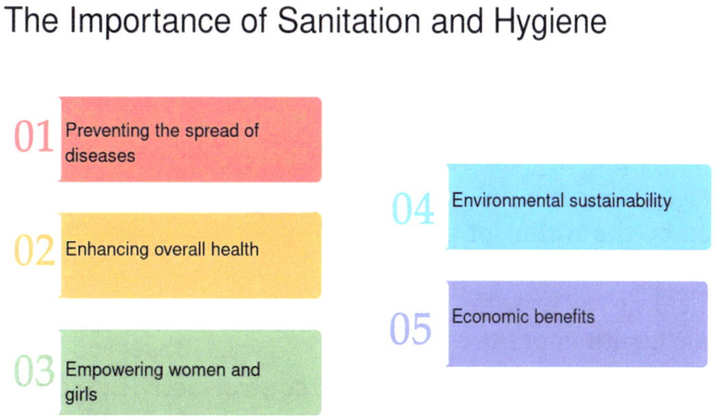

Figure 1.15. The importance of sanitation and hygiene.

Source: https://fastercapital.co/i/Social-entrepreneurship-sanitation--How-to-improve-sanitation-and-hygiene-through-social-entrepreneurship--The-Importance-of-Sanitation-and-Hygiene.webp.

1.5.2. Vaccination Strategies and Public Health

Vaccine policies are an important public health element not just in the prevention of infectious disease transmission but also in the promotion of overall community health. Effective vaccine campaigns are founded upon thorough planning, comprehensive public health education, and the integration of surveillance systems to monitor the incidence of diseases. One of the most important characteristics of these approaches is their ability to adapt to local conditions, particularly in developing countries, where infrastructural challenges could hinder the capacity to roll out vaccination campaigns. For instance, effective rabies control in a number of regions has established active mass vaccination as much more efficient than reactive approaches, particularly with enhanced surveillance activities. These findings remind us that without the proper detection systems in place, the potential success of vaccination efforts may be wasted, further supporting the need for continued investment in vaccination and surveillance to ensure continued control of disease (Townsend et al., 2013). With every new vaccine introduced and included in the immunization program, there will be a need to maintain a robust routine immunization program for long-term public good. Despite clear benefits imparted by vaccines towards alleviating morbidity and mortality, the focus on new vaccines at times leads to overemphasis and downplaying of ongoing immunization campaigns. This pendulum drift is generally supported by the whims of private healthcare systems, where profit incentives for manufacturers and healthcare providers take precedence over public health imperatives. The spread of anti-vaccine ideology contributes further complexity, generating confusion and disinterest among communities towards immunization. Hence, more properly regulating vaccination procedures in the private sector, particularly in developing nations, is inevitable to guarantee that the inherent purpose of vaccination, disease prevention, is not derailed by business (Baliga & baliga, 2008).

The relationship between effective vaccination strategies and public trust is inevitable for the maximum success of immunization policies. Public health initiatives must not only apprise communities of the immunization advantage but also engage with them to overcome ignorance in a scientific and sensitive manner. Building a trustworthy relationship between health professionals and the masses would serve to significantly increase the acceptance of vaccines. Further, incorporating civic participation into vaccination policy may instill an atmosphere of participatory politics where health interests take precedence over commercial interests.

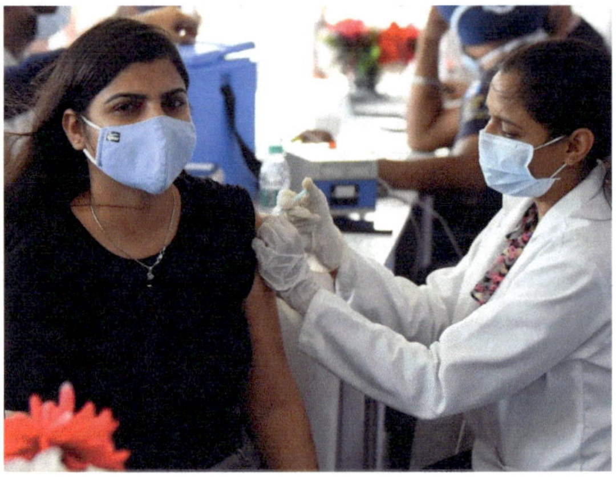

Figure 1.16. Vaccination strategies and public health.

Source: https://im.indiatimes.in/content/2021/Aug/bccl_61069505dec5b.jpg?w=1200&h=900&cc=1&webp=1&q=75.

As observed through successful rabies control activities demanding strict detection rates for surveillance, active interventions in combination with community mobilization and control can help transform vaccination from a simple medical intervention into a comprehensive public health strategy for addressing the complexities of disease control in diverse populations (Baliga & baliga, 2008; Townsend et al., 2013) (Figure 1.16).

1.5.3. Role of Healthcare Settings in Infection Control

Healthcare facility infection control is paramount in ensuring patient and staff health. Equipment and surfaces that have been in contact with pathogenic microorganisms become reservoirs that can cause HAIs. Infection control is therefore essential in the prevention of these risks. Refraining from careless violation of stringent hygiene precautions, , such as the regular disinfection of surfaces and equipment, is important in controlling microbial load. Further, hand hygiene protocols for healthcare professionals are at the center of preventing infection transmission in healthcare environments. The evidence shows that adherence to these processes significantly decreases the incidence of infections, enhancing patient care and saving healthcare costs associated with HAIs. However, the efficacy of these interventions is also largely dependent on continuous education, surveillance, and compliance by healthcare workers, as well as on the establishment of an organizational culture that is focused on infection prevention. The integration of mobile technology into the health care environment, desirable as it is, poses additional challenges to infection control. Current studies have also emphasized that single devices, i.e., cell phones, can carry extensive microbial contamination with the capability to serve as cross-contamination vectors in hospitals (Humphreys et al., 2012). Experiments have revealed that up to 86% of mobile devices surveyed in clinical settings had polymicrobial contamination, which precisely highlights the compelling requirement for effective cleaning and disinfection processes specific to such technology. The union of infection control and technological innovation necessitates the development of all-encompassing policies aimed at mitigating risks involved. Therefore, hospitals must implement not only rigorous disinfectant protocols for single-use equipment but also educate users on following the levels of hygiene in such equipment to lower the risk of infection transmission in seclusion.

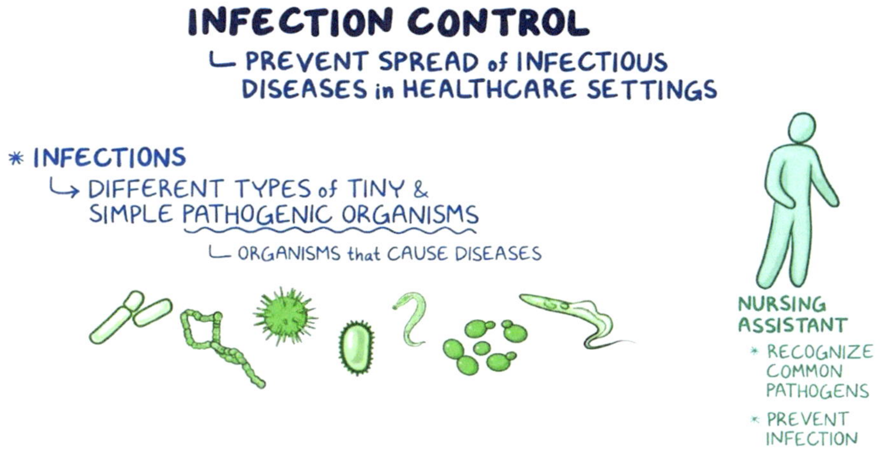

Figure 1.17. Infection control.

Source: https://www.osmosis.org/_next/image?url=https%3A%2F%2Fd16qt3wv6xm098.cloudfront.net%2FlFxYjREITIid15HQB5lVnVKuT9CNvOCV%2F_.jpg&w=3840&q=75.

Moreover, the creation and implementation of effective infection prevention and control measures should be based on a comprehensive understanding of antimicrobial resistance (AMR) in the healthcare environment. The efficacy of existing interventions against combating AMR is questionable and requires a firmer evidence base to facilitate informed decision-making (Dar et al., 2015). By examining fields , such as responsible antimicrobial use, improved surveillance systems, and rigorous infection control practices, healthcare facilities can implement policies that address region- and sector-specific needs. A One Health approach, focusing on interconnections between human, animal, and environmental health, is particularly vital in formulating proper and sensitive infection control policies. This approach enables a combined understanding of disease vectors and encourages cooperation among different agencies across various sectors, thus ultimately achieving maximum resistance of healthcare facilities to infectious agents (Figure 1.17).

Test Your Knowledge

1. What is the importance of good hygiene in preventing the spread of infectious diseases?
2. Why is infection control important in healthcare settings?

1.6. Emerging Infectious Diseases

Learning Outcome

1. Discuss the factors contributing to the emergence of new pathogens
2. Deal with case studies of recent outbreaks
3. Focus on global health implications and responses

Emerging infectious diseases pose huge risks to global public health and are of utmost significance in the medical microbiology arena. These diseases came into prominence since the 1950s, when the medical community for the first time noted the rising rate of new and emerging pathogens. The majority of them, typically of bacterial origin, are due to complex interactions between microbial evolution, environmental factors, and human behavior. The image of infectious diseases has greatly altered due to reasons , such as urbanization and climate change, which bring humans into contact with zoonotic pathogens more often that have their reservoir in animals. In addition, the development of new diagnostic technologies is central to the discovery and tracking of these pathogens, and thus increases our understanding of their significance to human health (Vouga & Greub, 2015). It is vital to allocate financial resources and analyze these intricacies as we work toward reducing the impact of emerging diseases on people worldwide. Tick-borne disease emergence shows the increasing prevalence of infectious pathogens. Emerging tickborne diseases placed an unprecedented burden on public health systems in recent years, rendering urgent attention to such dangers inevitable. Ticks are carriers that spread many infectious pathogens, and diagnosis and treatment become more challenging due to the potential of co-infection. The geographical range of such ticks is expanding based on climate change, land use change, and differential ecological tolerance among species. This widening results in a rising incidence of tick-borne illnesses in many regions in the United States in both the human and animal populations. Understanding the epidemiology of these diseases is essential, particularly when public health programs prepare to prevent and control their increasing diversity and pertinence. The fundamental burden of emerging infectious diseases extends beyond immediate health peril, encompassing societal implications like economic uncertainty and healthcare resource planning. As attested by the re-emerging and newly appearing diseases, response approaches have to be efficiently coordinated through microbiological investigation with clinical practice and epidemiological data. With emergent new pathogens, bringing forward peculiar problems like enhanced virulence and opportunistic infection, it is necessary to understand the relations between human populations and microbial forces. As remarked, multidisciplinary measures are required, and augmented international collaboration is essential for data collection and analysis. This collective knowledge will lead public health policy towards minimizing risks and maximizing preparedness to combat impending epidemics, ultimately protecting world health in an increasingly interconnected world (Vouga & Greub, 2015).

1.6.1. Factors Contributing to the Emergence of New Pathogens

Emerging pathogen discoveries have been a significant concern in the field of medical microbiology, with numerous factors driving the process. A primary impetus is the development of new diagnostic technologies that have increased our ability to detect and define emerging pathogens. Technological advances , such as enhanced culture methods, molecular methods, and mass spectrometry have revolutionized microbiology, making it simpler to detect previously undescribed or misclassified pathogens. This enhanced diagnostic capability allows for quicker action in response to outbreaks and more focused targeting of public health interventions, but also potentially exposes the health system to the uncertainty of evolving infectious agents. Furthermore, as more pathogens are identified by clinicians, the public health implications can be staggering, necessitating updated guidelines and methods of disease prevention and control. As such, ongoing innovation in diagnostic technology is necessary to grasp the landscape of new infectious diseases as outlined in (Greub et al., 2015). A second major factor for the development of new pathogens is the increasing contact between humans and animals, most often via zoonotic transmission. Climate change , such as deforestation, urbanization, and global warming, has also facilitated increased contact between wildlife reservoirs and human populations. These interactions allow disease-causing pathogens to be spread from animals to humans and new diseases to be formed. Emergence of antibiotic-resistant strains of bacteria, for instance, like *Escherichia coli* and *Staphylococcus aureus*, is due to shifts in agriculture as well as encroachment into habitats, and this goes a long way towards explaining the complex interplay between human activity and disease emergence. In addition, changes in human population, , such as population dynamics and migration, also enhance susceptibility to such infections. Understanding these trends is required for the prediction of outbreak occurrence, as well as the mitigation of risk factors for zoonotic infections, as emphasized in (Greub et al., 2015).

Finally, the development of antibiotic resistance also complicates the case of emergent pathogens. Antibiotic resistance data from nations like the Democratic Republic of Congo and Tanzania reveal sinister trends, particularly for multidrug-resistant organisms , such as Klebsiella pneumoniae and non-typhoid Salmonella. This has traditionally been exacerbated by the misuse of antibiotics both in veterinary medicine and human medicine, further complicating the battle against infection. This multi-dimensionality demands a coordinated one-health approach that inter-relates animal, human, and environmental health. Adhering to international guidelines and establishing clinical microbiology services enables health systems to better track and react to patterns of resistance, and thereby reduce the efficacy of such pathogenic agents. These actions are important in order to deal with the complexity of new diseases and properly implement public health policies.

1.6.2. Case Studies of Recent Outbreaks

Emergent MDRO outbreaks have confirmed the significant public health issues that these pathogens pose. For instance, in various hospital settings, rigorous infection control measures were used to prevent MDROs, which had considerable economic implications. A systematic review highlighted the costs of these strict interventions, ranging from €285 to €57,532 per patient with positive MDRO tests. Above all, most of such expenses resulted from interrupted admissions among patients, which constituted approximately 69% of the overall expenditure. This outbreak highlights the need for healthcare institutions to put effective measures in place while factoring in economic implications towards eliminating MDROs. Understanding such economic aspects remains crucial for subsequent policy formulations aimed at preventing outbreaks of MDROs and potentially reducing their occurrence within healthcare facilities (Birgand et al., 2015). The evolution of enterohemorrhagic *Escherichia coli* (EHEC) also raises important issues in medical microbiology, particularly in the wake of the notorious outbreak with strain O104:H4 in Germany in 2011. Not only was it the largest single strain to happen, but the outbreak was a reminder of the polymorphic nature of virulence factors because the strain shared certain characteristics of both EHEC and enteroaggregative *E. coli* (EAggEC). The hybrid nature renders epidemiological tracing challenging and emphasizes the process of tracking and monitoring outbreaks by public health authorities. The subsequent evolution of cases of hemolytic uremic syndrome (HUS) generated acute clinical and healthcare response requirements, and there was a requirement for an integrated monitoring and response approach to handle such pathogens in food chains and healthcare settings (Reu et al., 2012). Analysis of the foregoing outbreaks demonstrates the complexity of public health problems with infectious diseases. Tracing the source and transmission vectors for pathogens like MDROs and EHEC reveals loopholes in existing food safety and infection control measures. The need for strong surveillance systems and rapid response teams becomes critical, especially when new forms or strains abruptly emerge. These case studies present an urgent call for interdisciplinary research and concerted action between healthcare policymakers, medical microbiologists, and epidemiologists to develop robust strategies that can counter the impacts of future outbreaks. Placing highest importance on real-time sharing of data, clear communication, and reforms in universal healthcare can pave the way towards more robust public health infrastructures in the wake of burgeoning challenges from infectious diseases (Figure 1.18).

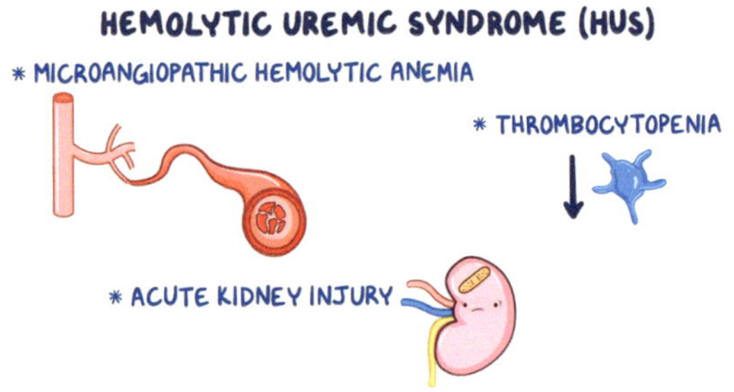

Figure 1.18. Hemolytic uremic syndrome (HUS).

Source: https://www.osmosis.org/_next/image?url=https%3A%2F%2Fd16qt3wv6xm098.cloudfront.net%2FFpgIN2EGTy6u2sqZ7jQqwDqPTBuOLrKD%2F_.jpg&w=3840&q=75.

1.6.3. Global Health Implications and Responses

The intricate relationship between global health and medical microbiology is underscored by the global issue of infectious disease, with profound implications for public health among health systems worldwide. Infectious diseases easily traverse borders, as has been seen in epidemics whose virulence propels them to global health crises instantaneously. One such example is the challenge offered by antimicrobial resistance (AMR), which undermines the efficacy of existing therapies and complicates disease management. International collaboration is required to address these challenges, through monitoring, investigation, and the development of new antimicrobial agents. As it is known that the healthcare environment keeps changing, the interventions should be adaptive in character. The use of a greater level of technology like machine learning and data analysis will better grasp epidemiological patterns and enable response measures, which consequently lead to improved health outcomes among various populations (Najar et al., 2025). Moreover, fraud and abuse of healthcare in healthcare systems exacerbate global health issues even further. Economical losses due to those false schemes can cost anywhere between 3% to 15% of total health expenditure, significantly reducing the effectiveness of the system and access to quality care. That financial cost might shift essential resources away from essential interventions and studies required for the fight against infectious conditions. Influential combat strategies in terms of legal reforms, proactive surveillance, and ethical training of healthcare workers are all crucial. Patient education also plays a crucial role in the development of a culture of accountability and transparency in healthcare settings. Understanding the complex nature, which involves several stakeholders, is at the heart of designing actionable interventions tailored to high-income countries and low- and middle-income nations (LMICs) (Najar et al., 2025). In recent years, the incorporation of digital solutions has brought new possibilities for enhancing public health education and engagement. The development of interactive digital tools, for instance, , such as MedMicroMaps, illustrates how technology may contribute to making learning more interactive for medical students and allied healthcare professionals. Such tools provide a better understanding of infectious diseases and evoke active participation in health discussions. Positive feedback from students indicates a growing appreciation for inspiring educational resources that illuminate and ready future generations of healthcare providers to adequately respond to worldwide challenges in health. Expanding their availability on multiple platforms can help to facilitate greater awareness and understanding of infectious diseases, eventually leading to improved worldwide health initiatives and responses. As community health literacy improves, the overall capacity to prevent and react to public health threats will inevitably be stronger, building a greater future amidst ongoing challenges.

Test Your Knowledge

1. What are the factors contributing to pathogen development?
2. Which are common multidrug-resistant organisms (MDROs)?

SUMMARY

In conclusion, scientific studies in medical microbiology have unveiled substantial details regarding the complicated relationship between microbial pathogens and host organisms. Rising secondary infections, particularly among critical care patients, underscore the significance of close monitoring and intervention strategies. There is evidence to suggest that Gram-negative bacteria, , such as *Klebsiella pneumoniae* and *Acinetobacter baumannii*, were common in secondary infections for COVID-19 patients and represent an alarming trend within intensive care units. These findings, as discussed in research , such as that found in (Prabil et al., 2024), consider the necessity for healthcare systems to prioritize monitoring microbial resistance patterns and infection prevalence, with strong consequences for patient outcomes within clinical contexts. In addition, the inclusion of multidisciplinary approaches within the analysis of microbial biofilms presents a significant area of future research and medical application. The recent surge of literature on the role of the COVID-19 pandemic and microbial biofilm demonstrates a rapidly expanding body of work that could introduce major breakthroughs in the treatment as well as prevention of infection. As observed in (Baliga & Baliga, 2008), there has been a recognition of the problems introduced by biofilms to microbial infections and drug resistance. By examining these intricate interactions among microorganisms in biofilms, researchers can design new solutions to combat recurring infection control and management issues across various medical specialties. The larger implications of such research extend beyond patient-level care and suggest a need for systemic overhauls in public health practice and policy. In light of the ongoing potential for emergent pathogens and the emergence of antibiotic resistance, there is a need to have research partnerships that bring together gaps in environmental science, medical microbiology, and epidemiology. This integrative approach might enhance our understanding of microbial interactions and their long-term implications for human health. Overcoming the challenge posed by microbial pathogens in actual and real terms, through multidisciplinary approaches, will not only augment clinical outcomes but also strengthen healthcare systems. Lastly, the dynamic nature of medical microbiology poses an urgent requirement for continuous research and responsive adjustment in order to guard public health.

On the clinical microbiological side, infectious disease and its etiological pathogen are key to understanding health patterns. A significant observation made is from the pathogenicity of pathogens during septicemia, particularly in leptospirosis. *Leptospira interrogans*, the causative spirochete for this disease, infects the human body through infected water and can spread through the bloodstream to other internal organs. Experiments have provided hints about how the pathogens enter endothelial and epithelial cells. Specifically, entry occurs by means of caveolae-mediated endocytosis using integrins and intracellular transport machinery to produce Lep-vesicles that are intact and do not fuse with lysosomes. This data sheds light on how leptospires exploit cell pathways for transcytosis, ultimately resulting in their persistence and transmission within the host, further informing disease dissemination (Li et al., 2019). The topic of nosocomial infections also brings attention to a significant problem in medical microbiology, particularly in intensive care units. A prevalence survey of nosocomial pathogens determined clustering of infections, which is influenced by patient placement and earlier colonization to a significant extent. Of special interest, pathogens , such as methicillin-resistant *Staphylococcus aureus* (MRSA) and *Pseudomonas aeruginosa* were shown to have distinct patterns of transmission relative to patient-bed movements. The study utilized clustering methods and structural equation modeling to identify risk factors associated with invasive pathogens, and it has indicated that previous nurse contact with contaminated patients is a critical predictor of transmission. This piece of information identifies infection control practice, , such as isolation practices, as crucial for preventing the spread of opportunistic pathogens in healthcare facilities (O'donnell et al., 2010). The emphasis on the consolidation of discussions on leptospirosis and nosocomial infection brings to mind the intricacy of microbial pathogenesis. The intricacy of the mechanisms employed by the pathogens for invasiveness and the dynamics of infection transmission in healthcare facilities call for holistic measures in disease management. Expanding on the role of health care practice, the intersection of staff mobility and patient contact seems instrumental in curtailing infection. Good microbiological research not only aids the tracing of the epidemiology of such pathogens but also assists in practice guidelines that optimize patient care. Through an integration of clinical experience and laboratory findings, the field of medical microbiology aims to enhance disease control and prevention and plays a crucial role in safeguarding public health against infectious risks (O'donnell et al., 2010; Li et al., 2019).

KEY TERMS FROM THIS CHAPTER

- Antimicrobial resistance
- Aspergillus fumigatus
- Biological organisms
- Clinical manifestation
- Cytoplasm
- Disease emergence
- Genetic adaptation
- Antiviral therapy
- Biofilm formation
- Biological science
- Clinical microbiology
- Diagnostic techniques
- Empirical antibiotic therapy
- Genetic makeup

CRITICAL THINKING QUESTIONS

1. **Which of the following is not considered a type of microorganism?**
   a. Bacteria
   b. Viruses
   c. Fungi
   d. Red blood cells
2. **Which microorganism is classified as a prokaryote?**
   a. Virus
   b. Bacteria
   c. Protozoa
   d. Fungi
3. **What is the primary step in the pathogenesis of infectious diseases?**
   a. Production of toxins
   b. Adherence of the microorganism to host cells
   c. Dissemination through the bloodstream
   d. Evasion of the immune system
4. **What is the most effective method for infection control in hospitals?**
   a. Hand hygiene
   b. Using antibiotics prophylactically
   c. Wearing gloves only
   d. Disinfecting floors once a week
5. **What is the first step in the pathogenesis of most infectious diseases?**
   a. Toxin production
   b. Damage to host cells
   c. Colonization of host tissues
   d. Immune system evasion

Short Answer Questions

1. What are the main differences between bacteria, viruses, fungi, and parasites in terms of cellular structure and replication?
2. Describe the mechanisms by which bacteria develop antibiotic resistance.
3. What is the significance of the bacterial capsule in pathogenesis?
4. What are the major classes of antimicrobial agents, and how do they target different microbial structures or processes?
5. Name three common bacterial pathogens responsible for hospital-acquired infections and their typical routes of transmission.
6. Explain how viruses differ from bacteria in structure and replication.
7. What are the key principles of infection control in healthcare settings to prevent the spread of infectious agents?

Answers to Critical Thinking Questions

1. (d) 2. (b) 3. (b) 4. (a) 5. (c)

REFERENCES

1. Dar, O. A., Hasan, R., Schlundt, J., Harbarth, S., Caleo, G., Dar, F. K., Littmann, J., Rweyemamu, M., Buckley, E. J., Shahid, M., Kock, R., Li, H. L., Giha, H., Khan, M., So, A. D., Bindayna, K. M., Kessel, A., Pedersen, H. B., Permanand, G., Zumla, A., ... Heymann, D. L. (2016). Exploring the evidence base for national and regional policy interventions to combat resistance. *Lancet (London, England)*, *387*(10015), 285–295. https://doi.org/10.1016/S0140-6736(15)00520-6(accessed on 13th June 2025).
2. Toutain, P. L., Ferran, A. A., Bousquet-Melou, A., Pelligand, L., & Lees, P. (2016). Veterinary Medicine Needs New Green Antimicrobial Drugs. *Frontiers in microbiology*, *7*, 1196. https://doi.org/10.3389/fmicb.2016.01196 (accessed on 13th June 2025).
3. Amos, G. C. A., Anastasi, E., Anyanful, A., Barber, M. F., Barnich, N., Beutin, L., Blango, M., et al. (2018). Virulence behavior of uropathogenic *Escherichia coli* strains in the host model *Caenorhabditis elegans*. https://core.ac.uk/download/188826801.pdf (accessed on 13th June 2025).
4. Anderson, J. G., Goudie, A. C., MacGregor, S. J., & Olateju, M. (2003). Inactivation of pathogens on food and contact surfaces using ozone as a biocidal agent. https://core.ac.uk/download/9020578.pdf (accessed on 13th June 2025).
5. Avci, O., Connor, J. H., Sevenler, D., Trueb, J., et al. (2017). Robust visualization and discrimination of nanoparticles by interferometric imaging. https://open.bu.edu/bitstream/2144/40114/4/Final_JSTQE_070116.pdf (accessed on 13th June 2025).
6. Baliga, Shantharam B and Baliga, Shrikala (2008) Vaccines: Propaganda and Practice. [Journal (On-line/Unpaginated)(accessed on 13th June 2025).
7. Bigeon, G., Copes, J. A., Giannuzzi, L., Pellicer, R., et al. (2014). The use of chloride, citric and ascorbic acid dip and packaged film to extend the shelf life of *Pejerrey (Odonthestes bonaerensis)* during storage at different temperatures. https://core.ac.uk/download/159289053.pdf (accessed on 13th June 2025).s
8. Birgand, G. J. C., Bourigault, C., Holmes, A., Iucet, D., et al. (2015). Measures to eradicate multidrug-resistant organism outbreaks: How much does it cost? https://core.ac.uk/download/77004407.pdf (accessed on 13th June 2025).
9. Borg, M. A. (2009). Addressing the challenge of antibiotic resistance in Maltese healthcare settings. Malta Medical Journal Volume 21 Issue 02 June 2009 https://core.ac.uk/download/46602217.pdf (accessed on 13th June 2025).
10. Bossy, R., Chaix, E., Deléger, L., & Nédellec, C., et al. (2017). Text-mining and ontologies: New approaches to knowledge discovery of microbial diversity. http://arxiv.org/abs/1805.04107 (accessed on 13th June 2025).
11. Boucherie, R. J., Hans, E. W., Hurink, J. L., Litvak, N., et al. (2009). A survey of health care models that encompass multiple departments. https://core.ac.uk/download/pdf/11471201.pdf (accessed on 13th June 2025).
12. Van Vaerenbergh, B., Koenen, F., Pauwels, K., Quanten, K., Boyen, F., Declercq, K., Desmecht, D., Thiry, J., & Herman, P. (2010). Methodology of the biological risk classification of animal pathogens in Belgium. *Revue scientifique et technique (International Office of Epizootics)*, *29*(3), 513–522. https://doi.org/10.20506/rst.29.3.1995(accessed on 13th June 2025).

13. Chiu, C. Y., & Miller, S. A. (2019). Clinical metagenomics. *Nature reviews. Genetics, 20*(6), 341–355. https://doi.org/10.1038/s41576-019-0113-7(accessed on 13th June 2025).

14. Coukell, A., Shore, C., Jungman, E., Talkington, K., Kothari, P., & Urahn, S. K. (2016). *A Scientific Roadmap for Antibiotic Discovery: A Sustained and Robust Pipeline of New Antibacterial Drugs and Therapies Is Critical to Preserve Public Health.* https://www.pew.org/en/research-and-analysis/reports/2016/05/a-scientific-roadmap-for-antibiotic-discovery https://core.ac.uk/download/75785719.pdf (accessed on 13th June 2025).

15. Daugherty, M. D., Geballe, A. P., Malik, H. S., Schaller, A. M., et al. (2016). Evolution-guided functional analyses reveal diverse antiviral specificities encoded by IFIT1 genes in mammals. https://core.ac.uk/download/323065418.pdf (accessed on 13th June 2025).

16. De Reu, K., De Zutter, L., Joris, A., Adelheid, V., Vanrompay, D., et al. (2012). Enterohemorrhagic *Escherichia coli* with particular attention to the German outbreak strain O104:H4. https://core.ac.uk/download/55755032.pdf (accessed on 13th June 2025).

17. Di Luca, M., Tavanti, A., Tkhilaishvili, T., Trampuz, A., et al. (2020). Antibacterial efficacy of two commercially available bacteriophage formulations, Staphylococcal bacteriophage and PYO bacteriophage, against methicillin-resistant *Staphylococcus aureus*: Prevention and eradication of biofilm formation and control of a systemic infection of *Galleria mellonella* larvae. https://core.ac.uk/download/288845816.pdf (accessed on 13th June 2025).

18. Diallo, G., Foguem, C., & Kamsu-Foguem, B. (2013). Conceptual graph-based knowledge representation for supporting reasoning in African traditional medicine. https://core.ac.uk/download/12044019.pdf (accessed on 13th June 2025).

19. Donoghue, H. D., Greenblatt, C., Lev, G., Matheson, C., et al. (2002). Confirmation of the presence of *Mycobacterium tuberculosis* complex-specific DNA in three archaeological specimens. https://core.ac.uk/download/1672393.pdf (accessed on 13th June 2025).

20. Dutta, A., Meijers, H., Ramani, S. V., & Frühauf, T. (2012). Determinants of the prevalence of diarrhea in adolescents attending school: A case study of an Indian village school. https://core.ac.uk/download/75783133.pdf (accessed on 13th June 2025).

21. Englund, S. (2002). Molecular biology techniques as a tool for detection and characterization of *Mycobacterium avium* subsp. *paratuberculosis*. https://core.ac.uk/download/11694594.pdf (accessed on 13th June 2025).

22. Li, Y., Li, K. X., Hu, W. L., Ojcius, D. M., Fang, J. Q., Li, S. J., Lin, X., & Yan, J. (2019). Endocytic recycling and vesicular transport systems mediate transcytosis of *Leptospira interrogans* across cell monolayer. *eLife, 8*, e44594. https://doi.org/10.7554/eLife.44594 (Retraction published Elife. 2020 Dec 03;9:e65227. doi: 10.7554/eLife.65227.)(accessed on 13th June 2025).

23. Generalov, I. I., Sencovich, S. A., & Zheleznyak, N. V. (2014). *Instructions for Laboratory Training in General Microbiology & Immunology*. https://core.ac.uk/download/80150439.pdf (accessed on 13th June 2025).

24. Gentile, G., & Micozzi, A. (2016). Speculations on the clinical significance of asymptomatic viral infections. https://core.ac.uk/download/98344656.pdf (accessed on 13th June 2025).

25. Gillen, A. L., Oliver, D., & Sherwin, F. (2010). Robert Koch, creation, and the specificity of germs. https://core.ac.uk/download/225131973.pdf (accessed on 13th June 2025).

26. Gow, N., Istel, F., Jenull, S., Lion, T., et al. (2017). Quantitative analysis of *Candida* cell

wall components by flow cytometry with triple-fluorescence staining. https://core.ac.uk/download/131024827.pdf (accessed on 13th June 2025).

27. Grelling, N., Liu, H., Nguyen, N. Y. T., Rosario, R., et al. (2018). Antimicrobial activities and mechanisms of magnesium oxide nanoparticles (nMgO) against pathogenic bacteria, yeasts, and biofilms. https://core.ac.uk/download/323067341.pdf (accessed on 13th June 2025).

28. Vouga, M., & Greub, G. (2016). Emerging bacterial pathogens: the past and beyond. *Clinical microbiology and infection : the official publication of the European Society of Clinical Microbiology and Infectious Diseases*, *22*(1), 12–21. https://doi.org/10.1016/j.cmi.2015.10.010 (accessed on 13th June 2025).

29. Harrington, J. (2024). A mixed methods pilot study to evaluate user engagement with MedMicroMaps: A novel interactive e-learning tool for medical microbiology. *Medical Science Educator, 34*, 753–757. https://www.semanticscholar.org/paper/0b2fb4738d6a24176acc4854e4feded0a27bd929 (accessed on 13th June 2025).

30. Hayatshahi, A., Heshmat, R., Nikoo, M. K., Qorbani, M., et al. (2012). Clinical microbiology study of diabetic foot ulcer in Iran; pathogens and antibacterial susceptibility. https://core.ac.uk/download/84432172.pdf (accessed on 13th June 2025).

31. Hejtmancik, K. E. (2025). A solid phase enzyme-linked immunosorbent assay for the antigenic detection of *Legionella pneumophila* (serogroup 1): A complement for the space station diagnostic capability. https://core.ac.uk/download/pdf/42833966.pdf (accessed on 13th June 2025).

32. Humphreys, P., Rout, S., Topping, A., White, C., et al. (2012). The cross-contamination potential of mobile telephones. https://core.ac.uk/download/9555607.pdf (accessed on 13th June 2025).

33. Huss, J. E., & Juengst, E. T. (2009). From metagenomics to the metagenome: Conceptual change and the rhetoric of translational genomic research. https://core.ac.uk/download/237182407.pdf (accessed on 13th June 2025).

34. Jacobson, M. (2003). Enteric diseases in pigs from weaning to slaughter. https://core.ac.uk/download/11694636.pdf (accessed on 13th June 2025).

35. Joseph, T. M., Mahapatra, D. K., Esmaeili, A., Piszczyk, Ł., Hasanin, M. S., Kattali, M., Haponiuk, J. T., et al. (2023). Nanoparticles: Taking a unique position in medicine. *Nanomaterials, 13*, 574–574. https://doi.org/10.3390/nano13030574 (accessed on 13th June 2025).

36. Koskella, B., & Lin, D. (2014). Friend and foe: Factors influencing the movement of the bacterium *Helicobacter pylori* along the parasitism-mutualism continuum. https://core.ac.uk/download/323080778.pdf (accessed on 13th June 2025).

37. Ludwig, D. (2018). Letting go of "natural kind": Toward a multidimensional framework of nonarbitrary classification. https://core.ac.uk/download/131213147.pdf (accessed on 13th June 2025).

38. Matee, M., Mshana, S. E., & Rweyemamu, M. (2013). Antimicrobial resistance in human and animal pathogens in Zambia, Democratic Republic of Congo, Mozambique and Tanzania: An urgent need of a sustainable surveillance system. https://core.ac.uk/download/pdf/18174800.pdf (accessed on 13th June 2025).

39. Najar, A., Alizamani, L., Zarqi, M., & Hooshmand, E. (2025). A global scoping review on the patterns of medical fraud and abuse: Integrating data-driven detection, prevention, and legal

responses. *Archives of Public Health, 83.* https://www.semanticscholar.org/paper/98115fd108aa341a9dcb55d862b16c8db5658a4d (accessed on 13th June 2025).

40. O'Donnell, A. G., Lanyon, C. V., Sheridan, E. A., Fridkin, M. D. F., Shirley, S. P., & Rushton, S. P. (2010). The transmission of nosocomial pathogens in an intensive care unit: A space–time clustering and structural equation modelling approach. https://core.ac.uk/download/9986795.pdf (accessed on 13th June 2025).
41. Prabil, A., Gandhi, M., & Vemuri, V. R. (2024). Retrospective assessment of secondary bacterial and fungal infections in COVID-19 patients at a tertiary care hospital in Navi Mumbai. *Journal of Medical Microbiology and Infectious Diseases.* https://www.semanticscholar.org/paper/20fa5dac2a9826ffe8da6e0fc099820a34c153f5 (accessed on 13th June 2025).
42. Townsend, S. E., Lembo, T., Cleaveland, S., Meslin, F. X., Miranda, M. E., Putra, A. A., Haydon, D. T., & Hampson, K. (2013). Surveillance guidelines for disease elimination: a case study of canine rabies. *Comparative immunology, microbiology and infectious diseases, 36*(3), 249–261. https://doi.org/10.1016/j.cimid.2012.10.008 (accessed on 13th June 2025).
43. Råsbäck, T. (2007). Laboratory diagnostics of *Brachy Spira* species. https://core.ac.uk/download/11695182.pdf (accessed on 13th June 2025).
44. Reynolds, L. A., & Tansey, E. M. (2008). *Superbugs and Super Drugs: A History of MRSA.* https://core.ac.uk/download/30696182.pdf (accessed on 13th June 2025).
45. Smith, A., Aspa, J., Austrian, R., Avery, T. M., Blake, D. P., Cecil, J. A., Robertson, C., et al. (2011). Death or survival from invasive pneumococcal disease in Scotland: Associations with serogroups and multilocus sequence types. https://core.ac.uk/download/110428.pdf (accessed on 13th June 2025).
46. Vitiello, A., Ferrara, F., Boccellino, M., Ponzo, A., Cimmino, C., Comberiati, E., Zovi, A., et al. (2023). Antifungal drug resistance: An emergent health threat. *Biomedicines, 11,* 1063–1063. https://doi.org/10.3390/biomedicines11041063 (accessed on 13th June 2025).
47. Walker, G. M. (2010). *Pichia anomala*: Cell physiology and biotechnology relative to other yeasts. https://core.ac.uk/download/228176756.pdf (accessed on 13th June 2025).
48. Wilcox, R E (1983). ECUT: Energy Conversion and Utilization Technologies program. Industry, university and research interest in the US Department of Energy ECUT biocatalysis research activity. (accessed on 13th June 2025).

MICROSCOPY AND STAINING TECHNIQUES

2

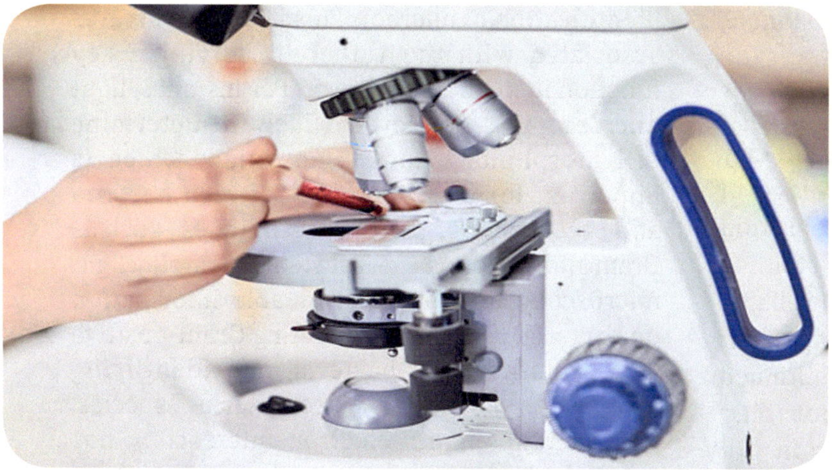

LEARNING OBJECTIVES

After studying this chapter, you will be able to:

1. Understand the fundamentals of light, electron, and fluorescence microscopy
2. Describe the Gram stain technique
3. Explain the acid-fast stain technique
4. Discuss about spore stain technique

Introduction

Medical microbiology relies on learning processes that foster the comprehension of microbial life. Among them is microscopy, which is an introductory tool that allows microscopic examination of cell structure and its nuances. Central to this is the use of various methods of microscopy, including light, electron, and fluorescence microscopy. Each of these modalities has unique strengths that can be used to achieve more insight into microbial morphology and function. For instance, such fine structural detail as is required for accurate diagnostics can be achieved using electron microscopy, beyond the ability of standard light microscopy. This is particularly important since accurate determination of the pathogen can lead to successful therapeutic regimens and better patient outcomes (Fazzan et al., 1953). In addition, staining techniques complement microscopic examination by providing distinct contrasts that emphasize distinct cellular morphology. The most prevalent staining protocols employed in microbiology are the Gram stain, acid-fast stain, and spore stain, each focusing on specific aspects of microbial cell characteristics. The Gram stain, for example, separates bacteria based on their cell wall composition into Gram-positive and Gram-negative groups related to virulence and resistance to antibiotics. Similarly, acid-fast stain is also an important diagnostic reagent in the detection of mycobacteria, such as the tubercle bacillus. Knowledge of the principles and applications of the above staining techniques allows microbiologists to draw a more realistic picture of microbial life, enabling diagnostic and therapeutic interventions (Heinaru & Naanuri, 2018).

Ultimately, the combination of microscopy and staining techniques in medical microbiology is important in advancing our knowledge of disease-causing agents. With the integration of high-resolution images with proper staining protocols, scientists and physicians can reliably test microbial specimens and learn important things about their biological behavior. Continued advancement in these protocols not only increases our sensitivity of observation but also enhances our capability to respond to newly arising infectious diseases. As we go on to examine them in more detail within this chapter, we shall observe the specifics behind their application and the main function they play in current medical microbiology (Fazzan et al., 1953).

Definition of Microscopy in Medical Microbiology

The scientific principle of microscopy in medical microbiology is intrinsic, in that it constitutes a fundamental tool for visualizing and investigating microorganisms. Microscopy describes various techniques that allow researchers and clinicians to magnify samples and examine the finer structure and cellular pattern not visible with the naked eye. This is particularly applicable in medical microbiology, where the identification of pathogenic agents can have significant implications in the diagnosis, treatment, and management of patients. Different types of microscopy, i.e., light, electron, and fluorescence microscopy, have specialized roles in medical discovery and clinical diagnosis, each with definite advantages in resolution, contrast, and visualization of dynamic cellular processes. The integration of these methodologies offers a balanced view of microbial biology, which allows advances in infectious diseases and immunology. Development in the field of microscopy has contributed to better identification of microorganisms and structures associated with them, thereby serving a key function in medical diagnosis. For instance, light microscopy is employed widely to determine cell morphology and organization, which is important for distinguishing between bacteria and other microorganisms. Techniques , such as Gram staining and acid-fast staining employ light microscopy to provide invaluable information on bacterial cell walls, separating Gram-positive and Gram-negative bacteria, and identifying acid-fast organisms like Mycobacterium species. On the other hand, electron microscopy has much better resolution, and ultrastructure details , such as organelles and viral particles, become crucial to identify in pathogenic processes. This multi-disciplinary approach is particularly significant in emphasizing the importance of microscopy as a basic tool in the diagnostic repertoire of medical microbiology. The application of fluorescence microscopy has enabled the ability to study of microbial behavior and interaction in real-time to a large extent. This technique utilizes fluorescent dye for labeling specific cell structures, allowing the study of live organisms and their physiological status. For example, techniques , such as live/dead staining may be employed to test for bacterial viability in probiotics and report on survival rates under various environmental conditions (Smith & Selby, 2017). Similarly, fluorescence microscopy can report on bacterial activity and persistence within biofilms that are normally resistant to conventional treatments Smith & Selby, 2017). Continuous advancement of microscopy techniques is of prime significance in medical microbiology as it not only aids in the identification of pathogens but also illuminates us regarding microbial pathogenesis and resistance mechanisms and thereby leads to improved therapeutic strategies and public health (Figure 2.1).

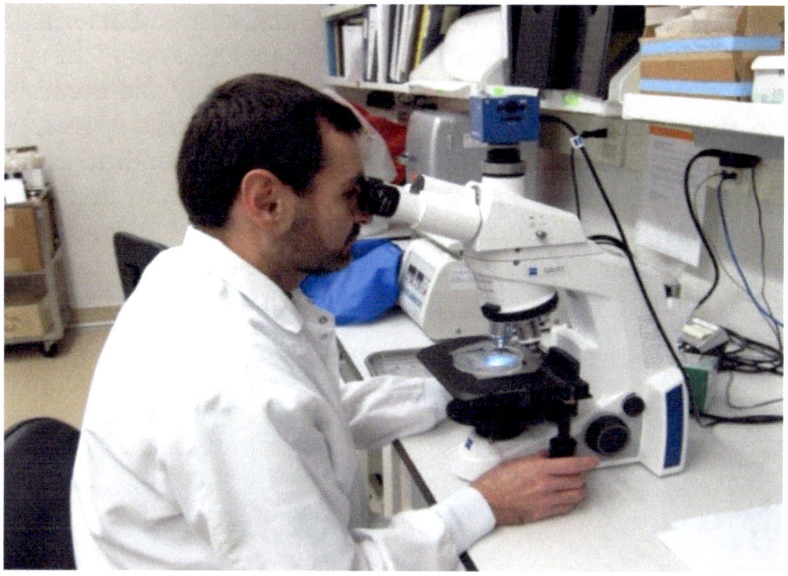

Figure 2.1. A microbiologist examines a specimen under a microscope at the New Mexico Department of Health Scientific Laboratory Division's mycology reference bench.

Source: https://www.nmhealth.org/image/about/sld/bib/gmb/ReferenceBench-Mycology-Microbiologist-Large.jpg.

Importance of Staining Techniques

Staining techniques are at the heart of the medical microbiology discipline and allow us to see microbial organisms that otherwise remain invisible. Using light microscopy, stains , such as the Gram stain give us key information on the physical properties of bacteria in order their division into Gram-positive and Gram-negative groups. This differentiation is not only significant for the detection of pathogens but also in guiding appropriate antimicrobial treatment. As a keystone technique, Gram staining can quickly inform clinicians about infection type and therefore, decide on treatments and improve patient outcomes. Also, the use of specific stains enhances contrast in microbial specimens to enable careful observation of morphologic structures, cell configurations, and potential pathogenesis-associated features of the cultured organisms. Fluorescence microscopy, complemented by certain fluorescent staining techniques, extends the usability of routine staining techniques by making it possible to identify specific microbial elements at a molecular level. Visualization of metabolism, subcellular organelles, and even molecules within cells is made possible through the use of fluorescent dyes and thus allows inference concerning microbial physiology and interaction. Techniques , such as flow cytometry and fluorescence-assisted cell sorting (FACS) are currently indispensable in microbial community analysis, particularly in the assessment of species-level heterogeneity. For instance, the application of FCM and FACS combined with fluorescent staining effectively distinguishes among cell states and types, e.g., vegetative and sporulation stages in bacteria , such as Pseudo*Clostridium thermosuccinogenes* (Smith & Selby, 2017). This advancement of the staining techniques improves not only our understanding of microbial ecology but also influences applied microbiological researches in such fields as biotechnological applications and infection control. Even specialty procedures like acid-fast stain and spore stain become significant by virtue of staining techniques, which are important for identification and investigation on specific microbial groups. Acid-fast staining is particularly important in mycobacterial identification since the organisms exhibit specific cell wall features that resist decolorization. This specificity is required in diagnosing infections , such as tuberculosis to ensure the timely and accurate interventions for treatments. Similarly, spore staining enables investigators to observe spores, which are essential survival structures formed by certain bacteria under unfavorable conditions. By applying staining techniques special for some microbial characteristics, researchers can illuminate the biology and pathogenicity of organisms, and eventually the establishment of diagnostics and therapeutics in medical microbiology (Heinaru & Naanuri, 2018). This emphasizes the focal role of staining techniques in both fundamental microbiological investigations and clinical practice (Figure 2.2).

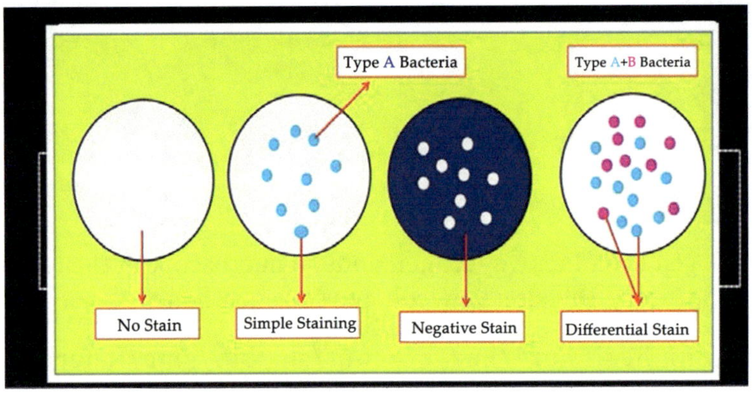

Figure 2.2. Staining.

Source: https://www.researchgate.net/publication/358978748_STAINING

2.1. Light Microscopy

Learning Outcome

1. Explain the principles of light microscopy
2. Describe the types of light microscopes
3. Understand the application of light microscopy in medical microbiology

Light microscopy, a key technique of medical microbiology, employs visible light and lenses to magnify samples in such a way that cellular architecture and microorganisms can be viewed. Light microscopy exploits the laws of refraction and transmission to provide perceptible detail of living as well as fixed samples. Light microscopy is particularly important in infectious condition diagnosis because it allows for instant visual examination of microbial shape and colony characteristics. Various light microscopy methods, , such as brightfield, darkfield, and phase-contrast microscopy, yield different observation conditions and enhance transparent specimen visibility. The ability to resolve structures of 0.2 micrometers allows clinicians and microbiologists to accurately classify pathogens, thereby necessitating prompt treatment and infection control practices that are of utmost importance in public health (Smith & Selby, 2017). In order to increase the diagnostic utility of light microscopy, staining is employed to achieve increased contrast between cells and their surroundings. Stains , such as Gram stain and acid-fast stain play pivotal roles in discriminating between bacterial groups based on cell wall structure. The Gram stain, for example, classifies bacteria into Gram-positive and Gram-negative groups and directs therapy regimens accordingly. Acid-fast staining, on the other hand, is extremely helpful in the detection of mycobacterial infections , such as tuberculosis. Staining not only allows the observation of the microorganisms but also provides critical information about their morphology and arrangement, which are critical for correct identification and further clinical practice. All these methods enhance the efficacy of light microscopy, thus making it a robust tool in microbiological diagnosis (Smith & Selby, 2017).

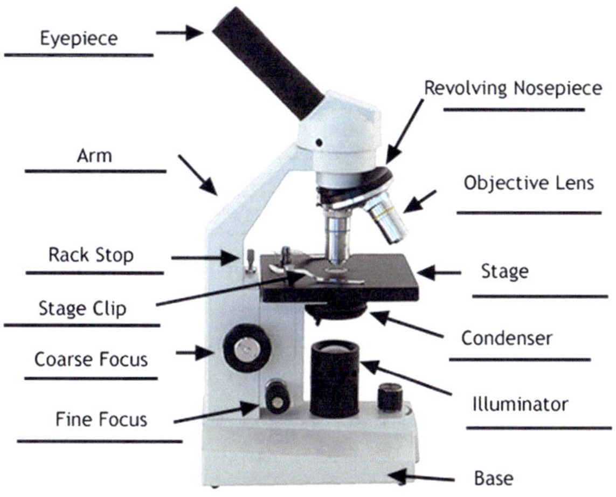

Figure 2.3. Parts of a light microscope.

Source: https://www.microscopeworld.com/Images/parts%20of%20a%20light%20microscope.jpg.

In addition, light microscopy is also found to be easily accessible and not highly expensive, which renders it a core technique in certain clinical laboratories. Equipment required, usually in the form of straightforward microscopes, is easily available in school environments, where students and novice health workers can learn by working on hands-on applications. With the Affordable Learning Georgia initiative that aims to enhance learning materials for students in microbiology, new lab manuals and instructional materials have also been developed to involve students in light microscopy. The resources enhance preliminary information required to excel in microbiological techniques and improve critical thinking and analytical capabilities through active learning practice (Smith & Selby, 2017). In this manner, light microscopy not only acts as a first-line diagnostic aid but also provides a learning environment for the cultivation of future healthcare professionals (Figure 2.3).

2.1.1. Principles of Light Microscopy

The principles of light microscopy form the basis of its primary contribution towards medical microbiology as a tool for visualization with microbial organisms. Utilizing visible light as the source of illumination, light microscopy allows for the investigation of samples via glass lenses that magnify the image for close scrutiny. The behavior of light when it interacts with the specimen is central to this, as it can be transmitted or reflected, thus delivering some level of contrast and transparency. Such an ability is most critical in microbiological diagnosis, where the characterization and identification of pathogens are dependent on accurate imaging methods. By manipulating light and lenses, light microscopy enables health science students to make significant observations of the structure and morphology of microorganisms, which enhances their understanding of microbial life and its relationship to human disease and health (McLaughlin et al., 2016).

One intrinsic component of light microscopy is its application in conjunction with varied staining techniques, which enable the optimization of the visibility of microorganisms. Stains , such as those applied in Gram staining and acid-fast staining are very common in laboratories to differentiate among microbial types based on the nature of their cell walls. The use of these stains allows for the observation of morphological characteristics, , such as form and arrangement, which is crucial in precise identification. Besides, the application of many stains can provide a complete picture of the microbial world, revealing information that is not readily obtainable in stained specimens. As stated in laboratory manuals, the integration of staining technique and light microscopy evidences the intersection of empirical practice and theoretical structure, driving students toward the level of competence needed for microbiological analysis (Heinaru & Naanuri, 2018).

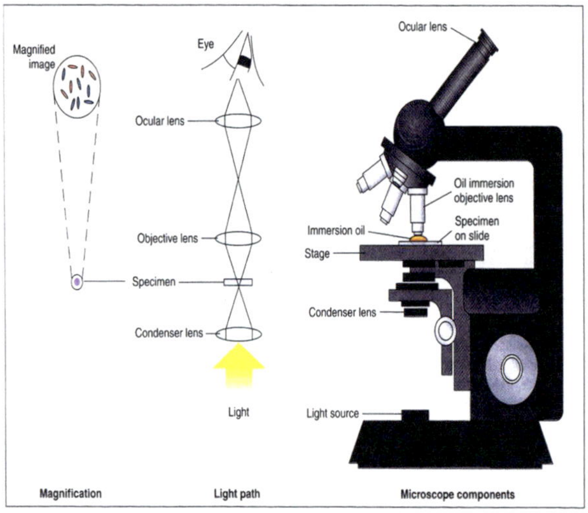

Figure 2.4. Principles of light microscopy.

Source: https://maharajacollege.ac.in/fileupload/uploads/66262999c7a7820240422091049principles%20and%20application%20of%20light%20microscope.pdf.

Additionally, light microscopy is not only about classical staining methods; it also acts as a stepping stone into viewing the full spectrum of sophisticated microscopy modalities available that advance the field of microbial inspection. Methods like fluorescence microscopy utilize the principles of light to observe specimens that fluoresce under certain wavelengths, enabling target-specific observation of microorganisms. Such advancement has extensive implications in clinical microbiology, particularly for pathogens that otherwise remain undiscovered with conventional staining protocols alone. Such a method makes it easier to learn the basics of light microscopy to equip students and practitioners with essential skills in scientific research, enabling them to navigate the complexities of microbial diagnosis and contribute meaningfully to clinical results in healthcare institutions (McLaughlin et al., 2016) (Figure 2.4).

2.1.2. Types of Light Microscopes

Light microscopy is a core facility of medical microbiology with many variants that are appropriate for various observation needs. The most basic but most popular type is the brightfield microscope, which employs visible light and combination lenses to magnify samples. It is particularly useful in staining procedures to view cell structures readily following Gram staining, acid-fast staining, and spore staining procedures. These techniques are important to the differentiation of microorganisms from their cell wall features and will ultimately be involved in diagnosis and treatment. The brightfield microscope, while strong, has resolution and contrast limitations that are potentially overcome through the use of other techniques to increase visibility in specimens. An important type of light microscope is the phase-contrast microscope, which enhances contrast of transparent samples without the need for complicated staining. By modifying the path of the light, phase-contrast microscopy allows for real-time viewing of living cells and cellular processes, particularly useful in microbiological research. This technique reveals subtle details invisible under conventional brightfield microscopy, and thus it is priceless for the observation of motility within microorganisms or for the analysis of cell-to-cell interactions within live cultures. Since clinical microbiology places greater emphasis on real-time imaging and insight into dynamic processes in cells, the phase-contrast microscope is an indispensable instrument, adding an extra dimension to conventional staining techniques for increased insight into microbial behavior. Lastly, the fluorescence microscope is an impressive advancement in light microscopy technology, where fluorescent dyes bound to biological samples are excited by precise wavelengths of light. This method is particularly convenient in the detection of certain microorganisms by targeted stains, e.g., in the application of immunofluorescence methods able to delineate types of pathogens based on immunological responses. Fluorescence microscopy enables the imaging of structures at the molecular level, thus enhancing our understanding of microbial cell biology and pathogenesis. This precision is crucial in medical microbiology, where the identification of pathogenic species from non-pathogenic strains can have a direct impact on treatment. Since it is possible to visualise cellular morphology with high sensitivity and specificity, fluorescence microscopy is an anchor-point in contemporary microbiological research, often supplemented with traditional staining techniques to completely illuminate microbial intricacies in clinical samples (Smith & Selby, 2017) (Figure 2.5).

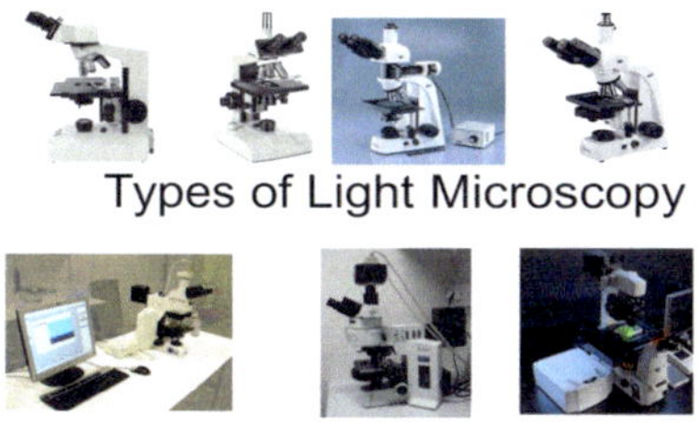

Figure 2.5. Types of light microscopes.

Source: https://slideplayer.com/4063226/13/images/slide_1.jpg.

2.1.3. Applications in Medical Microbiology

Microscopy and staining are essential to the identification and assessment of bacterial pathogens in medical microbiology. Light microscopy remains one of the cornerstones of preliminary evaluation of microbial specimens, as it allows one to observe morphology, motility, and spatial arrangements of bacteria. This simple technique is typically supplemented with staining techniques , such as the Gram stain, which differentiates bacteria according to cell wall content. The Gram staining technique is very crucial in clinical settings because it helps medical professionals determine the type of infection, whether Gram-positive or Gram-negative, and subsequently adjust antibiotic therapy accordingly. Consequently, the integration of light microscopy with effective staining techniques is critical in diagnosis and therapeutic approaches, and so helps in the timely control of infectious diseases (Heinaru & Naanuri, 2018). In addition, electron microscopy offers unrivaled resolution, and thus it is an important tool in the study of viruses and the ultrastructure of bacteria. Electron microscopy allows viewing of intricate cellular structures that are not readily visible using light microscopy. Electron microscopy offers important information on the assembly and morphology of pathogens at the molecular level and aids us in understanding how such organisms manage to avoid host defense and cause infections. In addition, fluorescence microscopy has enabled the detection of specific bacterial constituents, , such as proteins and nucleic acids. Through the use of fluorescent dyes or antibody labels, scientists can measure and locate specific targets within cells. Such specificity not only enhances the accuracy of diagnosis but also supports the development of novel antimicrobial strategies (Smith & Selby, 2017). Staining protocols, like the acid-fast stain and spore stain, play particularly important roles in identifying some resilient pathogens.

The acid-fast stain, for instance, is immensely helpful in diagnosing *Mycobacterium tuberculosis* since it colors the lipid waxy structures of the mycobacterial cell wall. This characteristic allows individuals to visually identify *M. tuberculosis* in clinical specimens and, consequently, make early diagnosis and treatment possible. Moreover, the spore stain is crucial for the identification of spore-forming bacteria like *Bacillus* and *Clostridium* species that are most often the etiological agent for severe infections. The awareness of spore viability and germination is also critical in bioterrorism readiness areas and food safety, where these microbes are a primary reason for impairment of health. Combined, these staining techniques enhance the analytical proficiency in clinical microbiology, the path to improved clinical outcomes (Heinaru & Naanuri, 2018) (Figure 2.6).

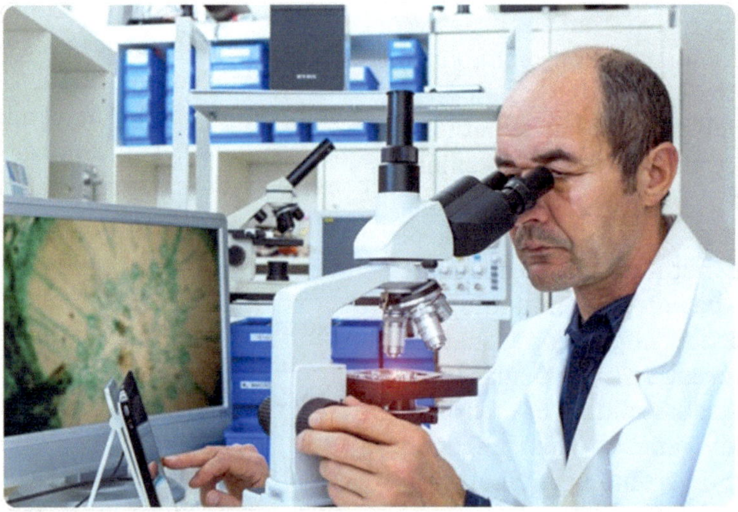

Figure 2.6. Microbiologist examining he characteristics of pathogens with the help of a light microscope.

Source: https://www.news-medical.net/image-handler/ts/20160614094952/ri/590/picture/2016/6/Light_microscopy_shutterstock_170882042.jpg.

Test Your Knowledge

1. What is the basic principle behind light microscopy, and how does it help visualize microorganisms?
2. What are the main types of light microscopes used in medical microbiology, and how do they differ?

2.2. Electron Microscopy

Learning Outcome

1. Discuss the principles of electron microscopy
2. Explain the types of electron microscopes
3. Focus on advantages and limitations of electron microscopy in microbiological studies

Electron microscopy (EM) is an essential breakthrough technology in clinical microbiology that provides unparalleled information on microorganism cellular structure. In contrast to standard light microscopy, which is limited by the boundaries of visible light wavelength, EM applies electron beams to achieve much higher resolutions, with the ability to observe structures at the nanolevel. This capability is of particular value to the analysis of subcellular structures, , such as membranes, organelles, and macromolecular complexes, which are all essential to understanding cell function and disease. Transmission electron microscopy (TEM) and scanning electron microscopy (SEM) methods permit a range of imaging strategies, enabling microbiologists to observe fine detail of organism morphology and surface topography essential for the diagnosis of disease and the mechanism of pathogen studies. One such critical advance in the application of electron microscopy is electron cryotomography (ECT), which optimizes the knowledge of microbial ultrastructure. It enables researchers to analyze thin samples, like tiny bacterial cells, in three-dimensional reconstructions with a near-native condition, thus eliminating the artifacts and distortions induced by standard fixation and staining. As focus has been geared toward new literature, ECT has provided valuable information on the spatial organization of cytoskeletal filaments, constituents of cell walls, and motility structures in bacteria, with minute details revealed that are inherent to the determination of biological mechanisms at a molecular level. Such innovations still render ECT more pertinent to microbiological research, suggestive of its capacity to demystify intricate cellular behavior and microbial species interactions (Jensen et al., 2009). Also, the combination of electron microscopy with advanced fluorescence techniques has opened up new frontiers in microbial pathogen research. Through the combination of the structural details of EM and the functional and dynamic information obtained by fluorescence microscopy, researchers are able to acquire a more integrated understanding of microbial behavior. This complementarity is especially relevant in infection mechanisms, where the understanding of both the morphology and physiological reaction of pathogens can give rise to improved therapeutic strategies. The improvement of new detection methods, as exemplified in evaluations of biological monitors, points to promising prospects for the utilization of sophisticated imaging techniques across a variety of disparate biological contexts. Such interdisciplinarity could be very significant in propelling forward our knowledge regarding microorganisms and thus directly affecting infection treatment and control (Smith & Selby, 2017).

2.2.1. Principles of Electron Microscopy

Electron microscopy is a powerful imaging technique that employs electrons rather than visible light to image specimens with nanoscale resolution. Electron microscopy is extremely valuable in microbiology where the delicate structural details of bacteria and viruses must be observed. As opposed to light microscopy, wherein the resolution is limited by the wavelength of visible light, electron microscopy achieves higher resolution with the use of an electron beam, allowing precise imaging of cellular structures. The standards of electron microscopy cover two main categories: transmission electron microscopy (TEM) and scanning electron microscopy (SEM), and each is used for a particular purpose. TEM is primarily used to observe thin specimens, and it produces well-defined internal structures, while SEM gives three-dimensional data on surface morphology. The unprecedented resolution offered by these methods enables microbiologists to study microbial structures at previously unattainable resolutions, and this adds depth to our understanding of microbial pathology and physiology. While electron microscopy offers insights that are unmatched, staining procedures remain at the heart of its utility, particularly in microbiological processes. Negative staining is a technique commonly used due to the ease and rapidity of use, producing contrast in samples that are otherwise hard to see. Negative staining allows for the observation of viruses and bacteria without heat fixation, which can warp or destroy the samples. By employing acidic dyes that are excluded from the surface of negatively charged cells, negative staining enhances contrast to allow morphology, size, and replication structures of specimens to be visualized clearly. Although the method is in decline now, the benefits for high-pressure laboratory conditions ensure that it is still a valid consideration by microbiologists. The integration of electron microscopy with negative staining has proven to be helpful in elucidating the structural features of microorganisms for clinical diagnosis, as testified by literature research work. Electron microscopy in combination with emerging monitoring techniques offers a better understanding of microbial behavior and interactions in advancing microbiological research. For instance, laser light scattering and fluorescence analysis are cooperative techniques to electron microscopy, supplementing detailed observation of samples. These will provide a multilevel insight into microbial characteristics, ranging from physical structure to functional behavior. With evolving laboratories fueled by rapid technological change, integration of various microscopic methods becomes inevitable for gaining firm scientific outcomes. Such integration, in addition to boosting analytical strength, also benefits clinical microbiology through more precise identification methods.

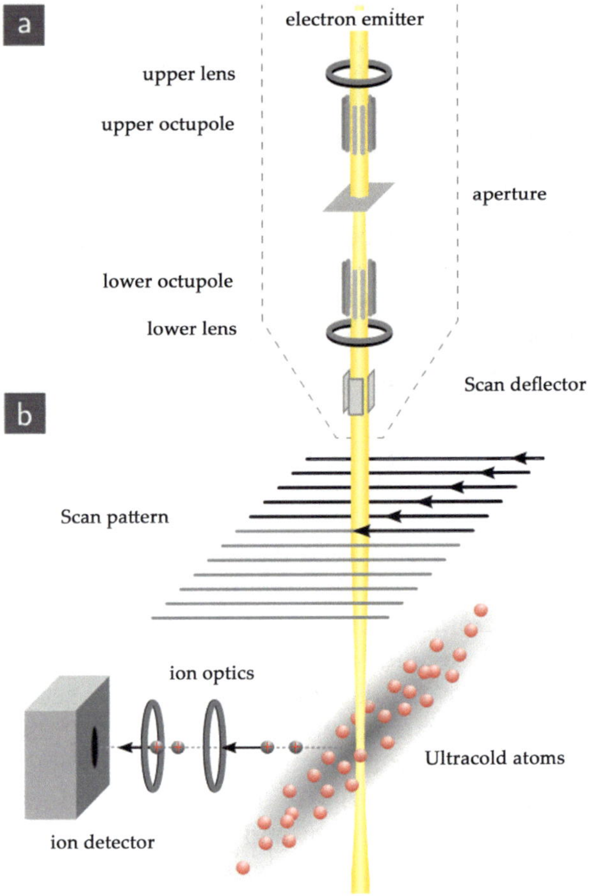

Figure 2.7. Working principle of the electron microscope. A schematic view of the electron column, represented by the dashed line, is shown in the upper half of the figure (a). A detailed description of the elements is given in figure (b) The column provides a focused electron beam which intersects a cloud of ultracold atoms prepared in an optical dipole trap. Electron impact ionization produces ions that are guided by ion optics towards a detector.

Source: https://www.researchgate.net/profile/Peter-Wuertz/publication/269908136/figure/fig6/AS:669015047426060@1536517025774/Working-principle-of-the-electron-microscope-A-schematic-view-of-the-electron-column.png.

The constant development and use of these approaches underscore their importance in today's microbiological research, yielding insights different from those produced by classical methods and thus informing better diagnostic and treatment practices (Figure 2.7).

2.2.2. Types of Electron Microscopes

Electron microscopy studies are at the core of medical microbiology with unrivaled resolution over the utilization of light microscopy. One of the principal types of electron microscope is the Transmission Electron Microscope (TEM), with atomic-level imaging of a sample being feasible through it. A TEM sends electrons through a thin sample, giving detailed information regarding cellular components , such as organelles, viruses, and even macromolecular complexes. This type of microscopy enables researchers to determine the structure and organization of microorganisms and thus enhance diagnostic precision. Secondly, the clear images captured through TEM enable us to understand the lifestyle of pathogens, which is crucial in designing effective treatments. As microbiologists continue to develop their methods, the capacity of TEM to view structures that were not visible in the past continues to remain a critical research tool in infectious disease research (Smith & Selby, 2017). In contrast, the Scanning Electron Microscope (SEM) has a unique but complementary function in microbiological research. SEM provides three-dimensional views by scanning the surface of a sample using a very narrow beam of electrons, allowing researchers to observe topographical characteristics and surface textures on nanometer levels. SEM is especially useful when observing the morphology of bacteria, fungi, and other microorganisms and provides information regarding their interaction with hosts and environments. The extent of information that is obtainable using SEM is vital in explaining the ways surface structures can be involved in pathogenicity, adhesion, and biofilm formation. This way, SEM enhances the understanding of microbial processes and mechanisms of infection and thus plays a central role in microbiological diagnosis and treatment strategies (Smith & Selby, 2017). SEM and TEM have transformed the practice of medical microbiology, yet their multifarious applications confirm the need to select the proper type of electron microscope based on specific research objectives. While TEM cannot dispense with elaborate intracellular investigation, SEM is better suited for surface structural investigations, bearing witness to the complementary nature of these machines. Both techniques provide different types of information, complementing each other in enhancing our overall knowledge concerning microorganisms and their role in disease. Thus, with advancing technology at all times, the application of electron microscopy in clinical and research settings remains at the forefront of advancing microbiological knowledge that will inform future diagnostic and therapeutic interventions (Smith & Selby, 2017) (Figure 2.8).

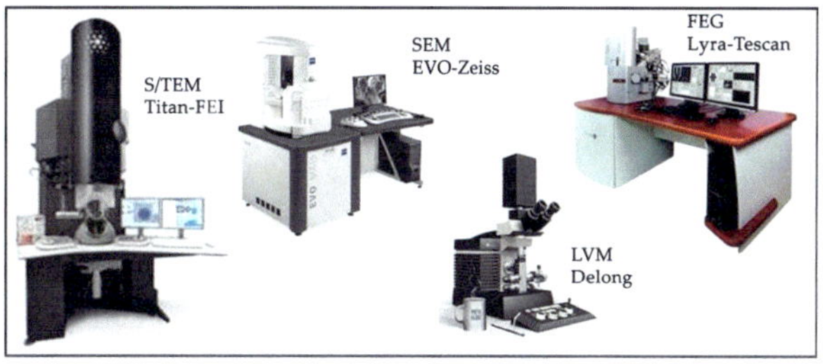

Figure 2.8. Examples of various types of electron microscopes.

Source: https://www.researchgate.net/profile/Daniel-Petlak/publication/267859158/figure/fig1/AS:650851236462600@1532186435468/Examples-of-various-types-of-electron-microscopes-3.png.

2.2.3. Advantages and Limitations in Microbiological Studies

Microbiological science benefits heavily from various methods of microscopy and staining, allowing observing and characterizing the microorganisms. The potential for real-time observation of living cells is a major advantage of light microscopy, as dynamic processes can be followed. It is also a widely accessible and cheap technique; hence, it is suitable for pedagogical uses and basic research. However, it is limited by having a lower resolution than electron microscopy, restricting the visualization of fine cellular morphology and minute pathogens. Electron microscopy, since it provides high-resolution images with informative details of microbial morphology, is plagued with some severe issues like the need for expert training and extremely costly operation. Thus, the choice of microscopy and staining technique has direct implications for the extent of microbial analysis, emphasizing the researcher's requirement to thoroughly consider the purpose of microbial research. As regards staining techniques, Gram staining remains a gem in microbial identification, providing information on cell wall structure and allowing discrimination between Gram-positive and Gram-negative bacteria. It is prized for its speed and simplicity, which are especially valuable for guiding initial treatment plans within the clinic. Nevertheless, it has some drawbacks; certain microorganisms, , such as those found in the Mycobacterium genus, resist Gram staining and require special techniques like the acid-fast stain to be correctly identified. Similarly, spore staining techniques can be invaluable in visualizing resting structures of bacteria, but may not precisely portray the living status of the organism.

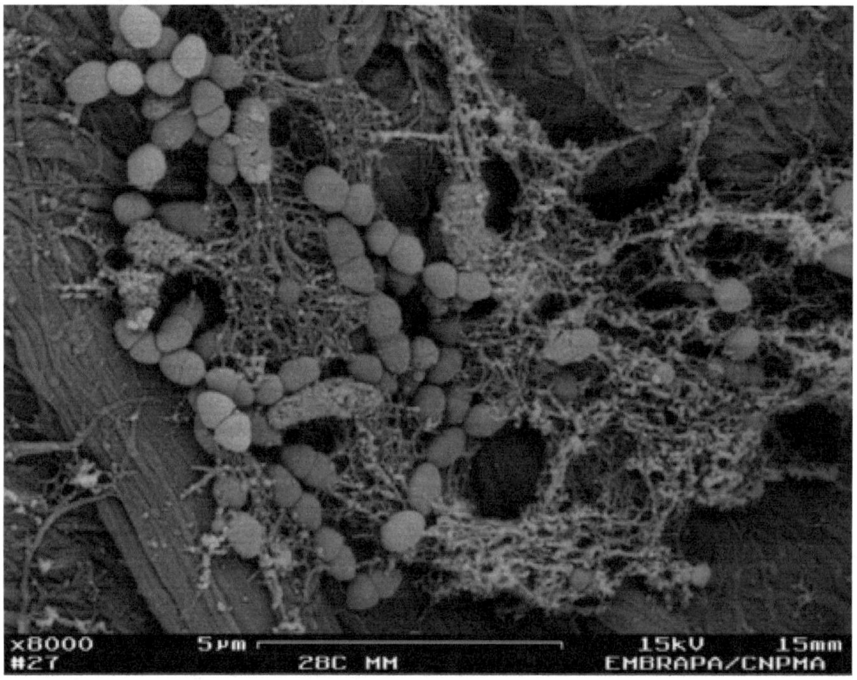

Figure 2.9. Scanning electron microscopy showing some bacteria capable of producing exopolysaccharides.

Source: https://www.researchgate.net/profile/Vanessa-Nessner-Kavamura/publication/225581731/figure/fig2/AS:302665314652161@1449172442327/Scanning-electron-microscopy-showing-some-bacteria-capable-of-producing.png.

Therefore, while staining techniques play a crucial role in directing microbiological investigations, their constraints necessitate the application of multi-mode technology where multiple techniques are utilized for exhaustive analysis. More advanced methodologies, including fluorescence microscopy and newer biofilm assessment techniques, are transforming microbiological investigations. Fluorescence microscopy complements the ability to selectively tag cell components, thereby allowing imaging of live microbial associations and complex behaviors. The method has been used to demonstrate microbial communities in biofilms that are determinant in environmental and clinical contexts. Interpretation of fluorescent signals, nonetheless, can be controlled by the choice of fluorophores as well as the intricacy of biofilm architectures. As has been pointed out in recent literature, the study of the physiology of biofilms and the various methods by which one would study such forms serves to emphasize the growth and issues within the field (Abràmoff et al., 2016). While new methods hold vast promise, ongoing debate concerning their strength and vulnerabilities acts to reaffirm the need for scientists to remain critically engaged with the methods employed in their microbiological studies, thereby advocating good scientific inquiry (Figure 2.9).

Test Your Knowledge

1. What are the primary differences between transmission electron microscopy (TEM) and scanning electron microscopy (SEM) in studying microorganisms?
2. How has electron microscopy contributed to the identification and characterization of viruses in medical microbiology?
3. What are the advantages of using electron microscopy over light microscopy for observing bacterial ultrastructure?
4. What are some limitations or challenges of using electron microscopy in routine clinical microbiology diagnostics?

2.3. Fluorescence Microscopy

Learning Outcome

1. Discuss the principles of fluorescence microscopy
2. Describe the types of fluorescent dyes and their applications
3. Explain the role of fluorescence microscopy in identifying specific microorganisms

Fluorescence microscopy is a novel technique in microbiology that enables researchers to visualize cellular components with great specificity and sensitivity. Fluorescence microscopy is founded on the principle of fluorescence, wherein fluorescent molecules absorb light at specific wavelengths and re-emit light at longer wavelengths. Scientists use fluorescent dyes and proteins to label specific structures or molecules in cells. This particularity makes fluorescence microscopy highly applicable in the study of microbial cells since it allows for differentiation between cell components, for instance, membranes, nuclei, and proteins, when exposed to ultraviolet light. Thus, this technique is essential in the study of microbes' interactions and activities in complex biological systems. One of the strong points of fluorescence microscopy in clinical microbiology is that it is capable of offering real-time images of dynamic processes in living cells. For instance, researchers have used the technique to view bacterial responses to antibiotics and thus gain a better understanding of microbial resistance mechanisms. Knowledge in this area is crucial, especially in the face of increased levels of multidrug-resistant strains, which pose serious threats to public health. With the aid of sophisticated fluorescent probes, scientists can observe how drugs impact the morphology and viability of microbes. Such a capability is important in designing effective treatments for bacteria that are resistant to antibiotics, making fluorescence microscopy a significant tool in current microbiological studies (Tahir et al., 2015).

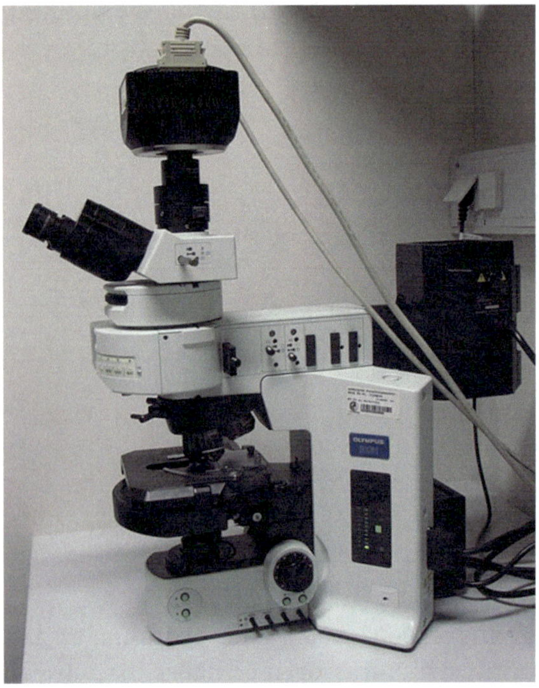

Figure 2.10. An upright fluorescence microscope (Olympus BX61) with the fluorescence filter cube turret above the objective lenses, coupled with a digital camera.

Source: https://upload.wikimedia.org/wikipedia/commons/thumb/d/dd/Olympus-BX61-fluorescence_microscope.jpg/500px-Olympus-BX61-fluorescence_microscope.jpg.

Fluorescence microscopy also enables research into microbial populations and their interactions within their native environment. With multiplex staining methods, researchers can investigate multiple microbial species simultaneously in biofilms or mixed cultures. This overview becomes indispensable to comprehending the synergistic and competitive relationships underlying microbial communities. Furthermore, the integration with automated image analysis makes it possible to analyze large sets of samples through high-throughput methods, further augmenting the power of fluorescence microscopy in experimental research. Through the display of these complex relationships, fluorescence microscopy participates in the development of novel antimicrobial treatments and directs approaches to combat biofilm-mediated infections, demonstrating its vital role in the advancement of medical microbiology (Heinaru & Naanuri, 2018) (Figure 2.10).

2.3.1. Principles of Fluorescence Microscopy

Fluorescence microscopy has emerged as a mainstay in clinical microbiology, providing unrivaled capability for resolving microscopic structures and processes at the cellular level. Varying from standard light microscopy, which is transmitted light-based, fluorescence microscopy uses specific wavelengths of light to cause fluorescent molecules within the sample to become luminescent. Fluorescence results in the release of light at longer wavelengths, allowing for greater contrast and selectivity of imaging. Fluorescence microscopy separates structures based on their intrinsic fluorescence or through the binding of fluorescent dyes to cellular components. These methods prove extremely useful for the identification of particular bacteria or pathogens by staining them with fluorochromes, thereby lighting them up against a black background. Visualization of these interactions in real time adds notably to our knowledge of microbial behavior and infectious processes. The technological foundation of fluorescence microscopy is dependent on several necessary elements, including light sources, filters, and detectors. The primary light source typically is a high-intensity lamp or a laser that emits chosen wavelengths of light, which excite the fluorophores within the sample. Filters are extremely significant; they are used to choose the light of excitation from the resulting fluorescence, as well as to prevent background noise that compromises the quality of the images. Fluorescence microscopes nowadays utilize advanced imaging technology, , such as computer analysis software and digital cameras, for quantification and documentation of fluorescence-level patterns. Not only does the technology allow better visualization, but also multi-channel imaging, whereby multiple fluorochromes are used together to explore cellular processes in parallel and thus set the stage for widespread microbiological studies. In clinical microbiology, visualization is not the sole application of fluorescence microscopy, but also diagnostic and research. For instance, it plays a crucial role in the determination of bacterial strains and their mechanism of pathogenicity by specific staining techniques. Fluorescence in situ hybridization (FISH) is particularly important in the detection and localization of specific nucleic acid targets within cells, generating information on microbial population dynamics and gene expression. The variety of fluorescence microscopy is shown by the various staining techniques used, for example, the Gram stain and acid-fast stain, which may be adapted into fluorescent techniques. Moreover, as researchers persist in trying to understand more of microbial life, methods of fluorescence microscopy are further enhanced, enabling new uses in diagnosing infections and microbial ecology studies. Hence, its principles and techniques are an integral component of contemporary medical microbiology research and diagnosis (Figure 2.11).

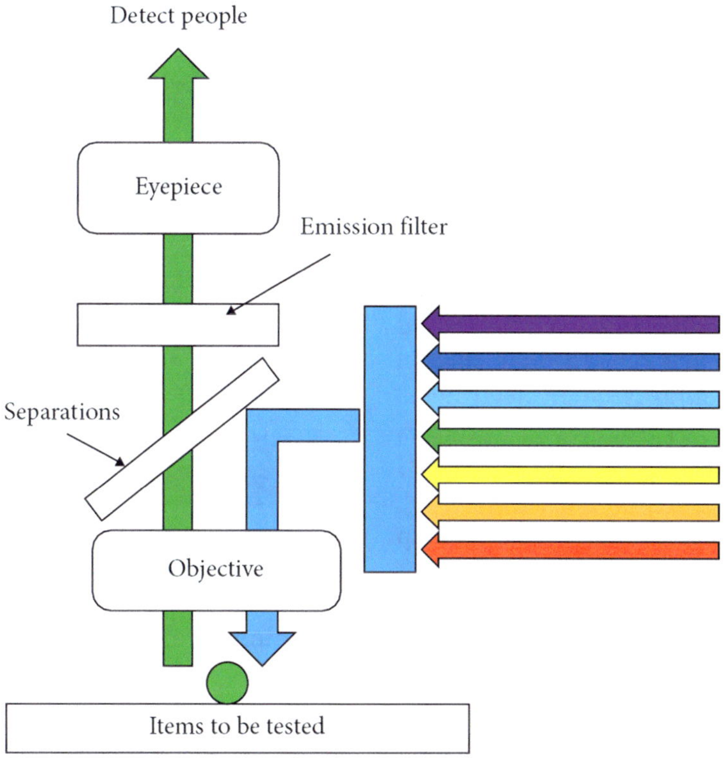

Figure 2.11. Schematic diagram of the fluorescence microscope principle.

Source: https://www.researchgate.net/publication/362650048/figure/fig2/AS:114312810854686 62@1663778795761/Schematic-diagram-of-fluorescence-microscope-principle.jpg.

2.3.2. Types of Fluorescent Dyes and Their Applications

Fluorescent dyes play a crucial role in microbiology as they enable visualization by fluorescence microscopy. Fluorescent dyes are light-absorbing at specific wavelengths and emit light at longer wavelengths, enabling specific identification of microorganisms. DNA-binding dyes like DAPI, which selectively stain nucleic acids, and membrane dyes like Dil, which target the lipid membrane, are the primary classes of fluorescent dyes. The use of these dyes is critical in the differentiation of live and dead cells, thus enhancing diagnostic accuracy. The use of these dyes not only enhances the imaging of microbial specimens but also enhances the efficacy of quantitative assays, thus providing the foundation for the sophisticated investigation of microbial pathogenesis and cellular dynamics within a culture setting, an innovation that is of significant importance in both clinical and research microbiology (Heinaru & Naanuri, 2018). But still another important class of fluorescent dyes is the conjugated polymers, which exhibit new properties beneficial in various applications for microbiology. These materials exhibit enhanced biocidal activity when they are loaded with bacterial cultures or attached to substrates. There are reports that certain cationic and anionic conjugated polyelectrolytes exhibit significant antibacterial effects, particularly when irradiated, which triggers reactive oxygen species leading to cell killing. This light exposure-biocidal efficacy relationship of these dyes proves their potential as dual-agent imaging and antimicrobials. The application of such fluorescent conjugated systems in tandem with advanced microscopy techniques, , such as Confocal Laser Scanning Microscopy (CLSM), facilitates thorough investigation of bacterial activity and treatment response at the cellular level (Corbitt, 2011). Expanding the application of fluorescent dyes, diverse applications have been discovered in a range of staining protocols used in microbiology and have impacted the diagnostics field significantly. For instance, fluorescently labeled antibodies are extremely specific to particular pathogens, such that they can be rapidly detected using techniques like fluorescence in situ hybridization (FISH). This method enables the identification of specific nucleic acid sequences within microbial populations and, thus, knowledge of microbial diversity and function within complex environments. Also, fluorescent stains may be used in combination with traditional techniques, , such as the Gram stain, to provide an overall analysis which includes morphology, as well as molecular identification. As fluorescent staining techniques continue to evolve, their synergy with modern microscopy will assist in making our understanding of microbiological processes more precise towards unparalleled diagnostic and therapeutic modalities in infectious disease (Heinaru & Naanuri, 2018) (Figure 2.12).

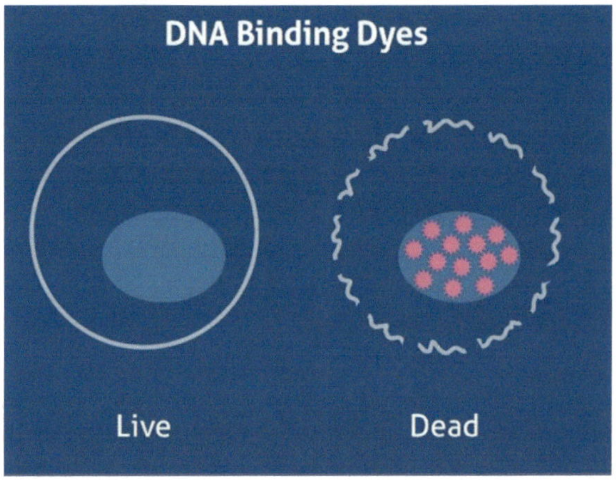

Figure 2.12. DNA-binding dyes.

Source: https://www.ptglab.com/media/5992/phantom-dye.jpg.

2.3.3. Role in Identifying Specific Microorganisms

Its use in detecting a single microorganism is the focal point of clinical microbiology. Light microscopes, via their capability to enlarge specimens 1,000 times, allow visibility of the morphology of the microbes, which is crucial for preliminary classification. In particular, Gram staining procedures capitalize on the differences in the cell wall architecture of Gram-positive and Gram-negative bacteria, so the organisms can readily be identified. This differential staining helps identify pathogens to categorize them, which is extremely important in identifying appropriate treatment regimens. Additionally, the visual cues obtained from light microscopy may guide further testing, , such as biochemical and serological tests, to make the diagnosis procedure more efficient in clinical settings (Heinaru & Naanuri, 2018). Through enabling rapid visualization of bacterial characteristics, microscopy is a potent first step in the identification of single microorganisms, which affects public health intervention as well as treatment protocols. Electron microscopy enables a novel way of microorganism identification at the nanoscale, particularly valuable in fine structure visualization beyond what light microscopy can offer.

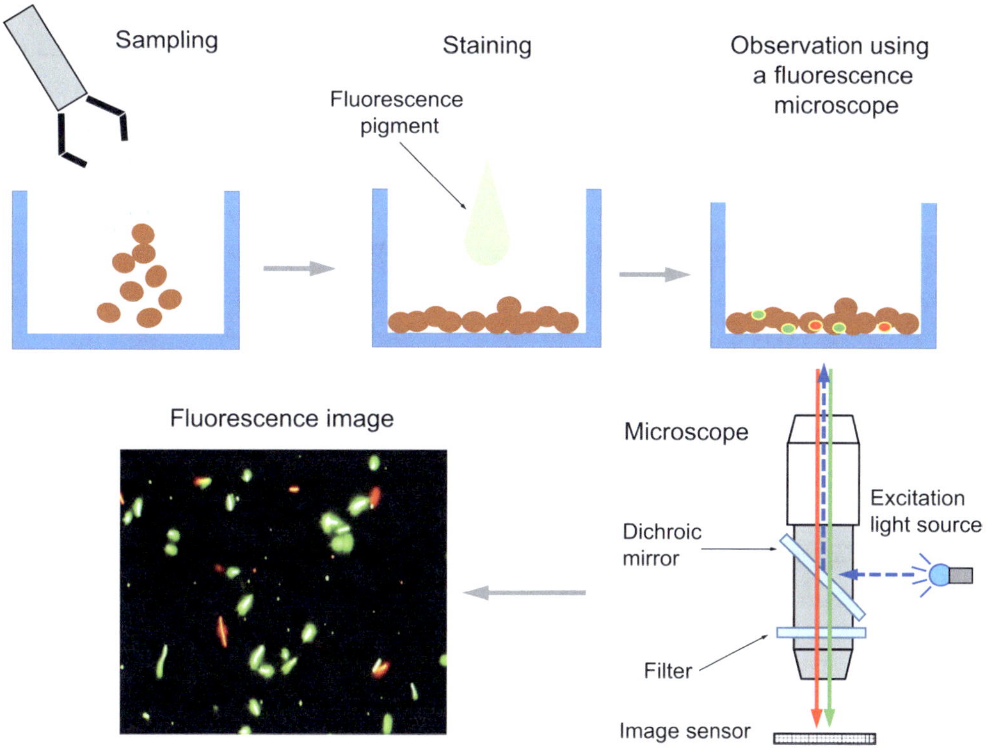

Figure 2.13. Schematic view of microorganism detection using a fluorescence microscope.

Source: https://www.researchgate.net/publication/362874271/figure/fig4/AS:1143128108672078 2@1664330902575/Schematic-view-of-microorganism-detection-using-a-fluorescence-microscope-The-sample-is.png.

This technique has unparalleled resolution, revealing intracellular organelles and surface details , such as appendages that are important for microbial differentiation. For instance, electron microscopy is able to identify viral particles clearly, providing information on morphology as well as structure. Fluorescence microscopy also complements the traditional techniques by utilizing specific stains that bind to unique microbial constituents, facilitating clear identification despite mixed populations. The combination of these techniques enhances diagnostic accuracy since it can determine subtle differences that express pathogen virulence or resistance mechanisms, which are required for particular therapeutic measures (Georgakopoulos et al., 2008). Lastly, new microscopy techniques enable the complete identification of microorganisms, which form the foundation of efficient disease control. Staining techniques also supplement the application of microscopy in the identification of specific microorganisms since they enhance contrast and facilitate the visibility of features pivotal to classification. Acid-fast staining is particularly important in the identification of Mycobacterium species like *Mycobacterium tuberculosis*, the causative agent of tuberculosis. The differential staining technique assists in making the characteristic lipid composition of specific bacterial cell walls discernible so that these can be detected in clinical specimens. Alternatively, spore staining is of particular significance in the identification of resistant spore-forming bacteria like *Bacillus* and *Clostridium* species, significant in food safety and infection control. Using various microscopy techniques, these staining methods provide valuable tools for both microbiologists and clinicians. By making systematic use of these approaches, laboratory researchers can effectively identify pathogens, and appropriate treatment measures can be begun, easing the burden of infectious diseases in health facilities (Heinaru & Naanuri, 2018) (Figure 2.13).

Test Your Knowledge

1. How does fluorescence microscopy enhance the visualization of microorganisms compared to traditional light microscopy?
2. What are fluorescent dyes and their applications?
3. What are some common applications of fluorescence microscopy in studying microbial physiology and interactions?

2.4. Gram stain Technique

Learning Outcome

1. Understand the historical background of the Gram stain
2. Discuss the procedure of the Gram staining process
3. Focus on the interpretation of Gram stain results

Gram stain is a fundamental microbiological method to classify bacteria into two general groups: Gram-positive and Gram-negative. The classification is based on the difference in the structure of the cell walls of bacteria, which reflects the capacity of bacterial cells to hold the crystal violet stain while staining. The staining process involves some essential steps: fixation, adding the crystal violet stain, iodine treatment, decolorization with alcohol or acetone, and safranin counterstaining. The differential response of bacteria to this staining process not only allows for identification but also assists in the comprehension of bacterial characteristics that are vital for diagnosis and treatment regimens. The process takes on a vital role in medical microbiology, whereby the Gram-positive vs. Gram-negative classification could decide on therapy and unveil the probable virulence determinants linked with several groups of bacteria. Evidence of the efficacy of Gram stains is brought forward by their application in clinical practice, where they have been employed to make the diagnosis of a number of infections (Smith & Selby, 2017). One research study at Tygerberg Academic Hospital referenced the employment of Gram-negative bacteria in cervico-facial sepsis patients. Despite evidence in Gram stain reports of gram-negative organisms, less than half were successfully cultured, showing the complex relationship between microbial viability and methods of staining. In the specific instance of 90 swabs of pus, 48 samples showed a Gram-negative stain, but only two cultured positive for Gram-negative organisms. This contrast highlights the value of confirming Gram stain by culture techniques, again stressing that although Gram stain is a rapid, valuable diagnostic tool, it cannot be relied on alone for positive pathogen identification, particularly in those cases with atypical clinical presentations. Furthermore, the Gram stain is not simply a diagnostic reagent and is a mainstay teaching technique in microbiology. Ease of use and effectiveness make it a routine part of the curricula for future microbiologists and medical doctors.

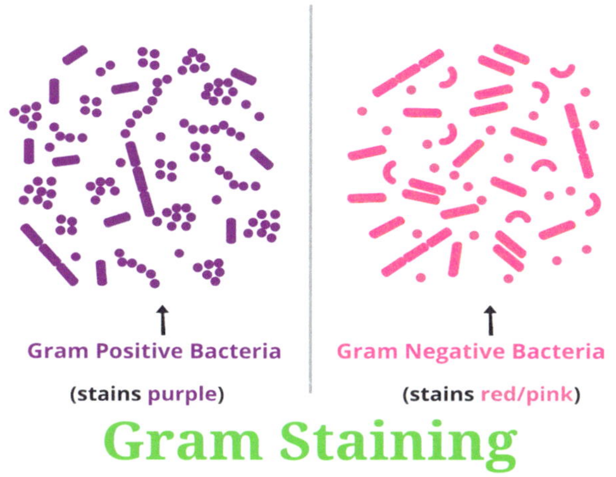

Figure 2.14. Gram staining.

Source: https://encrypted-tbn0.gstatic.com/images?q=tbn:ANd9GcQt4iOkj4ZWc2ffqrhba5ck5D5ypTZ4_P29xA&s.

An understanding of interpreting Gram stain results encourages a deeper understanding of microbial diversity and disease pathogenesis. In practice, recognition of limitations of the Gram stain, e.g., potential false positives or false negatives, also conditions practitioners to approach diagnostic challenges more intelligently. Because it plays a critical role in defining clinical outcomes and treatment regimens, ongoing research into Gram stain reports and their impact is an essential part of medical microbiology, and this is borne out in the findings at Tygerberg Academic Hospital, which underscored the importance of accurate bacterial identification in the management of patients (Barnard, 2019Barnard, 2019) (Figure 2.14).

2.4.1. Historical Background of the Gram stain

The Gram stain, a pivotal technique in medical microbiology, traces its roots to the late 19th century. Developed by the Danish bacteriologist Hans Christian Gram in 1884, this staining method emerged from Gram's investigation into the characteristics of bacterial cell walls. While examining lung tissue from patients who had died from pneumonia, Gram sought a way to differentiate between various bacterial species. His new approach used two cross-reacting dyes: crystal violet and safranin, and could identify bacteria depending on the nature of the cell walls. The fundamental technique established by him made it possible for subsequent scientists to categorize bacteria into Gram-positive and Gram-negative types, which significantly influenced the development of microbial identification and classification in clinical laboratories. The ease of availability of the Grams method encouraged its application in microbiological laboratories on a mass scale, ushering in a series of developments in clinical and research fields. By separating Gram-positive bacteria with a greater peptidoglycan layer to maintain the major dye and Gram-negative bacteria with an outer membrane accounting for a counterstaining effect, the Gram stain facilitated quick and effective identification of pathogens. This grouping was totally crucial for clinicians, as treatment, particularly with regard to the selection of antibiotics, was determined by it. As a result, Gram stain has not only influenced laboratory practice but has also been a vital component of epidemiological investigation and public health, aiding in the control and comprehension of infectious diseases. The Gram stain has evolved numerous times over the years without changing its basic principles. Current microbiologists are also supported by many of the refinements and variations of the initial procedure, most of which include digital imaging and high-power microscopy as part of more sophisticated staining procedures. Improvements in laboratory techniques, as well as the incorporation of staining techniques , such as the acid-fast stain and spore stain, have also broadened the scope of microbial diagnosis. Such is evident in instructional resources like the lab manual adapted for use in allied health courses, where additional staining procedures complement the Gram stain, which gives students a greater understanding of microbial identification and biochemical tests needed to determine unknown microorganisms (Generalov et al., 2014; Smith & Selby, 2017). Thus, historical significance is still preserved by the Gram stain, noting its place as a necessary element in medical microbiology.

2.4.2. Procedure of the Gram staining Process

Gram staining is a fundamental laboratory procedure in clinical microbiology to broadly categorize bacteria into two groups: Gram-positive and Gram-negative. Bacteria are classified on the basis of morphological diversity in the bacterial cell wall. The technique begins by making a bacterial smear on a microscope slide, followed by a heat-fixation step to adhere cells to the slide and destroy contaminating flora. Once the cells are corrected, the first stain, crystal violet, is employed. This first stain penetrates every bacterial cell and colors them purple, which is crucial as it serves as a point of reference for differentiation during subsequent steps. The function of crystal violet as a first dye cannot be overstated because it is what starts the process of differentiating bacteria based on cell wall properties (Smith & Selby, 2017). After the crystal violet is applied, the slide is then iodized, serving as a mordant.

The iodine complexes with the crystal violet, effectively sealing the dye within the cells, particularly in Gram-positive bacteria that have a thick peptidoglycan cell wall. Next, a decolorizer agent, typically ethanol or acetone, is applied, which exploits the structural differences found in bacterial cell walls. Gram-positive bacteria retain the violet-iodine complex due to their thick cell walls, while Gram-negative bacteria, whose walls are thinner and contain an outer membrane, release the complex and turn colorless by now. This critical process is significant because it demonstrates the significance of cell wall composition during Gram staining since it directly influences the observed color at this stage and also the identification of bacteria (Smith & Selby, 2017).

Finally, the decolorized slide is counterstained with safranin, which colors the otherwise colorless Gram-negative bacteria. This double staining allows for easy differentiation, whereby the Gram-positive bacteria will be purple and the Gram-negative bacteria pink in color. Under a microscope with the slide, clinicians are easily able to ascertain the type of bacteria present, which is essential to diagnosis and treatment. The consistency and reliability of Gram staining signify its extensive use in laboratories across the world. By the generation of informative preliminary data on microbial pathogens, the technique of Gram staining is a classic combination of microscopy and staining techniques to reassert its relevance in the practice of medical microbiology (Smith & Selby, 2017) (Figure 2.15).

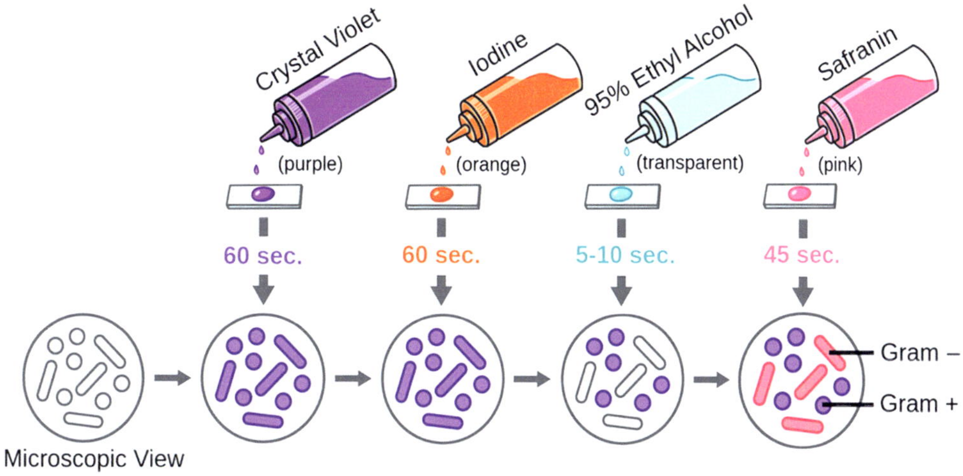

Figure 2.15. Workflow of Gram staining method.

Source: https://images.my.labster.com/bd7be05a-dd65-4273-a739-ff9801800aad/GRM_The_Gram_stain_procedure_overview_THEORY.en.x1024.png.

2.4.3. Interpretation of Gram stain Results

Gram stain is an essential diagnostic tool used in medical microbiology, which enables bacteria to be grouped into two groups immediately: the Gram-positive and Gram-negative. This grouping is according to the structural construction of the bacterial cell wall, primarily the thickness of peptidoglycan layers. Gram-positive bacteria do not resist the crystal violet stain, but they will be purple as seen under the microscope, while Gram-negative bacteria, with a thinner peptidoglycan layer overlaid by an outer membrane, do not retain the primary stain and are stained pink by the counterstain. These fundamental differences determine the primary identification of bacteria as well as subsequent therapeutic action, as Gram-negative bacteria are more resistant to antibiotics. Through proper interpretation of Gram stain tests, clinicians can initiate appropriate treatments, which affect patient care and treatment plans in medical microbiology to a large degree. Nevertheless, the reliability of Gram staining as a first-line diagnostic test is not unlimited. Variability may occur in microscopic examination due to preparation of the specimen, staining technique, or biological variation in bacterial populations. Studies that used an internal quality assurance (IQA) program highlighted these issues by reporting that the majority of results for Gram stains, close to 75.2%, were concordant with culture, leaving a large margin of error. Of the reported discrepancies, there were some cultures that had discrepant identification, in the form that while a Gram stain may report one type of microorganism, the culture would show differently. These findings emphasize the significance of combining Gram stain analysis with other diagnostic analyses, including culture and molecular testing, to enhance clinical utility and ensure that patient care is grounded on accurate laboratory results (Durussel et al., 2017).

Moreover, next-generation computerized image analysis technology can have the potential to revolutionize the interpretation of Gram stain reports. Traditional methods for image evaluation, as effective as they are, are susceptible to the nuances of human perception and inconsistency between technicians. The most recent innovations have proved that computer systems can evaluate Gram-stained slides with great accuracy, with sensitivity ranging from 66% to 99% and specificity from 78% to 99% in early working research. Utilizing algorithms trained on extensive datasets to interpret bacterial morphology not only offers the promise of standardization across laboratories but also allows for round-the-clock interpretation of samples. Such innovations could significantly improve diagnostic precision in clinical microbiology, addressing current limitations, and paving the way for more robust methodologies in the interpretation of Gram stain results (Hauser et al., 2011).

Test Your Knowledge

1. What is the purpose of performing a Gram stain in microbiology?
2. What are the main steps involved in the Gram staining procedure?
3. How can Gram stain results guide the initial choice of antibiotic treatment in bacterial infections?

2.5. Acid-Fast Stain Technique

Learning Outcome

1. Explain the importance of acid-fast staining in microbiology
2. Understand the procedure for acid-fast staining
3. Focus on clinical significance of acid-fast results

The Acid-Fast Stain technique is a critical medical microbiology technique for the staining of Mycobacterium species, , such as those responsible for causing tuberculosis. Unlike many bacteria, which are easily stained by common stains, the distinctive waxy lipid coating, mycolic acid, in acid-fast bacteria's cell walls prevents them from being stained using simple stains. Therefore, the Acid-Fast Stain achieves differential staining through a series of protocol steps , including carbolfuchsin utilization, heat, and acid-alcohol decolorization in order to efficiently distinguish acid-fast bacilli from non-acid-fast bacteria. This specificity is important in medical diagnosis so that rapid identification and proper treatment are possible, thereby facilitating the greater goal of effective public health intervention. As of the Acid-Fast Stain method, initial warming to permit penetration of the carbolfuchsin dye into the bacterial cell wall renders it an essential component of the procedure. When the acid-alcohol decolorization process is reached, acid-fast organisms hold the dye's red color, whereas non-acid-fast bacteria lose the color and are currently colorless. To provide a sharp contrast, methylene blue is employed as a counterstain to allow visualization of the non-acid-fast organisms blue against the vibrant color of the acid-fast stained cells. This dual-color presentation not only allows identification under the microscope but also gives a clear-cut characteristic of acid-fast bacteria; thus, it is useful in clinical microbiology where early diagnosis can make or break treatment and patient outcome. Implication of the Acid-Fast Stain method in clinical practice has widespread implications in the control of infectious diseases, particularly in the pathophysiology of chronic wounds and the interrelation between the latter and bacterial infection. Because chronic wounds are typically faced with wide microbial invasion, accurate identification of persistent acid-fast bacilli is necessary in addressing complications of poor healing and infection control. For instance, new developments in biopolymeric nanofibrous wound dressings with antibacterial agents illustrate the forward march in medicine towards enhanced delivery of wound care. By integrating the outcome of Acid-Fast Stain analysis, healthcare experts are able to develop targeted treatment modalities with the use of biohybrid nanofibers, thus curing both issues of bacterial infection as well as antibiotic resistance (Homaeigohar et al., 2020). This collaboration of staining techniques and novel materials opens up new research and therapy options in medical microbiology and indicates the vital role of the Acid-Fast Stain technique in medical microbiology (Figure 2.16).

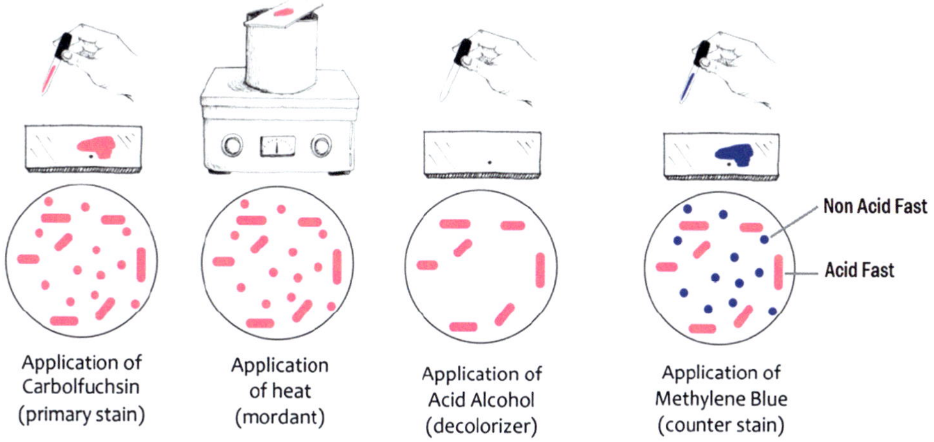

Figure 2.16. Acid-fast staining.

Source: https://biokimicroki.com/wp-content/uploads/2021/04/steps-of-acid-fast-staining-method-720x334.png.

2.5.1. Importance of Acid-Fast Staining in Microbiology

Acid-fast staining is a key procedure in microbiology, namely to identify and distinguish mycobacteria, the genus to which *Mycobacterium tuberculosis*, among other pathogens, belongs. Traditional staining procedures like Gram staining will not stain these microorganisms adequately due to the dense lipid composition of their cell wall, which does not allow penetration by traditional dyes. The acid-fast stain involves a specific method using heat and phenol to facilitate dye absorption, which ends in the identification of Gram-positive bacteria with acid-fast characteristics. The distinctive staining characteristic is critical to disease diagnosis and treatment, , such as tuberculosis, particularly epidemic cases, where it is most essential for public health measures because of the necessity of rapid and accurate identification. Besides, the use of acid-fast staining is not only for identification but also to determine the pathogenicity and resistance profile of mycobacterial species. The acid-fast *Bacillis* characteristic cell wall structure contributes to their survival against the environmental pressures and most of the antibiotics. The use of acid-fast staining techniques can yield not only a microscopic identification of the organisms but also information regarding their biochemical properties and potential problems in treatment. This type of information is crucial in clinical settings, where physicians rely on accurate diagnoses to inform treatment. Enhanced knowledge facilitated by acid-fast staining can aid in disease control, ultimately influencing patient outcomes and public health policy. Furthermore, the integration of acid-fast staining into routine laboratory practice is aided by extensive instructional materials, including laboratory manuals specifically designed for allied health students. These educational materials support enhanced understanding of microbiology procedures by providing crucial context and procedural details to students and professionals. For instance, materials developed from the OpenStax Microbiology textbook emphasize laboratory practice of acid-fast staining techniques while showing their applicability in the broader subject of medical microbiology. By establishing a hands-on learning setup, these materials can be able to enhance critical thinking and diagnostic skills, securing the invaluable role of acid-fast staining in preventing infectious diseases and enhancing the corpus of knowledge of future healthcare professionals (Smith & Selby, 2017) (Figure 2.17).

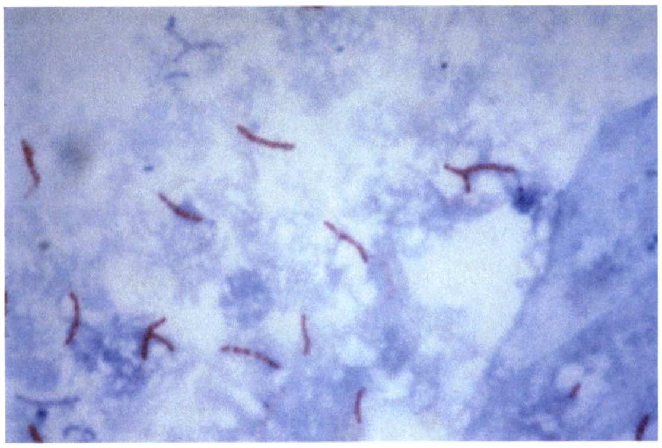

Figure 2.17. Microscopic visualization of the acid-fast bacteria *Mycobacterium tuberculosis*.

Source: https://upload.wikimedia.org/wikipedia/commons/thumb/7/71/Mycobacterium_tuberculosis_Ziehl-Neelsen_stain_02.jpg/1280px-Mycobacterium_tuberculosis_Ziehl-Neelsen_stain_02.jpg.

2.5.2. Procedure for Acid-Fast Staining

The acid-fast staining process is significant in microbiology for the detection and distinction among mycobacterial species, notably *Mycobacterium tuberculosis*, the agent of tuberculosis. The staining process is based on the ability of certain bacteria to resist carbol fuchsin dye retention even when followed by subsequent acid-alcohol decolorizing. A smear of a bacterium is initially made on a slide and fixed by passing it through the flame. The slide is then flooded with carbol fuchsin and heated, either by steaming over boiling water or by applying a heat source. This is an important step, as the heat causes the dye to penetrate the waxy cell wall of acid-fast organisms. Subsequently, the slide is washed with water and subjected to an acid-alcohol solution in order to decolorize any non-acid-fast bacteria, thus allowing for a differentiation between acid-fast and non-acid-fast organisms. After the decolorization process, a counterstain, most often methylene blue, is added to the slide. The counterstain produces color contrast, staining the non-acid-fast bacteria blue and leaving the acid-fast bacteria red due to them retaining the initial carbol fuchsin stain. This results in a good contrast differentiation that allows the observers ease of identifying Mycobacterium species in a light microscope. Good visualization depends not just on proper staining but also on good microscopy skills. Observations are usually made with an oil immersion objective that visually enlarges the organisms to a level where their morphology can be seen. These precise and standardized processes demonstrate the significance of staining procedures in medical microbiology, emphasizing the roles they play in infectious disease diagnosis and microbial pathogenesis research, as noted by laboratory supplies designed for allied health students (Smith & Selby, 2017). The significance of the acid-fast staining procedure goes beyond simple identification; it holds a basic role in epidemiologic research and public health surveillance. By identifying acid-fast bacilli correctly, healthcare professionals can make appropriate interventions and treatments for patients suffering from tuberculosis. The process is not only a laboratory process; it is an example of the application of microbiological principles in the clinical setting. Moreover, adaptations of this staining process have made it possible for its application in the detection of non-tuberculous mycobacterial infections, which have increased over the past few years. Thus, the acid-fast stain remains a standard-bearer of microbiological diagnosis, shaping individual health as well as population-based public health trends. With instructors developing teaching resources to assist students in such vital staining techniques (Smith & Selby, 2017), the applicability of such techniques to clinical microbiology gets progressively reinforced.

2.5.3. Clinical Significance of Acid-Fast Results

The acid-fast stain procedure is of supreme clinical importance in medical microbiology, especially for the diagnosis of mycobacterial infections, including tuberculosis (TB). The method takes advantage of the distinctive mycolic acid-containing cell walls of mycobacteria, which remain resistant to decolorization by acids after initial staining. This property allows discriminatory detection of such pathogens within clinical samples, and it forms the foundation of an active TB diagnosis, especially in low-resource environments where speed to result is extremely critical. Through microscopy, healthcare workers are able to visually identify the existence of acid-fast bacilli, with immediate therapeutic and public health measures to control the dissemination of infectious diseases caused by such microorganisms (Szewczyk et al., 2013). Further, the clinical application of acid-fast results extends beyond diagnosis. It represents a critical parameter employed in guiding treatment regimens as well as monitoring therapeutic responses in TB or other mycobacterial infections. The early identification of acid-fast results has an important bearing on patient management measures, such that clinicians are able to distinguish between drug-susceptible and drug-resistant mycobacterial strains. Progress in the past decades, including mass spectrometry techniques, allows for faster and more precise identification of mycobacterial species, which enhances the diagnostic value of acid-fast reports. The real-time data is crucial to facilitate appropriate treatment regimens that can cure TB effectively while avoiding transmission among vulnerable populations (Gow et al., 2017). With the global burden of tuberculosis and other mycobacterial infections still present, the clinical significance of acid-fast results becomes increasingly significant. Continued research and improvement of staining techniques, coupled with advances in molecular detection, will enhance public health monitoring and response to TB epidemic control. Consequences of correct acid-fast staining highlight the significance of medical microbiology in disease control and prevention.

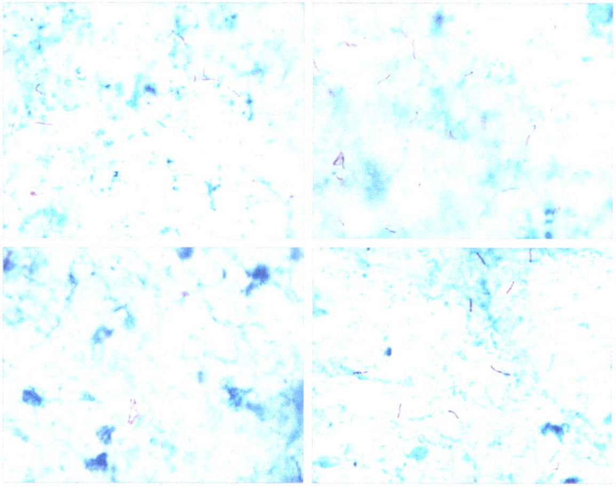

Figure 2.18. Acid-fast staining result under an oil immersion lens. Positive acid-fast stain results showed that among the pus, there were numerous rod-shaped *Mycobacterium tuberculosis* bacteria specifically stained red, while others were stained blue. Approximately 20 *Mycobacterium tuberculosis* bacteria could be seen in one view.

Source: https://www.researchgate.net/publication/345487922/figure/fig2/AS:11431281228934820@1710259015033/Acid-fast-staining-result-under-an-oil-immersion-lens-Positive-acid-fast-stain-results.tif.

More sophisticated diagnostic techniques, supplementing the traditional acid-fast method, have the potential for improved patient outcomes and to contribute to the global process of TB elimination as a public health problem. Future investigations need to focus on optimization of these procedures and examination of the extent of mycobacterial disease to enhance its use in the clinic (Szewczyk et al., 2013) (Figure 2.18).

Test Your Knowledge

1. What is the importance of acid-fast staining in microbiology, and which types of bacteria are typically identified using this technique?
2. Describe the main steps involved in the acid-fast staining procedure. Which primary stain, decolorizer, and counterstain are commonly used?

2.6. Spore Stain Technique

Learning Outcome

1. Present an overview of spore-forming bacteria
2. Understand procedure for spore staining
3. Explain the importance of spore staining in clinical diagnostics

The spore stain method is a significant technique applied in medical microbiology for the identification of endospore-forming bacteria , such as *Bacillus* and *Clostridium* species. These bacteria share the unique feature of encysted resting spores that enable them to withstand harsh environmental conditions , such as heat, desiccation, and chemicals. The staining of such resistant spores is traditionally achieved by the Schaeffer-Fulton method, assisted by malachite green to penetrate the hard spore coat and safranin as a counterstain to view the vegetative cells. This type of differentiation becomes essential in hospitals where pathogen detection from patient cultures can determine the direction of therapy. The clear visibility of spores above vegetative cells provides valuable information regarding bacterial life cycles, pathogenesis, and probable virulence, highlighting the significance of the spore stain procedure in diagnostics. In recent studies, the effectiveness of the spore stain procedures has been enhanced by comparative evaluation against other technologies, , such as the Calcofluor White M2R procedure for microsporidial spores. While the classical spore stain remains an indispensable reagent in *Bacillus* species identification, the added use of other staining techniques forms part of a more robust diagnostic system. Most importantly, double use of methods can circumvent vulnerability to problems with specificity inherent in single staining techniques, where misidentification would be counter to patient care. For instance, noting that the formation of discrete deep-blue equatorial or horizontal stripes in microsporidian spores would reduce false-positive yields highlights the requirement for the merger of different diagnostic approaches when working with clinical specimens. Thus, an efficient staining protocol enhances confidence in spore identification within microbiology laboratories. Further, the convolution of spore morphology, particularly of its protein assembly, highlights the complexity associated with the spore stain technique. The outer coat of the spore coat consists of numerous proteins that contribute to its strength and stability. This creates challenges for conventional microscopy. New developments in fluorescence microscopy, following on from genetic mapping of the spore coat, proteins have revealed spatially resolved structures of the spore coat, including a previously unappreciated glycoprotein outer layer called the spore crust. This growth of understanding into the structural composition of spores not only makes the utilization of the spore stain technique more rewarding but also enhances our understanding of bacterial survival mechanisms in unfavorable conditions. The technological advances in microscopy and molecular biology support the relevance of continued interaction between various approaches to methods in enriching diagnostic procedures and therapeutic interventions in medical microbiology (Smith & Selby, 2017) (Figure 2.19).

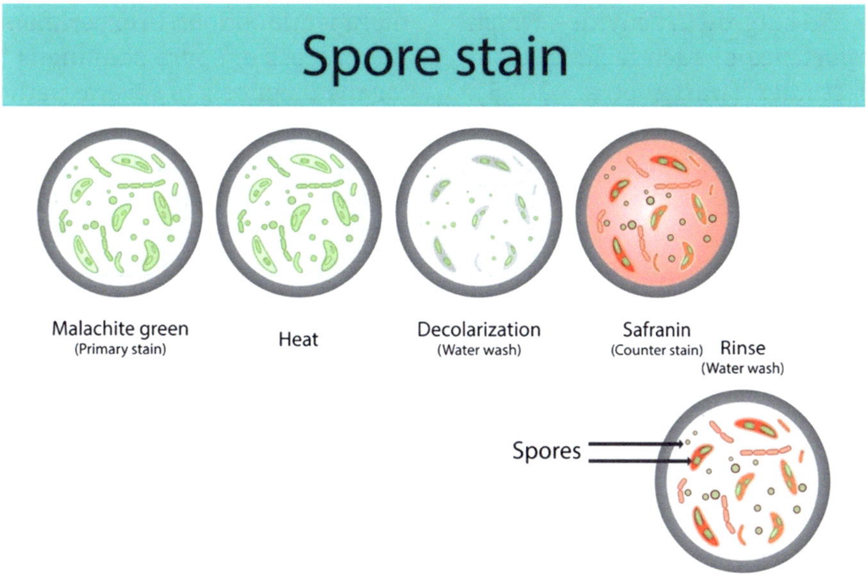

Figure 2.19. Spore stain.

Source: https://microbialnotes.com/wp-content/uploads/2022/11/Endospore-1.webp.

2.6.1. Overview of Spore-Forming Bacteria

The spore-forming bacteria are primarily classified under such genera as *Bacillus* and *Clostridium*, which have superb survival properties through the production of spores. The spores serve as a survival strategy against environmental pressure in the form of extreme temperatures and dehydration. When the environment is not supportive of bacterial growth, spore production enables the bacteria to enter a dormant state, which significantly enhances their survival properties in adverse environments. Microscopy plays a crucial role in the identification and characterization of these bacteria, and light microscopy is used most commonly. However, scientists are hindered by the inherent properties of light microscopy in imaging the spore morphology, thus the need for ancillary techniques that refine our understanding of such resilient microorganisms (Fazzan et al., 1953).

In addition, modern staining techniques provide crucial information relating to the identification of spore-forming bacteria. The spore stain, for instance, is designed to color bacterial spores visually with an efficiency that distinguishes them from vegetative cells. By heating and applying dyes, the process provides selective staining of the spores, which is a critical stage in the study of *Bacillus anthracis* and *Clostridium* difficile, two of the most virulent organisms in existence. The activity of such stains can also be tested under fluorescence microscopy, where researchers can measure spore viability and the germination outcome after being subjected to different conditions. As attested by certain investigations, growth factor manipulations, , such as L-methionine, during sporulation have a significant effect on spore resistance and outgrowth activities, which suggests the importance of such techniques in microbiological studies (Harris et al., 2015). It is of the most critical significance in public health and medical microbiology to know spore-forming bacteria. They can produce nasty infections and pose threats in a entire variety of environments, from food kitchens to hospitals. Not only does their spore-forming capacity hinder the sterilization process, but it also necessitates the use of specialized microscopic and staining procedures in order to be able to identify and study them effectively. The application of such techniques to investigate the morphology and viability of spores is important in the development of effective infection control measures as well as therapeutic interventions. As advances occur in technology, application of advanced microscopy and novel staining techniques will enhance our capacity to contend with the challenges presented by spore-forming bacteria in clinical and environmental environments (Fazzan et al., 1953).

2.6.2. Procedure for Spore Staining

The spore staining process is a significant technique of medical microbiology with the aim of distinguishing bacterial spores, which are typically resistant to regular staining. The principal goal of spore staining is the distinction of spores from vegetative cells on the basis of their particular structural differences. A significant process of staining is the Schaeffer-Fulton method employing malachite green as the principal stain. To start with, heat is used to initiate the penetration of the dye into the spores and washed out with water to remove excess dye. The process successfully stains the spores, which become green, while vegetative cells become a different color after counterstaining with safranin. Thus, the exact execution of this staining process is of utmost importance for accurate visualization and spore-forming bacteria detection, which dictates further clinical decisions in terms of diagnosis as well as therapeutic options. In experimental applications, the process of spore staining is highly valuable for the diagnosis of several pathogenic bacteria that can pose serious health issues. By way of example, *Bacillus* and *Clostridium* species are important examples of spore-forming bacteria that must be properly identified in the clinic. As has been argued in studies, routine diagnosis does not necessarily rely on normal techniques since spore identification is likely to call for special staining techniques for the purposes of establishing accuracy (Rahman et al., 2013).

The spore stain can also provide insights into the resistance of such microbes, especially in harsh environments where they remain viable without complete metabolism. Thus, the integration of spore staining into diagnostic strategies increases the likelihood of finding microsporidial infections, which are likely to be subjected to misdiagnosis when basic stains are employed singularly. The rationale behind the spore staining process is not limited to mere identification; it is an educational aspect that helps in understanding microbial morphology and behavior when observed under the microscope. Due to the depth of field and contrast limitations of the light microscope, spore staining techniques overcome such constraints (Fazzan et al., 1953). Such minor color variations better represent the physiology of the bacteria as well as the adaptive survival mechanisms that spores represent. The multistained images produced offer a greater insight into microbial interactions and resistance to the environment, thus more adequately equipping microbiologists with the tools needed for research and clinical applications. By this, spore staining is not just a component of a process but an integral part of learning the grander implications of microbial life and resilience in medical and pathogenic applications (Figure 2.20).

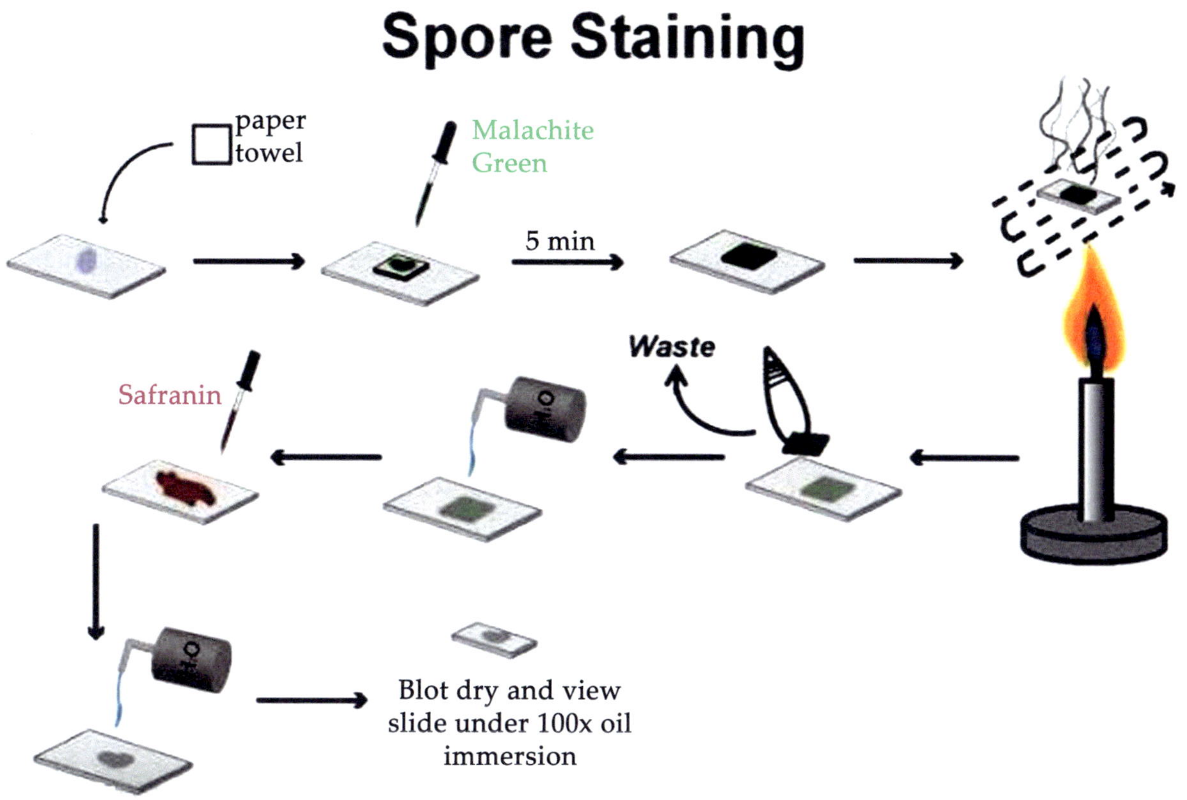

Figure 2.20. Spore staining procedure.

Source: https://i0.wp.com/microbeonline.com/wp-content/uploads/2015/05/Procedure-of-Spore-Staining.jpg.

2.6.3. Importance of Spore Staining in Clinical Diagnostics

The clinical significance of spore staining is emphasized by its ability to differentiate between spore-forming and non-spore-forming bacteria. Spores, produced by species within the genera *Bacillus* and *Clostridium*, are inherently very resistant to environmental stresses like desiccation and heat, and hence not stained effectively by routine staining procedures. Spore-forming staining, particularly through methods , such as the Schaeffer-Fulton technique, employs heat and differential dye treatment to effectively highlight the presence of spores. Early detection of spore-producing pathogens in clinical labs is crucial for accurate diagnosis and management, especially in life-threatening conditions involving *Clostridium* difficile or anthrax-producing *Bacillus anthracis*. Visualizing spores distinctly enhances the clinical microbiologist's skill for effective antimicrobial treatment and informs public health measures against epidemics of these deadly pathogens. In addition to their medical relevance, spores also play significant roles in environmental monitoring and biodefense. The spore-forming capacity of certain bacteria poses a possible risk in natural as well as human-made environments. Therefore, efficient spore staining techniques become not only a means for clinical diagnosis but also for environmental surveillance of contaminated environments. Investigation of the biocidal activity of various agents towards spores can be done through advanced staining techniques, as presented in research that associates photophysical properties of conjugated polyelectrolytes with antibacterial activity (Corbitt, 2011). These recognitions facilitate the development of specific decontamination protocols in health care settings as well as in the general population. Moreover, spore detection can influence biodefense strategic decision-making, linking clinical microbiology with overall safety concerns. Lastly, the pedagogical value of spore staining in microbiology must not be underrated. Incorporation of spore staining in the training laboratory enhances critical microscopic skills and analytical techniques among prospective microbiologists. Spore staining skill supports advanced concepts of pathogenicity processes and microbial resistance, which form the foundation of modern microbiology education. These fundamentals provide support to current research endeavors in understanding various microbial communities and interactions within ecological niches, thus influencing public health initiatives and infectious disease management. As the microbiology landscape is in evolution, incorporating advanced spore staining methods will further augment undergraduate and graduate programs through an appreciation for hands-on experience for microbial longevity as well as for pathogenicity (Generalov et al., 2016).

Test Your Knowledge

1. What is the purpose of performing a spore stain in microbiology?
2. Which bacterial genera are most commonly identified using the spore staining technique?
3. Describe the key steps involved in the spore staining procedure and the stains used.

SUMMARY

In concluding the discussion of microscopy and staining techniques in medical microbiology, it is evident that the techniques are important in accurate microbial identification and diagnosis. Light microscopy remains the most applied equipment in the lab since it provides valuable information regarding microbial morphology. However, its limitation necessitates other means of enhancing clarity and detail, hence the importance of various stains that are employed to view specific structures. Whereas light microscopy delivers a general image, the advent of advanced techniques, , such as electron and fluorescence microscopy, significantly expands the scope of investigation. These modalities allow for high-resolution imaging and selective identification of microorganisms, thereby resulting in more precise diagnoses. The use of multiple staining techniques also contributes to the precision and reliability of microbiological tests. For instance, the Gram stain and acid-fast stain are core methods for the differentiation of bacterial species based on cell wall characteristics. The Gram stain enables one to distinguish between Gram-positive and Gram-negative bacteria, while the acid-fast stain is utilized to identify Mycobacterium species. In addition, spore stain is critical to detect spores in certain bacterial genera, which can be critical in clinical applications. Interestingly, the synergistic effect of these techniques, in this instance the simultaneous application of Calcofluor White M2R and Gram-chromotrope Kinyoun modified, shows a novel approach to increasing specificity in the diagnosis of diseases , such as microsporidiosis, highlighting the results (Rahman et al., 2013). Lastly, the summation of this examination points out that continually advancing microscopy and staining techniques enhance not only our understanding of microbial life but also revitalize the field of medical microbiology. Advances in microscopy, despite inherent limitations, enable visualization of microscopic detail unprecedentedly (Fazzan et al., 1953). This ensures that clinical microbiologists are equipped with cutting-edge technology for more accurate and efficient diagnosis of infectious diseases. As research advances, having a multi-dimensional approach involving traditional along with novel methodologies will unveil avenues for enhanced diagnostic capability, leading to better patient outcomes in microbiological medicine.

Advances in microscopy and staining protocols form a fundamental aspect of medical microbiology because they provide scientists with the tools required to see and characterize microorganisms. Light microscopy represents a simple method that is widely employed due to the accessibility of equipment and simplicity. Through the utilization of visible light and lenses, practitioners are able to observe living samples under low to high magnifications. However, its limitation is its inability to identify smaller pathogens, hence the need to incorporate more sophisticated methods. Electron microscopy, for instance, has an advantage over light microscopy in the sense that it employs electron beams. This has much higher resolution and is therefore invaluable in investigating viral structure and subcellular features of bacteria, which are generally not identifiable by light microscopy (Heinaru & Naanuri, 2018). Consequently, electron microscopy has found a prominent role as a diagnostic and research tool in infectious diseases. Fluorescence microscopy enhances the advancements in light and electron microscopy by using fluorescent stains that bind particularly to cellular components. The technique permits visualization of specific microorganisms at the use of markers that emit light when stimulated by specific wavelengths of light. The particular strength of fluorescence microscopy is that it can label multiple cellular targets at once, enabling the study of complex interactions within microbial communities. Furthermore, new technologies, , such as Confocal Laser Scanning Microscopy (CLSM), provide higher precision by eliminating out-of-focus light, increasing image quality and depth. Recent research on the use of conjugated polyelectrolytes (CPEs) has indicated that they possess remarkable antibacterial activity, which is quantified by such advanced imaging techniques (Corbitt, 2011). The new technologies illustrate the continued revolution in microscopy that enhances the understanding of microbial pathogenesis and facilitates more efficient diagnostics. Staining procedures also contribute significantly to microorganism identification and characterization, including Gram staining and acid-fast staining, among the procedures that provide basic data regarding bacterial cell wall makeup. The Gram stain divides bacteria into Gram-positive and Gram-negative categories based on their cell wall composition, a critical parameter employed to inform treatment. This differential staining technique consists of a series of steps involving crystal violet staining, iodine treatment, decolorization, and counterstaining that yield valuable information about the composition and structure of the bacterial cells. Acid-fast staining is used, however, in specific to identify mycobacteria, which possess waxy cell walls that are resistant to the common staining processes. These classical methods, when applied in combination with the contemporary microscopy methods, provide revealing information on the morphology and function of microbes, underlining the critical interrelationship between the staining methods and microscopic examination in infectious disease diagnosis and comprehension.

KEY TERMS FROM THIS CHAPTER

- Acid-containing cell walls
- Acid-fast stained cells
- Acid-fast staining process
- Bacterial growth
- Bacterial responses
- Biofilm architectures
- Biotechnological applications
- Acid-fast stain
- Acid-fast staining
- Advanced fluorescence techniques
- Bacterial infection
- Biochemical tests
- Biofilm-mediated infections
- Cell morphology

CRITICAL THINKING QUESTIONS

1. Which type of microscopy uses a beam of electrons instead of light to visualize specimens?

a. Light Microscopy

b. Fluorescence Microscopy

c. Electron Microscopy

d. Phase-contrast Microscopy

2. What is the primary purpose of Gram staining in microbiology?

a. To measure the size of bacteria

b. To differentiate bacteria based on cell wall composition

c. To identify viruses

d. To observe live bacterial motility

3. In bright-field microscopy, why are stains often applied to samples?

a. To increase the fluorescence of the specimen

b. To kill the specimen

c. To increase contrast between the specimen and background

d. To focus the light source

4. Which microscopy technique allows visualization of live, unstained cells by enhancing contrast?

a. Electron Microscopy

b. Dark-field Microscopy

c. Fluorescence Microscopy

d. Phase-contrast Microscopy

5. Which staining technique is primarily used to differentiate Gram-positive and Gram-negative bacteria?

a. Gram stain

b. Acid-fast stain

c. Endospore stain

d. Negative stain

Short Answer Questions

1. What is the principle behind bright-field microscopy?
2. How does phase-contrast microscopy enhance the visualization of transparent specimens?
3. What are the main differences between electron microscopy and light microscopy?
4. Why is staining necessary in microscopy, and what are some common types of stains used?
5. Explain the difference between simple staining and differential staining techniques.
6. How does Gram staining differentiate between Gram-positive and Gram-negative bacteria?
7. What is the purpose of acid-fast staining, and which type of microorganisms is it primarily used to detect?
8. Describe the function of fluorescent dyes in fluorescence microscopy and give an example of their application.

Answers to Critical Thinking Questions

1. (c) 2. (b) 3. (c) 4. (d) 5. (a)

REFERENCES

1. Abdul Rahman, E. J., Hamat, R. A., Ithnin, N. R., M. S., et al. (2013). Comparison of Calcofluor White M2R fluorescence and modified Gram chromotrope Kinyon staining methods for the detection of microsporidia spores from stool samples. https://core.ac.uk/download/153821005.pdf (accessed on 13th June 2025).
2. Abee, T., Ganguly, J., Kranenburg, R. van, et al. (2025). Characterization of sporulation dynamics of *PseudoClostridium thermosuccinogenes* using flow cytometry. https://core.ac.uk/download/pdf/323105635.pdf (accessed on 13th June 2025).
3. Abràmoff, M. D., Costa, A. R., Lourenço, A., Azevedo, N. F., Brown, M. J., Bulut, F., Ceri, H., et al. (2016). Critical review on biofilm methods. https://core.ac.uk/download/55636361.pdf (accessed on 13th June 2025).
4. Georgakopoulos, D. G., Després, V., Fröhlich-Nowoisky, J., Psenner, R., Ariya, P. A., Pósfai, M., Ahern, H. E., Moffett, B. F., and Hill, T. C. J.: Microbiology and atmospheric processes: biological, physical and chemical characterization of aerosol particles, Biogeosciences, 6, 721–737, https://doi.org/10.5194/bg-6-721-2009, 2009. (accessed on 13th June 2025).
5. Ahmed, S., Alazazi, E. A., & Murtey, M. D. (2023). Negative staining: A forgotten technique in microbiology. https://core.ac.uk/download/590905589.pdf (accessed on 13th June 2025).
6. Altammar, K. A. (2023). A review on nanoparticles: Characteristics, synthesis, applications, and challenges. *Frontiers in Microbiology, 14*. https://doi.org/10.3389/fmicb.2023.1155622 (accessed on 13th June 2025).
7. Arendale, W. F., Kilgore, M. V., Jr., & Zahorchak, R. J. (2025). Definition of a near real time microbiological monitor for space vehicles. https://core.ac.uk/download/pdf/42821826.pdf (accessed on 13th June 2025).
8. Barnard, N. (2019). Prevalence of gram-negative infections in cervical-facial sepsis. https://core.ac.uk/download/289120735.pdf (accessed on 13th June 2025).
9. Bashir, A. (2025). Exploring the biological basis for *Salmonella* persistence in food manufacturing environments. https://core.ac.uk/download/78899101.pdf (accessed on 13th June 2025).
10. Bowe, C. (2025). Viability assessment of the probiotic spore former *Bacillus subtilis*: An investigation into the effect of *in-vitro* pig gastric conditions. https://core.ac.uk/download/46520249.pdf (accessed on 13th June 2025).
11. Corbitt, Thomas S.. "Antibacterial activity of conjugated electrolytes." (2011). https://digitalrepository.unm.edu/chem_etds/13 (accessed on 13th June 2025).
12. Driks, A., Eichenberger, P., Eskandarian, H. A., Gitai, Z., et al. (2010). A distance-weighted interaction map reveals a previously uncharacterized layer of the *Bacillus subtilis* spore coat. https://core.ac.uk/download/pdf/82224719.pdf (accessed on 13th June 2025).
13. Durussel, C., Greub, G., & Scherz, V. (2017). Internal quality assurance in diagnostic microbiology: A simple approach for insightful data. https://core.ac.uk/download/149207828.pdf (accessed on 13th June 2025).
14. Fazzan, F. P. (1953). Fluorescent staining of bacteria with auramine O. https://core.ac.uk/download/629903738.pdf (accessed on 13th June 2025).

15. Generalov, I. I. (2016). *Medical Microbiology, Virology & Immunology. Pt. 1. General Microbiology & Medical Immunology*. https://core.ac.uk/download/80150449.pdf (accessed on 13th June 2025).

16. Generalov, I. I., Sencovich, S. A., & Zheleznyak, N. V. (2014). *Instructions for Laboratory Training in General Microbiology & Immunology*. https://core.ac.uk/download/80150439.pdf (accessed on 13th June 2025).

17. Gow, N., Istel, F., Jenull, S., Lion, T., et al. (2017). Quantitative analysis of *Candida* cell wall components by flow cytometry with triple-fluorescence staining. https://core.ac.uk/download/131024827.pdf (accessed on 13th June 2025).

18. Harris, C. N. (2015). The efficiency of methionine as a radioprotectant of *Bacillus anthracis* for cell viability and outgrowth time after UVC and gamma irradiation. https://core.ac.uk/download/277528385.pdf (accessed on 13th June 2025).

19. Hauser, R. G. (2011). Digital image analysis of Gram-stained culture specimens. https://core.ac.uk/download/232768842.pdf (accessed on 13th June 2025).

20. Heinaru, E., & Naanuri, E. (2018). *Experimental Microbiology*. UNIVERSITY OF TARTU INSTITUTE OF MOLECULAR AND CELL BIOLOGY Chair of Genetics. ISBN 978-9949-77-911-6 (accessed on 13th June 2025).

21. Homaeigohar, S., & Boccaccini, A. R. (2020). Antibacterial biohybrid nanofibers for wound dressings. *Acta Biomaterial, 107*, 25–49. https://doi.org/10.1016/j.actbio.2020.02.022 (accessed on 13th June 2025).

22. Hushim, M. F. B., Khalid, A., Manshoor, B., Mohammed, Z., et al. (2016). Rapeseed oil spray development of diesel IDI spray nozzle under air movement influence. https://core.ac.uk/download/19162796.pdf (accessed on 13th June 2025).

23. Szewczyk, R., Kowalski, K., Janiszewska-Drobinska, B., & Druszczyńska, M. (2013). Rapid method for Mycobacterium tuberculosis identification using electrospray ionization tandem mass spectrometry analysis of mycolic acids. *Diagnostic microbiology and infectious disease*, *76*(3), 298–305. https://doi.org/10.1016/j.diagmicrobio.2013.03.025(accessed on 13th June 2025).

24. Jensen, G. J., & Li, Z. (2009). Electron cryotomography: A new view into microbial ultrastructure. https://core.ac.uk/download/4882547.pdf (accessed on 13th June 2025).

25. McLaughlin, S., & Petersen, J. (2016). *Laboratory Exercises in Microbiology: Discovering the Unseen World Through Hands-On Investigation*. https://core.ac.uk/download/217331732.pdf (accessed on 13th June 2025).

26. Smith, Molly and Selby, Sara, "Microbiology for Allied Health Students" (2017). Biological Sciences Open Textbooks. 15. https://oer.galileo.usg.edu/biology-textbooks/15(accessed on 13th June 2025).

27. Selby, S., & Smith, M. (2017). *Microbiology for Allied Health Students: Instructional Materials.* https://core.ac.uk/download/217306143.pdf (accessed on 13th June 2025).

28. Tahir, H. (2015). The effects of crude and pure green tea polyphenols on bacteria biofilm formation and endospore germination. https://core.ac.uk/download/352523693.pdf (accessed on 13th June 2025).

IDENTIFICATION OF MICROORGANISMS

3

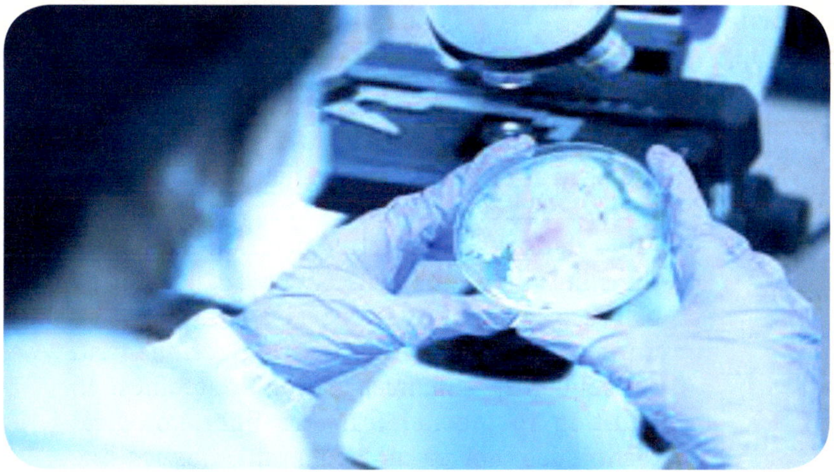

LEARNING OBJECTIVES

After studying this chapter, you will be able to:

1. Understand the concept of biochemical tests for the identification of microorganisms
2. Describe antigen-antibody techniques
3. Identify microorganisms by molecular diagnostics
4. Compare different types of identification techniques
5. Discuss clinical applications
6. Focus on future trends in microbial identification

Introduction

Microbial identification plays an important role in clinical microbiology in disease treatment and management. Through the identification of infecting pathogens, clinicians can adapt antimicrobial therapy to fight the pathogens efficiently. Microbial diagnostics have come a long way since the initial cultures that were easy to complicated systems that provide instant results. Such a transformation is particularly relevant as early detection of the pathogens completely alters the outcome in patients. Evolution of technology , such as ELISA, agglutination tests, and molecular diagnostics , such as PCR and RT-PCR, revolutionized microbial identification as a faster and more precise process in diagnostics, which is critical in the clinic. This chapter will try to discuss these techniques, providing a detailed description of their application and significance in contemporary microbiology. In the general context of microbial diagnosis, biochemical tests are the universal tools in the identification of the majority of microorganisms. These analyses generally entail the determination of metabolic potential, enzymatic function, and physiological characteristics of the organism, all of which continue to be relevant even with the age of molecular methods dominance. With all the increased sensitivity and specificity that have been attained through the implementation of advancements in molecular techniques , such as PCR and RT-PCR, microbial metabolism knowledge gained from biochemical analyses continues to be invaluable. Identification not only receives support in the metabolic processes of the pathogens, but also forms the foundation for the principle of designing accurate interventions. In addition, traditional biochemical test methods remain an affordable method, especially in resource-poor areas where newer molecular technology remains an unaffordable consideration.

The intersection of such methods reiterates the efficacy of a multidisciplinary strategy in infectious organism identification. The heterogeneity of microbial communities makes the identification and characterization of pathogens even more difficult. One should take into consideration that the majority of infections are caused by heterogeneous microbial populations of variable pathogenicity and drug susceptibility. Recent literature indicates that new molecular technologies, including advanced technologies like MALDI-TOF MS, hold great promise for better access to microbial diversity and resistance mechanisms. Challenges do remain; the complexity of such communities necessitates ongoing improvement in diagnostic methods. The ideal resolution would not only identify single species, but also indicate their dynamic relations in the host environment. As Sousa & Pereira, (2013) suggest, new-generation diagnostic agents are essential to remain in accordance with the constantly evolving landscape of infectious diseases in an attempt to better comprehend mechanisms of resistance and ultimately contribute to improved clinical decisions in antimicrobial therapy.

Importance of Microorganism Identification in Medical Microbiology

Accurate identification of microorganisms holds the topmost priority in medical microbiology because it has a direct impact on diagnosis, therapy, and control procedures of infectious diseases. Owing to the staggering variety of pathogens, traditional diagnostic procedures are inadequate to yield rapid and accurate results. This deficiency pinpoints the need to employ advanced techniques, such as biochemical tests, via which it becomes feasible to distinguish between microorganisms based on their metabolic characteristics. Moreover, antigen-antibody techniques like ELISA and agglutination are crucial in the direct antigen contact-based specific detection of pathogens, which enables rapid detection and better decision-making at the clinical level. Collectively, an amalgamation of these techniques supports a well-balanced understanding of microbial infections and consequently enhances patient outcomes. In addition to biochemical and immunological techniques, newer molecular diagnostics like PCR and RT-PCR have revolutionized pathogen identification completely. These methods provide unparalleled speed and accuracy, allowing healthcare professionals to detect microbial DNA or RNA with more specificity than the traditional culturing methods. Such advances are of particular significance in emergency clinical scenarios where quick identification can have a revolutionary impact on the approaches to treatment. For instance, the ability to rapidly diagnose infections caused by diarrhoeagenic *Escherichia coli* strains exemplifies the way molecular techniques allow for discrimination among the different pathogenic variants based on their genetic makeup. Consequently, the ongoing development of diagnostic methods underscores the need for rapid and correct identification processes to efficiently combat infectious disease threats, as supported by more recent developments in pathogen detection technology (Pavankumar & Sankaran, 2008).

In addition, understanding the genetic and phenotypic heterogeneity of microbial populations is critical to successful management of infection. Traditional diagnostic methods fail to fully do credit to such complexities in many cases, leading to incomplete identification of pathogens and suboptimal treatment outcomes. Molecular methods not only hasten identification procedures but also allow for assessment of microbial diversity, which hints at potential differences in pathogenicity and resistance patterns among strains. This highlights the crucial need for a next generation of diagnostic tools able to respond to microbial heterogeneity such that clinicians can make appropriately informed decisions for antimicrobial interventions. As highlighted, development of accurate identification techniques is critical not only for the understanding of microbial infection dynamics but also for the development of medical countermeasures to problems, such as resistance to antibiotics and persistent infections (Sousa & Pereira, 2013) (Figure 3.1).

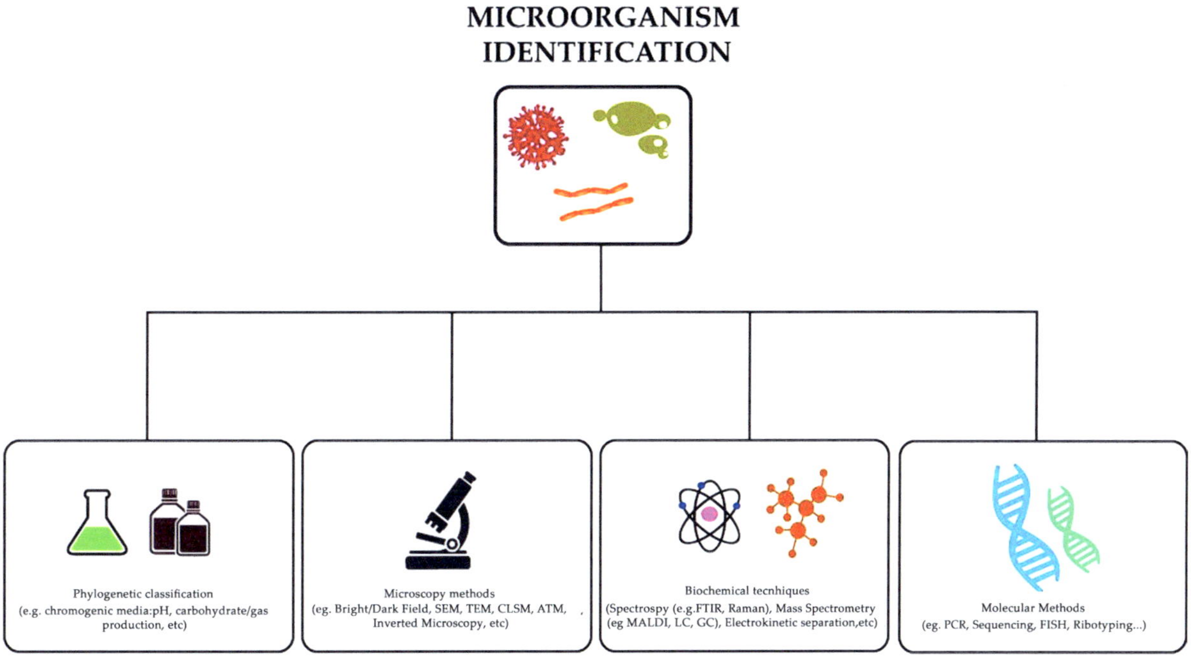

Figure 3.1. Microorganism identification.

Source: https://pub.mdpi-res.com/microorganisms/microorganisms-07-00130/article_deploy/html/images/microorganisms-07-00130-ag.png?1571525931.

Overview of Methods Used for Identification

Microorganism detection in clinical microbiology employs a wide range of methodologies, each with its own uses and advantages. One of the simple methods is the employment of biochemical tests, which analyze the metabolic profile of microorganisms. Such tests are applied to differentiate species based on the identification of enzymatic activities, such as sugar fermentation or the production of diagnostic metabolites. For example, the catalase test separates catalase-positive staphylococci from catalase-negative streptococci, showing the value of such tests. Although biochemical tests in general are to be desired, their requirement that the bacteria grow in culture may prevent the detection of fasidious bacteria or of organisms present in small numbers. Therefore, there is a growing need for the merger of quick and sensitive technologies to enhance the identification accuracy, as a reaction to the need for techniques that can handle the growing complexity of pathogenic microorganisms in clinical medicine. Antigen-antibody techniques, , such as enzyme-linked immunosorbent assays (ELISA) and agglutination tests, present an alternative technique of microorganism identification. ELISA is clinically preferred most due to its sensitivity and ability to identify several antigens in a sample simultaneously. ELISA quantifies the quantity of microbial antigens or host antibodies to infection, and it has been versatile enough to be applied in vaccine responses and serological surveys. The need to move towards multiplex assays is emphasized by the increasing demand for the detection of several pathogens at once, as witnessed in the study that reported the use of microarray immunoassays (MAIA) in the detection of antibodies against several viral antigens among children. These advancements go to show how crucial these techniques are in enhancing diagnostic regimes as they allow for timely and efficient treatment options. Over the last decade, molecular diagnostic techniques have transformed the methods of identification employed in medical microbiology, especially since the development of methods , such as polymerase chain reaction (PCR) and reverse transcription-PCR (RT-PCR). These procedures facilitate the amplification and detection of defined nucleic acid sequences with increased specificity and sensitivity that no conventional methods can match. The quick turnaround time with these molecular techniques is crucial in infectious disease control, particularly for the rapid detection of agents like SARS-CoV-2. Furthermore, the detection of pathogens from clinical specimens without the need for culturing them expands the diagnostic armamentarium, allowing for timely intervention in patient treatment. These technological innovations are identified in literature as fulfilling the exigent need for sophisticated diagnostic techniques that can adapt to the nuances of microbiological identification, particularly in respect to global health challenges posed by new and re-emerging pathogens (Pavankumar & Sankaran, 2008; Kazakova et al., 2019).

3.1. Biochemical Tests

Learning Outcome

1. Understand the definition and significance of biochemical tests
2. Describe common biochemical tests used in microbiology
3. Interpret biochemical test results

Biochemical tests have the first priority in microbiological identification in medical microbiology. Biochemical tests are designed to determine the biochemical activities of microorganisms and provide a reflection of their metabolic activity as well as of physiological properties. For instance, sugar fermentation, gas production, and utilization of various substrates can distinguish between very closely related bacteria. Such testing can include lactose fermentation or enzymatic synthesis of some enzymes like urease or catalase. These characteristics not only hold great importance in pathogen detection but also offer important information about their probable pathogenicity and virulence. Ongoing advances in rapid biochemical tests improve the speed of infection diagnosis, thereby making early intervention treatment and improved patient management feasible within healthcare facilities. Moreover, the integration of biochemical testing with more recent molecular techniques improves microbial identification. Though traditional biochemical testing is still an integral part of microbiology, the advent of molecular detection systems , such as PCR (Polymerase Chain Reaction), has revolutionized the velocity and precision of pathogen identification. Because molecular methods can amplify particular DNA sequences, molecular methods can confirm the presence of microorganisms that are not easily detectable with routine biochemical tests.

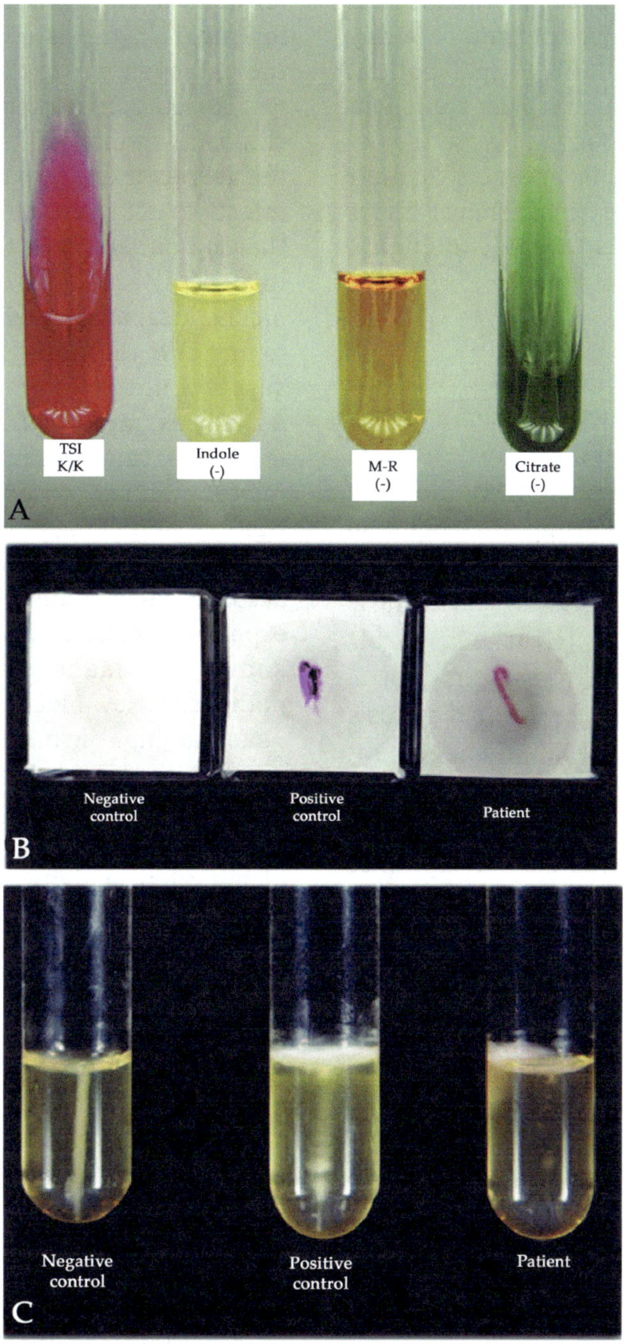

Figure 3.2. Biochemical tests (A), oxidase test (B), and motility test (C) for strain characterization.

Source: https://www.researchgate.net/publication/310812481/figure/fig3/AS:566127986462720@1511986838920/Biochemical-tests-A-oxidase-test-B-and-motility-test-C-for-strain.png.

Thus, biochemical tests and molecular diagnosis together provide an integrated method for pathogen detection, and hence, microbiologists are capable of confirming results and reducing rates of misidentification. This dual benefit maximizes laboratory efficiency, saving treatment time and validating pathogen targeting of therapeutic intervention. In addition to their application in the laboratory, biochemical assays also play significant roles in epidemiological surveillance and food safety.

For example, screening for some biochemical markers in foods can determine the presence of harmful bacteria , such as those that cause foodborne illness. As apparent from recent research, rapid detection methods of pathogens like *S. aureus* using PCR confirm the correlation between public health safety regulations and biochemical testing, particularly in food processing units (Hrušková et al., 2012). Such findings with pathogens like *E. coli* confirm the necessity for swift diagnosis and surveillance in outbreak management (Pavankumar & Sankaran, 2008). Its ability to detect and enumerate these microorganisms within a timely frame, aside from compliance with regulations, yields important information on pathways of microbial transmission and resistance patterns. This underlines the central place of biochemical tests as part of an integral system of microbial identification and public health conservation (Figure 3.2).

3.1.1. Definition and Significance of Biochemical Tests

Biochemical tests are useful tools for the identification and discrimination of microorganisms in clinical microbiology. Biochemical tests utilize specific biochemical properties of microbes, including enzymatic activities and metabolic processes, to generate a profile that can distinguish a single microbe from another. For instance, tests of carbohydrate fermentation can identify the presence of specific bacterial species based on their ability to ferment sugar. This is a step that not only allows for rapid diagnosis but also helps to establish the pathogenicity of the isolated microbes. The variety of biochemical tests available allows clinicians to make appropriate decisions about the correct therapy, particularly in the event of infection with severe health implications, and thereby underscores the value of these assays in best disease management. Application of biochemical tests extends beyond identification to include the ability to establish microbial susceptibility to antimicrobial medication. As an example, variations in biochemical measures can influence the susceptibility of microorganisms to antifungal medication, an issue of particular importance given the rising number of resistant strains. Quick detection and accurate susceptibility profiling are essential, especially where clinical settings are concerned about the management of opportunistic pathogens. New biochemical testing technology, , such as high-throughput screening, is in the pipeline to enhance sensitivity and specificity. Besides the promise of rapid diagnosis, these developments further give the complete picture of microbial activity, enabling a well-planned therapeutic regime essential in the battle against resistant infection, emphasizing the crucial role biochemical tests have to play in modern microbiological practice. With the evolving condition of medical microbiology, biochemical tests are now being linked with newer diagnostic devices. Techniques like clinical metagenomic next-generation sequencing (mNGS) are being used to augment the traditional biochemical analyses. mNGS provides the ability to examine highly sophisticated microbial communities from patient samples and provide data on microbial diversity, resistance mechanisms, and interactions with the host. Such a merger is applied to emphasize the strengths of biochemical assays and molecular diagnostics as a platform for enhancing overall diagnostic efficiency and accuracy. Use of such sophisticated techniques is not without problems, though, including the need for an efficient workflow and adequate laboratory staff training. To be capable of performing at their best, these issues must be addressed as they proceed further the implementation of the underlying principles introduced by biochemical tests to identify microorganisms efficiently, and hence their role even more important in the larger scheme of microbial diagnosis (Consortium OPATHY & Gabaldón, 2019; Chiu & Miller, 2019) (Figure 3.3).

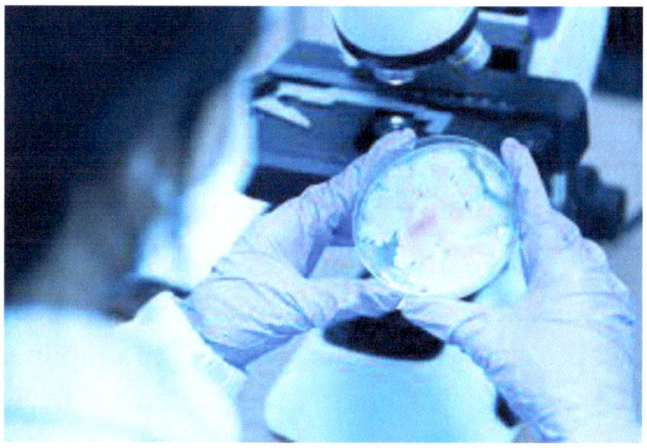

Figure 3.3. A laboratory technician examines microbial growth in a petri dish under a microscope, highlighting procedures used in microbiological analysis.

Source: https://encrypted-tbn0.gstatic.com/images?q=tbn:ANd9GcSSsTS3KEmIjAV3HN1t1p2PK5DjOr8oWbgwjlezfl4L9cTqnA0V7tlWYiFNKxE5adwEE3E&usqp=CAU.

3.1.2. Common Biochemical Tests Used in Microbiology

Biochemical testing is of central significance in microbiology since it is the foundation of identification and discrimination among microbial species. Routine, straightforward tests, , such as carbohydrate fermentation, simulation of enzymic activity, and gas production, are employed on a daily basis to identify bacteria. For instance, the increase in lactose as a carbon source can reflect the presence of coliform bacteria , such as *Escherichia coli*, while acid and gas production in a fermentation tube reflects the hydrolysis of sugars. These tests serve as the foundation for the detection of microbial species in clinical samples and guide the treatment protocol of infections. In addition, due to the constant foodborne pathogen threats, there is a demand for fast and accurate detection processes, hence the importance of continuous research in biochemical test procedures (Hrušková et al., 2012). With the increased complexity of microbial pathogenicity, understanding the biochemical basis of virulence is essential. Specific tests , such as the catalase test and the urease test, can be applied to differentiate between bacterial groups. Catalase-positive bacteria, for example, are separated from catalase-negative streptococci, aiding in the diagnosis of infections , such as strep throat as opposed to staph infections. Similarly, urease activity indicates the ability of bacteria, e.g., *Helicobacter pylori*, to survive in acidic environments, which is crucial in understanding their role in diseases like peptic ulcers. Such advancements enable the discovery of new pathogens and the mechanisms of virulence. As highlighted by recent studies on the ability of *Escherichia coli* to acquire virulence factors, incorporation of these biochemical tests into diagnostic programs is important to enable effective public health interventions (Pavankumar & Sankaran, 2008). Moreover, integration of biochemical tests with molecular diagnosis enhances the accuracy and speed of detecting microbes. Techniques like PCR complement traditional biochemical assays by precisely identifying specific nucleic acid sequences of disease-causing organisms. For example, PCR testing identifies enterotoxigenic *E. coli* (ETEC) strains responsible for causing acute foodborne disease. Collectively, this renders strong surveillance strategies in food safety and clinical diagnosis for timely intervention and prevention of disease outbreaks. Rapid advances in colorimetric, immunological, and nucleic acid assays not only increase specificity but also bypass the practical limitations of traditional methods. All this cumulatively forms a more complete four-dimensional vision of microbial physiology and infectious disease control of medical microbiology (Pavankumar & Sankaran, 2008) (Figure 3.4).

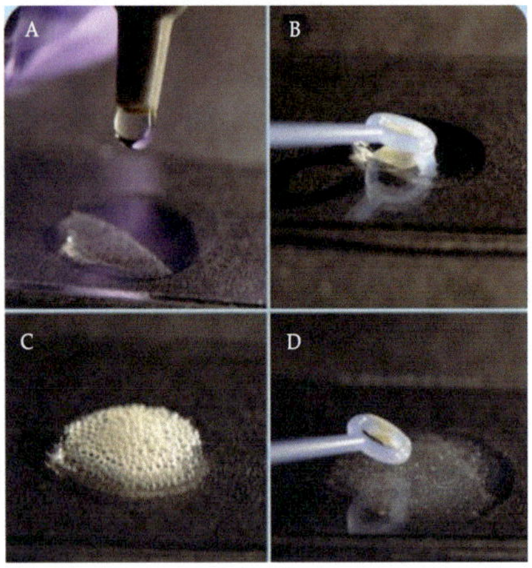

Figure 3.4. Catalase test. A. Apply one drop of 3% hydrogen peroxide on a microscopic slide. B. Transfer bacteria with a plastic loop to the H_2O_2 solution. C. Catalase positive bacteria produce gas (O_2) in form av bubbles which shows that the bacterium has catalase. D. Catalase negative bacteria does not have catalase and therefore, oxygen is not formed. Note the fragments of bacterial colonies, but there are no bubbles in the solutions.

Source: https://www.vetbact.org/images/terms/DSC_2460-76-81-99_H800.jpg.

3.1.3. Interpretation of Biochemical Test Results

The interpretation of biochemical test results is extremely critical in the identification of microorganisms in clinical microbiology. Biochemical tests have a tendency to use some metabolic characteristics to differentiate between bacterial species. For instance, carbohydrate fermentation tests examine an organism's ability to ferment carbohydrates and produce results that can determine a bacterium's species. The identification of enzymes , such as catalase or urease can further categorize these identifications. In particular, enzyme production analysis can separate pathogenic from non-pathogenic strains depending on whether or not such analysis will inform treatment. Furthermore, biochemical tests are often combined with serological assays to guarantee the robustness of diagnoses by providing a multi-dimensional approach to pathogen identification and disease mechanism insight. Also pushing the frontiers of microbiological diagnostics is the application of antigen-antibody techniques, , such as ELISA and agglutination tests, which are central in confirming biochemical test results. ELISA, in fact, utilizes antibodies' specificity for the detection of specific-pathogen antigens' presence.

This exercise finds its greatest relevance in the context of pathogens , such as the Japanese encephalitis virus, where quick detection is vital to ensure treatment success. Not only are these methods most efficient in diagnostics, but they are also employed for the quantification of infectious particles along with the measurement of immunological response (Gopinathan et al., 2017). Similarly, agglutination tests can provide fast and reliable results for the identification of various strains of bacteria, including enterotoxigenic *E. coli* (Pavankumar & Sankaran, 2008). But the validity of the interpretation is based on a sound acquaintance with these assays with an eye to the requirement for trained staff members in clinical diagnostic laboratories. Molecular diagnostics, , such as PCR and RT-PCR, enhance the interpretation of biochemical test results quite significantly by providing higher sensitivity and specificity than standard procedures. Molecular technologies can detect minute traces of microbial DNA, and hence, it is possible to identify pathogens that may be overlooked by biochemical tests alone. As an example, the application of RT-PCR for the identification of viral pathogens has transformed the clinician's approach to initial diagnosis, especially in instances where rapid intervention is required, e.g., viral encephalitis and acute foodborne infection (Gopinathan et al., 2017). Moreover, bringing together these molecular methods with biochemical tests facilitates the profiling of microbes in detail, bringing forth the possibility of targeted treatment. With the science of medical microbiology continuing to advance further, the connection between biochemical testing, antigen-antibody techniques, and molecular diagnosis underscores the significance of efficient interpretation of results promptly.

Test Your Knowledge

1. What is the purpose of performing biochemical tests in microbiology?
2. How does the catalase test help differentiate between bacterial species?

3.2. Antigen-Antibody Techniques

Learning Outcome

1. Give an overview of antigen-antibody interactions
2. Understand the enzyme-linked immunosorbent assay (ELISA) technique
3. Describe agglutination tests and their applications

Among the various methods applied in microorganism identification, antigen-antibody techniques have been a cornerstone of medical microbiology. These techniques utilize the specific interactions between antigens, typically microbial proteins, and antibodies from the immune system of hosts. Serological methods are applied primarily in the diagnosis of infectious diseases, including bacterial, viral, fungal, and parasitic, and also non-infectious diseases of oncological or endocrine nature. In addition, serological studies continue to be relevant due to the rapid and reliable identification capability they offer, enabling prompt medical intervention. These resulting products of the immunobiotechnology for these serological diagnostics fall under the broad category of immunobiotechnology, still emphasizing their important roles towards safeguarding public health and enhancing clinical outcomes in disease treatment (Gorshunov et al., 2019).

One of the widely recognized antigen-antibody techniques utilized in clinical laboratories is the enzyme-linked immunosorbent assay (ELISA). This method allows antigens or antibodies to be quantitatively assayed in a sample, and thus provides a better insight into the infection status or immune status of an individual. ELISA is characterized by its sensitivity, specificity, and ability to process large series of samples at a time and is therefore particularly useful for epidemiological surveys and screening programs. Further, advances in this technique have expanded its application in clinical diagnosis and research to allow it to be adapted to meet varied pathogen detection needs. Regular updates and validation of the protocols applied in ELISA ensure that they are in line with high-quality standards, thus enhancing diagnostic accuracy and reliability in microorganism identification along with their implications in patient treatment (Gorshunov et al., 2019). In relation to traditional methods, molecular techniques , such as Polymerase Chain Reaction (PCR) and reverse transcription-PCR (RT-PCR) have revolutionized detection and identification of microorganisms through their ability to provide quick results alongside high sensitivity. Such techniques allow targeted DNA or RNA sequences to be amplified, which can be employed in the identification of microbial pathogens even in the absence of measurable amounts present and even without the requirement of prior culturing. As suggested in recent reviews, the increased frequency of opportunistic infections places a special emphasis on improved, faster and more efficient diagnostic reagents to detect not only the etiological pathogens but also patterns of drug resistance. Thus, the union of antigen-antibody techniques and molecular diagnostics is a critical advance in medical microbiology that offers upgraded diagnostic reagents with which efficient disease management and therapy are possible.

3.2.1. Overview of Antigen-Antibody Interactions

These interactions are fundamental to the immune response and are the basis for most of the diagnostic techniques used in medical microbiology. Antigens, which can be proteins or polysaccharides on the surface of a pathogen, induce the production of antibodies, specialized glycoproteins secreted by B cells. This is a specific binding that occurs by means of non-covalent forces like hydrogen bonding and van der Waals interactions, resulting in the formation of an antigen-antibody complex. These not only serve as a defensive action against infection but are also applied within the laboratory, where they allow for the identification of microorganisms by means of antigen-antibody techniques like enzyme-linked immunosorbent assays (ELISA) and agglutination. In the scenario of bacterial pathogens, antigen-antibody interaction yields insight into mechanisms of disease and identification of infecting agents. Diarrhoeagenic *Escherichia coli*, for instance, has diverse virulence factors that can be effectively identified through immunological methods regulated by antigen-antibody interactions. The precision of such methods has been enhanced with increased sophistication of molecular diagnostics so that practitioners have been able to detect pathogens with unprecedented specificity and sensitivity. The rapid identification of such microorganisms in clinical samples and food safety contexts underscores the importance of these interactions. Through extensive reviews presented on *E. coli* pathogenesis, incorporating these detection technologies gives depth to pre-and post-harvest food safety interventions, thus playing a significant role in public health programs (Pavankumar & Sankaran, 2008).

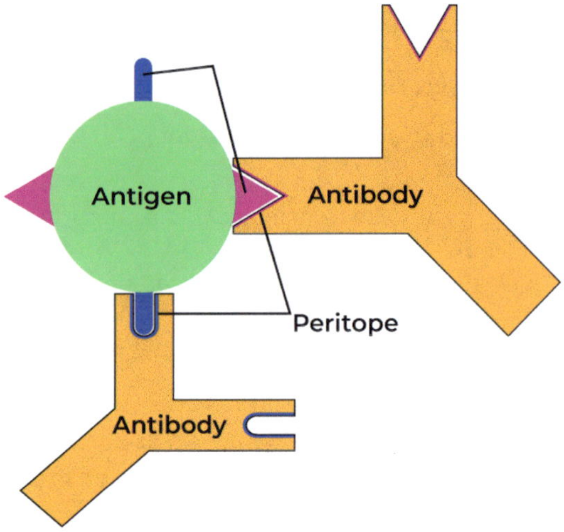

Figure 3.5. Antibody-antigen interaction.

Source: https://media.geeksforgeeks.org/wp-content/uploads/20240222114011/Antibody-Antigen-Interaction-1.png.

Moreover, while traditionally culturing techniques have been applied in diagnosis, recent developments have revealed the utility of antigen-antibody reactions in determining the microbial heterogeneity in infection conditions.

Molecular methods like PCR and ELISA offer quick identification of different strains of the pathogen from mixtures of microbes, hence ruling out issues of the heterogeneous population of microbes. It is important to recognize the genetic heterogeneity of pathogens, particularly in view of the varied mechanisms followed by such pathogens to evade the host immune system. As outlined in recent publications, the advancement in diagnostics is required to keep pace with the evolving nature of microbial infections, as it attests to the inherent significance of antigen-antibody reactions in delineating and managing infectious disease (Sousa & Pereira, 2013) (Figure 3.5).

3.2.2. Enzyme-Linked Immunosorbent Assay (ELISA)

Enzyme-Linked Immunosorbent Assay (ELISA) is currently a routine procedure in medical microbiology for the detection and quantification of microorganisms. ELISA allows the detection of various pathogens from clinical specimens by typical antigen-antibody interactions, with enhanced diagnostic accuracy. The validity of the technique lies in its sensitivity, specificity, and adaptability, permitting its use in a variety of applications, from serological surveys to vaccine efficacy surveillance.

In comparison to the traditional culture methods, which are prone to being time-consuming and labor-intensive, ELISA facilitates early diagnosis, and therefore early medical intervention. Through antibody detection against pathogens, ELISA offers a critical benefit of unsealing the window to past infection or current immunity. Through this, ELISA is a landmark contribution towards infectious disease control worldwide, highlighting innovation in diagnostic practice (Sousa & Pereira, 2013). Moreover, the application of ELISA in clinical laboratories is complemented by its standardization and automation capability. This capability allows for high-throughput screening of samples, which is a critical feature where there is a necessity to react fast, for instance, in situations of an epidemic outbreak. Its capability to process samples in parallel not only keeps the workflow streamlined but also renders results statistically significant. In addition, developments in ELISA technology, , such as the advent of multiplex assays, have further enhanced its applicability by allowing for the simultaneous detection of multiple pathogens and their biomarkers from a single sample. This capability for multiplexing addresses the multifaceted nature of infectious diseases, where co-infection makes diagnosis and treatment challenging. Thus, ELISA not only meets the demands of today's time to detect pathogens but also aligns with the shifting patterns of medical diagnosis according to precision and effectiveness (Akter et al., 2024).

As research and development are ongoing, ELISA is also evolving continuously by incorporating new materials and technology to make it more effective. The combination of ELISA platforms with nanotechnology has been shown to be promising for enhancing sensitivity and specificity, which can revolutionize pathogen identification precision. It is essential that microbial communities become more heterogeneous and antibiotic-resistant, necessitating new approaches for their efficient identification. Existing studies that evaluate the performance of ELISA against new emerging pathogens demonstrate its adaptability to new health scenarios while revealing challenges associated with microbial heterogeneity. This interactive play of traditional and novel techniques in microbial diagnostics heralds the central role ELISA plays in advancing public health outcomes. As scientists continue to refine these techniques and bridge the gaps, the future of ELISA is to be part of the fight against infectious disease (Sousa & Pereira, 2013) (Figure 3.6).

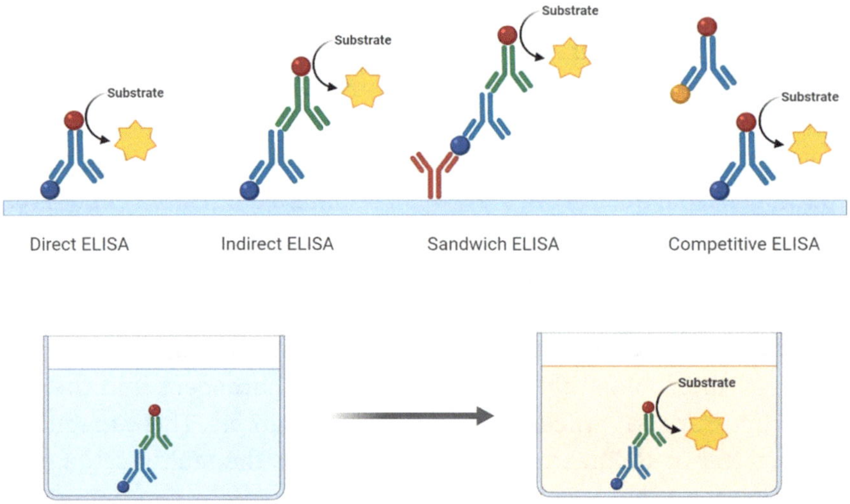

Figure 3.6. ELISA Diagram.

Source: https://microbenotes.com/wp-content/uploads/2022/05/ELISA-Diagram.jpeg.

3.2.3. Agglutination Tests and Their Applications

Agglutination tests are a significant component of diagnostic microbiology, employing the ability of some antibodies to interact with antigens, leading to visible clumping of particles. Agglutination tests belong to a category of antigen-antibody reactions and are an essential tool in the identification of microorganisms responsible for infectious diseases. For instance, blood grouping and the diagnosis of most diseases rely heavily on agglutination processes. Their rapid performance and simple interpretation render them well-liked in hospital and field settings. Moreover, the integration of agglutination tests into health systems increases the efficiency of disease detection, especially where other technologies are not feasible, , such as in resource-poor environments, indicating their adaptability to respond to varying health care demands. Application of agglutination tests extends beyond the simple identification of the pathogen; they are also significant in serological studies, infectious as well as non-infectious diseases. They are able to identify the state of immunity of a person through the measurement of antibodies in serum and the detection of pathogens through their respective antigens. Agglutination techniques are significant in epidemiological studies as they enable health workers to trace outbreaks and chart disease patterns efficiently. Their utility is demonstrated by ongoing advances in immunobiotechnology that enhance the specificity and sensitivity of serological tests, thus enhancing diagnostic accuracy. It becomes particularly pertinent to disease control and surveillance public health programs, pointing to the way these older techniques remain at the heart of current clinical medicine, as they retool to meet modern demands (Gorshunov et al., 2019). In microbial diagnostics, agglutination tests are complemented by more advanced techniques , such as ELISA and molecular diagnostics by PCR and RT-PCR. Nevertheless, the simplicity and frugality of agglutination tests maintain their place in routine laboratory diagnostics. As health systems become increasingly conscious of the importance of rapid and precise diagnostics, agglutination tests are central instruments in laboratories. Their progress is also aided by clinical metagenomic next-generation sequencing (mNGS), which allows for comprehensive analyses, but agglutination remains central at the point-of-care level for prompt decision-making. Combining the traditional and modern approaches, agglutination tests significantly assist in enabling timely diagnoses and treatment measures in medical microbiology (Chiu & Miller, 2019). Thus, they depict an amenable blend of conventional practices and newer technological advances, attesting to their applicability in the continuous quest for improved health outcomes (Figure 3.7).

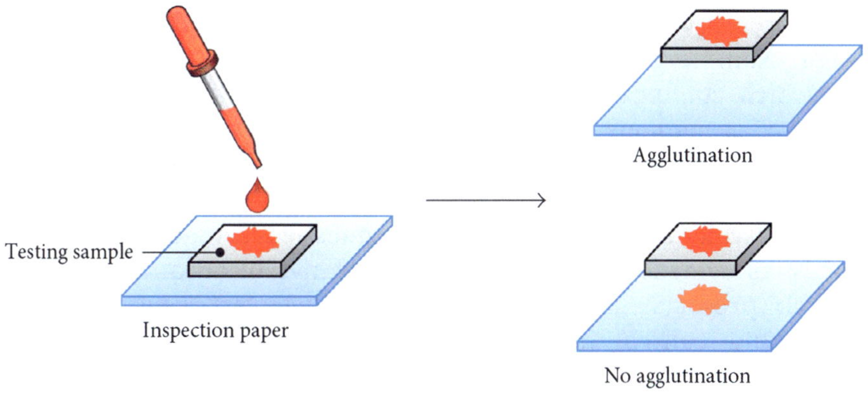

Figure 3.7. A schematic diagram of the blood agglutination test.

Source: https://www.researchgate.net/publication/326152115/figure/fig2/AS:1086429253906436@1636036327481/A-schematic-diagram-of-the-blood-agglutination-test.jpg.

Test Your Knowledge

1. What is the principle behind the antigen-antibody reaction?
2. How does an ELISA test detect the presence of an antigen or antibody in a sample?
3. Why is the specificity of the antibody important in antigen-antibody techniques?

3.3. Molecular Diagnostics

Learning Outcome

1. Introduce molecular diagnostic techniques
2. Describe the polymerase chain reaction (PCR) methodology
3. Discuss reverse transcription PCR (RT-PCR) and its relevance

The evolution of molecular diagnostics has greatly revolutionized medical microbiology. Polymerase Chain Reaction (PCR) and Reverse Transcription PCR (RT-PCR) are spearheading this revolution, which allows for rapid and precise identification of microorganisms. These methods employ the specific amplification of nucleic acids to allow the identification of even trace levels of pathogen genetic material in clinical samples. The design of the assay is modifiable to identify particular sequences of genes in various pathogens, enabling not only diagnosis but also disease activity and therapeutic response monitoring. Molecular diagnostics is thus now a part of clinical practice, enhancing our ability to initiate timely and effective therapeutic regimes. During the recent decades, the quickly growing field of marine biotechnology has resonated with the growth of molecular diagnostics by revealing new infectious agents and expanding the need for advanced diagnostic technologies. Advances toward augmenting research funding in the field have provided impetus to the design of advanced rapid diagnostic tools. These advances comprise fully automatic systems that can perform real-time PCR and multiplex analyses, enhancing diagnostic accuracy while shortening time-to-results. For example, immunoassays using biosensors, which combine traditional immunology and molecular methods, are a cost-efficient alternative. Both emphasis on classical methods and novel molecular techniques reflect the need for an interdisciplinary approach to identifying microbes, as evident in a number of applied research projects intended to improve diagnostic and control infectious diseases in different populations (Ince et al., 2009). Application of molecular diagnosis in the clinical setting reflects the increasing trend towards specificity and efficiency in pathogen identification. The techniques are more sensitive compared to traditional biochemical tests, which rely on the growth and phenotypic characteristics of microorganisms and sometimes result in delayed diagnosis. Molecular techniques can also detect a large number of pathogens, , such as bacteria, viruses, and fungi, simultaneously, thereby making the process of diagnosis in clinical microbiology laboratories more optimal. Since research grants to develop rapid diagnostic devices have been rising exponentially, the field is poised to be propelled to exponential growth, with academia and industry stakeholders being urged to collaborate. Such breakthroughs are a critical step to the improved identification and control of infectious diseases and are indicative of the significant nexus of developing technology and public health (Ince et al., 2009).

3.3.1. Introduction to Molecular Diagnostic Techniques

Molecular diagnostic methods have transformed the practice of medical microbiology with the ability to detect microorganisms using sensitive and specific methods. They utilize the pathogen genetic material to identify infectious agents quickly and characterize them. Among the most common methods employed are PCR and RT-PCR, which amplify nucleic acid sequences to enable the identification of bacteria and viruses. The utility of such methods is brought into perspective by the exigency for rapid diagnostic tests in clinical practice, especially during outbreaks or pandemics when timely detection is able to dramatically improve patient outcomes and limit disease spread. Ndao, (2009) recognizes stagnation in traditional diagnostic techniques, bridging the gap with the imperative of advanced molecular approaches that deliver fast results without the expense of precision. PCR and RT-PCR not only speed up diagnostics but also enhance the possibilities for detection of genetic markers of antibiotic resistance or virulence factors in disease-causing organisms. Since they are aimed at particular DNA or RNA structures, these methods have the potential to distinguish between closely related microorganisms to which traditional culture techniques are blind. This specificity is important for the design of effective therapy and an understanding of the epidemiology of infectious disease.

Furthermore, advances in microfluidic and "Lab-on-Chip" technology are making point-of-care diagnosis possible, thus being of tremendous use in both high- and low-resource settings. Such technologies can fill diagnostic capacity gaps across the world, as articulated in reports from recent reviews looking at the need for optimized diagnostic strategies, particularly for diseases like tuberculosis and other mycobacterial infections. (Eda et al., 2012) Despite the much-heralded benefits of molecular diagnostics, the challenges still persist in terms of accessibility, expense, and interpretive difficulty. Such sophisticated techniques are not only technologically complicated but also require massive training of laboratory personnel. With the further establishment of molecular diagnostics, additional research is being focused on their further firmness and reliability, particularly in the management of emergent pathogens. In addition, the use of these advanced methods in combination with conventional techniques may offer a multi-level approach to microbial identification, balancing speed with cost-effectiveness and reliability. The emphasis on the design of new assays based on DNA or protein markers also highlights the promise of molecular diagnostics for the ongoing battle against infectious diseases, as medical microbiology keeps pace with the evolution of microbial hazards (Ndao et al., 2009) (Figure 3.8).

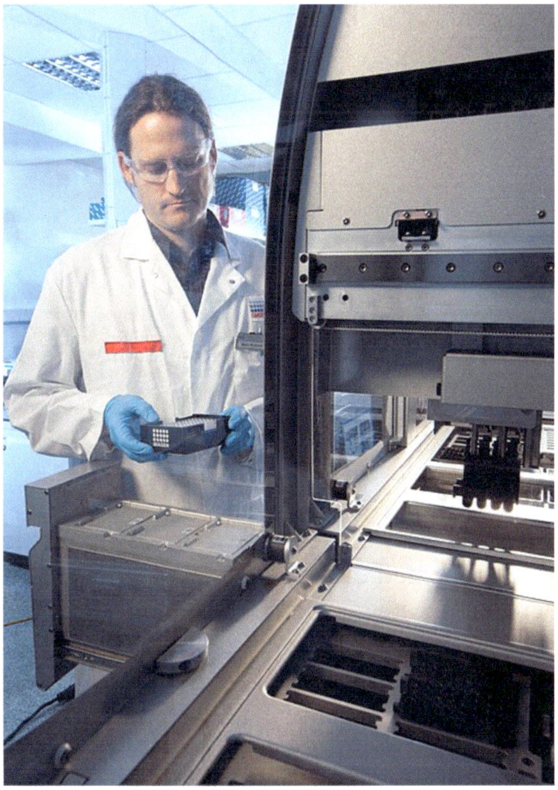

Figure 3.8. Specialist using an automation platform for molecular diagnostic tests.

Source: https://upload.wikimedia.org/wikipedia/commons/thumb/a/ad/Molecular_diagnostics_qia_symphony.jpg/500px-Molecular_diagnostics_qia_symphony.jpg.

3.3.2. Polymerase Chain Reaction (PCR) Methodology

The Polymerase Chain Reaction (PCR) method is a revolutionary method in molecular diagnosis of medical microbiology. PCR is a method by which specific DNA sequences are exponentially amplified, and hence, the presence of microorganisms that could be present in minute quantities could be identified. Its sensitivity is higher than that of routine culture methods, which are of low sensitivity and require longer incubation periods, thereby resulting in a delay in diagnosis and treatment. For instance, in systemic fungal infections, conventional culture techniques are positive in only around 50% of the patients (Consortium OPATHY & Gabaldón, 2019). By circumventing the need for culture before detection, PCR is a quick and effective aid to identify infectious agents, significantly enhancing patient outcomes while reducing healthcare expenses through the prevention of delayed diagnosis. Another important advantage of PCR is that it can identify a broad category of microorganisms , including bacteria, viruses, and fungi. The ability to develop specific primers enables the amplification of target sequences from diverse species, and targeted detection becomes possible. PCR-based molecular diagnostics is increasingly at the core of the identification of antimicrobial resistance, which is emerging as an increasingly significant issue in clinics. Such resistance calls for quick and correct diagnostic methods to inform proper treatment decisions. Recent studies point towards the utility of PCR-based techniques in managing antifungal treatments, where confirmed species identification is necessary for starting the right therapy (Consortium OPATHY & Gabaldón, 2019). This accuracy in microbial identification thus increases the efficacy of treatment regimens, with improved recovery rates among infected patients. Despite having a number of benefits, PCR technology is not unproblematic. There are still problems with standardization and validation between different clinical environments that jeopardize the reliability of the results. While PCR is very sensitive, false positives can be generated because of contamination or the presence of non-viable organisms, leading to the risk of unjustified therapeutic actions. These limitations must be solved if PCRs are to be implemented on a routine basis in general clinical practice. Yet, the ongoing development of PCR technology, for instance, the unfolding multiplexing opportunities and real-time PCR, holds the potential to enhance diagnostic sensitivity and efficiency. As these technologies evolve further, they complement and in some cases excel over traditional approaches, further cementing PCRs essential role in medical microbiology and infection control in the future (Franco-Duarte et al., 2021) (Figure 3.9).

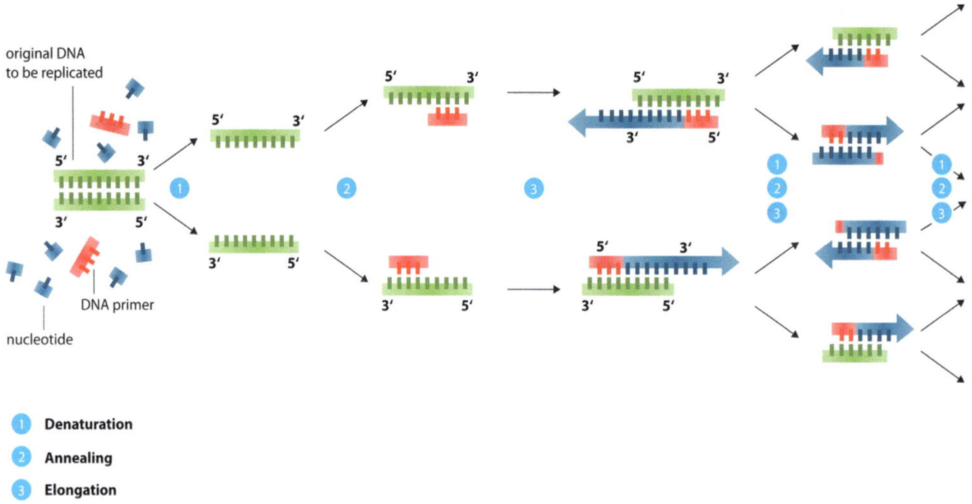

Figure 3.9. Polymerase chain reaction (PCR).

Source: https://cdn1.byjus.com/wp-content/uploads/2021/10/pcr.png.

3.3.3. Reverse Transcription PCR (RT-PCR) and Its Relevance

The advent of Reverse Transcription PCR (RT-PCR) has revolutionized the field of molecular diagnostics, especially in the detection of microorganisms in medical microbiology. The method facilitates amplification of RNA to identify viral and bacterial pathogens, if any, in a clinical sample. RT-PCR is particularly significant in the context of viral infections, e.g., caused by retroviruses and other RNA viruses, where accurate quantitation of the viral load is critical to treat the patient. Unlike traditional culture methods, which are sometimes time-consuming and sometimes may provide inconclusive information, RT-PCR combines unmatched specificity and sensitivity, serving as an anchor for rapid diagnostic testing of infectious disease agents, e.g., foodborne pathogens like enterotoxigenic *E. coli* and enterohemorrhagic *E. coli*, of particular public health concern (Pavankumar & Sankaran, 2008). RT-PCR also plays a crucial role in explaining pathogenic processes and microbial genetic diversity. Noticeably, bacterial pathogens exhibit extensive genetic and phenotypic diversity, which complicates diagnosis and treatment (Sousa & Pereira, 2013). RT-PCR not only allows for the detection of specific RNA sequences of virulence factors but can also be employed to study the expression of such factors under various conditions of environment or stages of infection. Such insight plays a key role in the formulation of targeted interventions and the explanation of microbial population behavior in the host. The precision and adaptability of RT-PCR make it an important tool in the ongoing struggle of microbial identification and treatment of infection. As technology becomes more advanced in RT-PCR, it is more and more being paired with other identification techniques to further enhance the power of microbial identification. For instance, the combination of RT-PCR with high-throughput sequencing tools allows for extensive investigation of microbial communities, thus allowing researchers to witness interaction and adaptation in intricate detail. This combination narrows the distance between the traditional diagnostic practices and sophisticated molecular techniques, ensuring improved patient outcomes as well as public health reactions. In addition, the rapid advancement of RT-PCR technologies means future applications may include multiplex assays capable of identifying multiple pathogens or their variants in one assay, consistent with the growing threat of antibiotic resistance and the need for targeted therapeutic strategies in clinical microbiology (Sousa & Pereira, 2013) (Figure 3.10).

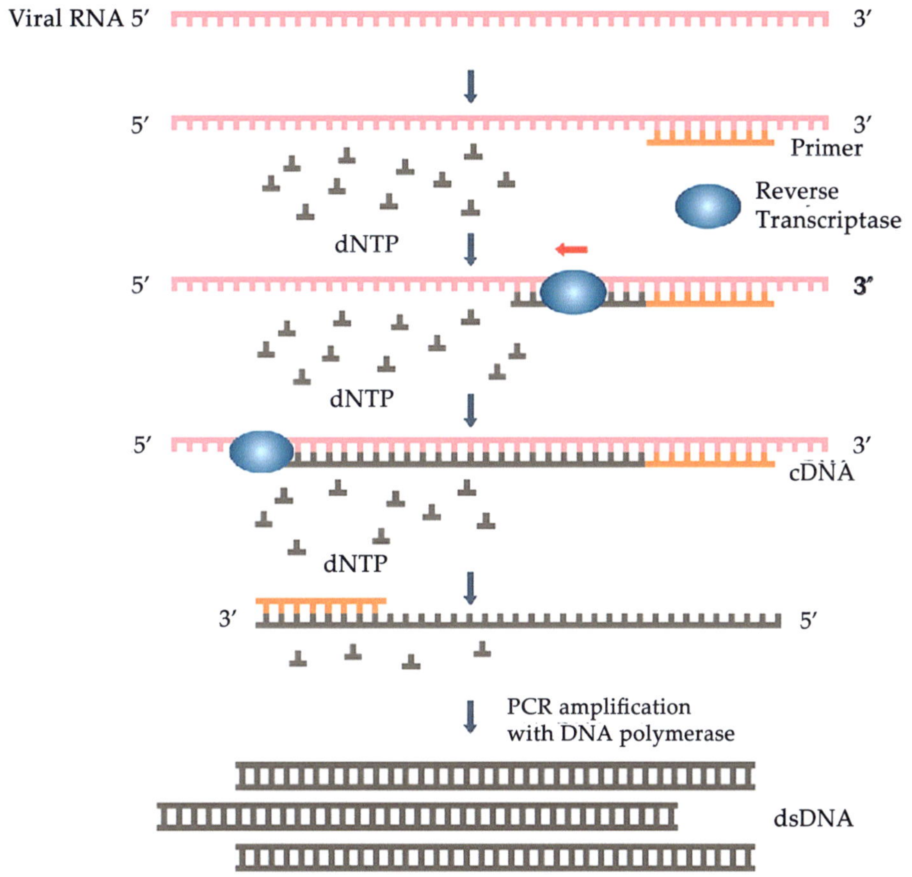

Figure 3.10. Reverse transcription-polymerase chain reaction (RT-PCR). The RT-PCR creates a cDNA copy of a specific segment of the viral RNA, which is converted to dsDNA that is exponentially amplified.

Source: https://www.researchgate.net/profile/Janet-Sasso/publication/341062500/figure/fig1/AS:886309807742979@1588324133823/Reverse-transcription-polymerase-chain-reaction-RT-PCR-The-RT-PCR-creates-a-cDNA-copy.png.

Test Your Knowledge

1. What are the molecular techniques used for the identification of microorganisms?
2. What does RT-PCR stand for and what is the purpose of RT-PCR?

3.4. Comparison of Identification Techniques

Learning Outcome

1. Understand the strengths and weaknesses of biochemical tests
2. Explain the advantages and limitations of antigen-antibody techniques
3. Discuss the efficacy of molecular diagnostics in pathogen identification

In medical microbiology, the identification of microorganisms is a critical step in making an accurate diagnosis and treatment. There are a number of methods available, each dealing with a particular aspect of species identification, of which biochemical testing, antigen-antibody interactions, and molecular diagnostics are the most prominent ones. Biochemical tests are traditional but effective tools to differentiate species based on metabolic characteristics. For instance, lactose fermentation can be applied to distinguish Enterobacteriaceae strains. While easy, this test cannot distinguish between highly related strains or aberrant forms and requires more sophisticated techniques for effective identification.

Antigen-antibody assays, particularly enzyme-linked immunosorbent assay (ELISA) and agglutination assays, have increased the speed and specificity of microorganism identification. ELISA is used extensively in the detection of pathogens by means of specific antigen-antibody interactions that allow for the detection of infections like viral hepatitis and HIV. Agglutination tests are also useful for a rapid test of pathogen presence in clinical samples based on visible clumping as a marker of infection. Although these methods are very advantageous in terms of speed and specificity, they are dependent on the quality of the antibodies used and cross-reactivity, so caution must be used when conclusions are drawn. Molecular diagnoses like polymerase chain reaction (PCR) and reverse transcription-PCR (RT-PCR) represent the current best technology in the identification of microorganisms with unmatched specificity and sensitivity.

These methods are capable of direct detection of microbacterial RNA or DNA and are therefore invaluable for the diagnosis of infections caused by fastidious and slow growers. The recent developments have highlighted the versatility of molecular techniques since, for instance, the use of dried blood spots to analyze nucleic acid has the advantage of avoiding sample transport and storage issues, as demonstrated in studies on diagnostics of tropical infectious disease (Abdelwhab et al., 2013). However, although such methods are promising, they are not without limitations, some of which are the potential for contamination and failure to sufficiently validate against gold standards, strikingly affirming ongoing development and comparison of identification techniques in medical microbiology. The use of varied methodologies keeps an integrative approach to pathogen identification, which increases clinical outcomes and public health processes overall (Pavankumar & Sankaran, 2008).

3.4.1. Strengths and Weaknesses of Biochemical Tests

Biochemical tests are a cornerstone in microorganism identification, particularly in medical microbiology, with numerous strengths that enhance diagnostics. One of the greatest strengths of biochemical tests is their ability to differentiate between very similar species based on metabolic properties, enzyme activity, and nutrient utilization patterns. This specificity is crucial in identifying causative pathogens of infections, thereby informing appropriate treatment interventions. In addition, most biochemical tests are simple to perform and can yield fast results, which is paramount in clinical settings where timely interventions can significantly improve patient outcomes. For instance, biochemical tests, including glucose fermentation and indole production, can be done within a short time, which enables practitioners to start empirical therapy awaiting confirmatory results. Such rapid turnaround helps clinical decision-making, especially in the situation of acutes (Duarte et al., 2016). While they are strong, biochemical tests also have a few flaws that it makes it difficult to apply them to diagnose microbial infections. One of the big weaknesses is the potential for incorrect identification based on non-specific reactions or biochemical overlap between organisms. For instance, certain bacteria may exhibit unusual biochemical reactions; the differentiation process becomes complicated and the ensuing treatment decision is inapplicable. Moreover, the sensitivity and specificity of biochemical tests can vary significantly based on the particular method or reagents used. In some cases, such tests could be under-refined incubation conditions and extended periods, delaying diagnosis in life-threatening situations. Therefore, using biochemical tests exclusively would delay pathogen identification accurately, and it is essential to integrate these methods with other methodologies, , such as molecular diagnostics (Tinsley et al., 2010). Moreover, the emergence of highly advanced methods, , such as molecular diagnostics, has increased the limits of standard biochemical tests. The common occurrence of antibiotic-resistant microorganisms necessitates the use of more sensitive methods that are capable of identifying and characterizing microorganisms precisely at the genetic level. Molecular methods, e.g., PCR, have higher sensitivity and specificity which allows them to identify the pathogens even at low concentrations. This evolution reverses the diagnosis, questioning whether it is time to end the reliance on biochemical tests. Since biochemical tests are advantageous by virtue of their expense and ease, their own limitations must be taken into account within the larger context of microbiological diagnosis. Consequently, there is a clear need for having a multidisciplinary intervention that unites the speed and ease of biochemical tests with the power of molecular methods to further improve pathogen detection and control interventions (Duarte et al., 2016).

3.4.2. Advantages and Limitations of Antigen-Antibody Techniques

Antigen-antibody techniques are central to the diagnosis and detection of many microorganisms in clinical microbiology. One major advantage of such techniques, e.g., Enzyme-Linked Immunosorbent Assay (ELISA) and agglutination assays, is that they are rapid to perform, and the resulting rapidity of the reports can facilitate immediate therapeutic interventions. These techniques are based on the antigen-specific antibody binding, allowing specific pathogen detection, , such as viral diseases, bacterial diseases, and fungal diseases. For instance, ELISA can quantify the antibody or antigen concentration in a sample, allowing for effective disease incidence monitoring and response monitoring. Such specificity, however, raises diagnostic accuracy, which results in enhanced patient management and clinical outcomes. However, while these techniques have many advantages, their success is heavily reliant on the quality of reagents, and that can vary significantly between different uses. Despite their advantages, antigen-antibody techniques have intrinsic constraints that could impinge on diagnostic utility. One of these limitations is cross-reactivity, where antibodies adhere to similar antigens present in other pathogens or host tissues and result in false-positive reactions. Also, the assays are often reliant on the presence of antibodies, which, at the initial stages of infection when early detection is crucial, may be undetectable. This flaw is doubled in situations where there are chronic antibody responses, as in some infections in which detection is not coordinated with the current disease. Furthermore, the sensitivity and specificity of these procedures may be inadequate for less common pathogens. For example, development of rapid diagnostic tests for tropical infections , such as dengue fever, has highlighted significant loopholes in clearly distinguishing between a variety of febrile illnesses, emphasizing the need for improved methodologies of antigen-antibody testing (Alirol et al., 2013).

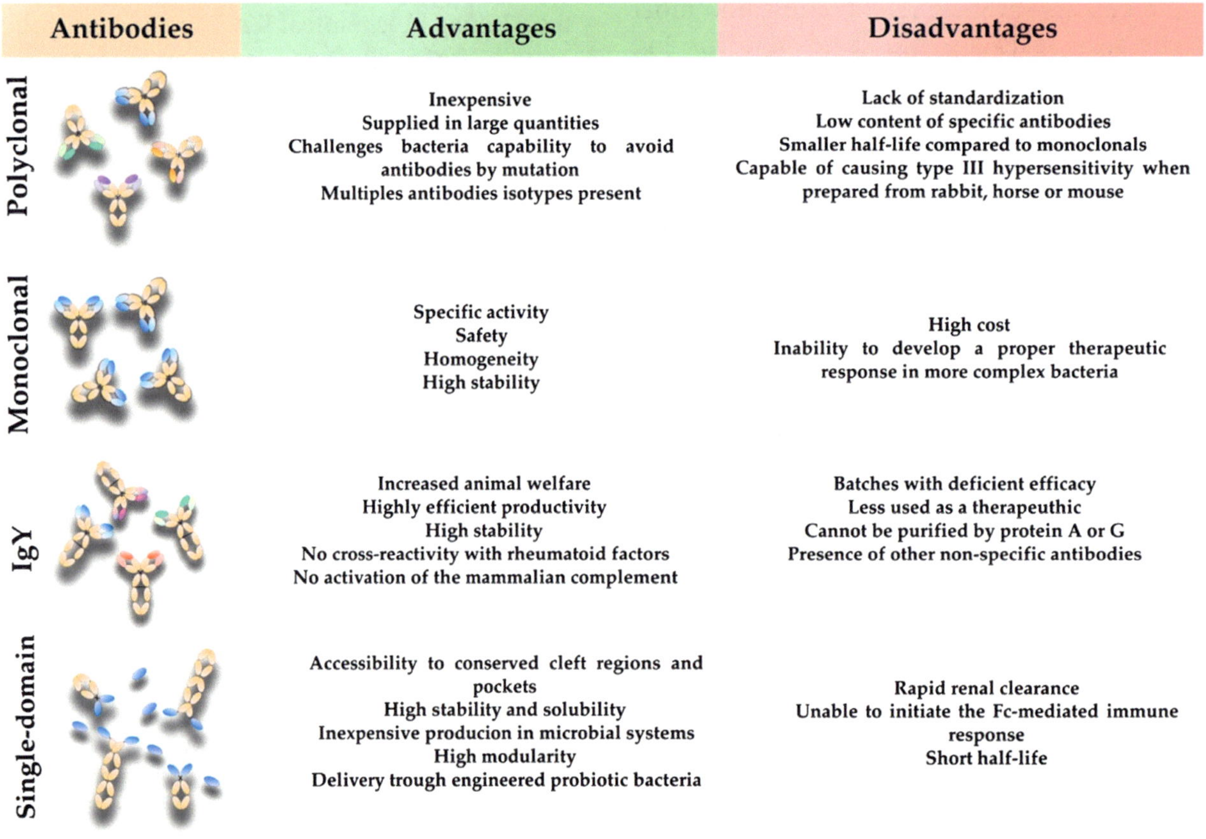

Figure 3.11. Main advantages and disadvantages of the four types of antibodies.

Source: https://www.researchgate.net/publication/364763049/figure/fig4/AS:11431281217055393@1705020301656/Main-advantages-and-disadvantages-of-the-four-types-of-antibody-formats-discussed-in-this.tif.

The evolving nature of microbiological diagnostics leads to increased need to address the limitations that involve antigen-antibody methods. New advancements in high-throughput technologies, including next-generation sequencing and proteomic approaches, have been promising in increasing diagnostic accuracy and speed, particularly for those with antifungal resistance (Consortium OPATHY & Gabaldón, 2019). These techniques may have more sensitive detection qualities, which are particularly critical with opportunistic infections where traditional immunological techniques are not sufficient. Despite such emerging innovations, the effective implementation of novel diagnostic strategies in the clinical context hinges on the resolution of certain challenges, including cost-effectiveness and availability in low-resource environments. Ultimately, complementary consideration of the advantages of antigen-antibody techniques combined with emerging molecular diagnostics can provide access to better surveillance and control of infectious diseases in a wide range of populations (Figure 3.11).

3.4.3. Efficacy of Molecular Diagnostics in Pathogen Identification

Molecular diagnostics have revolutionized pathogen identification with unparalleled specificity and sensitivity of microbial detection. The traditional methods based on culturing and biochemical testing are no longer adequate because of the limitations of time and expert personnel involved. Molecular methods , such as polymerase chain reaction (PCR) detect pathogen-specific nucleic acid sequences to diagnose infection irrespective of clinical symptoms. This early identification is precious when it comes to control of outbreaks and containment of disease, proving the efficacy of molecular diagnostics in clinical usage. The focus on inclusion of such technologies into standard processes can also deliver increased patient advantage through early interventions, which becomes essential in case of the emergence of new pathogens as well as antibiotic resistance. The progressive development of various molecular diagnostic methods continues to enhance their application in clinical microbiology. Methods , such as quantitative PCR and reverse transcription PCR (RT-PCR) not only permit pathogen detection but also quantify viral load, which provides information concerning disease severity and progression. Implementation of these molecular techniques coincides with the current trend in personalized medicine, allowing for individualized therapeutic regimens based on the specific pathogen causing an infection.

Furthermore, the greater reliance upon speed diagnostics enhances decision-making in the clinic, where quick action is necessary. This versatility of molecular diagnostics, combined with their growing popularity among clinical practitioners leans toward a shift from traditional practices to more efficient and accurate pathogen identification techniques, thus improving overall disease care. Molecular diagnostics being introduced into agricultural practices is just as important, particularly in the management of plant pathogens. Early and accurate identification, as noted with recent agronomic research, can contribute significantly to reducing crop losses due to disease. For instance, application of molecular techniques allows for oomycete disease pathogen detection prior to observable symptoms, with the potential to institute preventive measures early enough to contain nascent outbreaks.

Molecular diagnostic output also informs better practice in disease control, including intervals for rotation and varietal selection, further maximizing agricultural yield. As indicated by the increasing interest in fast point-of-care diagnostics in various fields, the scope of molecular approaches extends far beyond the traditional bounds, opening a new paradigm in medical microbiology as well as plant disease management, thus facing the larger dimensions of prevention of disease (Abd-Elmagid et al., 2016; Heilek et al., 2016) (Figure 3.12).

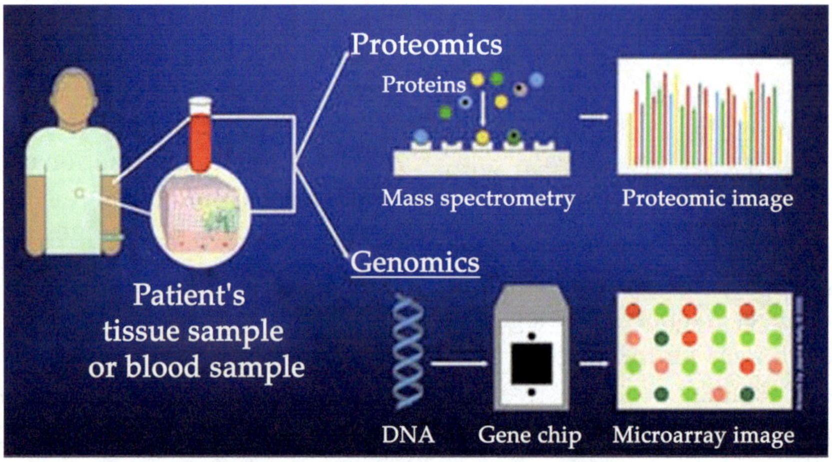

Figure 3.12. Molecular diagnostics uses techniques , such as mass spectrometry and gene chips to capture the expression patterns of genes and proteins.

Source: https://upload.wikimedia.org/wikipedia/commons/d/de/Molecular_Diagnostics.jpg.

Test Your Knowledge

1. What are the strengths and weaknesses of biochemical tests?
2. What are the advantages and disadvantages of biochemical tests?

3.5. Clinical Applications

Learning Outcome

1. Explain the role of identification techniques in clinical settings
2. Understand the impact on treatment decisions and patient outcomes
3. Discuss the case studies illustrating successful identification

In a clinical setting, the detection of microorganisms needs to be accurate to achieve successful control over disease. Advanced diagnostic techniques, including biochemical tests and antigen-antibody reactions like ELISA, have revolutionized the ability to detect specific pathogens on time. Biochemical tests, for instance, that work to study the metabolic functions of bacteria can result in primary information about their identification, hence allowing for targeted therapeutic intervention. Furthermore, the use of antigen-antibody techniques enhances specificity, allowing for quicker decision-making in a clinical setting. Particularly for foodborne pathogens , such as *Escherichia coli*, quick diagnosis and strain characterization, as emphasized in current studies, has become a critical component of pre- and post-harvest food safety protocols as well as clinical practice. This union of diagnostic methods ultimately helps to bring about improved patient outcomes through the ability to provide early and accurate treatment plans (Pavankumar & Sankaran, 2008). Molecular diagnostics, or polymerase chain reaction (PCR) and reverse transcriptase PCR (RT-PCR), are significant advancements in microbial identification, providing sensitivity and specificity unmatched by other methods. These techniques are imperative in detecting genetic material of pathogens, thereby facilitating clinicians to diagnose infections that may not be easily detectable using traditional techniques. As Sousa & Pereira (2013) surmise, the rapid technological progress in the identification of bacteria emphasizes such advanced methodologies keeping pace with the intricacies of microbial diversity and pathogenicity. The ability to differentiate distinct strains and characterize microbial populations enhances infection dynamics knowledge, tailoring antibiotic therapies to the unique genetic fingerprint of causative pathogens. By means of these molecular techniques, practitioners can refine treatment regimens, ultimately improving patient and population health care. Further, inclusion of methods like mass spectrometry in clinical settings has broadened the scope of microbial analysis. Methods like MALDI-TOF MS allow rapid identification of microbial species from colonies directly and have greatly shortened turnaround times. Though molecular techniques have given us a quantum leap in our diagnostic prowess, these also point towards the complexity of microbial communities and their resilience to environmental variations, including resistance to antimicrobials. As the literature suggests, heterogeneity in microbial populations complicates pathogen detection, and dynamic diagnostic paradigms are therefore needed to manage this diversity (Sousa & Pereira, 2013). Future advancements therefore, must address these challenges to further our understanding of microbial processes and hone therapeutic practice so that medical microbiology can continue to innovate and expand patient care within a constantly evolving paradigm of infectious diseases (Figure 3.13).

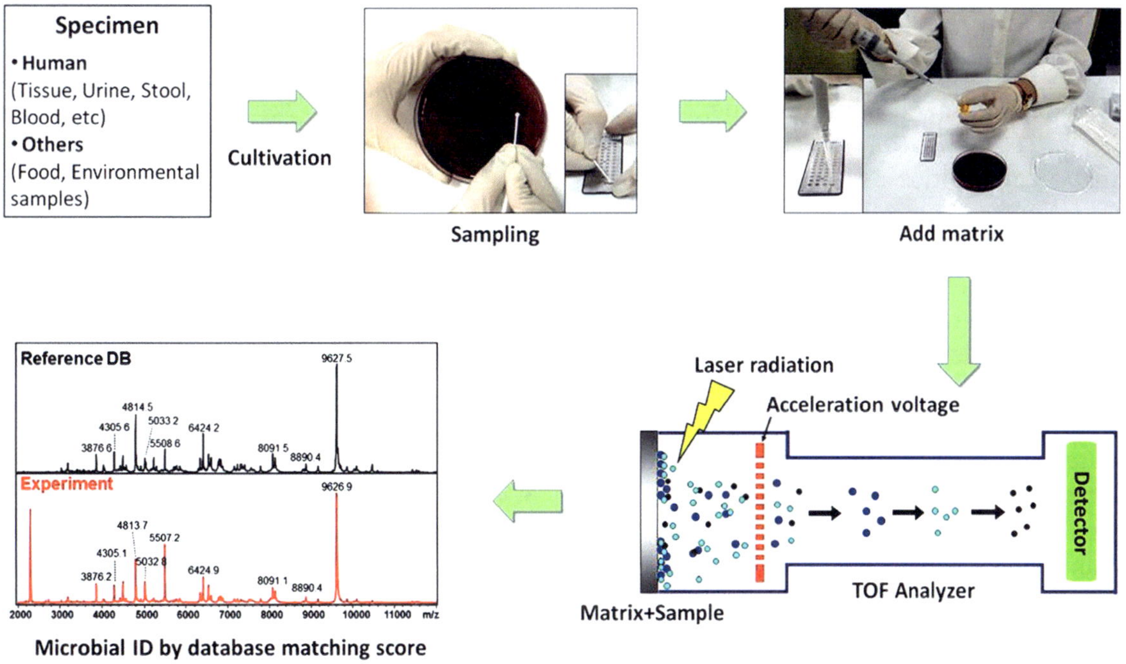

Figure 3.13. Workflow for microbial identification using MALDI-TOF MS.

Source: https://www.researchgate.net/profile/Kyoung-Soon-Jang/publication/322752329/figure/fig1/AS:599271690735618@1519888913670/Workflow-for-microbial-identification-using-MALDI-TOF-MS.png.

3.5.1. Role of Identification Techniques in Clinical Settings

Introduction of identification techniques in the clinical setup is a major breakthrough in infectious diseases and other conditions management and diagnosis. Biochemical tests, antigen-antibody tests like ELISA, and new molecular diagnostics have transformed laboratory practice by providing accurate and timely results. Biochemical tests allow for the identification of microorganisms based on metabolic features, leading to efficient pathogen detection. These approaches are also particularly valuable in choosing the appropriate therapeutic interventions since they minimize the delay time between patient evaluation and treatment. For instance, the use of these approaches in the identification of clinically significant species, e.g., bacterial pathogens, can have a direct impact on therapy choices so that patients receive optimum antimicrobial therapy with the ability to reduce the formation of antibiotic resistance. Aside from these, antigen-antibody techniques , such as enzyme-linked immunosorbent assays (ELISA) and agglutination tests supplement the diagnostic capabilities of clinical laboratories. These immunosassays provide a level of sensitivity and specificity that are necessary for the diagnosis of infection, even in low pathogenic burden. These assays not only serve well in the detection of infectious agents but also in monitoring disease progression and response to therapy. Particularly, ELISA has emerged as a chief technique in serological testing that has enabled clinicians to measure immune responses to specific pathogens, thereby influencing the treatment of patients. The potential uses of such techniques extend even to screening for new infectious diseases and the discovery of biomarkers in chronic conditions, warranting the importance of immunodiagnostic methods in current clinical microbiology. Molecular diagnosis, including methods like polymerase chain reaction (PCR) and reverse transcription PCR (RT-PCR), is an advancement in the detection of microorganisms. These techniques provide unmatched sensitivity and specificity and can detect pathogen genetic material within clinical samples. Clinicians can quickly diagnose microorganisms by using PCR, which can take hours, remarkably speeding up diagnosis. Uses of RT-PCR for RNA viruses become increasingly common during outbreaks, demonstrating the method's crucial role in public health interventions. Moreover, integration of molecular strategies in clinical labs enables us to better comprehend microbial genetics and resistance mechanisms, thereby informing therapy choices. With the problems regarding emerging pathogens and antibiotic resistance continuing to increase, the application of methods of identification, and particularly molecular diagnostics, is increasingly contributing to ensuring effective and timely treatment of patients (Jiang et al., 2007; Achan et al., 2022) (Figure 3.14).

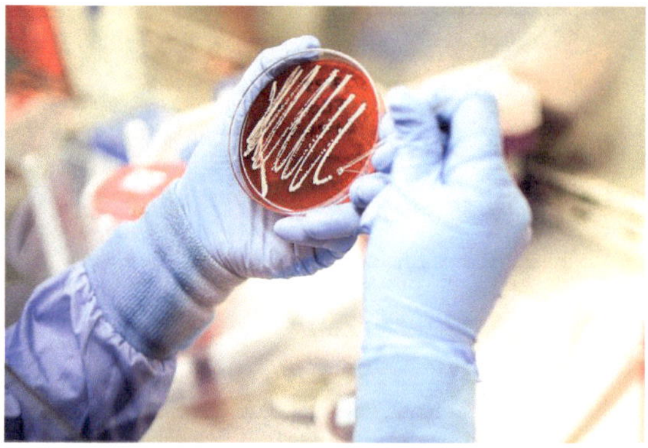

Figure 3.14. Role of identification techniques in clinical settings.

Source: https://criver.widen.net/content/bqcsxzkotr/jpeg/MS-001536.jpg?w=640&h=426&keep=c&crop=yes&color=fffffff&quality=80&u=tgoadr.

3.5.2. Impact on Treatment Decisions and Patient Outcomes

The identification of microorganisms in clinical microbiology directly impacts patient treatment and patient outcomes, primarily by employing diagnostic methods. Biochemical testing, for instance, separates microbial types according to metabolic properties. By developing accurate organism profiles, healthcare providers are able to provide successful antimicrobial treatments against target pathogens, reducing the risks of unsuccessful treatment. In infections due to bacteria, rapid identification is inversely related to improved patient outcomes because early treatment may forestall complications. Additionally, proper microbial identification promotes more rational use of antibiotics, which finally has an intrinsic role to play in the control of antibiotic resistance, an important public health problem of the current age. This accuracy in diagnosis not only influences the success of treatment but also optimizes total healthcare efficiency as well as patient satisfaction. Antigen-antibody techniques, including ELISA and agglutination tests, are also of significant relevance in patient outcome and treatment planning. These tests facilitate rapid detection of pathogens with the recognition of specific antigens in causative organisms or antibodies due to such infections. These tests enable physicians to make intelligent decisions, often before the onset of advanced disease, because of the rapidity of their results. As an illustration, in viral infections , such as HIV, early diagnosis through these tests allows for early treatment with antiretroviral therapy to significantly improve the long-term health status of patients. Monitoring therapeutic responses through serological tests also assists in modulating therapeutic interventions such that patient care is adaptive and efficacious. Incorporation of these antigen-antibody techniques thus underscores the role of accurate diagnostics towards optimizing patient management. Moreover, the evolution of molecular diagnostics, particularly PCR and RT-PCR, has revolutionized the face of medical microbiology, with significant impacts on treatment and patient outcomes. These procedures enable the rapid detection of microbial genetic material within a few hours, which can be priceless in acute care. They are highly specific and sensitive towards good decision-making, particularly where traditional practice will be expected to fail, e.g., polymicrobial infections or immunocompromised hosts. Furthermore, the ability to identify resistance genes using molecular methods allows clinicians to prioritize their treatment regimens to be successful against probable resistant strains, thereby increasing therapeutic effectiveness. As presented in the literature, advances in laboratory medicine, e.g., molecular diagnostic methods, highlight the need for accurate identification of microorganisms and contribute to enhanced quality of patient care and treatment results (Consortium OPATHY, & Gabaldón, 2019).

3.5.3. Case Studies Illustrating Successful Identification

In the medical microbiology clinical laboratory, accurate pathogen identification is critical for effective treatment and infection control. One of the most significant case studies is the development of a new antigen-capture enzyme-linked immunosorbent assay (ELISA) to detect *Francisella tularensis*, the causative agent of tularemia. In the research, a murine monoclonal antibody (mAb) against the bacterial lipopolysaccharide (LPS) was employed to enhance diagnostic sensitivity. Through various antibody subclasses, researchers identified that a switch to IgG1 and IgG2b mAbs increased the sensitivity of the assay with reduced background noise caused by self-association in IgG3. This innovative method not only made detection easy but also placed greater emphasis on characterizing the importance of antibodies in increasing antigen-antibody interaction, leading to timely and accurate clinical diagnosis of suspected tularemia cases (Nualnoi et al., 2017). Yet another significant advancement is noted when it comes to melioidosis, as researchers have developed an immunoassay for the specific discrimination between typical and atypical LPS strains of *Burkholderia pseudomallei*. Using antibody mAbs designed for targeted detection, the study was able to achieve a high success rate of 98.8%. This is a significant example as it emphasizes the importance of proper differentiation in demarcating the epidemiology of melioidosis. Furthermore, in vivo data have shown that the capsule polysaccharide (CPS) of B. *pseudomallei* has a short half-life in serum and is cleared primarily through urine. These findings not only pave the way for non-invasive diagnostic sampling but also for a possible biomarker of therapeutic response (Nualnoi et al., 2017). The construction of point-of-need diagnostic devices illustrates yet another crucial area of successful pathogen identification, this time for foodborne pathogens. Current conventional diagnostic methodologies are slow and limited to food samples taken post-production, something which plays a key role in necessitates the development of rapidly detectable techniques. Recent advances involving the application of molecular methods, biosensors, and microfluidics make it possible rapidly, sensitively, and specifically identify pathogens throughout all stages of food processing. As highlighted in a recent review, acceptance of portable devices into the food industry is essential for public health due to the fact that they enable real-time pathogen detection without the extensive lag times associated with conventional methods. The use of low-cost detection techniques with nucleic acid amplification processes represents a vital milestone in enhancing food safety and has greater implications for medical diagnostics as well (Figure 3.15).

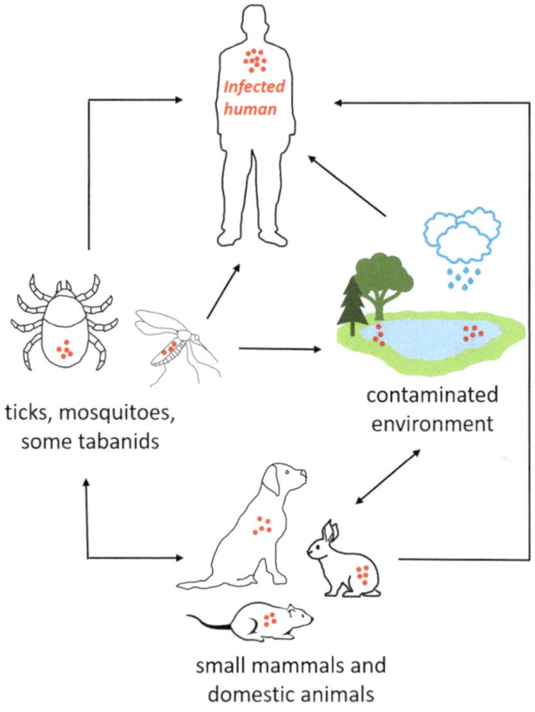

Figure 3.15. Transmission vectors and pathways of *Francisella tularensis* subspecies.

Source: https://www.researchgate.net/publication/380151011/figure/fig3/AS:11431281261177847@1721440588848/Transmission-vectors-and-pathways-of-Francisella-tularensis-subspecies.png.

Test Your Knowledge

1. What is the role of identification techniques in clinical settings?
2. How does the identification of microorganisms in medical microbiology fundamentally impact treatment decisions and patient outcomes?

3.6. Future Trends in Microbial Identification

Learning Outcome

1. Understand the advances in technology and their implications
2. Focus on the integration of artificial intelligence in diagnostics
3. Discuss the potential for rapid and accurate identification methods

The future of microbial identification promises a drastic transformation as technological developments continue to redefine the field of medical microbiology. Historically, microbial identification relied heavily on conventional techniques that entailed culture methods and biochemical tests, which, while enlightening, are time-consuming and labor-intensive. Introduction of molecular diagnosis through technologies , such as polymerase chain reaction (PCR) and real-time PCR (RT-PCR) has significantly accelerated the identification process which is both more sensitive and specific now. Moreover, newer developments , such as MALDI-TOF mass spectrometry present a new era that can identify microbial species on the basis of protein profiling. As pointed out by Sousa & Pereira (2013), there is nonetheless a fundamental need for advanced methods that can establish microbial heterogeneity in complex populations with high accuracy, thus enabling clinicians to take well-informed antimicrobial therapy. Next-generation sequencing (NGS) is another frontier for the identification of microorganisms since it enables researchers to examine entire genomes with speed and accuracy. NGS technology not only offers the identification of the target microorganisms but also their genetic diversity and potential virulence factors, as pointed out in studies on pathogenic *Escherichia coli* strains (Pavankumar & Sankaran, 2008). This aspect is important in clinical cases in which the determination of the pathogenesis of infections will dictate the treatment protocol. In addition, NGS can be supplemented with traditional methods to give a better insight into the microbial dynamics within the host organisms. With the improvement in technology and its cost-effectiveness, it is expected that NGS will become standard equipment both in clinical microbiological laboratories as well as in public health. In addition to these technologies, the development of rapid diagnostic tools should progress to improve microbial identification efficiencies. As reflected in recent research, there is a necessity for creating user-friendly, affordable, and effective assay methods that are suitable for facilitating screening of microorganisms across various environments, including clinical, environmental, and food safety (Sousa & Pereira, 2013). These methods could be immunological assays that involve colorimetric detection or more sophisticated nucleic acid tests suitable for high-throughput screening. These technologies will not only accelerate diagnostic procedures but also find significant roles in food safety and outbreak response measures, particularly for pathogens like *E. coli*. In shedding more light on infectious diseases through the solutions of the challenges of microbial identification using integrated and holistic approaches, the future of microbial diagnostics will definitely provide more illumination into infectious diseases and result in improved patient outcomes.

3.6.1. Advances in Technology and Their Implications

Emerging technologies have revolutionized the identification of microorganisms, particularly in clinical microbiology. While traditional approaches often take hours and require high resources, molecular diagnostics have been an effective solution. Techniques , such as polymerase chain reaction (PCR) and reverse transcription PCR (RT-PCR) have significantly improved the detection of pathogens, increasing speed along with accuracy in healthcare settings.

Not only do these molecular technologies enable the rapid amplification of specific DNA sequences, but also allow the identification of different strains of pathogens, which is crucial in the targeting of the right treatment interventions. Moreover, by providing accurate genetic information, these technologies enhance knowledge of microbial pathogenesis and therefore direct public health strategies and individualized patient care. The ability to rapidly detect pathogens in clinical specimens is a revolutionary development in medical microbiology that has major patient-outcome implications. Concurrent with these developments, technical progress in antigen-antibody methods, including enzyme-linked immunosorbent assay (ELISA) and agglutination tests, has further enhanced the range of diagnostic options. These immunologic methods provide an efficient method for the detection of pathogens by identifying particular antibodies or antigens. ELISA, with high specificity and sensitivity, has become the norm in serological tests, enabling the detection of infections yet undetectable using molecular methods. Moreover, the ease and repeatability of the tests make them suitable for use in large-scale screening in any environment, from clinical laboratories to field-based diagnoses. Such a method is welcomed in conjunction with molecular diagnostics in order to offer a multi-faceted approach to detect pathogens. Thus, their integration into diagnostic processes is essential for effective epidemiological surveillance and control, ultimately contributing to reducing the healthcare system burden caused by infectious diseases. Technological innovations in expanding analytical capacity, , such as molecular mass spectrometry (MALDI-TOF MS), also offer a novel method of microorganism identification with accuracy and efficiency. By the examination of microbial protein profiles, MALDI-TOF MS provides rapid and accurate identification, invaluable in clinical microbiology. Though the method has numerous limitations, challenges remain, especially the full characterization of microbial diversity. As pointed out in recent reports, molecular methods may lack addressing the complex dynamics of microbial communities, which are most likely to lead to clinical infections and exhibit variable sensitivity to treatment. Hence, the need for ongoing innovation in diagnostic methods is of greater significance. Developing new diagnostic platforms that can capture this microbial diversity has the potential to provide significant insight into pathogenicity, antibiotic resistance, and the formation of effective infection control systems, ultimately with improved medical decision-making in antimicrobial therapy (Pavankumar & Sankaran, 2008; Sousa & Pereira, 2013) (Figure 3.16).

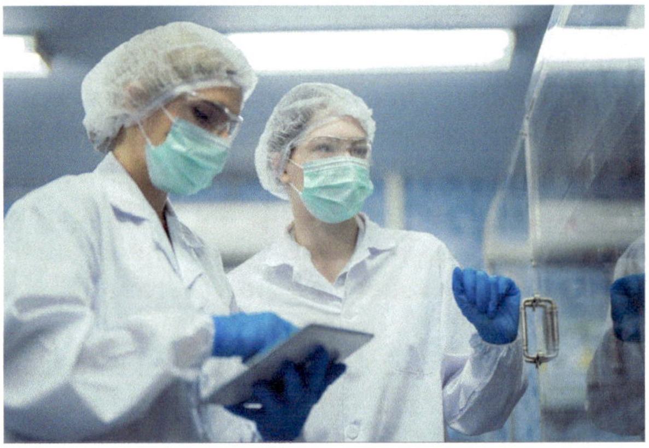

Figure 3.16. Advances in technology and their implications.

Source: https://www.susupport.com/media/2205/download/Costs-monoclonal-antibody-production.jpg?v=1&inline=1.

3.6.2. Integration of Artificial Intelligence in Diagnostics

The use of artificial intelligence (AI) in the diagnostic procedure has revolutionized the practice of medical microbiology, particularly in the identification of microorganisms. Traditional methods, , such as biochemical tests and antigen-antibody tests, have traditionally been time-consuming and prone to human error. The advent of machine learning algorithms has enabled more accurate and less time-consuming diagnoses by identifying patterns within large datasets. According to early studies, AI platforms can significantly reduce levels of human error, enhance clinical outcomes, and improve long-term patient monitoring (Dutta et al., 2022). In the context of infectious diseases, early detection has the potential to radically alter treatment outcomes, highlighting the sheer potential of AI in enhancing diagnostic potential. Another important area in which AI has a significant contribution is the enhancement of biosensor technology for the detection of microorganisms. The COVID-19 pandemic stimulated demand for biosensor platforms that offer rapid, cheap, and precise diagnostics, leading to home testing and point-of-care systems (Consortium OPATHY, & Gabaldón, 2019). AI techniques are essential when it comes to optimizing these biosensors so that they can analyze physiological data in a more comprehensive manner. These smart sensors utilize advanced machine learning algorithms for real-time analysis and detection, effectively decentralizing traditional lab tests and providing in-situ diagnostic capability.

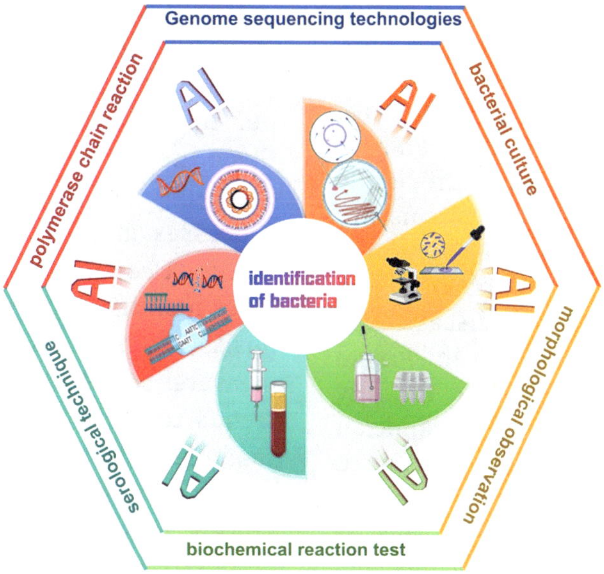

Figure 3.17. Artificial intelligence facilitates the diagnosis of bacterial infectious diseases.

Source: https://www.frontiersin.org/files/Articles/1449844/fmicb-15-1449844-HTML-r1/image_m/fmicb-15-1449844-g002.jpg.

As a result, clinicians are able to make faster treatment choices, thereby improving patient outcomes and streamlining healthcare processes. Moreover, AI-driven molecular diagnostics, particularly PCR and RT-PCR tests, benefit from the use of advanced algorithms that provide improved accuracy in identifying pathogens. With its ability to process advanced genetic information faster, AI is capable of streamlining primer design, detecting mutations, and analyzing results with accuracy. Such a feature is essential when confronting the hurdles posed by novel infectious diseases, where evolution is fast and real-time surveillance and detection are necessary. Besides, with ever-improving machine learning technologies, they are able to learn continuously from new data, making diagnostics even more efficient, with improved and speedier microbial identification in the future. This way, the use of AI positions itself as a keystone for modern medical microbiology, crafting diagnostics for decades to come (Figure 3.17).

3.6.3. Potential for Rapid and Accurate Identification Methods

The necessity for rapid and accurate identification tools in clinical microbiology is at the heart of enhancing diagnostic methodology and patient treatment. Conventional methods, , such as biochemical testing and antigen-antibody reactions, while being precise, involve long incubation periods which compromise critical clinical decision-making. In contrast, molecular diagnostic technology like PCR and next-generation sequencing offers a new paradigm where detecting various pathogens from clinical samples is made feasible with fast detection. These approaches not only prolong turnaround times but also improve diagnostic accuracy by ensuring that even low-abundance microbial organisms are sufficiently identified. Given that healthcare systems are increasingly interested in timely interventions, the use of rapid identification methods becomes imperative in managing infectious diseases and aligning appropriate treatments to individual patient requirements. This ability for rapidity and precision is a game-changer for a clinician in clinical microbiology, with the potential to broadly enhance patient outcomes and public health intervention. Emerging methods , such as clinical metagenomic next-generation sequencing (mNGS), underscore the game-changing nature of rapid identification techniques in medical microbiology. In allowing detailed examination of microbial and host genetic material, mNGS overtakes the limitations of existing diagnostics. Such a technology innovation not only allows for the detection of disease-causing microorganisms with unprecedented speed but also provides data on patients' microbiome and immune status. Consequently, this cross-disciplinary approach allows for accurate diagnosis of infectious diseases even in failures of conventional tests. However, bringing mNGS into the clinic demands breaking hurdles of daunting magnitude, including the need for robust data analysis and interpretation pipelines. Through overcoming these issues, the medical community can harvest mNGS's maximum potential in order to improve diagnostic processes and lead by example in curtailing infectious diseases as documented in the literature (Chiu & Miller, 2019).

Furthermore, the rapid detection of pathogenic microorganisms plays a significant role in public health emergency response, as per the literature (Rajapaksha et al., 2018). Given the growing menace of re-emerging and emerging infectious diseases, identification processes directly influence the efficiency of outbreak control measures. The application of quick identification techniques not only enables healthcare providers to implement controlling measures speedily but also to monitor resistance trends towards antimicrobials. Given the fact that infections tend to spread quickly, especially in a clinical setup, the development of simplified but efficient diagnostic kits is imperative. The addition of biochemical assays, antigen-antibody techniques, and molecular diagnostics adds a strong foundation for the identification of pathogens to keep pace with the complexity of contemporary infectious diseases. The success of these methods again points to the urgency required to prioritize advances in identification techniques that ultimately benefit individual patients and public health infrastructure in general.

Test Your Knowledge

1. What are recent advancements in technology for the identification of microorganisms?
2. What innovative diagnostic techniques can be developed to improve the rapid and accurate identification of pathogenic bacteria?

SUMMARY

In summarizing this investigation into the identification of microorganisms in medical microbiology, it is clear that an interdisciplinary method involving biochemical tests, antigen-antibody assays, and molecular diagnostics is crucial. The versatility of the methods increases the diagnostic precision and efficiency of identifying different pathogens. Methods like ELISA and agglutination offer critical tools for the identification of precise antigen-antibody interactions, hence ensuring the identification of infecting agents. As highlighted in experiments like the iMALDI assay, these technologies can push the boundaries of specificity and sensitivity so that clinical diagnosis can be prompt as well as precise (Jiang et al., 2007). The convergence of these different methodologies strengthens the epidemiological foundation of infectious diseases and ultimately assists in effective therapeutic strategies. Moreover, enhanced molecular diagnostics, i.e., PCR and RT-PCR, have revolutionized the field of pathogen detection quite immensely. Their ability to amplify tiny quantities of nucleic acids allows for rapid detection of microbial agents even under challenging clinical conditions. The applicability of the methods is underscored by their use in the detection of pathogenic organisms responsible for severe health threats, e.g., antibiotic-resistant organisms. The comparative speed and accuracy of PCR techniques over traditional culture techniques render them indispensable in modern medical microbiology. As shown by ongoing research advancement, e.g., confirmation of magnetic detection methods, conjugation of new technologies continues to detect pathogens more specifically and sensitively (Duarte et al., 2016).

In the long term, microorganism identification in the future lies in the successful integration of these diverse methodologies into a single diagnostic system. By optimizing biochemical testing, antigen-antibody techniques, and molecular diagnosis, clinicians can improve patient outcomes through accurate and timely diagnosis. As we focus further on advancing into the era of personalized medicine, these strategies will be optimized not only to further our understanding of microbial pathogenesis but also to direct evidence-based treatment regimens. Researchers must continue to innovate and refine these diagnostic techniques to maintain the pace of microbial infections evolving and remain focused on patient care as the top priority for medical microbiology. The journey to full microbial identification has been fraught with failures and triumphs, with each advance bringing new developments into the field.

Microorganism identification in medical microbiology is characterized by various methods critical in the diagnosis of infection and food safety. One key area is the application of biochemical tests with the ability to differentiate organisms based on metabolic activities. Biochemical tests , such as fermentation tests and enzyme activity assessments, provide valuable information regarding the pathogenic potential of species like *Escherichia coli*. Specifically, *E. coli* presents diverse pathogenic patterns from enterotoxigenic to enterohemorrhagic types, which present varying detection and treatment challenges. Molecular diagnostics have also further enhanced the identification process through assays presenting simplicity and low cost with high specificity and sensitivity. Integration of such molecular approaches into microbiological routine can potentially enhance surveillance and control activities for foodborne pathogens (Pavankumar & Sankaran, 2008). Antigen-antibody techniques, including enzyme-linked immunosorbent assays (ELISA) and agglutination tests, are also very important for the identification of pathogens. Employing these techniques enables the detection of some antigens or antibodies, which in turn results in successful diagnosis of infections caused by certain microorganisms. In the determination of biotype, as is the situation with *Yersinia ruckeri*, antigenic characterization gives distinct cut-out serotypes, which is valuable in the creation of specific vaccines and control measures. These strategies not only assist in the diagnosis of infections but also in the acquisition of knowledge regarding the epidemiology of diseases by revealing potential outbreaks or endemic characteristics. The integration of antigen-antibody strategies with biochemical and molecular diagnostics therefore, yields a fuller paradigm for the monitoring of microbial threats as well as optimizing public health yield (Tinsley et al., 2010).

As new trends emerge in the discipline of medical microbiology, integration of different identification approaches remains crucial for continued advancement. The ongoing development of molecular diagnostics, coupled with traditional biochemical and immunological techniques, encourages an integrated approach for microbial identification. The synergy enables the practitioners to respond quickly and accurately to pathogen outbreaks, thus safeguarding public health. Furthermore, ongoing research on the pathogenicity of microorganisms, particularly those emerging with evolving nature after environmental changes, is important to stay ahead of forthcoming infectious diseases. Adequate understanding and application of these techniques will foster greater diagnostic capability and facilitate the work of endeavors worldwide in combating microbial diseases effectively.

KEY TERMS FROM THIS CHAPTER

- Agglutination tests
- Antibiotic resistance
- Antifungal resistance
- Antigen-antibody interactions
- Biochemical assays
- Biochemical tests
- Carbohydrate fermentation
- Catalase-negative streptococci
- Catalase-positive staphylococci
- Co-infection
- Diagnostic testing
- ELISA
- Enzymatic activities
- Enzymatic function

CRITICAL THINKING QUESTIONS

1. **Which of the following biochemical tests is commonly used to identify bacteria that ferment lactose?**
   a. Catalase test
   b. Coagulase test
   c. Indole test
   d. MacConkey agar test
2. **The catalase test differentiates between which two major groups of Gram-positive cocci?**
   a. *Streptococcus* and *Staphylococcus*
   b. *Escherichia* and *Pseudomonas*
   c. *Salmonella* and *Shigella*
   d. *Bacillus* and *Clostridium*
3. **In antigen-antibody techniques, which method is commonly used for detecting specific microbial antigens in a sample using fluorescent-labeled antibodies?**
   a. Immunofluorescence
   b. ELISA
   c. Western blot
   d. Agglutination
4. **What is a major advantage of antigen-antibody techniques over biochemical tests?**
   a. They are less expensive
   b. They identify microorganisms based on metabolic activity
   c. They are faster and more specific for certain pathogens
   d. They require large quantities of bacteria
5. **Which of the following correctly compares identification methods?**
   a. Biochemical tests are more rapid than molecular tests
   b. Molecular methods like PCR offer higher sensitivity and specificity than traditional methods
   c. Antigen-antibody techniques are more accurate than sequencing for all microbes
   d. Culture methods are always preferred over molecular methods

Short Answer Questions

1. What are the main methods used to identify microorganisms in the laboratory?
2. What is the role of biochemical tests in microorganism identification? Give an example.
3. How can molecular techniques like PCR aid in microbial identification?
4. What is the significance of using selective and differential media in microbial identification? Provide an example of each.
5. What is the principle behind antigen-antibody reactions in the identification of microorganisms?
6. Explain how the enzyme-linked immunosorbent assay (ELISA) is used to detect microbial antigens or antibodies.
7. Why might antigen detection tests be preferred over culture methods in certain clinical situations?

Answers to Critical Thinking Questions

1. (d) 2. (c) 3. (a) 4. (c) 5. (b)

REFERENCES

1. Abd-Elmagid, A., Adams, J., Adhikari, R., Ali-Shtayeh, M. S., Altschul, S., Arap, S., Arcate, G., et al. (2016). Diagnostic tests and their application in the management of soil- and water-borne oomycete pathogen species. https://core.ac.uk/download/76977879.pdf (accessed on 13th June 2025).
2. Abdelwhab, E. M., Abe, H., Adam, M., Al-Harthi, H., Al-Tukhi, M., Alam, M., Anderson, R., et al. (2013). An overview of the clinical use of filter paper in the diagnosis of tropical diseases. https://core.ac.uk/download/42631176.pdf (accessed on 13th June 2025).
3. Achan, B., Baguma, A., Itabangi, H., Mboowa, G., et al. (2022). Laboratory diagnosis of candidiasis. https://core.ac.uk/download/539671413.pdf (accessed on 13th June 2025).
4. Akter, M., Hussain, S. B., Lucky, S., Sharmin, S., Sejuti, S., et al. (2024). Development of novel nanostructured biosensors for rapid detection of pathogens in clinical diagnostics. https://core.ac.uk/download/620838435.pdf (accessed on 13th June 2025).
5. Alirol, E., Bottieau, E., Chappuis, F., d'Acremont, V., et al. (2013). Rapid diagnostic tests for non-malarial febrile illness in the tropics. https://core.ac.uk/download/pdf/17182914.pdf (accessed on 13th June 2025).
6. Consortium OPATHY, & Gabaldón, T. (2019). Recent trends in molecular diagnostics of yeast infections: from PCR to NGS. *FEMS microbiology reviews*, *43*(5), 517–547. https://doi.org/10.1093/femsre/fuz015(accessed on 13th June 2025).
7. Chiu, C. Y., & Miller, S. A. (2019). Clinical metagenomics. *Nature reviews. Genetics*, *20*(6), 341–355. https://doi.org/10.1038/s41576-019-0113-7 (accessed on 13th June 2025).
8. Duarte, C. M. P. C. (2016). Portable "lab-on-chip" platform for bovine mastitis diagnosis in raw milk. https://core.ac.uk/download/61490319.pdf (accessed on 13th June 2025).
9. Dutta, G., Shukla, R. P., & Verma, S. (2022). Machine learning-enabled biosensors in clinical decision making. https://core.ac.uk/download/621168588.pdf (accessed on 13th June 2025).
10. Eda, S., Hickling, G. J., & Wadhwa, A. (2012). Opportunities for improved serodiagnosis of human tuberculosis, bovine tuberculosis, and paratuberculosis. https://core.ac.uk/download/pdf/8740257.pdf (accessed on 13th June 2025).
11. Eesti Arsti toimetus. (2022). 16th Baltic Congress in Laboratory Medicine. https://core.ac.uk/download/574544557.pdf (accessed on 13th June 2025).
12. Fortina, P., Kricka, L. J., Park, J. Y., & Polsky, T. G. (2015). The future of laboratory medicine–A 2014 perspective. https://core.ac.uk/download/54509579.pdf (accessed on 13th June 2025).
13. Franco-Duarte, R., Mendonça, A., Sampaio, P., Santos, J., et al. (2021). Fungal infections diagnosis–Past, present and future. https://core.ac.uk/download/541292208.pdf (accessed on 13th June 2025).
14. Gadjanski, I., Giouroudi, I., Kavanaugh, D., Knežević, N., et al. (2019). Point-of-need DNA testing for detection of foodborne pathogenic bacteria. https://core.ac.uk/download/553569098.pdf (accessed on 13th June 2025).
15. Gopinathan, R. (2017). To study the evaluation of conventional culture methods and serodiagnosis methods for clinically diagnosed as meningoencephalitis in patients admitted in Thanjavur Medical College Hospital with special reference to Japanese encephalitis. https://

core.ac.uk/download/288215595.pdf (accessed on 13th June 2025).

16. Gorshunov, Y. V., Komar, A. G., & Motronenko, V. V. (2019). Serological methods in modern biotechnologies and their bioanalytical standardization. https://core.ac.uk/download/323528090.pdf (accessed on 13th June 2025).

17. Heilek, G. (2016). Nucleic acids–The use of nucleic acid testing in molecular diagnostics. https://core.ac.uk/download/322425829.pdf (accessed on 13th June 2025).

18. Hrušková, V. (2012). Foodborne *Staphylococcus aureus*: Identification and enterotoxin production in milk and cheese. https://core.ac.uk/download/30310825.pdf (accessed on 13th June 2025).

19. Ince, J., & McNally, A. (2009). Development of rapid, automated diagnostics for infectious disease: Advances and challenges. https://core.ac.uk/download/30633630.pdf (accessed on 13th June 2025).

20. Jiang, J. (2007). Immune tandem mass spectrometry (iMALDI) assay for clinical diagnostics. https://core.ac.uk/download/210600831.pdf (accessed on 13th June 2025).

21. Kazakova, A. (2019). Multiplex diagnostics: Development of serological dual-mode multiplex microarray immunoassay and analysis of influenza and respiratory syncytial virus disease burden in early childhood. https://core.ac.uk/download/275894270.pdf (accessed on 13th June 2025).

22. Ndao, M. (2009). Diagnosis of parasitic diseases: Old and new approaches. https://core.ac.uk/download/pdf/8366774.pdf (accessed on 13th June 2025).

23. Nualnoi, T. (2017). Detection and *in vivo* fate of surface-expressed bacterial polysaccharides. https://core.ac.uk/download/622257603.pdf (accessed on 13th June 2025).

24. Pavankumar, A.R. i Sankaran, K. (2008). Primjena novih metoda kontrole patogenih oblika bakterije Escherichia coli. *Food Technology and Biotechnology, 46* (2), 125-145. Preuzeto s https://hrcak.srce.hr/24397 (accessed on 13th June 2025).

25. A. M. Sousa, M. O. Pereira IBB – Institute for Biotechnology and Bioengineering, Centre of Biological Engineering, University of Minho, Campus de Gualtar, 4710–057 Braga, Portugal (2013). A prospect of current microbial diagnosis methods. Microbial pathogens and strategies for combating them: science, technology and education (A. Méndez-Vilas, Ed.). https://core.ac.uk/download/55632035.pdf (accessed on 13th June 2025).

26. Rajapaksha, P., Elbourne, A., Gangadoo, S., Brown, R. R., Cozzolino, D., & Chapman, J. (2018). A review of methods for the detection of pathogenic microorganisms. *The Analyst, 144*, 396–411. https://doi.org/10.1039/c8an01488d (accessed on 13th June 2025).

27. Seaman, W., & Whitehouse, J. H. (2001). Florida marine biotechnology: Research, development and training capabilities to advance science and commerce. https://core.ac.uk/download/11016354.pdf (accessed on 13th June 2025).

28. Tinsley, J. (2010). Studies on the pathogenicity of *Yersinia ruckeri* biotype 2 to rainbow trout (*Oncorhynchus mykiss*, Walbaum). https://core.ac.uk/download/77035128.pdf (accessed on 13th June 2025).

HOST-MICROBE INTERACTIONS AND PATHOGENESIS

4

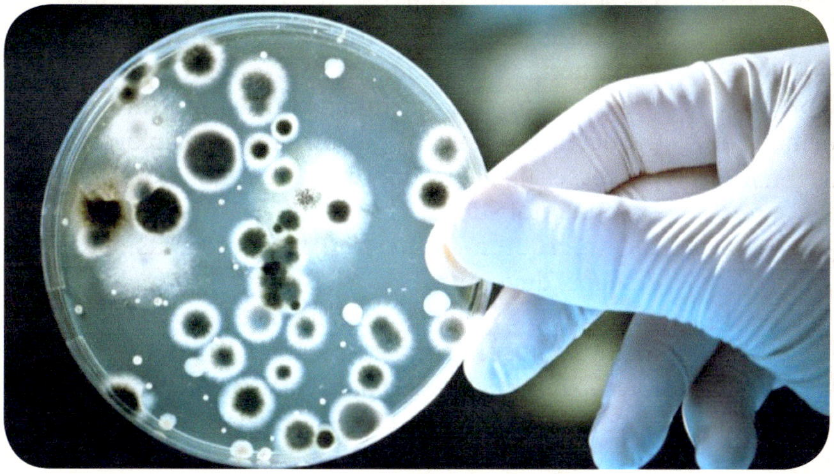

LEARNING OBJECTIVES

After studying this chapter, you will be able to:

1. Explain the types of microbes involved in host interactions
2. Discuss the mechanisms of pathogenesis
3. Understand host immune response to microbial infections
4. Describe the factors influencing host-microbe interactions
5. Deal with therapeutic approaches to combat pathogenesis

Introduction

The intricate relationship between microbes and hosts is a theme of research in microbiology, particularly in relation to unraveling pathogenesis. The intricate interaction encompasses various mechanisms leading to either health or disease states, thereby highlighting microbial regulation of host physiology. Recent research accentuates the central role of microbial communities, or microbiomes, in host homeostasis and their participation in destabilization of this process and the onset of disease states. Elucidation of the cellular and molecular mechanisms that influence these interactions will uncover new insights into the etiology of many diseases, including inflammatory bowel disease and infection. Efforts to describe these interactions have increased, as proven through major conferences that bring together leading scientists to discuss advances in the field, again evidencing the significance of this research field (Barret et al., 2012). Host-microbe complexity is exemplified through the bidirectional effects that microbes have on host immunity. Pathogenic microbes can employ specific pathways to evade detection and destruction, thus ensuring their survival and proliferation in the host. In contrast, beneficial microbes enhance immune function, thus protecting against infections and promoting overall well-being.

A classic example can be seen in inflammatory bowel diseases , such as ulcerative colitis and Crohn's disease, which occur as a result of dysregulated interactions between the gut microbiome and the immune system of the host. Researchers are now employing systems biology approaches to unravel the intricate dynamics of such interactions, integrating information from various layers of biology, including genetic and epigenetic components, to develop novel therapeutic strategies for the correction of these dysregulations (Polytarchou et al., 2014).

The understanding of host-microbe interactions is not a theoretical concern but is important in healthcare and disease control. The studies that increasingly appear in this area are able to lay the groundwork for new interventions on microbial processes with potential applications both in the prevention and treatment of infectious disease and chronic disease. This requires multi-disciplinary investigation, including microbiology, immunology, and computational biology, to comprehensively canvass these interactions and effects.

As new breakthroughs in technology continue to shed light on the intricate networks that govern host-microbe interactions, it is ever more crucial to develop a more nuanced understanding of those dynamics. Ultimately, the battle to decipher the mysteries of host-microbe interactions promises to transform our paradigm of pathogenesis and therapeutic development in the years ahead.

Definition of Host-Microbe Interactions

Clarifying host-microbe interactions is pivotal to the comprehension of the complex dynamics between microbial populations and host organisms. Host-microbe interactions are very diverse, from mutualism, where both the microbe and host benefit, through to parasitism, where the microbe kills the host. Such interactions are generally inseparable from the host immune response and from the microbial metabolic processes that can control health and disease conditions. New research illustrates the wide-ranging impact of microbial communities, particularly within the gut, on many physiological processes like digestion, immune regulation, and even mental status. Through these interactions, the microbiome can trigger homeostasis or disease development, again highlighting the value of a symbiotic microbial community to maintain host health. The research of these host-microbe interactions is particularly critical when it comes to pathogenesis, where pathogenic microbes utilize host mechanisms to gain access and cause disease. A careful observation of these dynamics provides evidence that certain microbes possess well-developed virulence factors that enable them to thrive and multiply in the host. For example, pathogens are able to hijack host cell signal transduction or evade host immune recognition, allowing them to survive and damage tissues (Cadwell & Debnath, 2017). In addition, understanding the mechanisms by which microbes interact with the host not only sheds light on infectious disease pathogenesis but also informs therapeutic strategies, , such as probiotics, to re-engineer the microbiota to fight pathogens. This intricate interaction presents a challenge to researchers to disentangle the specific routes of host-microbe interactions for advancing microbial pathogenesis studies. Furthermore, the role of the gut microbiome in host well-being highlights the importance of microbial function and diversity in disease prevention. Gut microbiome consists of a highly diverse collection of microbial species, each possessing a distinctive functional repertoire that is central to host well-being (Lynch et al., 2019). The microbial network may lead to dysbiosis when it changes, and this dysbiosis is implicated in various chronic disorders, including autoimmune diseases, obesity, and nonalcoholic fatty liver disease (NAFLD). Research using next-generation sequencing technologies has begun unraveling the complexities of such microbial communities towards their metabolic end products and their implication in disease and health. By emphasizing the multiscalar nature of host-microbe interactions, researchers are in a better position to understand how the microbiome can be used for therapeutic intervention, thereby closing the gap between bench research and clinical applications of disease regulation linked with microbial dysbiosis (Figure 4.1).

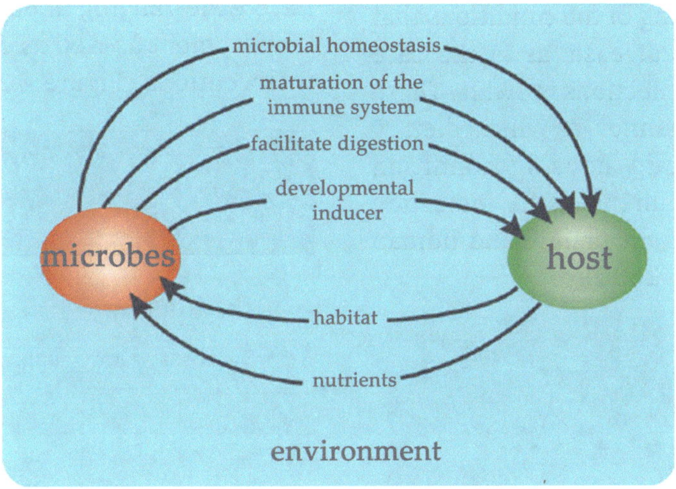

Figure 4.1. Schematic view of the interactions between host organisms and their microbiota.

Source: https://www.researchgate.net/profile/Sebastian-Fraune/publication/44669997/figure/fig6/AS:277155461255169@1443090419297/Schematic-view-of-the-interactions-between-host-organisms-and-their-microbiota.png.

Importance of Studying Pathogenesis

Pathogenesis must be comprehended, particularly in how the relationship between microbes and hosts leads to and aggravates most diseases. Examining the mechanisms of infection causation, evasion of killing by the host, and disease causation by pathogens can lead researchers to identify targets for therapy. Pathogenesis does not only encompass the microbes themselves but also the hosts' reaction to the invaders, and this may, in turn, complicate the disease process even more. For instance, ulcerative colitis and Crohn's disease are two forms of inflammatory bowel disease caused by intricate dynamics involving genetic susceptibilities, immune responses, and interactions with the gut microbiome. As hypothesized in contemporary research, systems biology is a technique for investigating inflammatory bowel disease that seeks to integrate numerous omics data to de-mystify mechanisms of pathogenicity at the molecular level and, as a byproduct, design new therapeutics (Polytarchou et al., 2014).

Additionally, exploring the intricacies of host-microbe interactions provides sophistication to our understanding of public health challenges and can lead to improved prevention. The global occurrence of antibiotic-resistant pathogens justifies the need to explore new strategies in combating infectious diseases. Knowledge of the processes whereby enteric disease-causing pathogens like *Brachyspira hyodysenteriae* and *Lawsonia intracellularis* work provides researchers with the ability to design targeted interventions that will disrupt these processes. Effective prophylaxis involves a thorough understanding of the conditions that predispose animals to disease, as is the case with studies of enteric infections in swine. These studies indicate the manner in which dietary manipulation and group housing condition animals to develop certain infections, indicating the longer implications for animal and human health (Jacobson et al., 2003).

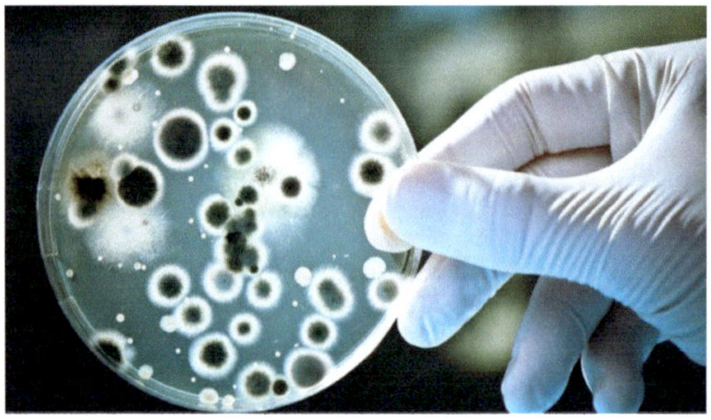

Figure 4.2. A gloved hand holds a petri dish showing diverse fungal and bacterial colonies, illustrating microbial growth patterns in a laboratory setting.

Source: https://asm.org/getmedia/752a7290-80c0-417a-b816-16a6301e2d58/pathogenesis_feature.jpg?width=874&height=491&ext=.jpg.

Secondly, advances in diagnostic technology are at the core of pathogenesis studies. Breakthroughs , such as the polymerase chain reaction (PCR) technologies have made us more able to detect pathogens accurately and sensitively and hence in time for intervention. Model construction for sequential disease pathogenesis monitoring allows improved understanding of infection response by the host, in addition to pathogenesis mechanisms employed by microbes. Such studies improve knowledge about specific disease processes but also further the profession of microbiology through the provision of novel information on how host-microbe interaction dynamics evolve. As researchers unravel the intricacies of pathogenesis, the knowledge obtained will have wide-ranging implications for therapeutic development as well as enhanced public health interventions (Figure 4.2).

4.1. Types of Microbes Involved in Host Interactions

Learning Outcome

1. Discuss about dynamic interplay between bacteria and their hosts
2. Understand viruses and their reliance on host cells for replication and survival
3. Explain how Fungi play a pivotal role in host-microbe interactions

The human microbiome is a complex society of microbes, , such as bacteria, viruses, fungi, and archaea, with each playing a vital role in host interaction and potentially governing health or disease. Bacteria are the most numerous and diverse of these and have specific taxa occupying specific locations in the body, , such as the gut, skin, and mouth. The gut microbiota, in particular, has been of significant interest due to its intimate connection with many of the physiological processes, , such as digestion, metabolism, and immunity. Not only do these microorganisms help in acquiring nutrients, but they also interact with immune cells of the host to create a symbiotic community necessary in the upkeep of homeostasis. Dysbiosis, or imbalance of the microbial community, can lead to pathologies like inflammatory bowel disease (IBD), in which complex relationships among genetic, immune, and microbial factors mediate the course and severity of disease, as outlined in recent studies (Polytarchou et al., 2014).

In addition to bacterial communities, viruses, particularly bacteriophages, have become increasingly important for host-microbe interactions. Bacteriophages infect and regulate bacterial populations, thus influencing the overall microbial composition within the gut. Such viral interaction guarantees bacterial diversity and stability, indicating the fine balance of the microbiome. Furthermore, research implies that such viral particles can transfer genes to bacteria through horizontal gene transfer, increasing microbial resiliency or virulence. Among host interactions, the viral component is used to change the pathogenic potential of bacterial groups and is currently known for its role in diseases , such as IBD. Unveiling these interactions between bacteria and their virus equivalents is essential for the development of therapeutic measures with a goal of modulating the microbiome towards improved health (Polytarchou et al., 2014). Fungal microbes, less well defined than their bacterial cousins, also have significant roles to play in host interaction. The mycobiome, or fungal component of the microbiome, has the ability to influence host immune function and play key roles in metabolic regulation. Recent research has shown that some fungi have been able to communicate with gut-residing bacteria, manipulating their function and developmental patterns as well as modulating host signals. Such interaction discloses a multilayered system of communication in the microbiome with fungi as intermediaries of bacterial influence on host health. The gut-brain axis, a bidirectional system of exchange between the gut microbiota and the central nervous system, discloses how modification of microbial composition can trigger neurological and psychological responses in similarly similar fashion. As emphasized in research investigating this axis, there is evidence that microbial homeostasis disturbances are involved in many disorders, again emphasizing the importance of knowing the types of microbes involved in host interaction.

4.1.1. Bacteria

The dynamic relationship between the bacteria and hosts is central to unlocking host-microbe interactions and the mechanisms of pathogenesis. Bacteria , such as *Yersinia pseudotuberculosis* possess specific structures known as adhesins, which facilitate their attachment to the host tissue. Not only do the virulence factors cause the colonization of the bacteria, but they also regulate the immune responses of the hosts. In research that was conducted, it was proven that the multivalent adhesion molecule (MAM) in *Y. pseudotuberculosis* is essential for effective binding and host phagocytic uptake, particularly in immune cells like hemocytes in the *Galleria mellonella* model. Of importance, disruption of such interaction will invariably increase pathogenic effects since diminished phagocyte association is accompanied by more aggressive bacterial clearance but also triggers unwarranted immune reactions that can adversely affect host viability, bespeaking a fragile balance between bacterial adhesion and defense mechanisms of the host (Coates et al., 2021).

Research on the role of bacterial pathogenesis extends beyond adhesion to encompass broader considerations of microbial interaction with host physiology. The Vibrio genus, for instance, illustrates this multiplexed interaction, in its case employing its type VI secretion system (T6SS). This system has been employed to modify intestinal motility in larval zebrafish, shedding light on how bacterial activity leads to cellular damage and consequent activation of immune responses. By inducing tissue damage, Vibrio suppresses optimal gut functioning, causing macrophages to migrate out of their typical midgut habitat to areas that are damaged. These movements emphasize the effect of bacterial-induced pathology on host cellular dynamics, and therefore underpin the need for additional research into how pathogenic bacteria influence intestinal motility and gut health as a whole (Ngo et al., 2024).

These complex relations are critical to understanding to develop strategies that can reduce bacterial infection and its pathological effects. The two-faced nature of bacteria to be pathogens and immunomodulators of host immune response is an indication of host-microbe interactions. The capacity of bacteria to strongly modulate host physiological activities through the secretion of virulence factors dictates that such mechanisms are given precedence in advancing therapeutic approaches. Further research that defines how certain bacterial components, e.g., MAM and T6SS, influence host immunity and gut motility is thus vital in this context. This information not only broadens our understanding of bacterial pathogenicity but also provides new avenues to redress host homeostasis compromised by pathogenic infection (Figure 4.3).

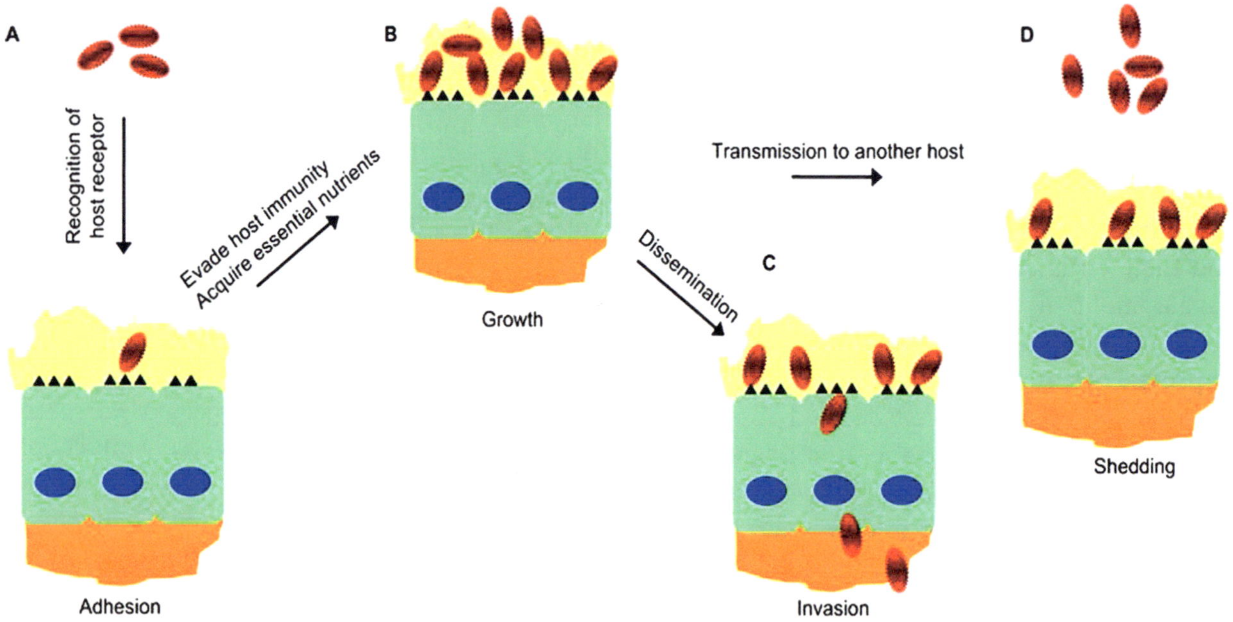

Figure 4.3. Major requirements for successful infection of human hosts by pathogenic bacteria. (A) Once bacteria enter the host, they need to adhere to mucosal surfaces by recognizing specific receptors on host cells. (B) The bacteria must be able to evade host immune mechanisms for survival (e.g., complement system, antibody) and acquire the necessary nutrients for the growth and expansion of the population (e.g., iron). (C) Once the population size has expanded to a certain level, bacteria can disseminate to other tissues/organs from the initial infection site by intracellular invasion through molecular interactions with host receptors or other means. (D) Some bacteria may be released into the surrounding environments and transmitted to another human host.

Source: https://www.researchgate.net/publication/277782368/figure/fig3/AS:271778094252054@1441808355789/Major-requirements-for-successful-infection-of-human-hosts-by-pathogenic-bacteria-A.png.

4.1.2. Viruses

Viruses are a strange group of pathogens that defy traditional definitions of life since they have to rely on host cells to survive and reproduce. Viruses are distinct from bacteria or fungi in that they lack cellular components or metabolic processes and thus have to rely completely on the processes of their hosts. This characteristic requires viruses to become engaged in complex host-microbe interactions that can lead to a variety of outcomes, ranging from benign infection to fatal disease. The host's immune response plays a key role in defining the course of a viral infection, often leading to a dynamic interaction in which the virus must escape both innate and adaptive immunity.

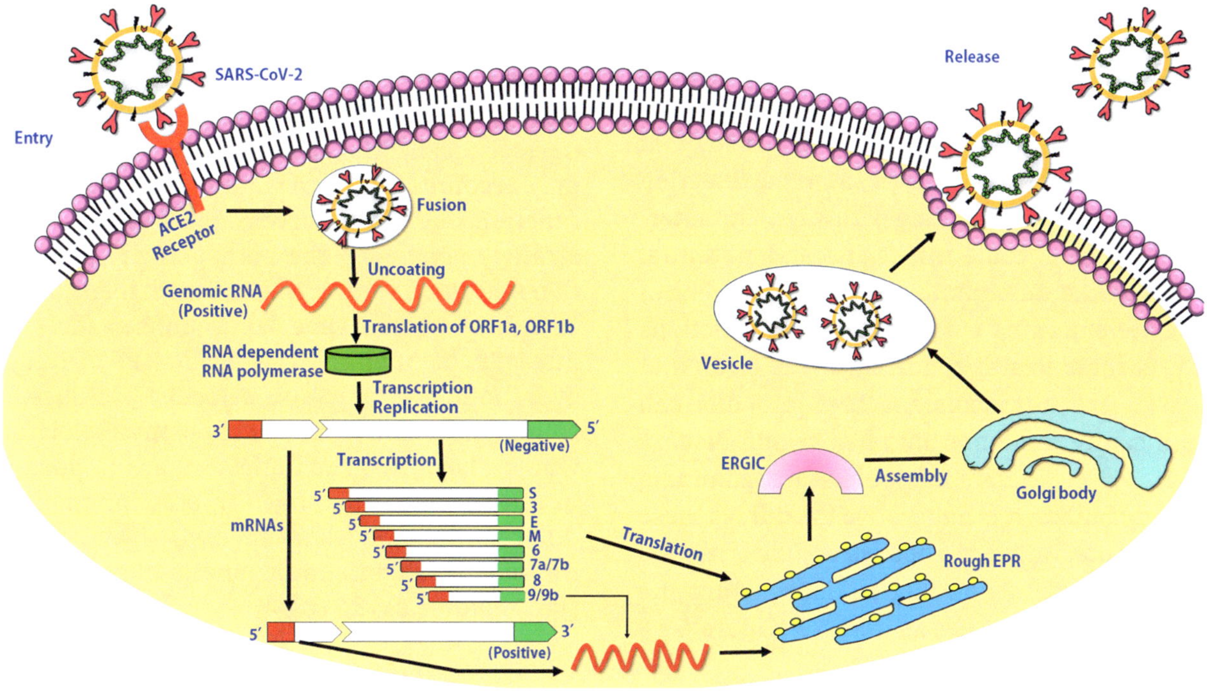

Figure 4.4. Pictorial representation of viral-host interaction and replication of the virus SARS-CoV-2.

Source: https://www.researchgate.net/profile/Ashish-Mishra-31/publication/344281686/figure/fig3/AS:936659797417985@1600328506238/Pictorial-representation-of-viral-host-interaction-and-replication-of-the-virus-SARS-CoV-2.png.

Understanding these interactions is critical to unraveling the mechanisms of viral pathogenesis, as viruses have evolved various mechanisms to subvert host cellular processes and immune responses and thereby cause various clinical manifestations and disease processes. The virulence of viruses typically entails their ability to exploit host cellular processes to replicate and grow. Recent research has emphasized the role of autophagy in such pathways, where viruses exploit autophagic processes to facilitate replication, as evidenced by recent revelations on autophagy-associated proteins (ATGs). The proteins are not only vital for degrading cellular content but also in viral replication and egress. These findings are evidence of the double role of autophagy as both a cell protective process and a contributor to viral pathogenicity. The intricate relationship calls for further extensive research to detail the mechanisms that determine these interactions, facilitating a better comprehension of how viruses can manipulate host pathways for their advantage, possibly leading the way to new therapeutic approaches to control viral infections. Besides, it is not only about replication but also their effect on the immune functions of the host, as well as the potential for the creation of long-term infections. Some viruses are capable of inducing immunomodulatory effects, hence altering the capacity of the hosts to react appropriately to other pathogens. This is a phenomenon that can especially be observed among viruses that utilize mechanisms to escape immune detection or hijack immune signaling pathways, ultimately resulting in chronic infections and potential sequelae like autoimmune diseases. In light of the now emerging evidence of viral infections with chronic health conditions, it is clear that viruses are not transient invaders but can significantly influence host health and disease states. While researchers persist in examining these dynamics, it is imperative to address these from an integrative perspective to fully grasp the host-virus interaction implications within the context of pathogenesis as a whole (Figure 4.4).

4.1.3. Fungi

Fungi play a major role in host-microbe interactions, both as disease agents and as beneficial symbionts. Their ability to occupy a variety of host environments, ranging from plants to animals, attests to their adaptability and evolutionary success. Through approaches , such as the secretion of effector proteins, fungi are able to manipulate the immune response of the host to permit infection. This manipulation is the complex cooperation of host recognition processes, where some fungal proteins are recognized by host receptors. Some recent work has proposed the concept of effector-triggered defense (ETD) that is distinct from the traditional models of pathogen-associated molecular pattern (PAMP)-triggered immunity (PTI) and effector-triggered immunity (ETI). Unlike PTI, a general response to the presence of fungi, ETD is a more sophisticated interaction induced by the detection of particular fungal effectors, and thus a more discriminative response to specific fungal diseases (Avrova et al., 2014). The ability of fungi, , such as the maize anthracnose pathogen *Colletotrichum graminicola*, to secrete effectors aimed at the host nucleus emphasizes their pathogenic potential. The work found a specific effector protein, CgEP1, that plays a crucial role in disease development in maize and possesses nuclear localization functions. The effector not only accounts for the regulation of host cellular functions but also serves as an evolutionary strategy enhancing the pathogenicity of fungi. Gene research verifies that the most likely origin of CgEP1 was from gene duplications in ancestral lineages, highlighting the dynamism of fungal evolution over time. This selective pressure, in conjunction with evidence of positive selection, would show that such effectors are important in effective host-pathogen interactions among different Colletotrichum species, which justifies the role of fungi in pathogenesis in agriculture (Jaramillo et al., 2016).

It is important to comprehend the pathogenic processes of fungal pathogenesis for effective design of control methods in agriculture. The double-edged sword of fungi as pathogens and non-pathogens due to their beneficial nature complicates this dynamic, with some fungi being essential to the health of plants and nutrient acquisition. Molecular interaction between fungi sheds light on the mechanisms by which they can coexist in plant systems and also be pathogenic concurrently. Research through studies on effector proteins and their modes of action can yield new routes for biotechnological interventions in enhancing host resistance. Besides, elucidating the interactions deciphers further how the fungi influence ecological processes, such that their importance is not only shown in disease mechanisms but also in sustaining ecosystem balances. Such insights thus have the potential to inform future agriculture operations and management plans (Avrova et al., 2014) (Figure 4.5).

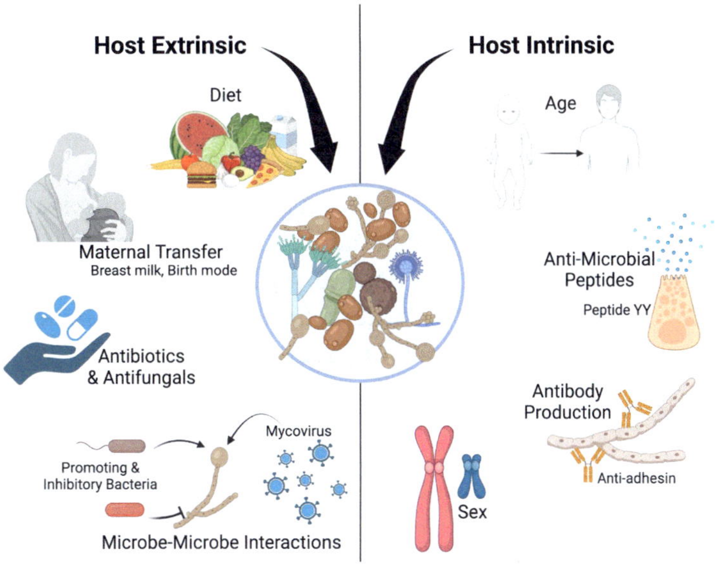

Figure 4.5. Host intrinsic and extrinsic factors that can influence fungal composition and function.

Source: https://www.cell.com/cms/10.1016/j.chom.2024.09.010/asset/724ce5e8-5339-4038-80b6-1d39e07d21d1/main.assets/gr2_lrg.jpg.

Test Your Knowledge

1. What are the main categories of microbes that interact with a host, and how do their interactions differ?
2. Give one example each of a bacterium, virus, fungus, and parasite that commonly interacts with the human host, and briefly describe the nature of each interaction.

4.2. Mechanisms of Pathogenesis

Learning Outcome

1. Explain how adherence and colonization represent critical steps in the establishment of host-microbe interactions
2. Understand the invasion of host tissues by pathogenic microbes
3. Focus on evasion of the immune response

Pathogenesis mechanisms are intricate processes that account for the way pathogens engage with host organisms to establish infection and disease. An important aspect of such interactions is the ability of pathogenic microbes to hijack host cellular processes to their advantage. For instance, it has been found through research that certain bacteria, like Vibrio, utilize specialized secretory systems, like the type VI secretion system (T6SS), to secrete effector proteins into host cells. These proteins can induce cell death or disrupt the function of the cells normally, providing the bacteria with a niche in the host organism. Specifically, the VgrG-1 protein's actin cross-linking domain (ACD) plays a critical role in inhibiting intestinal motility in larval zebrafish, illustrating how bacterial pathogenesis can induce large-scale physiological alteration in the host, resulting in disease pathology and underscoring the complexity of host-microbe interactions (Ngo et al., 2024).

Beyond that, symbiotic microbes' metabolic activities also significantly influence host health and disease processes. *Bacteroides thetaiotaomicron* (*B. theta*), a representative human gut symbiont, exemplifies this relationship through its end products of metabolism. Its organic and amino acids modulate host nutrition as well as immune response. Metabolomics has indicated that metabolites , such as acetate and formate can engage in dose-dependent communication, modulating other secreted metabolites that engage in pathogenesis and nutrient acquisition. This metabolic interaction emphasizes the way the host microbiota are able to regulate their own pathways in response to microbes, demonstrating that it is not a static interaction in which the host and microbes continue to adapt to each other's metabolic requirements (Buan et al., 2020).

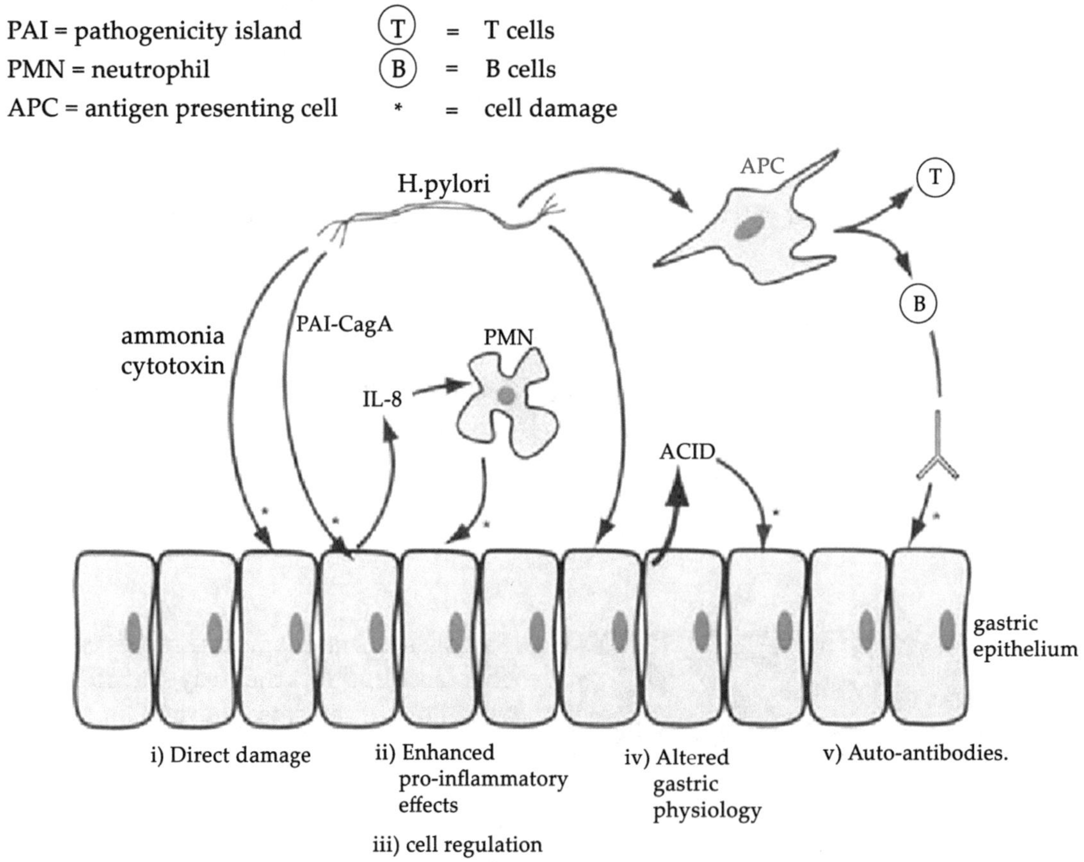

Figure 4.6. Overview of mechanisms of pathogenesis of disease caused by *Helicobacter pylori.*

Source: https://www.researchgate.net/publication/11399401/figure/fig4/AS:642485286080512@1530191837175/Overview-of-mechanisms-of-pathogenesis-of-disease-caused-by-Helicobacter-pylori.png.

Understanding mechanisms , such as pathogenesis is crucial for formulating targeted therapeutic protocols that can neutralize infectious diseases. Therapies that disrupt microbial adhesion, block effector delivery, or modify host responses to microbial metabolites can provide new therapeutic opportunities. As our knowledge becomes better, the identification of distinctive pathways and interactions responsible for the host-microbe environment will allow precision medicine approaches, enhancing our ability to rebalance dysbiotic disorders brought on by pathogenic microbes. By shedding light on the mechanisms employed by commensal microbes as well as pathogens, future research can provide a way for new interventions that utilize the inherent functioning of the microbiome to promote host robustness and health (Buan et al., 2020; Ngo et al., 2024) (Figure 4.6).

4.2.1. Adherence and Colonization

Adherence and colonization are central mechanisms in host-microbe relationship development, and the results profoundly affect infectious disease pathogenesis. The microbes use various specialized structures like pili, fimbriae, and adhesins to bind to host tissue, an activity that is important for survival and later colonization. Effective adherence not only sustains microbial viability in different niches but also abolishes host defenses, allowing the pathogen to evade elimination mechanisms.

Particularly, competitive interactions of microbial colonization also suggest the balance between commensal and pathogenic organisms, whereby healthy microbes can repress pathogen colonization and growth by mechanisms , including competition for nutrients and excretion of inhibitory metabolites. This is important since it can indicate therapeutic strategies that aim to restore normal microbiota and prevent pathogenic infection. Besides mere attachment, the action of adherence extends to host immune response modulation. Commensal microbes play a critical role in molding the immune system and maintaining homeostasis. For instance, skin microbiota consists of intricate microbial communities that affiliate with the host to hinder the colonization of virulent pathogens, , such as *Staphylococcus aureus*, most pertinent in diseases , such as atopic dermatitis (AD). There has been evidence presented that loss of microbial diversity on the skin correlates with increased disease severity and pathogen colonization.

Therapeutic use of commensals , such as *Staphylococcus* hominis, in particular, has been seen to have potential in reducing *S. aureus* load and alleviating AD symptomology. This underscores that attempts to maintain microbial diversity as a preventative measure must be taken to control and suppress disease exacerbation due to pathogen colonization (Gallo et al., 2019). New advances in the study of host-microbe interactions, particularly through the use of human intestinal organoid (HIO) cultures, illuminate the complexity of colonization and adhesion. These systems enable researchers to study the pathogenesis of enteric pathogens as well as commensal microbes within physiologically relevant conditions. HIOs provide for a sophisticated realization of how some microbial interactions dictate health versus disease, information that traditional cell lines and animal systems were not capable of providing. Notably, the application of HIO technology leaves room for exploring therapeutic avenues against microbial pathogenesis, complementing vaccine and target therapeutic development. As the research continues in place, HIOs can further enhance our comprehension of mechanisms of microbial colonization and relevance to host well-being (Adeniyi-Ipadeola et al., 2023) (Figure 4.7).

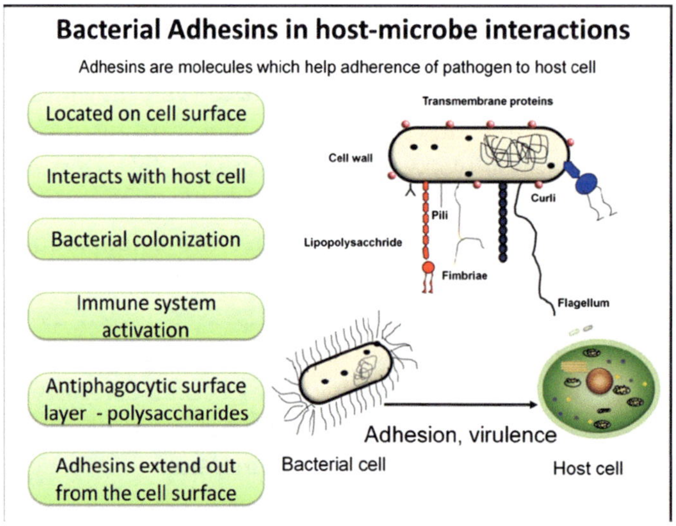

Figure 4.7. Bacterial adhesins in host-microbe interactions.

Source: https://www.researchgate.net/profile/Sanjiv-Kumar-25/publication/319710923/figure/fig1/AS:614112463708160@1523427229104/Bacterial-Adhesins-in-host-microbe-interactions.png.

4.2.2. Invasion of Host Tissues

Host tissue invasion by pathogenic microbes is a central feature in understanding host-microbe interactions and pathogenesis. Effective invasion may begin with pathogens adhering to host cells, aided by virulence factors known as adhesins. These attachment proteins enable bacteria to adhere to epithelial surfaces, penetrating the mucosal lining and mechanical barriers. To illustrate, *Yersinia pseudotuberculosis* employs a multivalent adhesion molecule (MAM) to bind host cells and consequently enhance its colonization ability. Microbes' ability to get a foothold in host tissue forms the background for subsequent pathogenic activities, , such as evading the immune system and causing additional tissue damage, and points out the importance of adhesion to the general pathogenicity of these microbes. After they are bound, pathogenic bacteria employ multiple strategies to invade host tissues and exploit cellular machinery for replication. During invasion, pathogens like *Yersinia pseudotuberculosis* are actively engaged in interaction with host immune cells, , such as phagocytes, to gain access into internal tissues. Microbial adhesin-host phagocyte interaction is capable of either mediating uptake as a mechanism of evasion or triggering inflammatory cascades resulting in tissue destruction. Actually, loss of essential adhesins, , such as *Y. pseudotuberculosis* MAM, does not necessarily translate into reduced pathogenicity. It was found that in certain models, phagocyte association loss has the unexpected consequence of maximizing elimination of bacteria but inducing overreaction in the immune response, thus with augmented mortality. This complex dynamic illustrates that the interplay between microbial adhesion and immune system activation is a critical determinant of host-pathogen interaction outcomes. In addition, tissue invasion leads to more than straightforward infection; the outcomes reach into the host's immune system far beyond. The dynamics of microbes invading and interacting with the immune system following invasion may bring about deleterious consequences to the host, including over-inflammation and tissue destruction. Of greatest interest has been the induction of humoral immune reactions, , such as melanin production, in situations where pathogens successfully evade phagocytosis. In *Y. pseudotuberculosis*, increased levels of melanin have been correlated with reduced clearance of pathogens and increased phagocyte death upon hyperactivation of host defenses. Such complex interactions are a prime example of the twofold role played by microbial invasiveness as an impetus for pathogenesis, deserving a greater understanding of the host and microbe elements that cooperate to determine infection outcomes as well as the general disease progression (Brown et al., 2014) (Figure 4.8).

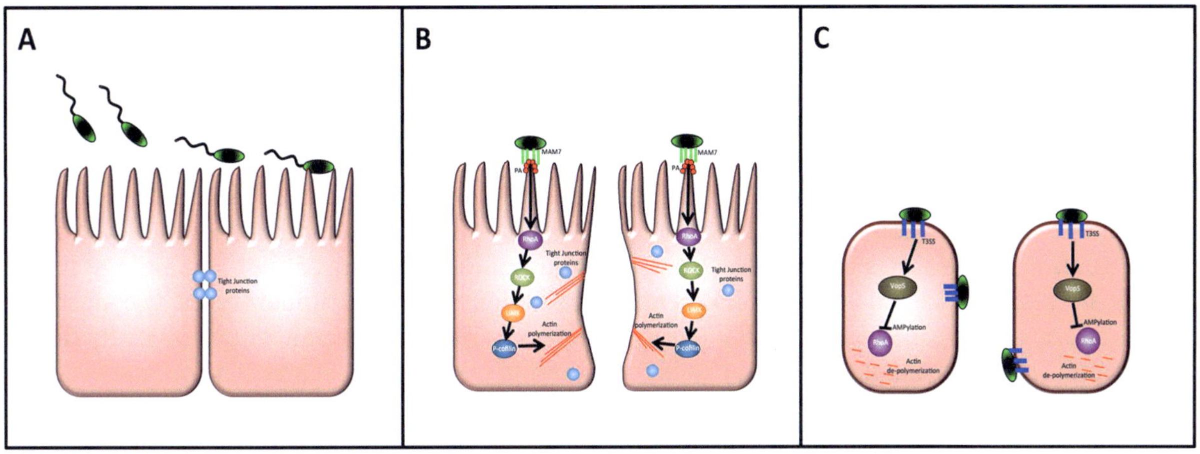

Figure 4.8. Adhesion molecule compromises epithelial barrier integrity and accelerates T3SS effector-mediated tissue damage during infection. (A) Flagella-driven, highly motile *V. parahaemolyticus* (green) reach the gut epithelium and attach to the cell surface. (B) MAM7 (green) binding to PA (red) on the epithelial surface leads to RhoA activation (purple). (C) These MAM7-mediated events increase the surface area accessible to *V. parahaemolyticus*, thus increasing the efficacy of T3SS (dark blue) effector transfer.

Source: https://www.researchgate.net/profile/Anne-Marie-Krachler/publication/279919274/figure/fig1/AS:616376960024577@1523967127241/Multivalent-Adhesion-Molecule-7-compromises-epithelial-barrier-integrity-and-accelerates.png.

4.2.3. Evasion of the Immune Response

The host-microbial pathogen interaction is characterized by a complex interplay of mechanisms of immune evasion necessary for microbial survival and pathogenesis. A paradigmatic example can be observed with the malaria parasites, and most prominently *Plasmodium falciparum*, which employs antigenic variation as a mechanism of immune evasion. This mechanism allows the parasite to alter its surface proteins and therefore evade immune detection by antibodies produced from previous infections. Progress in genome sequencing in recent times has enhanced our understanding of P. falciparum's evolutionary dynamics and how selective pressures shape its genetic constitution and enhance its immune-evading capabilities. As scientists dig deeper into population genomics, they discover specific gene regions that are subject to strong selective pressures and that inform their functional purposes in immune evasion and toward applications for the development of targeted therapies and vaccines (Kirchner et al., 2016).

In addition, other pathogens, including flaviviruses, depict sophisticated countermeasures toward host immunity defense, i.e., the type I interferon response. Flaviviridae family members , including Zika virus and dengue virus, have evolved mechanisms that actively suppress interferon signaling pathways, thereby lowering the host's antiviral state. This provides these viruses with stable antiviral infection, which in most instances culminates in severe disease outcomes. By their interference with interferon-driven immune responses, they demonstrate a sophisticated level of host cellular process recognition, which determines their pathogenic potential. Investigation of these molecular processes has become essential, especially in light of the absence of effective antiviral treatments against several flaviviral infections. Such research is significant not just for the knowledge of viral pathogenesis but also for informing the development of novel therapeutic approaches that reverse these evasion processes (Clark et al., 2017). In short, immune evasion is the pivotal nature of host-microbe interactions with a decisive influence on the pathogenesis of infectious disease. Pathogens like Plasmodium falciparum and flaviviruses are the paradigm for the creative and complex mechanisms deployed to evade host immunity. Unraveling such strategies is pivotal in the progress of medical research in maximizing disease control and therapy. The more we understand the genetic and molecular mechanisms of immune evasion, the more likely it is that we can create more effective vaccines and treatments. This focus on host-pathogen interactions not only yields a better understanding of the pathobiology of such pathogens but also underscores the necessity for continued surveillance and investigation in the fight against global health threats posed by infectious disease.

Test Your Knowledge

1. How do pathogens adhere to and colonize host tissues? Describe the role of adhesins and provide one example of a pathogen that uses this mechanism.
2. What strategies do pathogens use to invade host tissues, and how does this invasion contribute to disease progression?

4.3. Host Immune Response to Microbial Infections

Learning Outcome

1. Explain how Innate immunity serves as the body's first line of defense against invading pathogens
2. Understand Adaptive immunity for host defense
3. Understand the role of inflammation

Host immune response to microbial infection involves a complex interaction comprising various aspects of innate and adaptive immunity. The initial contact between the host and the pathogen activates innate immunity, which is the body's first defense against the infection. It includes the activation of phagocytic cells , such as macrophages and neutrophils, as well as the release of pro-inflammatory cytokines, which bring in more immune cells to the infected site. These responses are not only effective for killing the pathogens but also for sending a signal to the adaptive immune system, leading to a more specific response. Enhanced communication among immune cells at this time is paramount for the mounting of an effective defense system that reduces microbial load and, eventually, terminates the infection. As the immune response progresses, adaptive immunity becomes the focus, with activation of T and B lymphocytes. T cells develop into cytotoxic cells to directly kill infected host cells, while B cells produce antibodies that adhere to particular pathogens, neutralizing them and marking them for other immune cells to destroy. This adaptive immune response is fundamental in the development of immunological memory, which continues to be active long after infection removal, enabling quick and robust immunity against subsequent infections by the same microorganism. Innate and adaptive immune coordination ensures that immediate and long-term responses are mounted, highlighting the importance of intense host immune reactions in the control of microbial infections. Such an insight may also lead to novel therapeutic approaches aimed at the enhancement of immunity. Microbial dysbiosis or an imbalance of the microbial population may have a significant impact on the host immune system and make one susceptible to many infections and diseases. For instance, diminished diversity of commensals, as observed with atopic dermatitis (AD), has been linked with susceptibility to pathogenic infections, specifically by pathogens like *Staphylococcus aureus*. In healthy hosts, commensals have a regulatory role, stimulating the immune system and excluding pathogen colonization via competition for substrates and immunomodulation. It has been shown by studies that microbial balance restoration through the addition of beneficial microorganisms can be employed to alleviate immune-mediated conditions like AD, which implies that understanding host-microbe interactions will drive the development of new therapeutic strategies focused on microbial communities to enhance host defense and treat infections more effectively (Gallo et al., 2019).

4.3.1. Innate Immunity

Innate immunity is the first line of defense of the body against invading pathogens, an immediate but nonspecific defense crucial to limit infection. This machinery involves physical barriers, i.e., the skin and mucous membranes, and cellular components like phagocytes and natural killer (NK) cells. Even the skin itself is not a passive barrier; it harbors an active microbiome that engages with host immune mechanisms. For instance, symbiotic skin commensals play a crucial role in regulating the outgrowth of pathogenic bacteria and hence averting potential infection. In establishing harmony on the skin surface, innate immunity demonstrates the intricate relationship between microbe and host, suppressing the colonization of pathogens like *Staphylococcus aureus* and triggering disease mechanisms (Gallo et al., 2019). Thus, an understanding of the interaction between innate immune responses and microbial communities is essential in finding effective means of controlling infectious diseases. Innate immunity also calls for the understanding of its role in regulating both inflammatory responses as well as the adaptive immune system. The components of innate immunity are charged with pattern recognition receptors (PRRs) that identify pathogen-associated molecular patterns (PAMPs), thus precipitating an instant immune response. This process of identification begins the activation of many immune cells, including dendritic cells and macrophages, to induce inflammation and further recruit adaptive immune components. These interactions are important, particularly in the modulation of the immune responses during the initial stages of pathogen exposure. The dialogue of commensals with the innate immune system also illustrates how microbial influences can regulate immune development in early life and affect susceptibility to diseases like asthma and atopic dermatitis in adulthood (Gallo et al., 2019). By comprehending such interactions, scientists are able to devise therapeutic interventions that promote innate immune function while maintaining microbiome stability. In addition, innate immunity has a function that extends beyond mere protection against infection, as it plays a crucial part in the maintenance of homeostasis in the host.

As a part of the immune system, innate responses support tissue integrity and facilitate wound repair following injury or infection. Cooperative action among immune cells , such as neutrophils and macrophages, effectively clears out dead cells and pathogens to enable tissue repair and regeneration. In disorder, such as atopic dermatitis, research has demonstrated that cutaneous microbiome dysregulation can lead to dysregulation of innate immune function, exacerbating disease severity (Gallo et al., 2019). The fine balance between maintaining microbial diversity and supporting vigorous innate immunity implies that future targeted therapies could be realized by restoring microbial equilibrium to alleviate inflammation. Ultimately, expanding our understanding of innate immunity in the context of host-microbe interactions is critical to the development of new strategies against a variety of pathologies (Figure 4.9).

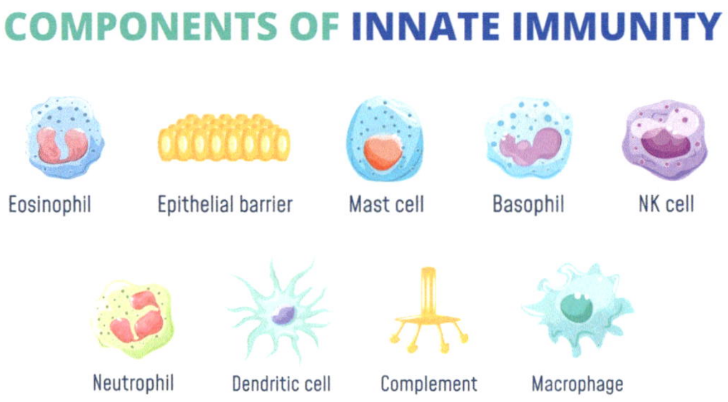

Figure 4.9. Components of innate immunity.

Source: https://www.biocode.org.uk/wp-content/uploads/2021/11/Blog-Thumbnail-Components-of-Innate-Immunity.png.

4.3.2. Adaptive Immunity

Adaptive immunity is an integral part of host defense, working by a complex response capable of differentiating between self and non-self antigens. Unlike the innate immune system, which offers immediate but non-specific defense, adaptive immunity develops gradually to allow immunological memory. This involves the activation of lymphocytes, specifically T and B cells, which are in charge of recognizing particular pathogens. It begins with antigen presentation when antigen-presenting cells (APCs) take up and present foreign antigens. It activates T helper cells, which activate B cells to secrete highly specific antibodies. These antibodies neutralize the pathogens, marking them for destruction by other immune cells, thus underlining the adaptive-immune microbial interaction between the host. In addition, the adaptive immunity is of paramount importance during microbial infections, as in the case of atopic dermatitis and asthma, which could be modulated by microbial interactions. The skin, as a major host-environment interface, contains a rich microbiome that is capable of modulating innate and adaptive immune responses. Studies have shown that crosstalk between commensals of the skin and the immune system has a substantial effect on disease severity. For example, decreased diversity of the cutaneous microbiome is associated with a higher abundance of pathogenic bacteria like *Staphylococcus aureus*, which may amplify adaptive immune responses. It is also necessary to learn about these dynamics, as treatment strategies aimed at balancing the microbiome will aim to provide an improved immune response and minimize chronic inflammatory disease related to dysregulated adaptive immunity (Gallo et al., 2019).

Beyond human health, however, a knowledge of adaptive immunity is significant in veterinary medicine as well, with regard to enteric disease in livestock. For example, studies on adaptive immune mechanisms in pigs provide insights into pathogens , such as *Lawsonia intracellularis* and *Brachyspira hyodysenteriae*, whose incidence leads to complex host responses. It is by the development of diagnostic methods, for example, PCR, that enhanced detection of such pathogens and their interfaces with the host immune system has been achieved. Host-microbe interactions in pigs reflect the influence of environmental determinants, such as diet components and housing, on disease susceptibility. Immune response analysis in pigs may contribute to better insight into adaptive immunity to enteric health and more effective prophylactic intervention against these pathogens (Jacobson et al., 2003) (Figure 4.10).

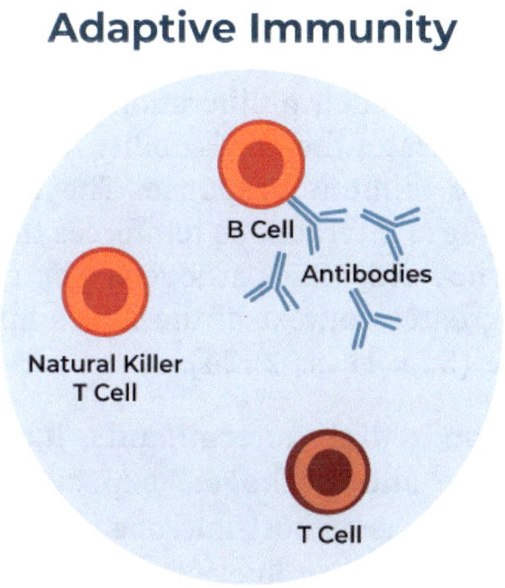

Figure 4.10. Adaptive immunity.

Source: https://media.geeksforgeeks.org/wp-content/uploads/20240220100851/Adaptive-Immunity.png.

4.3.3. Role of Inflammation

Inflammation is a key host protective response in host-microbe interactions, with both defensive against pathogens and potentially pathogenic functions. When microbial pathogens are encountered, the immune system mobilizes inflammatory responses that are meant to trap and eliminate such pathogens. This is attended by immune cell migration to the site of infection, release of pro-inflammatory cytokines, and activation of a variety of molecular cascades of signaling. However, chronic inflammation can have pathological effects, as chronic exposure to inflammatory mediators has the capacity to induce tissue damage and promote disease. In asthma and atopic dermatitis, for instance, an abnormal inflammatory response is observed, highlighting the two-edged sword of inflammation in host-microbe interactions. Hence, understanding the balance between protective and harmful inflammation is important in the development of therapeutic interventions that can control the immune response without weakening host defense. The role of the microbiome in modulating inflammation contributes to the complexity of host-microbe interactions. The cutaneous microbiome regulates immune homeostasis by having pathogen-laden microbial communities residing on the skin. It acts by inhibiting the colonization of pathogenic bacteria , such as *Staphylococcus aureus* and integrity of the epidermal barrier. Dysbiosis, or microbial imbalance, is responsible for causing inflammatory skin illnesses, with lower microbial diversity correlating with increased severity of disease in conditions , such as atopic dermatitis. Notably, restorative therapies that restore microbiome homeostasis, , such as the administration of therapeutic commensal bacteria, have been promising at lowering inflammation and improving clinical outcomes in patients. These observations highlight the significant role of the microbiome in modulating inflammation and indicate potential avenues for future therapeutic intervention against inflammatory disease (Gallo et al., 2019). Current studies have also shed light on the interplay between autophagy and inflammation, further augmenting our knowledge of host-microbe interaction. Autophagy, the cellular mechanism responsible for intracellular protein degradation and recycling, plays a role in modulating inflammatory pathways and is itself modulated by inflammatory pathways. The discovery of autophagy-related proteins (ATGs) has been a key to unlocking their multidimensional roles, far exceeding traditional autophagy. These proteins are involved in immune signaling control, trafficking of phagocytosed material, and replication of viral particles. Of particular interest is the interaction between autophagy and inflammation, where enhanced autophagic activity lessens overactive inflammatory responses. Dysregulated autophagy, conversely, exacerbates inflammation and causes autoimmune diseases. As the dynamics of such sophisticated molecular interactions become more comprehensible, they promise to explain methods of targeting inflammatory pathways in an effort to treat a variety of diseases (Cadwell & Debnath, 2017).

Test Your Knowledge

1. What are the key components of the innate immune system, and how do they provide the first line of defense against microbial infections?
2. What is the role of inflammation in the immune response to infection? Include both protective effects and potential harmful consequences.

4.4. Factors Influencing Host-Microbe Interactions

Learning Outcome

1. Describe the term host genetics
2. Understand microbial virulence factors
3. Discuss how environmental factors play a crucial role in shaping host-microbe interactions

Understanding of host-microbe interaction determinants is crucial for comprehending the complexity of microbial pathogenesis. The most significant determinant is microbiota composition, which varies greatly with host individual factors like immune status and genetics. Host immune systems regulate the microbiome to support the growth of helpful microbes while restraining the development of harmful microbes. This interaction is particularly intense when the body is infected and pathogens evolve complex mechanisms to evade the immune system. For instance, intracellular pathogens can hijack host cell function to create an appropriate environment for their proliferation and survival, which complicates the host's ability to generate an effective immune response. The dynamic nature of these interactions reinforces the need to study not only the pathogens per se, but also the greater context of the host's immune landscape (Soni et al., 2024).

Environmental determinants like diet, medication, and pathogen exposure have significant effects on host-microbe interactions. As an illustration, antibiotics may result in a disruption of normal microbiota, leading to dysbiosis and having the potential to trigger opportunistic infections or chronic disease. Similarly, the ingredients of food can modulate the density and diversity of the gut microbiota, which in turn affects the host's immunological reactions. Colonization of the gastrointestinal tract and skin of ultra-high-risk hosts, , such as very preterm infants, begins in utero and is greatly affected by gestational age and exposure to the environment (Underwood & Sohn, 2017). These factors contribute to modulating the host's immune responses, which have long-term health effects, for example, susceptibility to infections like necrotizing enterocolitis and sepsis. Understanding these factors underscores the potential for therapy to re-establish or augment a normal microbiota in high-risk groups. In addition, where microbes reside within the host significantly influences the outcome of host-microbe interactions. Different tissues contain unique microenvironments that are supportive or inhibitory to the growth and survival of microbes. By way of example, intracellular pathogens have developed invasion mechanisms for penetrating some cell types, enabling them to evade immune surveillance but utilize the hosts' resources for their reproduction. Such specificity is important in pathogenic success and is difficult in terms of diagnosis and treatment. The complexity of such interactions calls for advanced approaches, such as integrated host microbiome single-cell genomics, to have an adequate understanding of the significance of microbial persistence within the host (Soni et al., 2024). Ultimately, realizing the multi-faceted nature of host-microbe interactions can lead to more directed therapies and prevention measures, and hence improved clinical outcomes in disease-causing infection as well as other microbial disorders.

4.4.1. Host Genetics

This intricate interaction between host genetics and the microbe plays a pivotal role in ascertaining host susceptibility or resistance against various pathogens. The host-to-host genetic variations may have a significant impact on immune processes and the entire microbiome profile. For instance, single-nucleotide polymorphisms (SNPs) within genes that are involved in immune responses determine the capability with which the organism can resist infections. Therefore, certain genetic types can cause heightened susceptibility to disease that is otherwise manageable or suppressed by robust microbial load. Host population genetic diversity, in this case, is a significant stimulus that dictates pathogenesis outcome and possibly the reason why other hosts suffer severe effects following microbial infection, while others remain asymptomatic or recover quickly. Besides, understanding the genetic basis of host-pathogen interactions aids in the determination of predictive biomarkers of disease outcome. Host genetics also assists in informing treatment approaches, particularly in the development of personalized medicine therapies. For example, the discovery of specific alleles with enhanced immune functions can assist clinicians in making choices regarding appropriate vaccinations or treatment regimens in response to an individual's genetic background. Additionally, research on the genetic factors influencing microbiome composition has provided evidence that certain microbes may thrive in genetically predisposed hosts and thus form hostile or welcoming environments for pathogenic microbes. Therefore, the intersection of host genetics and microbial ecology is providing new avenues for intervention in infectious disease management, resulting in improved public health outcomes. In addition, advances in genomic technologies in recent years have allowed us to gain more insights into the complexities involved in host genetics associated with microbial interactions. Genome-wide association studies (GWAS) and high-throughput sequencing enable researchers to investigate the associations between variations in host genes and their effects on microbiome assembly and function. This emerging field provides evidence of how microbial community impacts host gene expression that can modulate immune responses and susceptibility to disease. With every successive advance, researchers can uncover the intricate networks directing host-microbe interactions, presenting an intricate picture of pathogenesis. The promise of translating these genetic results into clinical significance underscores the importance of ongoing research on host genetics as a basis for understanding host-microbe interactions and disease outcomes, as underscored in studies documenting the germane challenges facing modern health systems (Baldin et al., 2014; Jiang et al., 2016) (Figure 4.11).

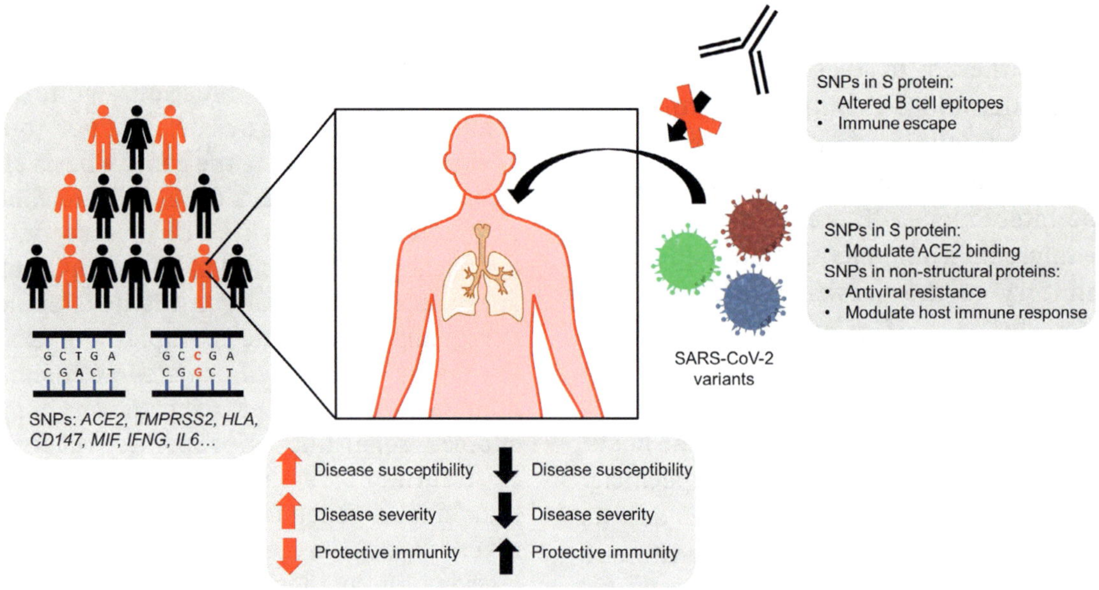

Figure 4.11. The impact of host genetics and viral variation on SARS-CoV-2 infection and COVID-19 severity.

Source: https://www.researchgate.net/profile/Stephen-Crooke/publication/342906119/figure/fig1/AS:1143128146488404 8@1748267655436/The-impact-of-host-genetics-and-viral-variation-on-SARS-CoV-2-infection-and-COVID-19.png.

4.4.2. Microbial Virulence Factors

An understanding of microbial virulence factors is essential to unravel the complex host-microbe interactions and pathogenesis. These virulence factors, like toxins, adhesins, and invasion proteins, are involved in facilitating the pathogen to colonize the host environment and eventually result in disease. Toxins, for example, disrupt cellular processes and induce damage to host tissue, which facilitates the spreading of the pathogen in the host. Adhesins play a key role in facilitating microbes to adhere to epithelial surfaces, a critical step toward colonization. The virulence determinants not only play a critical role in the microbes' survival but also in evading the host immune systems, which indicates that an effective understanding of these mechanisms is of key importance in formulating therapeutic approaches (Jiang et al., 2016). Recent years have seen developmental progress in microbiological research that has shed light on the intricate signaling networks and gene regulatory pathways governing the expression of virulence factors. Most such mechanisms are regulated by the host environment, where microbes react to host signals in order to be maximally virulent. For instance, the expression of some virulence genes may be induced by host factors to maximize expression so that pathogens can modify and survive in diverse tissues. This kind of interaction between microbial virulence factors and host immunity highlights the dynamic nature of disease pathology, and it is suggested that successful infections often depend on finely coordinated interactions between the pathogen and host (Barret et al., 2012). Further, investigations of microbial virulence factors are critical in the exploration of putative drug targets. Through the identification of how these factors operate, researchers are able to create new strategies against combating infection. Immunological methods that induce high levels of immunity against specific virulence factors are highly promising because they may effectively prevent disease by eliminating the pathogen before it can establish infection. In addition, drugs that target specific virulence factors can have the capability to inactivate pathogens in order for the host immune system to fight them effectively. Overall, enhancing the knowledge of microbial virulence factors is imperative to advancing public health interventions and clinical efficacy in infectious disease (Jiang et al., 2016) (Figure 4.12).

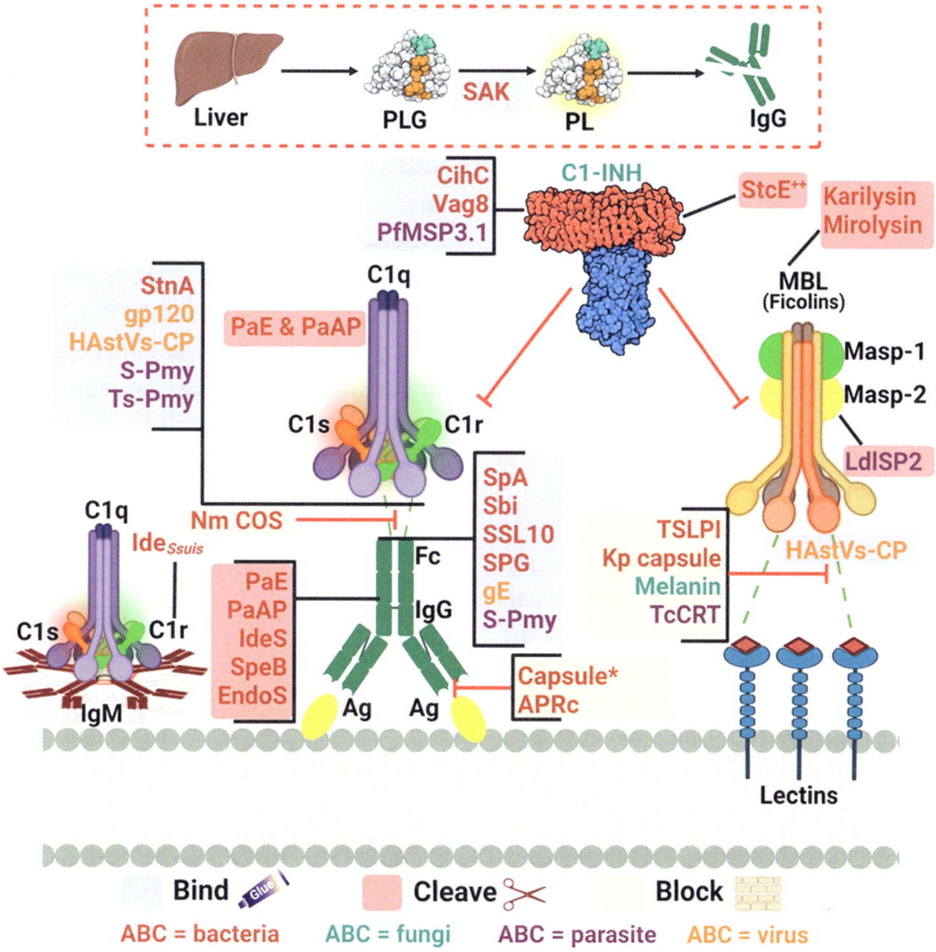

Figure 4.12. A schematic diagram showing microbial virulence factors involved in targeting the initiation phase of the complement system.

Source: https://www.researchgate.net/publication/377528084/figure/fig2/AS:11431281254832017@1719306791433/A-schematic-diagram-showing-microbial-virulence-factors-involved-in-targeting-the.tif.

4.4.3. Environmental Factors

Environmental factors are an important component in modulating host-microbe interactions, with emphasis on pathogen emergence and disease susceptibility. Under various production conditions, enteric disease in wean pigs has suddenly increased, leading to an appreciation of how these situations result in host predisposition to infection. For example, some factors like group-housing management and composition of diet, , such as the soybean meal level in feed, can influence the intestinal microenvironment so as to enhance the possibility of infection caused by pathogens like *Lawsonia intracellularis* and *Brachyspira hyodysenteriae*. Such types of observations point to the importance of maintaining control over environmental stress factors to avoid disease outbreaks in livestock, thus contributing to better animal welfare and enhanced agricultural yields (Jacobson et al., 2003). In disease in humans, the contribution of environmental stimuli to the modulation of host disease susceptibility, and among these conditions, inflammatory bowel disease (IBD), has been of foremost interest. Recent years have seen the implicating of dietary exposures as prominent environmental stimuli influencing gut microbiota, particularly in genetically predisposed humans. Increasing incidence of IBD may be accounted for, in part, by diet, and this points toward the need for increased investigation into how specific nutrients might modulate host interactions with microbial communities. Research in this field indicates three topics of interest: diet as a causative factor, its role in controlling disease, and the assessment of nutritional status. Through the understanding of these dimensions, host-microbe interactions can be understood better, ultimately providing improved prevention and control approaches to IBD among the affected population (Allan et al., 2017).

Furthermore, the intricate interaction between microbial communities and environmental factors can drive pathogenesis in other disease contexts. For instance, the composition of the microbiome can be altered by environmental stimuli , such as pollution, antibiotic treatment, and nutritional changes that are crucial to disease mechanism elucidation. Environmental stressors may disrupt microbial balance, which could cause dysbiosis, a disturbance in which the pathogenic microbes proliferate unchecked, causing disease to occur. This indicates how an interdisciplinary approach to the examination of pathogenesis is necessary, where the environmental, microbial, and host parameters converge. Through the recognition of environmental relevance in host-microbe interactions, researchers can design more useful therapeutic interventions as well as public health practices to reduce the prevalence of infectious and chronic diseases equally (Jacobson et al., 2003).

Test Your Knowledge

1. How can host genetic factors influence susceptibility or resistance to microbial infections? Provide one example.
2. What are microbial virulence factors, and how do they enhance a pathogen's ability to cause disease? Mention two common types.
3. In what ways can environmental factors impact the outcome of host-microbe interactions?

4.5. Therapeutic Approaches to Combat Pathogenesis

Learning Outcome

1. Describe antibiotics and antimicrobial agents
2. Understand vaccination strategies

The host-microbe interaction is complex, often leading to pathogenesis that requires novel therapy. An important area of investigation is the development of drugs that can specifically target and neutralize the activity of pathogenic causes. As the knowledge in understanding the molecular mechanisms of various pathogens, , such as viruses and bacteria, has evolved, researchers have begun developing therapies that not only inhibit the replication of these agents but also assist in the host's immune system. For instance, therapeutic strategies against exosomes playing a role in HIV pathogenesis have gained popularity. It has been observed through research that HIV employs exosomal pathways to spread and create neurocognitive dysfunction of the infection. A mechanism that disrupts the viral RNA sorting into exosomes has the ability to prevent this pathogenic dissemination, thus showing the potential of targeted exosomal therapeutics for treating complex infectious diseases (Patters et al., 2018).

Nanotechnology has brought new ways through which the antimicrobial agents can be delivered effectively. Nanoparticles (NPs) have been shown to possess unique properties that can facilitate the targeted delivery of therapeutic molecules with fewer side effects on normal tissues. Chitosan-alginate nanoparticles, in particular, have been found to be highly effective against cutaneous pathogens , such as Propionibacterium acnes, a cause of acne pathogenesis. These NPs, besides interfering with the bacterial cell membrane through direct antimicrobial activity, possess anti-inflammatory activity that can curb the inflammation response triggered by the infection. Encapsulation of formulated therapy , such as benzoyl peroxide, in these nanoparticles enhances their therapeutic activity, offering improved results compared to the conventional form. This novel delivery vehicle shows how nanotechnology can transform the treatment model for pathogenically aggravated dermatologic conditions (Blecher-Paz et al., 2013). Researching therapeutic interventions in combat against pathogenesis also involves re-examining existing treatment regimes and optimizing their efficacy with combination therapy. For instance, the introduction of antiretroviral therapy (ART) for the management of HIV has been pivotal in viral suppression, but several patients continue to present with chronic symptoms, including HIV-associated neurocognitive disorders. Research into exosomes in mediating such pathophysiology points towards the necessity for multi-modal treatment capable of targeting the virus and the secondary effects of infection. The development of adjunct therapies aimed at targeting the transport of exosomes and their impact can potentially significantly improve the prognosis of patients. By bridging the knowledge gap between traditional pharmacological treatment and cutting-edge technologies, including ones based on nanotechnology and targeted molecular methods, researchers can create comprehensive therapeutic platforms to better overcome infectious disease pathogenesis barriers in various diseases (Blecher-Paz et al., 2013).

4.5.1. Antibiotics and Antimicrobial Agents

The intricate host-microbe association is a predominant factor that influences the effectiveness of antimicrobial drugs and antibiotics. Biofilm development, particularly in certain pathogens , such as *Pseudomonas aeruginosa*, is a serious challenge for hospitals nowadays. Biofilms are capable of adhering to biotic surfaces like lung epithelial cells, thus resisting therapy very efficiently. Research indicates that antibiotics are less potent in inhibiting biofilms in natural environments compared to in vitro conditions.

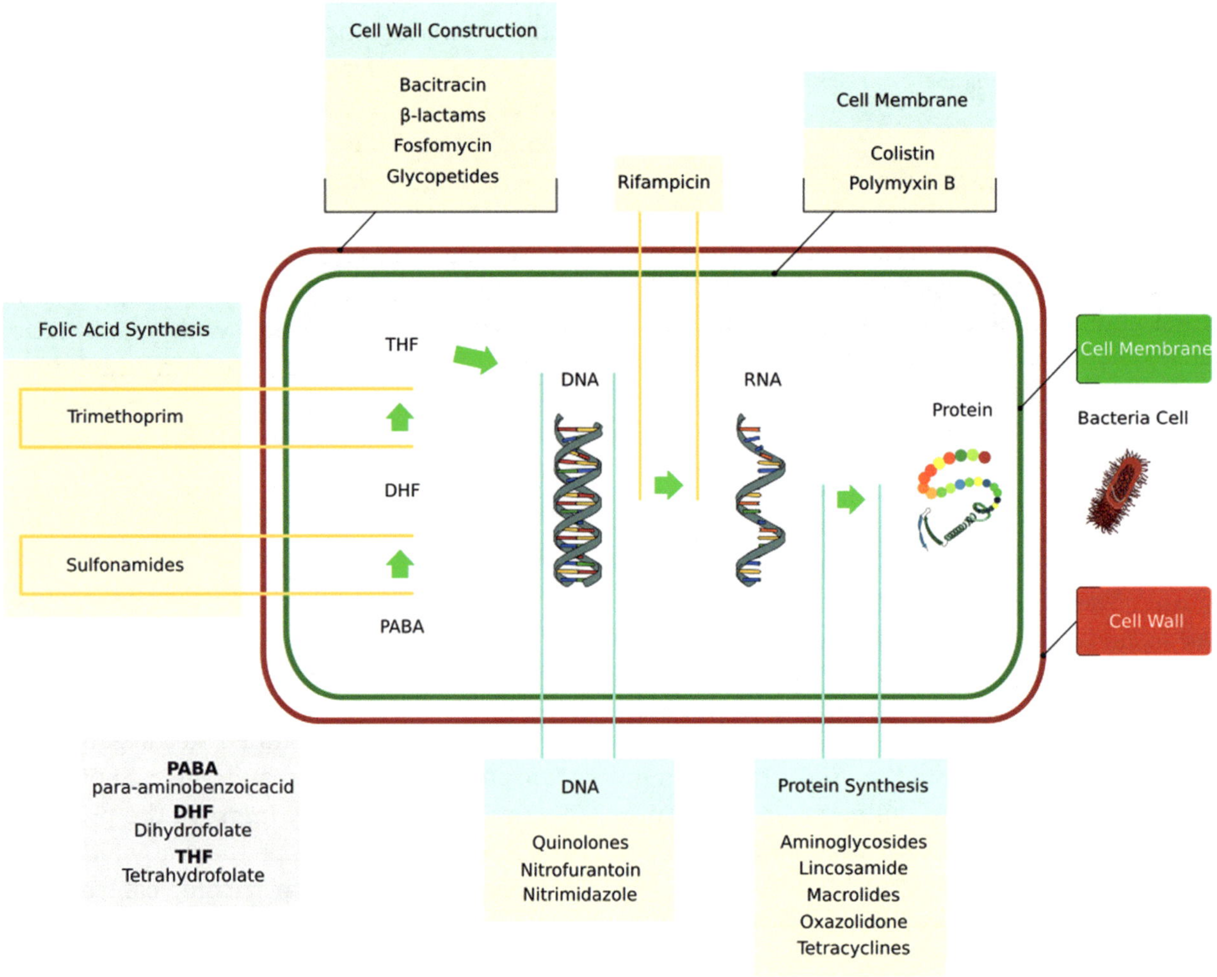

Figure 4.13. Molecular targets of antibiotics on the bacterial cell.

Source: https://upload.wikimedia.org/wikipedia/commons/thumb/0/08/Antibiotics_action.svg/1024px-Antibiotics_action.svg.png.

More specifically, the biofilm-inhibitory activity of most antibiotics is modulated by host factors as well as microenvironmental conditions, and therefore, it becomes necessary to include host-microbe interactions in the assessment of drug efficacy (Coenye et al., 2017). An understanding of these dynamics is important for the development of more potent antimicrobial therapies to combat chronic infections that can arise as a result of biofilm establishment. Further, the respiratory microbiome of patients with long-term diseases, , such as cystic fibrosis (CF), illustrates how interaction within communities can establish dynamics of changes in the efficacy of antibiotics. In CF, the lung environment tends to be colonized by a diverse number of microbial species, both commensal and pathogens. Conventional antibiotics against such bacteria fail to produce desired effects due to the complex interaction between bacteria in the lung microbiome. Mechanisms such as degradation of antibiotics, alteration of the bacterial cell wall, and matrix component synthesis play a crucial role in drug penetration (Coenye et al., 2019). These interspecies interactions can either form a protective barrier against antibiotics or, conversely, make bacteria even more vulnerable to them. Such a nuanced understanding of microbial dynamics is the basis for the necessity of rationally designing treatment regimens that maximize antibiotic efficacy. Given the limitations of traditional antibiotic therapy, there is increasing interest in finding other forms of therapy and new antimicrobial drugs. One of the more promising of these is the development of synergistic therapy by combining antibiotics with anti-biofilm peptides or other adjuvant molecules. For instance, studies have proven that co-administration of DJK-5 anti-biofilm peptide and tobramycin greatly enhances inhibition of *Pseudomonas aeruginosa* binding to biotic as well as abiotic surfaces (Coenye et al., 2017). The two-pronged strategy targets not just the pathogens but also the protective process offered by the biofilm formation. In the background of the evolving microbial resistance, the integration of such novel approaches may substantially improve treatment outcomes for chronic infection and reveal new host-microbe interaction mechanisms in the pathogenesis scenario (Figure 4.13).

4.5.2. Vaccination Strategies

dentification of vaccine strategies lies at the core of understanding the complexities of host-microbe interactions and pathogenesis. Vaccines are a proactive defense mechanism that enable the immune system to recognize and combat pathogens efficiently. These immune-mediated therapies take advantage of the body's intrinsic ability to develop immunity through either live attenuated, inactivated pathogens, or subunit vaccines containing major antigens. Not just in engineering but also in how they interact with the host microbiome, which has a significant part to play in shaping immune responses. Research has indicated that an appropriately regulated microbiome can improve the efficacy of vaccines by regulating immune signaling and cytokine release, thus allowing for an efficient adaptive immune response. These interactions emphasize the importance of insight into microbiome dynamics in the design and implementation of vaccination strategies, particularly in diverse populations with variable microbiome composition. Utilization of advanced vaccination strategies requires an understanding of new ideas, such as mechanisms of disease tolerance, in addition to traditional immune responses. Disease tolerance refers to the host's capacity to decrease the damaging effects of infection without necessarily eradicating the pathogen itself. Such an approach paves the way for new vaccine designs that not only aim at pathogen clearance but also enhance the host's own defense mechanism to reduce disease severity. For example, research indicates that immunologically induced resistance mechanisms and disease tolerance could complement each other to enhance therapeutic outcomes in vulnerable individuals. By the discovery and manipulation of these mechanisms, researchers can create vaccines that not only provide active protection but also predispose the host to resistance against a range of infectious agents, exhibiting an integrated approach to managing host-microbe interactions in pathogenesis. Recent discoveries in the use of cytokines, namely interferon-lambda (IFN-λ), reveal new hopeful vaccination strategies against enteric viruses. IFN-λ is a central immune molecule of the innate immunity with solid antiviral activity that could be used in vaccination. Importantly, its role in infection regulation through virus-host relationship modulation emphasizes the importance of host-derived molecules in vaccine strategies. The therapeutic potential of recombinant IFN-λ also resides in regulating both intestinal well-being and pathogen load, setting it up for incorporation into chronic viral infection vaccine platforms. With increasing research indicating the interaction between the immune system, the microbiome, and the behavior of pathogens, the development of vaccines utilizing these dynamic interactions, e.g., cytokine modulation, can significantly enhance our ability to combat infectious diseases effectively (Gozzelino et al., 2014).

4.5.3. Probiotics and Microbiome Modulation

The contemporary understanding of probiotics transcends their traditional role as dietary supplements; they are now also recognized for their capacity to alter the gut microbiome and influence host health and disease trends. Probiotics, which are live microbial organisms that impart health benefits when administered in adequate numbers, possess the capacity to restore or enhance gut microbiota function and diversity. Several studies have established that probiotics might mitigate the effects of gastrointestinal disorders, , such as irritable bowel syndrome and nonalcoholic fatty liver disease (NAFLD), by reshaping the composition of microbiomes. Because the gut microbiome has many more functional genes than the human genome, its metabolic products and host interactions are important for maintaining homeostasis.

This intricate interaction between the microbiome and probiotics is the hallmark of an understanding of much pathology, as any imbalances in these interactions can potentially result in adverse health outcomes (Lynch et al., 2019). In addition to their function in the upkeep of gastrointestinal health, probiotics play a role in regulating the brain-gut-microbiome axis, a delicate network through which gut microbiota and neurological activity are integrated. It has been established in vitro that gut microbes possess the capability to modulate brain function through immune, endocrine, and neural mechanisms, establishing a bidirectional network of communication between the central nervous system and microbiome. This dynamic interaction can be disrupted in obesity and psychiatric illness, where alterations in gut flora increase symptoms and pathophysiology. Consequently, probiotic supplementation to modulate the microbiome can be a potential therapeutic opportunity for these diseases by re-establishing optimal interaction along these tracts and improving metabolic parameters (Martin et al., 2018). The fact that probiotics can influence gut microbiota and, in turn, brain and behavioral health serves to further establish their potential as a disease prevention and management tool. The implications of probiotic use for the modulation of the microbiome indicate the need for rigorous clinical trials to identify effective strains and dosages specific to given health issues. Despite the favorable benefits associated with the use of probiotics, individual variation in response and the complexity of interaction among microbiomes make the use of probiotics challenging. Dietary, lifestyle, genetic, and existing condition factors can strongly interact with the efficacy of probiotics in the modification of populations of gut microbiota. Accordingly, all future studies must focus on customized approaches considering such factors to achieve the highest possible level of therapeutic intervention. In establishing a more specific knowledge base of host-microbe interaction and the specific mechanisms through which probiotics exert their effects, scientists can better utilize their potential for the restoration of microbiome balance, ultimately for disease control and overall well-being (Martin et al., 2018; Lynch et al., 2019) (Figure 4.14).

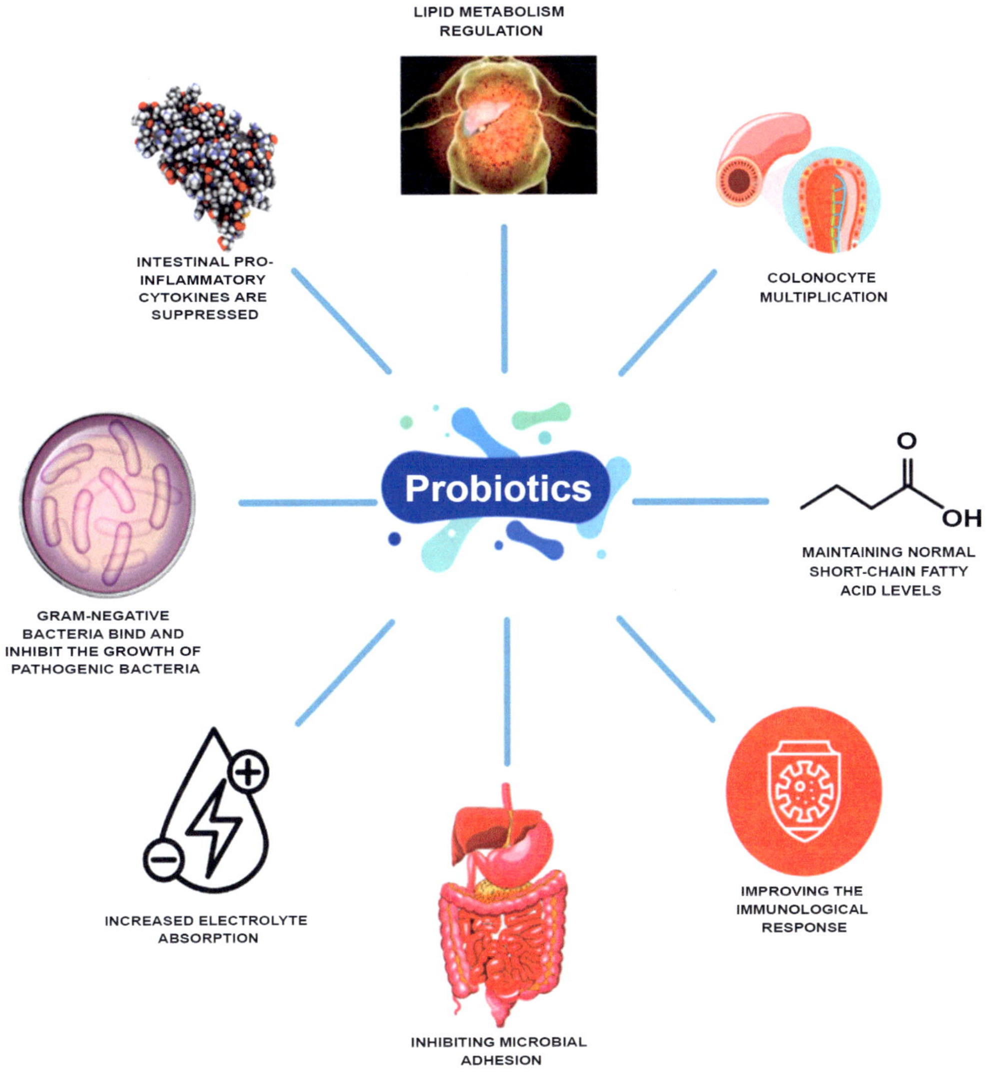

Figure 4.14. Action mechanisms of probiotics.

Source: https://www.mdpi.com/microorganisms/microorganisms-12-00234/article_deploy/html/images/microorganisms-12-00234-g001.png.

Test Your Knowledge

1. How do antibiotics and other antimicrobial agents work to eliminate pathogenic microbes?
2. What is the principle behind vaccination strategies, and how do vaccines help prevent infectious diseases at both individual and population levels?
3. How can probiotics and microbiome modulation contribute to the prevention or treatment of infections?

SUMMARY

The intricate host-microbe interactions play a central role in unraveling the complexity of pathogenesis. From a systems biology point of view, researchers can unravel the intricate dynamics of the interaction between pathogens and host elements to reveal the underlying drivers of disease like inflammatory bowel disease (IBD). By integrating information from genetic, epigenetic, and microbial levels, it is possible to identify crucial regulators within IBD interactome. Such an approach focuses on not only attacking pathogens but also on the hosts molecular environment, opening up for novel therapies that are personalized to the patients individual biological context, as presented in recent discoveries of IBD pathogenesis (Polytarchou et al., 2014).

Also, the research into autophagy-related proteins (ATGs) has revealed novel pathways between host defenses and microbial interactions. Groundbreaking studies posit that ATGs play functions beyond canonical autophagy mechanisms to include vital processes like immune signaling and inflammation. This finding is crucial in how the host is able to modulate populations of microorganisms without breaching homeostasis. Knowledge of such interactions will enable us to know more about inflammatory disease and other human diseases and suggest that successful disentangling of such interactions is crucial for developing focused therapeutic interventions that can override the adverse effects of dysregulated host-microbe interactions (Cadwell & Debnath, 2017).

Lastly, studies on host-microbe interactions are necessary to further develop the field of pathogenesis and give feedback in planning new therapeutic strategies. In an understanding of the sheer magnitude of complexity within these interactions, there are active roles played by both parties, the host and microbial inhabitants, in disease creation and health preservation. Future research should therefore continue to be aimed at the integration of disparate biological data so that a more complete understanding of pathogenesis may be gained. With researchers accessing the findings of these studies, it may well recognize biomarkers and treatments applicable to everyone, which could bring hope for illnesses previously thought to be intractable (Polytarchou et al., 2014; Cadwell & Debnath, 2017).

Understanding the interactions between microbes and the host is significant to comprehending the mechanisms of pathogenesis. Recent studies demonstrate the complexity of these interactions, particularly in diseases , such as inflammatory bowel disease (IBD), including ulcerative colitis (UC) and Crohn's disease (CD). IBD affects millions of people in the United States and is found to result from intricate interactions between the host's genetic and epigenetic characteristics and the microbiome. By applying a systems biology approach, researchers are able to integrate molecular and cell-level information, providing greater insight into the pathogenesis of IBD. By identifying key regulators or hubs in the IBD interactome, potential therapeutic targets are unveiled, which can be utilized to develop more efficient treatments according to individual patient profiles (Polytarchou et al., 2014).

Also impressive is the work on viral infection and host metabolism, , such as with Cricket paralysis virus (CrPV) in silkworm and Drosophila cells. The disparate metabolic patterns in persistently infected versus acute infection stages provide an interesting perspective for understanding host-microbe interaction. In the persistently infected Bm5 cells, high levels of glucose and glutamine were found, whereas these metabolites significantly decreased during pathogenic phases. Conversely, S2 cell acute infection had a drop in critical metabolites preceded by their recovery with the initiation of pathogenesis. This contradictory trend emphasizes investigating the changes in metabolism with various types of infection to drive home the fact that the infection stage is a major determinant of host-microbe outcome (Meeus et al., 2020). Together, these findings validate the necessity for careful examination into the delicate interactions of host-microbe and their implications in disease causation. Through integration of information from both microbiome studies and viral pathogenesis, more comprehensive models can be constructed, shedding light on therapeutic strategies that pursue cause-dependent cure. The incorporation of high-throughput data not only enriches our understanding but also provides an entrance to innovative therapeutic approaches towards controlling and, in fact, reversing the deleterious effects of pathogenic microbes. As research evolves further, solutions to these complex interplays will be pivotal to the formulation of effective interventions and fine-tuning patient care in infectious and inflammatory disorders.

KEY TERMS FROM THIS CHAPTER

- Antibiotic-resistant pathogens
- Antimicrobial activity
- Atopic dermatitis (AD)
- Autophagy-associated proteins (ATGs)
- Autophagy-related proteins (ATGs)
- Beneficial symbionts
- Biofilm development
- Cellular dynamics
- Computational biology
- Disease pathogenesis
- Disease pathology
- Disease process
- Disease susceptibility
- Disease-causing pathogens

CRITICAL THINKING QUESTIONS

1. **Which of the following types of microbes is most commonly involved in pathogenic interactions with the host?**
   a. Algae
   b. Viruses
   c. Protozoa
   d. Lichens
2. **What is the term for the ability of a microbe to cause disease?**
   a. Infectivity
   b. Pathogenicity
   c. Virulence
   d. Immunogenicity
3. **Which mechanism is commonly used by bacteria to adhere to host cells?**
   a. Endospore formation
   b. Capsule production
   c. Fimbriae or pili
   d. Toxin secretion
4. **What type of toxin is released only when bacterial cells lyse?**
   a. Endotoxin
   b. Exotoxin
   c. Enterotoxin
   d. Neurotoxin
5. **Which factor does NOT influence host-microbe interactions?**
   a. Microbial virulence factors
   b. Host genetic makeup
   c. Environmental conditions
   d. Gravitational force

Short Answer Questions

1. What are the main types of microbes involved in host-microbe interactions? Provide examples for each type.
2. How do commensal microbes differ from pathogenic microbes in their interaction with the host?
3. Describe the key steps involved in microbial pathogenesis from colonization to disease manifestation.
4. What are some common virulence factors used by pathogenic bacteria to establish infection?
5. What are some mechanisms by which viruses evade host immune responses?
6. How do host genetic factors influence susceptibility to microbial infections?
7. Discuss the impact of environmental factors on the outcome of host-microbe interactions.

Answers to Critical Thinking Questions

1. (b) 2. (b) 3. (c) 4. (a) 5. (d)

REFERENCES

1. Adeniyi-Ipadeola, G., Nwanosike, H., & Ramani, S. (2023). Human intestinal organoids as models to study enteric bacteria and viruses. https://core.ac.uk/download/643777105.pdf (accessed on 13th June 2025).
2. Allan, P., Fiorino, G., Gatti, S., Gerasimidis, K., et al. (2017). Research gaps in diet and nutrition in inflammatory bowel disease: A topical review by D-ECCO Working Group (Dietitians of ECCO). https://core.ac.uk/download/84340703.pdf (accessed on 13th June 2025).
3. Amos, G. C. A., Anastasi, E., Anyanful, A., Barber, M. F., Barnich, N., Beutin, L., Blango, M., et al. (2018). Virulence behavior of uropathogenic *Escherichia coli* strains in the host model *Caenorhabditis elegans*. https://core.ac.uk/download/188826801.pdf (accessed on 13th June 2025).
4. Armijos Jaramillo, V. D., Díaz Mínguez, J. M., Echeverria, M. de L. M., Rech, G. E., et al. (2016). A fungal effector with host nuclear localization and DNA-binding properties is required for maize anthracnose development. https://core.ac.uk/download/159287034.pdf (accessed on 13th June 2025).
5. Avrova, A., Bai, Y., Balesdent, M. H., Belfanti, E., Berruyer, R., Bhattacharjee, S., Bonardi, V., et al. (2014). Effector-triggered defense against apo plastic fungal pathogens. https://core.ac.uk/download/29842450.pdf (accessed on 13th June 2025).
6. Baldin, C., Brakhage, A. A., Castanheira, S., Di Pietro, A., et al. (2014). Fungal model systems and the elucidation of pathogenicity determinants. https://core.ac.uk/download/25497497.pdf (accessed on 13th June 2025).
7. Baldridge, M. T., & Lee, S. (2017). Interferon-lambda: A potent regulator of intestinal viral infections. https://core.ac.uk/download/84911326.pdf (accessed on 13th June 2025).
8. Barret, T., Brackman, G., Brown, P., Bush, K., Cascales, E., Corrigan, R. M., Costerton, J. W., et al. (2012). Socializing, networking and development: A report from the second 'Young Microbiologists Symposium on Microbe Signaling, Organization and Pathogenesis.' https://core.ac.uk/download/9839329.pdf (accessed on 13th June 2025).
9. Bell, L. C. K., & Noursadeghi, M. (2018). Pathogenesis of HIV-1 and *Mycobacterium tuberculosis* co-infection. https://core.ac.uk/download/151187028.pdf (accessed on 13th June 2025).
10. Blecher-Paz, K., Champer, J., Friedman, A. J., Kim, M., et al. (2013). Antimicrobial and anti-inflammatory activity of chitosan-alginate nanoparticles: A targeted therapy for cutaneous pathogens. https://core.ac.uk/download/323078644.pdf (accessed on 13th June 2025).
11. Brown, A. J. P., Brown, G. D., Chen, K., Drummond, R. A., et al. (2014). *Candida albicans* colonization and dissemination from the murine gastrointestinal tract: The influence of morphology and Th17 immunity. https://core.ac.uk/download/29151197.pdf (accessed on 13th June 2025).
12. Buan, N. R., Carr, S., Cashman, M., Catazaro, J., et al. (2020). Metabolic feedback inhibition influences metabolite secretion by the human gut symbiont *Bacteroides thetaiotaomicron*. https://core.ac.uk/download/334984789.pdf (accessed on 13th June 2025).
13. Cadwell, K., & Debnath, J. (2018). Beyond self-eating: The control of nonautophagic functions and signaling pathways by autophagy-related proteins. *The Journal of cell biology, 217*(3), 813–822. https://doi.org/10.1083/jcb.201706157(accessed on 13th June 2025).

14. Cavalieri, D., Godaly, G., Hagberg, L., Hedges, S., Schappert, K. T., & Shahin, R. (2016). Subversion of host innate immunity by uropathogenic *Escherichia coli*. https://core.ac.uk/download/80494906.pdf (accessed on 13th June 2025).
15. Clark, J. J., Cumberworth, S., Donald, C. L., Kohl, A., et al. (2017). Inhibition of type I interferon induction and signaling by mosquito-borne flaviviruses. https://core.ac.uk/download/80697084.pdf (accessed on 13th June 2025).
16. Coates, C. J., Krachler, A. M., Lim, J., Monteith, S., et al. (2021). Defective phagocyte association during infection of *Galleria mellonella* with *Yersinia pseudotuberculosis* is detrimental to both insect host and microbe. https://core.ac.uk/download/373291081.pdf (accessed on 13th June 2025).
17. Coenye, T., Crabbé, A., Davis, R., De La Fuente-Nùñez, C., et al. (2017). Antimicrobial efficacy against *Pseudomonas aeruginosa* biofilm formation in a three-dimensional lung epithelial model and the influence of fetal bovine serum. https://core.ac.uk/download/84047108.pdf (accessed on 13th June 2025).
18. Coenye, T., Crabbé, A., Tavernier, S., Vandeplassche, E., et al. (2019). Influence of the lung microbiome on antibiotic susceptibility of cystic fibrosis pathogens. https://core.ac.uk/download/227040537.pdf (accessed on 13th June 2025).
19. Coleman, F. T. (2016). Influence of macrophage NF-kappaB activation on pneumococcal pneumonia. https://open.bu.edu/bitstream/2144/14597/10/Coleman_bu_0017E_11688.pdf (accessed on 13th June 2025).
20. Gallo, R. L., Irvine, A. D., Kong, H. H., Luger, T., et al. (2019). The microbiome in patients with atopic dermatitis. https://core.ac.uk/download/323064499.pdf (accessed on 13th June 2025).
21. Gozzelino, R., Soares, M. P., & Weis, S. (2014). Tissue damage control in disease tolerance. https://core.ac.uk/download/84064289.pdf (accessed on 13th June 2025).
22. Huitema, E., Kulagina, N., Monteiro Amaro, T. M., Motion, G., et al. (2015). Nuclear processes associated with plant immunity and pathogen susceptibility. https://core.ac.uk/download/30663567.pdf (accessed on 13th June 2025).
23. Polytarchou, C., Koukos, G., & Iliopoulos, D. (2014). Systems biology in inflammatory bowel diseases: ready for prime time. *Current opinion in gastroenterology*, *30*(4), 339–346. https://doi.org/10.1097/MOG.0000000000000081 (accessed on 13th June 2025).
24. Jacobson, M. (2003). *Enteric Diseases in Pigs from Weaning to Slaughter*. https://core.ac.uk/download/11694636.pdf (accessed on 13th June 2025).
25. Jiang, H., & Wang, D. (2016). The microbial zoo in the *C. elegans* intestine: Bacteria, fungi and viruses. https://core.ac.uk/download/212858942.pdf (accessed on 13th June 2025).
26. Martin, C. R., Osadchiy, V., Kalani, A., & Mayer, E. A. (2018). The Brain-Gut-Microbiome Axis. *Cellular and molecular gastroenterology and hepatology*, *6*(2), 133–148. https://doi.org/10.1016/j.jcmgh.2018.04.003 (accessed on 13th June 2025).
27. Kirchner, S., Power, B. J., & Waters, A. P. (2016). Recent advances in malaria genomics and epigenomics. https://core.ac.uk/download/46580201.pdf (accessed on 13th June 2025).
28. Lynch, S. V., Sharpton, S. R., Terrault, N. A., Yong, L., et al. (2019). Gut microbial metabolism and nonalcoholic fatty liver disease. https://core.ac.uk/download/323065660.pdf (accessed on 13th June 2025).

29. McCullers, J. A. (2013). Do specific virus–bacteria pairings drive clinical outcomes of pneumonia? https://core.ac.uk/download/pdf/82071893.pdf (accessed on 13th June 2025).

30. Meeus, I., Smagghe, G., Swevers, L., Van Meulebroek, L., et al. (2020). Metabolomic analysis of cricket paralysis virus infection in *Drosophila* S2 cells reveals divergent effects on central carbon metabolism as compared with silkworm Bm5 cells. https://core.ac.uk/download/322827688.pdf (accessed on 13th June 2025).

31. Ngo, J. (2024). An actin cross-linking effector of the *Vibrio* type six secretion system increases intestinal motility through macrophage redistribution. https://core.ac.uk/download/613868205.pdf (accessed on 13th June 2025).

32. Patters, B. J. (2018). The role of exosome transport of viral agents in persistent HIV pathogenesis. https://core.ac.uk/download/234018970.pdf (accessed on 13th June 2025).

33. Underwood, M. A., & Sohn, K. (2017). The Microbiota of the Extremely Preterm Infant. *Clinics in perinatology*, *44*(2), 407–427. https://doi.org/10.1016/j.clp.2017.01.005 (accessed on 13th June 2025).

34. Soni, J., & Pandey, R. (2024). Single cell genomics-based insights into the impact of cell-type specific microbial internalization on disease severity. https://core.ac.uk/download/615303706.pdf (accessed on 13th June 2025).

35. Uehara, A., Ansari, A. A., Dang, A. T., Thurman, A. R., Dang, A. T., Dale, B. A., Shacklett, B. L., et al. (2013). Transcription profiling reveals potential mechanisms of dysbiosis in the oral microbiome of rhesus macaques with chronic untreated SIV infection. https://core.ac.uk/download/323071203.pdf (accessed on 13th June 2025).

BACTERIAL STRUCTURE AND GENETICS

5

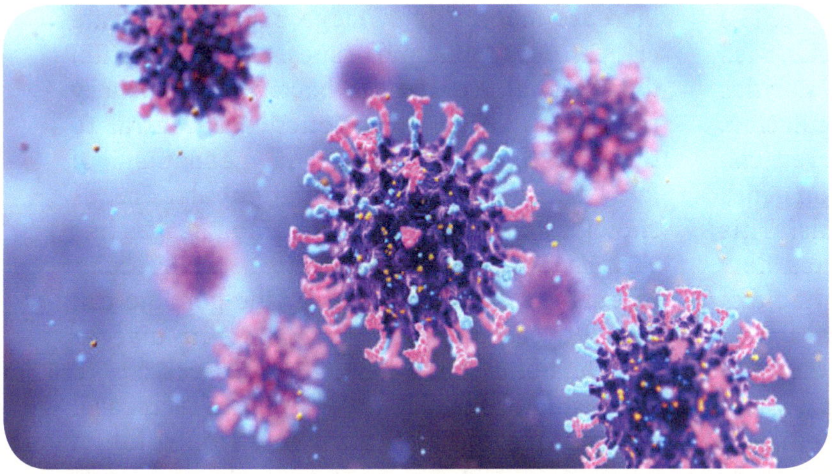

LEARNING OBJECTIVES

After studying this chapter, you will be able to:

1. Understand the basic structure of bacteria
2. Describe bacterial cell types
3. Discuss genetic material in bacteria
4. Explain the basics of bacterial reproduction
5. Define gene regulation in bacteria
6. Focus on applications of bacterial genetics

Introduction

In microbiology, the study of the structure and genetics of bacteria is a basis for cellular life. Being unicellular, bacteria possess a large range of structural attributes important in survival and adaptability. One of the significant structures of bacteria, the cell wall, varies between species and influences not only shape but also the interaction of the organism with the environment. For instance, Gram-positive and Gram-negative bacteria may be distinguished based on their cell wall structure, which also dictates bacterial antibiotic sensitivity and overall pathogenicity. Such complexity requires thorough research, particularly in light of the functions of bacterial genetics in medicine, biotechnology, and ecology. Further, the bacterial genetic makeup shows an amazing adaptability to withstand the environmental brunt, which speaks volumes of their applicability. Bacterial genomes can convert into various traits, from antibiotic resistance to metabolites, that are often acquired through horizontal gene transfer processes like transformation, transduction, and conjugation. The genetic adaptability enables bacteria to develop very rapidly under selective pressure. Understanding the intricacies of bacterial genetics not only adds to our knowledge of evolutionary biology but also has utilitarian applications in the development of new therapies against resistant bacteria. The application of plasmids—naturally occurring plasmid DNA molecules found in bacteria—shows how genetic elements can be employed for purposes , such as recombinant protein production, showing the intersection of bacterial anatomy and genetic engineering. The study of specific bacterial genetic elements, such as the nod-box in Rhizobium species, clarifies mechanisms of gene expression regulation. In particular, the nod-box is a conserved cis-acting sequence that regulates nodulation genes in response to environmental signals. This specificity is important as it illustrates how bacterial organisms respond to their habitats via intricate systems of regulation. As shown in research on the regulatory role of the nod-box, these mechanisms can produce a variety of patterns of expression required for efficient symbiosis with host plants. Investigation of these genetic and structural models allows for an increased understanding of bacterial life, setting the stage for applied uses in agriculture and environmental control, thus informing the interconnection of bacterial structure and genetics within higher biological systems.

Importance of Studying Bacterial Structure and Genetics

Understanding the cell structure and genetics of bacteria is crucial for many areas of application,, such as medicine, agriculture, and biotechnology. The structure of the bacterial cell acts as a determinant of how these microorganisms interact with host organisms and environments. An illustrative example is how the composition of the bacterial cell wall as Gram-positive or Gram-negative profoundly impacts drug resistance to antibiotics and pathways of infection. By the study of these structural differences, scientists can plan targeted therapies that block the pathogens' capability to stay alive in host tissue. Moreover, the understanding obtained from bacterial genetics allows researchers to design these microbes for biotechnological applications, , such as the production of biofuels or biodegradable plastic, enhancing the utilization of sustainable technology in industry. By proceeding step-by-step to the investigation of bacterial structure and genetics, we not only increase medical knowledge but also alleviate critical environmental issues. The population dynamics of evolution in bacteria, particularly their adaptability to genetics, are central to their ecological success. The mechanism of fast diversification in bacterial populations, as shown by the evolution of specific lineages like Wrinkly Spreader in *Pseudomonas* fluorescens, reveals the way mutations in the genome can provide competitive advantages in diverse environments. Such flexibility is necessary to understand bacterial activity within terrestrial environments and clinical infection. Biofilm development is one such example of genetic impacts on community function and ecological interactions, ensuring long-term colonization and resistance to treatments. Studying such genetic processes unravels the mechanism along key processes, , such as biofilm formation and resistance to drugs, which are of immense importance in bacterial infection treatment and exploring beneficial bacterial characteristics for industrial purposes (Jerdan et al., 2020). Beyond their medical and ecological value, studies on the structure and genetics of bacteria are important for the advancement of marine biotechnology and related sciences. Since there is increased interest in the marine environment as a reservoir of novel bacterial species and biopharmaceuticals, information about the genetic makeup and structural capacity of these organisms allows us to harness their new features optimally. Research on bacterial strains allows us to uncover potential collaborations between academia and industry, thereby optimizing funding opportunities as well as collaborative work in biotechnology research (Seaman & Whitehouse, 2001). Molecular tools that have been derived from genetic research also allow us to enhance our ability to engineer bacteria for specific goals, including bioremediation or nutrient cycling in oceanic ecosystems. Overall, studying bacterial structure and genetics in detail promotes innovative methods of resolving different issues, thereby highlighting the applicability of this course in today's scientific research (Figure 5.1).

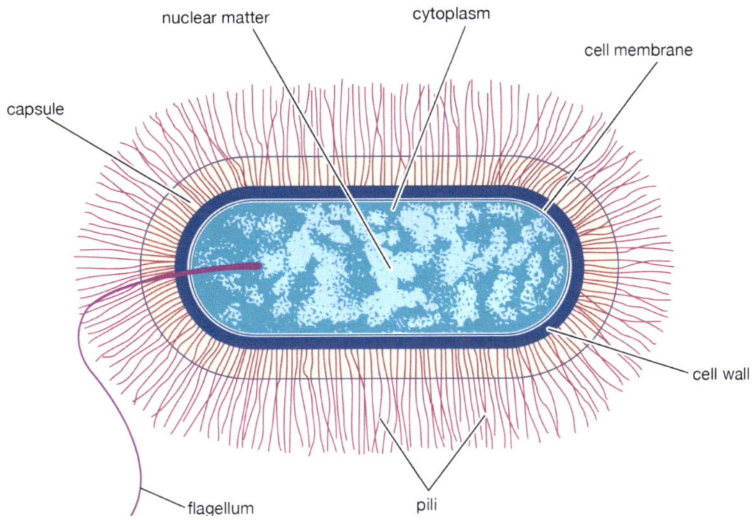

Figure 5.1. Bacterial structure.

Source: https://plantlet.org/wp-content/uploads/2020/10/drawing-structure-cell-bacillus-type.jpg.

5.1. Basic Structure of Bacteria

Learning Outcome

1. Understand cell wall composition and function
2. Describe plasma membrane characteristics
3. Discuss cytoplasm and its components

The general architecture of bacteria is characterized by their separate cellular organization, which in essence makes them different from eukaryotic cells. The keystone of the bacterial architecture is the cell membrane, covering the cytoplasm and fundamental cell components. Not only is the membrane a protective wall, but it also regulates nutrient intake and the expulsion of waste to maintain homeostasis inside the cell. Along the membrane, many bacteria possess a peptidoglycan-based rigid cell wall. This structure not only provides shape and support but also serves as a crucial component to resist osmotic pressure, which is a vital feature for organisms' survival in various environments. The simplicity of the structure in bacteria mirrors their efficiency and versatility, enabling them to exist in all sorts of ecological niches, from soil to the human body, and highlighting their evolutionary significance in the microbial realm. Within the cytoplasm, bacteria include essential genetic material, typically organized in a single, circular chromosome devoid of membrane sheath, characteristic of eukaryotes. This genome structure allows for efficient replication and transcription in order to rapidly react to environmental stress. Plasmids are present in most bacteria: small, round DNA molecules that exist independently of the chromosome. Plasmids can contain genes that transfer desirable traits , such as antibiotic resistance, demonstrating how they allow bacterial adaptability and evolution. Further, the presence of ribosomes, which are crucial for protein synthesis, also signifies the multidimensional nature of the genetics of bacteria in that these organelles translate genetic information into beneficial proteins. Overall, the intricate structure of genetic information within bacteria signifies their functional capabilities as well as evolutionary adaptability. The surface characteristics of bacterial cells, including flagella and pili, are significant in enabling their interaction and adaptation in their environment. Flagella, a long whip-like appendage, enables locomotion, as bacteria travel in various environments in search of nutrients or optimal conditions. Motility is important for survival because it enables bacteria to move away from harmful conditions or migrate towards useful resources. Pili, short hair-like structures, enable adhesion to surfaces and enable conjugation, a form of genetic transfer. This interaction is crucial for the exchange of genetic characters, particularly those related to antibiotic resistance, and underscores the significance of such structures in bacterial evolution and genetics. The joining of these external features with the cell's machinery results in a highly adaptive organism, one that is robust and capable of survival and growth over a broad variety of ecological niches, justifying the need for knowledge of bacterial form in the overall scheme of bacterial genetics.

5.1.1. Cell Wall Composition and Function

The robustness of bacterial cells is also because of their cell wall morphology, which is primarily made up of peptidoglycan, a sugar and amino acid polymer. This unique morphology develops hardness and organizes bacteria and also serves as an immune shield against external stress factors, , such as osmotic pressure. In Gram-positive bacteria, the cell wall has a thick peptidoglycan layer, which holds up to crystal violet dye in the Gram staining, making these bacteria purple. Gram-negative bacteria have a thinner peptidoglycan layer located between an inner and outer membrane, with the result being a pink color upon staining. The differences in cell wall structure influence not only the physical characteristics of these organisms but also their antibiotic sensitivity, with certain antibiotics preventing the formation of the peptidoglycan layer, which demonstrates the vital role it plays in bacterial cell survival. The cell wall is also crucial to the pathogenicity of certain bacteria. Most pathogens exploit the architecture of their cell wall to resist host immune mechanisms or to enhance infection. For instance, the presence of some surface antigens, like lipopolysaccharides in Gram-negative bacteria, may induce severe inflammatory reactions from the host as well as play a role in adhesion to tissues of the host. Second, structural differences in cell walls can also lead to antibiotic resistance, where mutations or the acquisition of resistance genes enable bacteria to modify their peptidoglycan layer such that normal treatments fail. This flexibility not only highlights the evolutionary significance of the structure of bacterial cell walls but also demands pressing public health and imminent infectious disease therapy issues, justifying further investigation into targeted therapies that circumvent these resistance mechanisms, especially in relation to increasing antibiotic resistance globally. Further, the intricate interaction of cell walls of bacteria with their function in microbiomes is the best example of the need for an overarching knowledge of bacterial structure. For instance, the function of the cell wall in homeostasis and its decisive role in interaction with eukaryotic cells is a highly relevant topic of study in research on microbiomes. These recent workshops have attempted to investigate the character of healthy gut microbiomes and the implications for human health, shedding some light on the role bacterial structure, i.e., their cell walls, has in mediating host interactions and overall well-being. The complex dynamics here highlight the significance of cell wall structure in shedding light on broader questions of microbial disease and health dynamics. As more research continues to show, unlocking the functional potential tied to cell wall variation in bacterial communities may become key information for the development of novel therapeutic methods to manage dysbiosis and maintain microbial balance in human health (McBurney et al., 2019) (Figure 5.2).

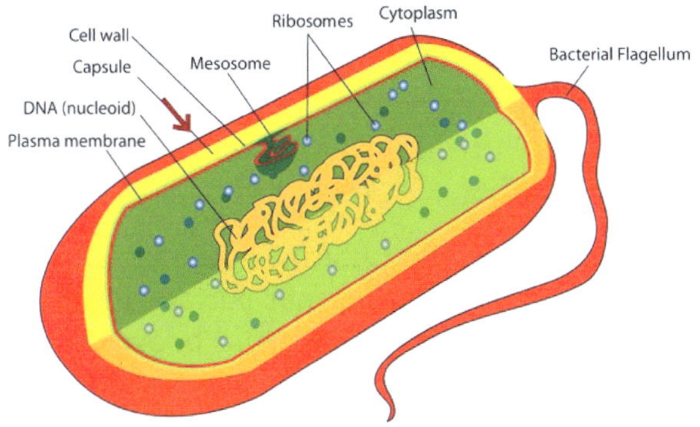

Figure 5.2. Bacterial cell structure.

Source: https://i.ytimg.com/vi/4DYgGA9jdlE/hq720.jpg?sqp=-oaymwEhCK4FEIIDSFryq4qpAxMIARUAAAAAGAElAADIQj0AgKJD&rs=AOn4CLDia-7NpwGUfPENvIBkoxVXx-9Szw.

5.1.2. Plasma Membrane Characteristics

The plasma membrane is an elementary characteristic of the bacterial structure that plays a critical role in the maintenance of cellular integrity and mediating interactions between the cell and the outside environment. At the structural level, it is primarily composed of a bilayer of phospholipids that is selectively permeable to permit survival-required nutrients but not toxic substances. This selective permeability is critical for bacterial cell viability and effectiveness, given that they survive in most instances in environments that constantly change. Besides, the addition of varying proteins to the membrane also facilitates its performance, like the transport proteins that are charged with the movement of molecules across the bilayer. Not only does this dynamic structure facilitate cellular homeostasis but also enables the reaction of bacteria to external stimuli, a characteristic crucial to their capacity to adapt and evolve according to the accounts of recent studies towards microbial resilience. In addition to its general role in substance transport and environmental communication, the plasma membrane also has a specific role in signaling pathways and energy production in bacterial cells. Proton gradients in the plasma membrane are employed by a majority of bacteria to generate ATP, a function entirely reliant on the integrity of the membrane. This is directly applicable to those bacterial groups that respire or ferment, where the plasma membrane's ability to support varying electron transport chains is of direct significance in terms of energy yields. Recent research on membrane composition, such as the identification of specific lipid types that influence membrane fluidity, holds significant potential for contributing to bacterial growth and survival approaches. This research expands the plasma membrane's functional diversity from being a physical barrier to a responsive entity following metabolic needs and environmental stress. Moreover, the plasma membrane plays a significant role in determining bacterial cell shape and division and establishing its properties directly into corresponding structural and genetic features. The membrane structure must be specifically engineered to maintain the shape of cells, which will determine overall function and gene expression. For instance, during cell division, the plasma membrane plays a critical role in genetic material segregation in order that each daughter cell receives an accurate and complete copy of genetic information. This relationship between genetic stability and membrane integrity underscores a broader evolutionary trend where structural adjustments facilitate successful reproduction and survival within bacterial populations. The ramifications of such findings are legitimate; as recognized within existing research, understanding of plasma membrane characteristics may eventually mean enhancements in preventing bacterial infections and enhancing agricultural resistance against pathogens, i.e., root-knot nematodes recognized within agricultural research that can significantly affect the performance of crops (Kaloshian et al., 2019). Thus, the plasma membrane emerges as a central player in the ballet between structure, function, and genetics in bacteria, with opportunities for further research and exploration in microbial biology (Horowitz et al., 1954) (Figure 5.3).

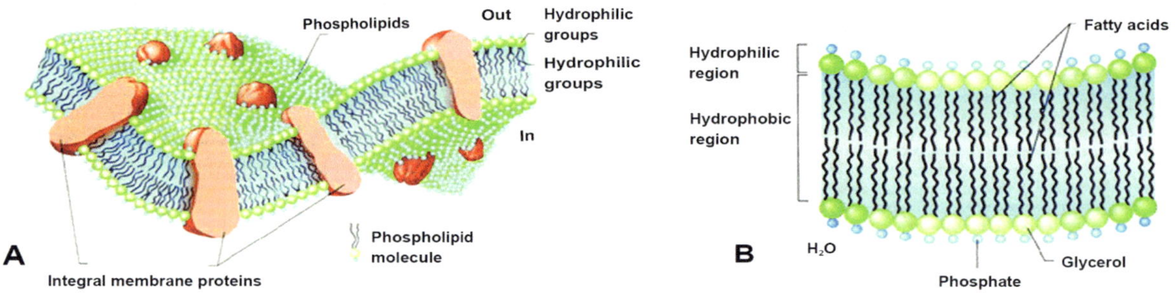

Figure 5.3. Schematic structure of a bacterial phospholipid bilayer membrane. (A) Cytoplasmic membrane showing the lipid molecules and transmembrane proteins. The inner surface faces the cytoplasm and the outer part faces the environment. (B) Detailed view of the lipid bilayer.

Source: https://www.researchgate.net/profile/Julius-Lipp/publication/27336292/figure/fig7/AS:669391620427785@1536606807787/Schematic-structure-of-a-bacterial-phospholipid-bilayer-membrane-A-Cytoplasmic.png.

5.1.3. Cytoplasm and Its Components

Cytoplasm is a crucial medium within bacterial cells where important biochemical reactions occur. It comprises a jelly-like substance known as cytosol and contains many macromolecules, soluble ions, and metabolic enzymes that are necessary for cell operation. In this regard, ribosomes, which are responsible for protein synthesis, float freely and play a central function in translating genetic code into proteins that can act. This dynamic medium not only maintains metabolic functions but also enables orchestration of cellular functions, highlighting the role of cytoplasmic content in the maintenance of bacterial existence. The cytoplasm is further pivotal in functions , such as cell division and reaction to environmental stimuli, highlighting the multicategory function of the cytoplasm in the overall construction of the bacterial structure and genealogy. In addition to ribosomes, the cytoplasm holds other inclusions and granules that serve as reservoirs of nutrients, storage of energy, and structural components. Polyhydroxybutyrate granules, for instance, supply carbon and energy storage, while magnetosomes, made up of magnetically orienting iron oxides, assist in geomagnetic orientation. Such inclusions enable bacteria to be better suited for various environmental conditions, allowing them to survive and function optimally. Moreover, the positioning of nucleoid regions, where the bacterial chromosome is located, reinforces the importance of cytoplasmic structure to gene regulation and replication. The structural organization of genetic material within the cytoplasm plays a vital role in successful transcription and translation since it facilitates fast transport of genetic information and proteins involved within the cell, guiding fundamental processes associated with bacterial genetics. Recent studies of engineered bacteria illustrate the function of the cytoplasm in the display of active enzymes that could be used to enhance biotechnological usefulness. For instance, research has shown that *Escherichia coli* bacteria, under specific oxidative cytoplasmic environments, are capable of significantly amplifying glycosyltransferase production, essential enzymes in glycoprotein formation (Carroll et al., 2009). This illustrates the versatility and capacity of the cytoplasms for improvement through microbial engineering. Furthermore, understanding how DNA is packed in bacterial cells provides insight into the structural integrity of cytoplasmic genetic material, as observed with stresses and forces upon phage infection (Molineux et al., 2010). Studying such details enables scientists to manipulate bacterial operations, resulting in genetic engineering and synthetic biology advancements (Figure 5.4).

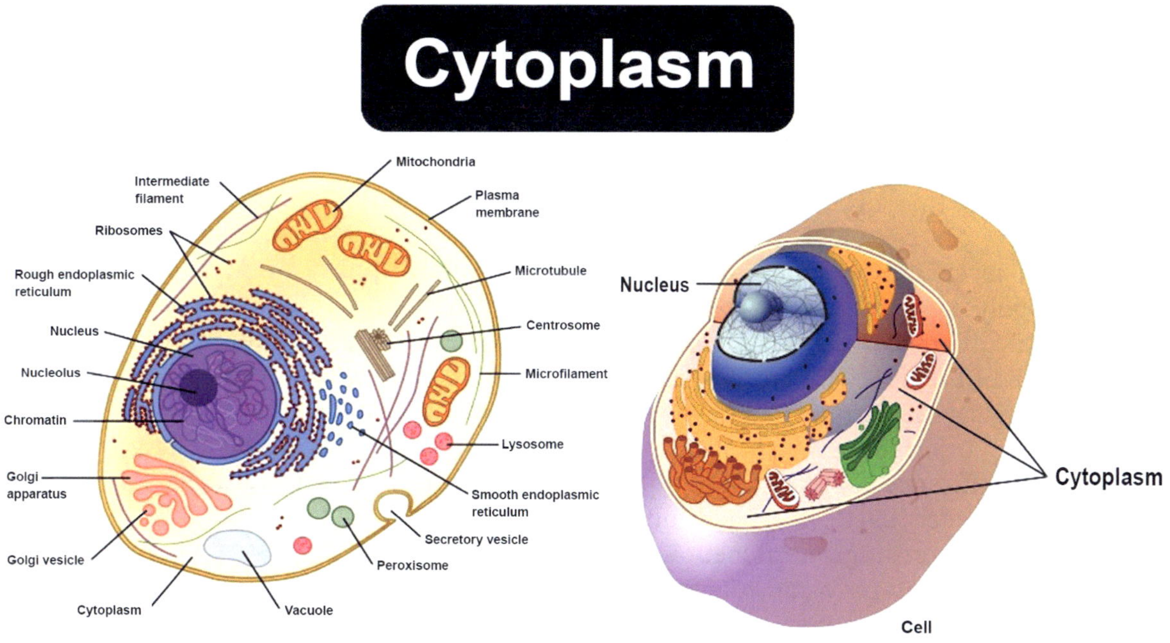

Figure 5.4. Cytoplasm.

Source: https://biologynotesonline.com/wp-content/uploads/2021/11/Cytoplasm.jpg.

Test Your Knowledge

1. What are the primary chemical components of the bacterial cell wall, and how do they contribute to its function?
2. What are the main functions of the bacterial plasma membrane, and how does its structure support these functions?
3. Describe the components found in the bacterial cytoplasm and their roles in cellular processes.

5.2. Bacterial Cell Types

Learning Outcome

1. Differentiate between Gram-positive and gram-negative bacteria
2. Understand the shapes of bacteria
3. Describe specialized structures of bacteria

The diversity of cell types in bacteria is at the heart of characterizing their genetic and structural features. Bacteria are basically grouped into two big categories: Gram-positive and Gram-negative, depending on the nature of their cell walls. Gram-positive bacteria contain a thick peptidoglycan layer, which retains the crystal violet stain used in Gram staining, hence appearing purple during microscopic observation. On the other hand, Gram-negative bacteria possess a less electron-dense peptidoglycan layer and an outer membrane made of lipopolysaccharides, fuchsia-staining. The structural difference influences not only the interaction of bacteria with antibiotics but also their ecological adaptability and infectivity. The structural differences emphasize the evolutionary significance of bacterial cell types, illustrating how such bacteria have evolved to occupy various ecological niches while maintaining cellular integrity and function. In addition to structural variations in cell walls, cell types of bacteria are also extremely varied in terms of genetic organization and replication mechanisms. Bacterial DNA from chromosomes typically remains a single circular unit, as opposed to linear chromosomes that are usually present in eukaryotic cells. Additionally, plasmids or small circular pieces of DNA can be found in most bacteria and can contain genes that are advantageous for survival, such as antibiotic resistance genes. Recent studies have shown principal bacterial DNA repair mechanisms comparable to eukaryotic mechanisms, including non-homologous end-joining mechanisms. This indicates the sophisticated genetic regulation bacteria possess, not just maintaining genomic integrity but also allowing them to evolve quickly in response to environmental stresses and selection pressures due to pathogenicity and antibiotic exposure, making them evolutionarily robust (Bowater et al., 2006). The functional implication of the different forms of bacterial cells extends beyond structural differences and genetic arrangements. Bacterial cell types specialize in being important to how the bacteria interact with the host environment, particularly immunity. For instance, it has been demonstrated that certain groups of bacteria, e.g., the bacteria in the healthy murine middle ear, possess unsuspected cellular heterogeneity and functional specialization upon exposure to pathogens. In such environments, innate immune responses take center stage, with varying cell types, including monocytes and epithelial cells, each with unique immune gene expression patterns. Such cell diversity ensures effective and rapid response to infection, and thus it is inferred that the interaction between bacterial cell types and host immunity constitutes a vital research interest (Draf et al., 2020). Being aware of these dynamics is critical for furthering our understanding of bacterial behavior under both health and disease conditions.

5.2.1. Differences Between Gram-positive and Gram-Negative Bacteria

The Gram-negative vs Gram-positive bacteria difference is a fundamental principle of microbiology involving primarily their cell wall structure and composition. Gram-positive bacteria possess a thick peptidoglycan layer that retains the crystal violet stain used during the Gram staining procedure, exhibiting a purple color when observed using a microscope. This peptidoglycan layer is made up of up to 90% of their cell wall content, which is held accountable for their hardness and endurance to environmental pressures. Gram-negative bacteria possess a peptidoglycan layer that is thinner in thickness, typically composing 10-

20% of their cell wall, which they place between an outer membrane and the plasma membrane. The outer membrane contains lipopolysaccharides (LPS), which induce strong immune responses in hosts, typically leading to the virulence of the organisms.

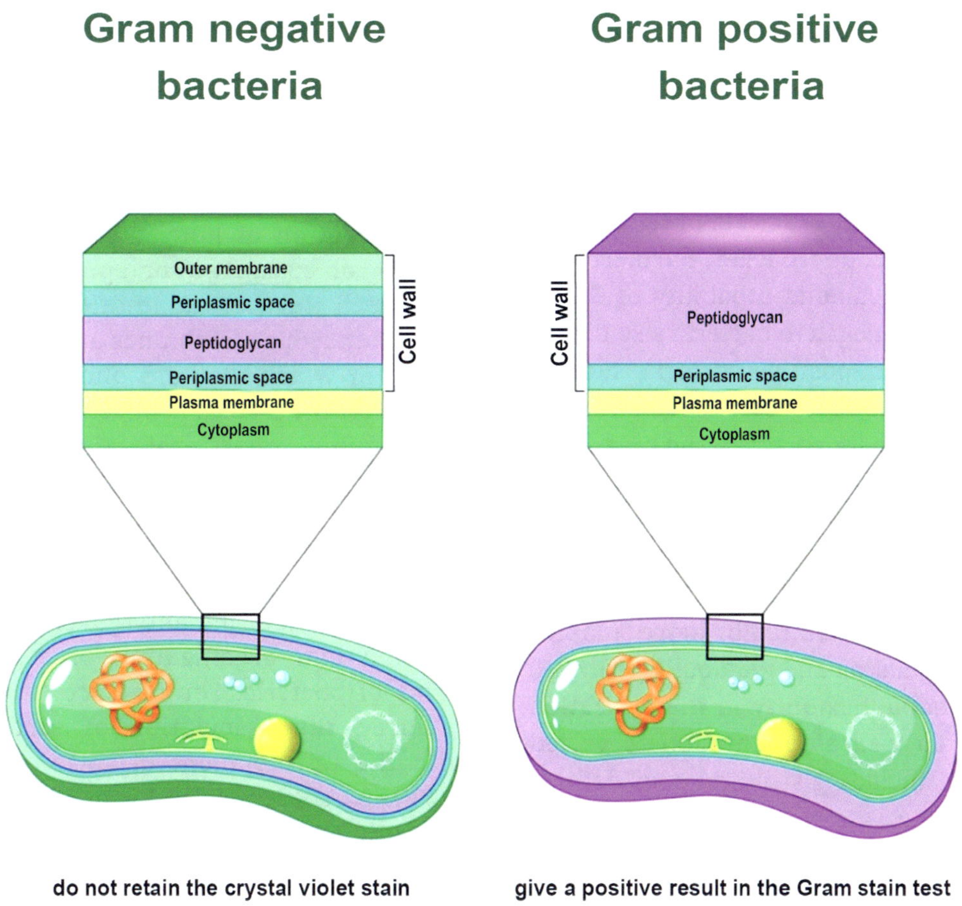

Figure 5.5. Gram-positive vs. Gram-negative bacteria.

Source: https://blogger.googleusercontent.com/img/b/R29vZ2xl/AVvXsEi4fKbB4e7SjWWIkHh8VeAl4934sFxiF2bSpgxq6PICwkb2IQKMnlKCWwgAm-aXdPwQxcjLBhRwV45uQLaIhp_huIqMJXsHwAhXmzpry7piPcHw1JHFgEpcUzgY25odA_A4tANrpwWdgC90FR8tm9VCC1OQk56cxEgP5T3wOOVZoeXw9LmqcQYRNeCfBRU/s1000/Differences%20Between%20Gram%20Positive%20And%20Gram%20Negative%20Bacteria.jpg.

This fundamental cell wall composition difference lies at the heart of their antibiotic susceptibility and general pathogenicity. These structural differences have implications that go beyond their identification; they are key factors in the interaction of these bacteria with their surroundings. For instance, the resilience of Gram-positive bacteria makes them survive in more inhospitable conditions than the Gram-negative counterparts, which are at times more sensitive to physical damage and desiccation. Additionally, the outer membrane of Gram-negative bacteria serves as a protective shield for countless antibiotics, thus necessitating special treatment approaches in order to treat infections caused by such bacteria. For example, it is difficult to treat infections caused by organisms like Campylobacter jejuni, *E. coli*, and *Salmonella* enteritidis because they are Gram-negative, as evident from differential testing methods like ozonation, which can effectively inactivate such pathogens (Anderson et al., 2003). Having the ability to understand such differences will be crucial in order to make sound antimicrobial approaches. Furthermore, the genetic and metabolic capability of Gram-positive and Gram-negative bacteria also differs tremendously. Gram-positive bacteria, such as *Staphylococcus* and *Streptococcus* species, have a less complicated genetic structure and can readily acquire genes conferring them advantages, such as resistance to antibiotics, via horizontal gene transfer mechanisms, such as transformation and transduction. On the other hand, Gram-negative bacteria are defined by more complex networks of regulation and metabolic pathways in order to enable flexibility in the utilization of nutrients as well as adaptation to varied environments, including stressful ones defined by ecological pressures (Baldwin et al., 2019). This adaptability helps them survive in various habitats, including plant-microbe-based ones, where some interactions help nurture their growth and environmental stress tolerance. It is therefore vital for both academic purposes and real-world applications in medicine and environmental management to thoroughly understand the various differences between these two types of bacteria (Figure 5.5).

5.2.2. Shapes of Bacteria: Cocci, Bacilli, and Spirilla

Bacterial morphology, which is separated into three categories—cocci, bacilli, and spirilla—are fundamental components in bacterial shape that play a significant role in their ecological niche and interaction. Cocci are round-shaped bacteria that can either be free or in various aggregations, such as pairs (diplococci), chains (streptococci), or clumps (staphylococci). This flexibility allows cocci to survive in diversified environments and their abundance and importance in both pathogenic and symbiotic conditions. Bacilli are rod-shaped bacteria, and they will be found in chains due to their nature of binary fission. The structure of bacilli is very crucial for the structural aspects, as structure aids in the absorption of nutrients and locomotion. Spirilla, of corkscrew or spiral morphology, present a further adaptation, locomotion through mucous membranes and other viscous media, in which they are often implicated in playing essential roles in infection and recycling of nutrients. Apart from simple taxonomy, bacterial morphology has been the subject of study as a foundation for understanding the genetic determinants governing the ensuing morphologies. Environmental conditions and genetic determinants govern the overall function and organization of the different forms of bacteria. For instance, studies have explored the association of certain genes with the development of cocci, bacilli, and spirilla's characteristic form. The regulation of peptidoglycan synthesis—a determinant in cell wall stability—is a key component of this relationship. Various forms impart survival advantages in varying ecological niches; thus, their genetic correlation is instrumental to addressing bacterial diversity and evolution. Recent studies indicate that environmental factors—, such as nutrient levels, temperature, and soil depth—can have significant effects on bacteria's morphological diversity in natural habitats, further illustrating how structure and genes are intimately connected (Wheeler, 2017).

Detection of morphological differences among bacterial shapes holds particular significance in the laboratory, allowing identification and examination of unusual species. Practical application, like that stressed in microbiology teaching, integrates experience-based learning with studying these shapes to offer a better understanding of bacterial physiology and behavior (Ahern et al., 2020). Through active laboratory methods, students gain information about the implications of bacterial morphology for their ecological role, whether it is for their interaction with host organisms or for their role in biogeochemical cycles. Finally, the morphologies of bacteria are not merely descriptive features but also critical elements of their genetic and functional topography, offering entryways for investigation and elucidation in numerous areas of scientific inquiry. This integration of morphology and genetics emphasizes the value of bringing these ideas together to understand the intensity and richness of bacterial existence (Figure 5.6).

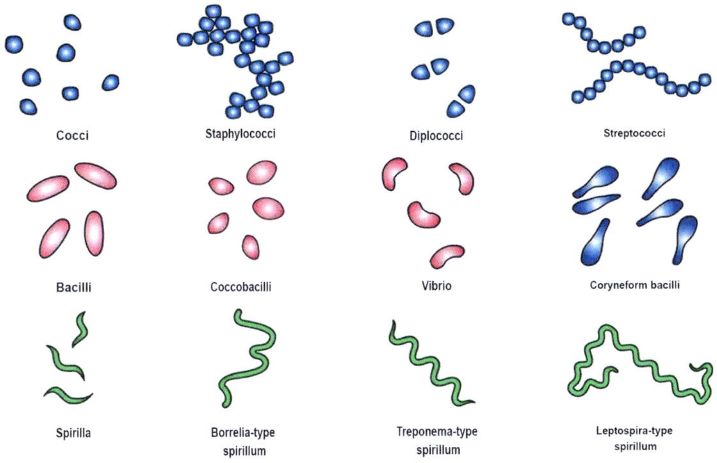

Figure 5.6. Shapes of bacteria.

Source: https://i0.wp.com/microbeonline.com/wp-content/uploads/2021/05/Basic-morphologies-of-various-bacteria.png?ssl=1.

5.2.3. Specialized Structures: Flagella and Pili

The organization and function of specialized structures, such as flagella and pili are the foundation of the knowledge of bacterial motility and diverseness. Flagella are long, whip-like structures that facilitate swimming in fluid environments, a crucial adaptation for survival and colonization. The structures work through a motor system located in the cell envelope of the bacterium, which can spin rapidly and propel the organism forward. In spirochetes, whose periplasmic flagella are unusual, the flagellar hook, which is largely made of the FlgE protein, has a fundamental role in bonding the motor to the filament. The hooks are defined by their resilience in unpleasant conditions, thus affirming their centrality in the provision of motility in hostile environments. This new structural design was used to emphasize the evolution of motility strategies for bacteria, which have allowed them to be ecologically successful in a wide variety of niches (Cockayne et al., 2014). Pili, as opposed to flagella, are utilized for functions beyond motility, like adhesion and biofilm development. These short hair-like structures play a critical role in bacterial adhesion to surfaces, like host tissues, enhancing the bacterias infective ability. Fimbriae, which are a type of pilus, are an excellent illustration of this property of adherence, since they allow bacteria to adhere to specific receptors and thus colonize. Pilus structural and functional variations illustrate the adaptability of bacteria to environmental forces. Current genomic studies indicate that specific types of pili can emerge depending on ecological and evolutionary needs. Through such systems, pili not only contribute to the physical existence of bacteria but also influence their mechanisms of genetic exchange, thereby contributing significantly to genetic diversity and evolution (Taoka et al., 2020). The interaction between pili and flagella is an interesting aspect of bacterial mobility and contact with their environment. While flagella more broadly augment locomotion, pili often allow surface interaction of equal relevance to survival. Such a dual function allows bacteria to cope with complexity in their worlds, whether to swim towards food sources or to attach stably to surfaces. Beyond this, the molecular configuration of such structures, namely the proteins constituting flagella and pili, is presently an object of investigation. Understanding of the stability and interactions of such proteins, such as covalent cross-linking of FlgE in the hook of the flagellum, is already revealing the underlying mechanisms of bacterial versatility and motility. Broadly, the specific structures of flagella and pili are just part of the greater concepts of bacterial genetics and structure, interlacing the physical and genetic machinery whereby these organisms are able to thrive (Cockayne et al., 2014) (Figure 5.7).

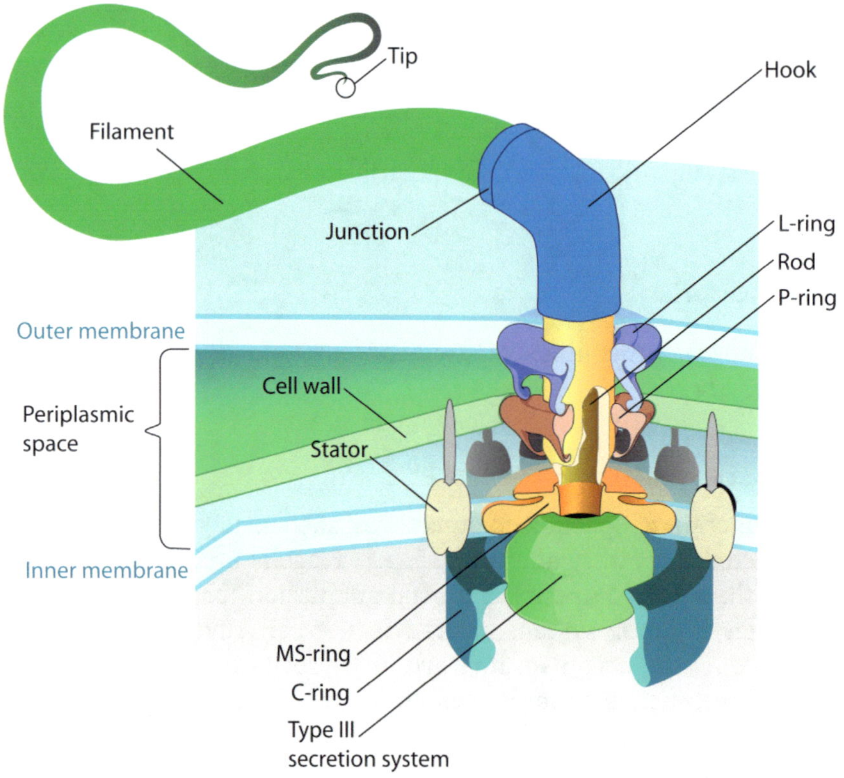

Figure 5.7. Structure of bacterial flagellum.

Source: https://upload.wikimedia.org/wikipedia/commons/thumb/4/40/Flagellum_base_diagram-en.svg/1024px-Flagellum_base_diagram-en.svg.png.

Test Your Knowledge

1. What are the common shapes of bacteria, and how are these shapes classified?
2. What is the structure and function of bacterial flagella, and how do they contribute to bacterial motility?
3. What roles do pili play in bacterial cells, and how do they differ from flagella?

5.3. Genetic Material in Bacteria

Learning Outcome

1. Understand the structure of bacterial DNA
2. Explain plasmids and their role in genetic diversity
3. Compare between bacterial and eukaryotic genetic material

The bacterial genetic material is composed mainly of deoxyribonucleic acid (DNA), which is different from that in eukaryotic organisms. DNA in prokaryotic cells is in the form of one circular chromosome that resides in an area called the nucleoid. The structural arrangement provides for effective regulation and replication mechanisms that are necessary in the rapid growth characteristic of bacterial life. Watson and Crick's DNA model is responsible for elucidating the double helix shape, in which the complementary base pair basis of genetic fidelity on replication is emphasized. Each DNA strand is a template for the synthesis of its complement, where genetic information is copied and inherited correctly. This intrinsic property of DNA not only facilitates the transmission of characteristics but is also behind the process of genetic variation by mutation and horizontal gene transfer, thus a pivotal process in bacterial evolution and adaptation (Horowitz et al., 1954). In addition to the chromosomal DNA, a majority of bacteria have extrachromosomal DNA structures known as plasmids. These DNA molecules that are ring-shaped can vary in size and typically will carry genes that provide extra advantages to the host bacteria, , such as resistance against antibiotics or toxin production. Plasmids play an important role in the flexibility of bacteria because genes can be exchanged among cells through mechanisms like conjugation, transformation, or transduction. This horizontal gene transfer mechanism plays a significant role in spreading traits quickly within bacterial populations that demonstrate the dynamic nature of bacterial genetics. Also, some types of plasmids that integrate into chromosomal DNA result in the development of new functions and metabolic capabilities, thereby enhancing the adaptation possibilities of bacteria in different habitats (Boutry et al., 2008). Bacterial genetic material not only consists of chromosomal and plasmid DNA but also mobile genetic components like transposons and insertion sequences. These play an important role in the enablement of genetic diversity and versatility among bacterial populations. Transposons can move from one locus to another within the genome, perhaps altering gene expression and allowing the development of antibiotic resistance. Their ability to undergo genomic rearrangements underscores the flexibility of bacterial genetics and the selective forces exercised by stresses from the environment and therapeutic intervention. Since bacteria evolve constantly in response to selective pressures, understanding these genetic events is required for effective treatment design and management of antibiotic resistance. Overall, the complex interaction of various forms of genetic material in bacteria illustrates the complexity of their genetic structure and the interactive nature of their genetic landscape (Horowitz et al., 1954).

5.3.1. Structure of Bacterial DNA

The structure of bacterial DNA is largely characterized by its unique double-stranded configuration, which differs sharply from the linear eukaryotic organism DNA. Bacterial DNA typically resides in a single, circular chromosome that is compacted in the nucleoid region of the cell. This allows maximum genetic information storage as well as ensuring that essential genes become readily available during replication and transcription events. Moreover, the close packaging allows for swift adaptation and survival of bacteria in fluctuating environments. Understanding this structure is valuable since it illuminates scientists regarding prokaryotic gene expression and regulation processes, which could be divergent from eukaryotic systems, to offer insights into genetic engineering and synthetic biology applications. Other than the single circular chromosome, most bacteria also possess plasmids—small, circular DNA molecules that can replicate autonomously. Plasmids are typically known to possess genes that confer advantageous traits, , such as antibiotic resistance, which is a prevalent issue in public health. The presence of plasmids introduces a second tier of genetic diversity that allows bacterial populations to evolve at a high rate in response to selective pressures like antibiotic treatment. This figure is most relevant while considering the extrapolation to pathogen control, as disease-causing bacteria tend to mobilize plasmids in order to acquire and disseminate resistance genes through mechanisms of lateral gene transfer. The dynamic interaction between chromosomal and plasmid DNA is the essence of bacterial genetics and survival strategies to successfully exist in environments.

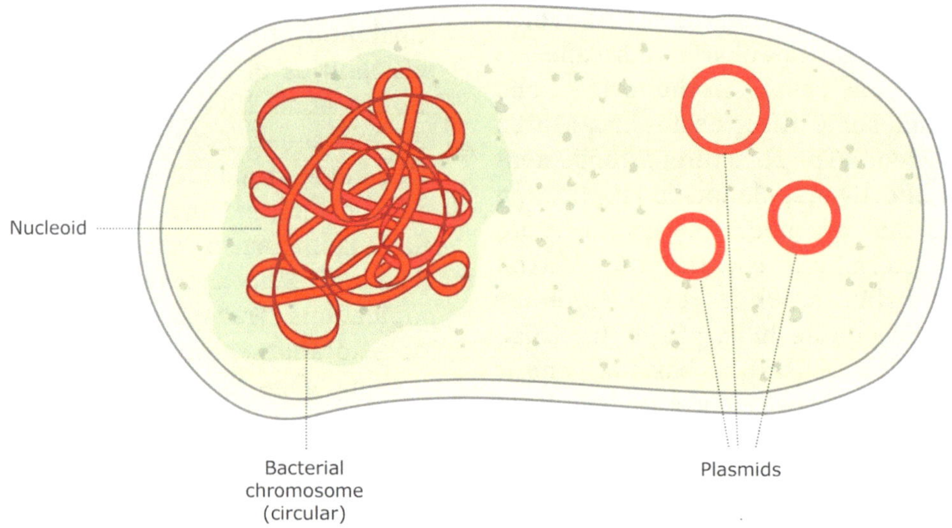

Figure 5.8. Bacterial DNA.

Source: https://www.sciencelearn.org.nz/_next/image?url=https%3A%2F%2Fwww.datocms-assets.com%2F117510%2F1722387675-enzymes_bacterialdna.jpg%3Fw%3D1840%26h%3D920&w=1920&q=85&dpl=dpl_3rhusQfrbXYfrm8BSLwuTDgVSr8n.

Moreover, the topological organization of bacterial DNA is a critical determinant of its functional potential. DNA's supercoiling allows for tighter packaging, facilitating more effective arrangement of genetic material within the dense cellular regime of bacteria. This structural manipulation aids not only the physical shielding of DNA but is also critical for gene expression control. Supercoiling can regulate the accessibility of certain genes, influencing the transcriptional machinery's ability to initiate gene expression. As seen in studies of pathogenic microbes, the supercoiling dynamic is significant for defining how bacteria adapt to respond to environmental stresses and adjust to changing conditions, thus giving insight into broader evolutionary tendencies within the microbial community (Hofvander et al., 2004; Emmett & Rabadan, 2014) (Figure 5.8).

5.3.2. Plasmids and Their Role in Genetic Diversity

Plasmids are central to bacterial genetic diversity because they serve as gene transfer vehicles between strains and species. They are extrachromosomal DNA molecules that can potentially transport a range of genes, including those that confer antibiotic resistance, virulence determinants, and metabolic capabilities. The ability of plasmids to self-replicate independently of the bacterial chromosome allows for a rapid spread of beneficial traits, particularly under conditions of selective pressure, , such as the presence of antibiotics. Plasmid transmission is often facilitated by processes , such as conjugation and transduction, which facilitate horizontal gene transfer (HGT), thereby enhancing genetic diversity in bacterial populations. Here, plasmid research not only highlights their importance in bacterial adaptation but also their contribution to the creation of new strains that have the ability to escape treatment and control measures(Haaber et al., 2017).

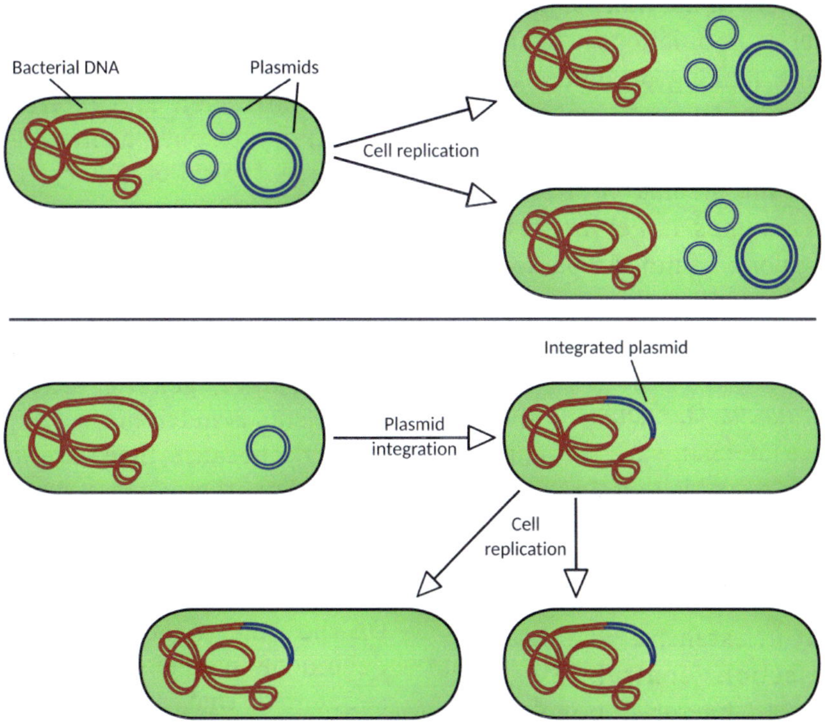

Figure 5.9. There are two types of plasmid integration into a host bacterium: Non-integrating plasmids replicate as with the top instance, whereas episomes, the lower example, can integrate into the host chromosome.

Source: https://upload.wikimedia.org/wikipedia/commons/thumb/4/42/Plasmid_replication_%28english%29.svg/1024px-Plasmid_replication_%28english%29.svg.png.

Structural plasmid diversity has a very significant contribution towards the evolutionary dynamics of bacterial populations. Plasmids are extremely diverse and changeable in size, so as to their origin and function as well, for some plasmids there are genes essential for the survival of those bacteria that live in specific environments, e.g., plasmids that enable nitrogen fixation in rhizobia. For instance, the vast amount of DNA within *Sinorhizobium meliloti* up to 45% of its genome indicates the diversity. Multiplicity of several plasmids assists the bacterium to adapt to changing conditions and form symbiotic associations with legumes. Interestingly, the conjugative character of most plasmids assists in the transfer of favorable traits across species and contributes to genetic diversity. Such complexity is particularly pertinent in the wake of the rapid response of bacterial populations to changes in the environment, making plasmids critical parameters in ecological and evolutionary studies (Lagares et al., 2014). Moreover, the role of plasmids in the mediation of bacterial genetic diversity assumes larger importance in the context of public health. As pathogenic bacteria acquire plasmids carrying antibiotic resistance genes, the prognosis in terms of treatment becomes unfavorable. In bacteria, such as *Staphylococcus aureus*, the ability to quickly develop resistance mechanisms through the mechanism of plasmid acquisition threatens the effectiveness of existing antibiotics. It has been established through studies that mechanisms, such as conjugation and transduction have the potential to result in extensive gene transfer, complicating infection control. By their multiplication within bacterial populations, these mobile genetic elements create a situation with rapidly evolving genetic patterns that are resistant to traditional treatment approaches. It is crucial to understand mechanisms of plasmid-mediated gene transfer and their significance for bacterial genetics in order to come up with new approaches towards inhibiting the development of antibiotic-resistant pathogens (Haaber et al., 2017) (Figure 5.9).

5.3.3. Comparison with Eukaryotic Genetic Material

The distinction between bacterial and eukaryotic genetic material is marked by enormous structural, organizational, and functional dissimilarities that emphasize the divergent evolution of these two lines of life. Bacterial genomes are found in a single circular chromosome, usually with additional smaller plasmids, that may contain additional genetic information that can encode for advantageous traits , such as antibiotic resistance. On the other hand, eukaryotic DNA is condensed into a number of linear chromosomes within a membrane-bound nucleus. Such compartmentalization allows for eukaryotic gene expression and interaction to a larger regulatory extent, facilitating diverse cellular activities typical of eukaryotes but uncommon in prokaryotes. Since bacteria lack this nuclear organization, they have paired transcription and translation in order to respond to environmental cues instantly, a big difference from the distinct transcription and translation in eukaryotic cells. Furthermore, genetic content in eukaryotic organisms is much more complicated, and that is partly because there are introns present in genes. Eukaryotic genes typically contain non-coding introns breaking up coding sequences, which need a sophisticated splicing process in RNA processing to produce functional mRNA. On the other hand, bacterial genes are often devoid of introns, having continuous coding sequences that are translated directly into proteins without splicing. This spartan genomic architecture results in greater gene expression efficiency in bacteria, allowing them to adapt quickly to new surroundings. In eukaryotes, complex organization of regulatory sequences and introns results in a higher degree of genetic regulation, which is crucial to the formation of multicellular organisms with advanced structures, allowing specialized function in various tissue types. These differences have implications beyond structural differences; they may influence evolutionary dynamics and adaptability between eukaryotic and bacterial organisms. For instance, bacteria can pass on genetic information via horizontal gene transfer, which, under selective pressure, , such as from antibiotic treatment, can increase exponentially genetic variation and adaptability. This is a divergence from the vertical inheritance of eukaryotes, which is mainly seen, with genetic change happening mainly through mutation and recombination during sexual reproduction. Such diversity is encoded in their genomic structures, e.g., recent research indicating long-range variations in guanine-cytosine content (GC%) of eukaryotic genomes that could reveal evolutionary forces shaping genetic stability and variation, as discussed in (Bernardi et al., 2004). Understanding these genetic variations not only enhances our appreciation of bacterial diversity but also directs the development of specificity-based therapeutic applications that exploit these variations in the treatment of bacterial infection rather than eukaryotic disease.

Test Your Knowledge

1. What is the structure of bacterial DNA, and how is it organized within the bacterial cell?
2. What are plasmids, and how do they contribute to genetic diversity in bacterial populations?

5.4. Bacterial Reproduction

Learning Outcome

1. Understand the concept of asexual bacterial reproduction through binary fission
2. Describe genetic exchange mechanisms
3. Discuss the impact of reproduction on bacterial evolution

Bacterial growth is mostly defined by binary fission, a process where a bacterial cell of single nature splits into two daughter cells that are identical to each other. This process is useful for the rapid expansion of populations, which enables bacteria to survive in various environments. Each division usually happens every 20 minutes under ideal conditions and results in exponential growth that can rapidly consume available resources. Genetic material is precisely duplicated during this process so that every new cell inherits a complete copy of the parent genome. The simplicity of binary fission also works to highlight the simple nature of bacterial structure, in which the absence of sophisticated mitotic equipment is compensated for by efficient replication and segregation of genetic material. This rapid replicating strategy is one of the principal mechanisms of bacterial evolution and adaptability and facilitates rapid adaptation to environmental stress and the creation of genetic diversity by mutation and horizontal gene transfer. Genetic exchange between populations of bacteria is significant in their evolutionary mechanisms. Although binary fission dominates bacterial reproduction, mechanisms like transformation, conjugation, and transduction create genetic diversity. Transformation involves the uptake of free DNA from the environment, which allows bacteria to acquire new traits through cell lysis. Conjugation, in the majority of instances facilitated by plasmids, involves cell-to-cell contact and guarantees the transfer of genetic information between two bacteria. Transduction is a process through which bacteriophages transmit DNA from bacterial cell to bacterial cell. These mechanisms augment the genetic machinery involved in adapting, more crucial when bacterial populations are subject to selective pressures, such as antibiotic resistance. For instance, the operation of these processes of genetic transfer enables bacteria to rapidly evolve mechanisms that ensure their survival and growth, not only in terms of structure, but also ecologically within niches. The connected relationships between bacterial reproduction and environmental fitness underscore the importance of gene regulation and evolutionary rates of mutation for bacteria. It has been discovered that scaling gene content in prokaryotic genomes not only reflects differences in lifestyle but also adaptations energized by spontaneous mutation rates and evolutionary pressures. The RAevol model has clarified that such scaling laws arise from selective pressures for robustness, which ultimately decide bacterial genome size and architecture (Adami et al., 2010). Moreover, the role of virus satellites, i.e., staphylococcal pathogenicity islands (SaPIs), illustrates the complexity of host-virus interactions in bacterial reproduction. Such satellites are capable of exerting selective pressures on helper viruses to favor coevolution and genetic variation in bacterial populations (Buckling et al., 2015). Such evolutionary dynamics indicate not only the plasticity of bacteria but also have great bearing in uncovering bacterial structure and genetics in a rapidly changing environment.

5.4.1. Asexual Reproduction Through Binary Fission

Asexual reproduction through binary fission is a simple mechanism in which bacteria make copies of their genetic material and replicate successfully. Asexual reproduction enables one bacterial cell to divide into two daughter cells, both genetically the same. Before division, the bacterium's DNA is replicated and each of the daughter cells obtains a complete set of genetic information. This is a mechanism preferred in dynamic settings where population growth is crucial for survival. The rapid transmission of genetic material by binary fission demonstrates the spartan nature of bacterial genomes, which tend to be a single circular chromosome with no major non-coding regions. This sparseness is indicative of how bacterial structure is bound closely to their reproductive processes, such that rapid adaptation and evolutionary rebound can be achieved against ecological pressures. Its high efficiency is a critical contributing factor to the rapid population growth typical of bacterial species. Bacteria double with extremely short doubling times, often within 20 minutes, given optimal conditions for growth. The exponential increase has the capability of swift colonizing suitable niches, outcompeting other organisms. But with its mode of reproduction are certain constraints. Mutations can occur during DNA replication and introduce genetic variation even in so-called identical offspring. More significantly, even in controlled conditions, around 10% of the *E. coli* cultures exhibit size and volume variation following binary fission, indicating the presence of random manufacturing defects even under homogeneous replication conditions (Bois et al., 2019). Thus, while binary fission ensures rapid reproduction of bacteria, it also allows for genetic diversity to ensure adaptation. Acknowledging the implications of binary fission and its resultant genetic diversity becomes critical if we take a look at evolutionary patterns and population dynamics. Asexual reproduction by this method can have consequences for larger ecological and evolutionary processes, especially if acted upon by environmental forces. For instance, in the face of abrupt change, the rapid doubling by binary fission can lead to wholesale changes in community composition and ecosystem structure as bacteria stream into new areas to exploit resources before others are able to move. Investigations of such dynamics become more critical in the face of Anthropocene Epoch conditions, when human activity alters environmental conditions on a significant scale. Evolutionary biology and physics understanding, as indicated in recent research, aims to explain potential pathways of bacterial response during epochs of extinction and recovery periods, with reference to the multifaceted interaction between bacterial form, genetics, and their role in regulating ecological stability (King et al., 2015) (Figure 5.10).

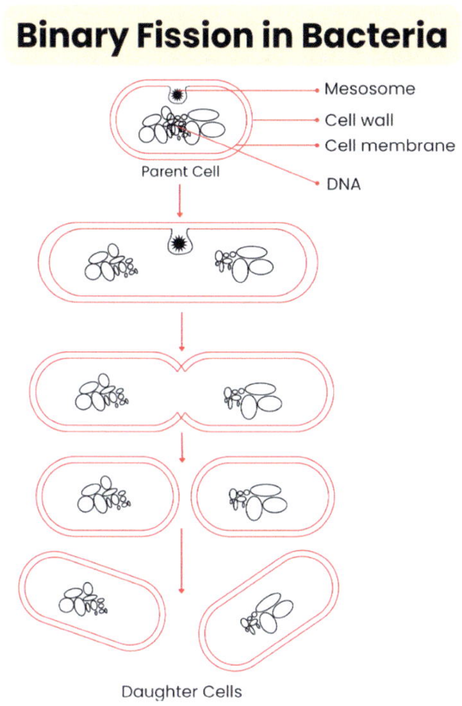

Figure 5.10. Binary fission in bacteria.

Source: https://www.vedantu.com/seo/content-images/28212b8d-5ee8-4d81-a002-8925dd8f15fd_1.png.

5.4.2. Genetic Exchange Mechanisms: Transformation, Transduction, and Conjugation

In bacterial genetics, transformation, transduction, and conjugation are three main mechanisms of genetic exchange. All these methods are crucial in the maintenance of genetic variation in bacteria populations to allow them to evolve and adapt to environmental factors. Transformation is achieved through free uptake of DNA by a competent cell from the environment, which could lead to a change in the phenotype. This activity is an example of how bacteria acquire useful traits, , such as resistance to antibiotics, from their environment rather than being accomplished by virtue of vertical gene transfer. Transformention aids bacterial evolution and adaptation to hostile environments significantly through the promotion of genetic diversity. Transduction is yet another important genetic transfer process involving bacteriophages, which are viruses that infect bacteria. In the process, a bacteriophage can transfer genetic material from one host bacterium to another in error while replicating. Horizontal gene transfer in this way aids in the transmission of genes encoding virulence or antibiotic resistance. Recent studies have placed greater importance on the process of transduction in transmitting genes, particularly between pathogens , such as *Staphylococcus aureus*.

This microbe has some excellent adaptations since it can inherit antibiotic resistance genes, demonstrating just how efficient transduction is as a mechanism of genetic transfer, especially in medical usage, where time is a factor (Haaber et al., 2017). Conjugation, the third genetic exchange process, is unique in that cell-to-cell contact is necessary and the transferring of plasmids; circle-shaped DNA molecules that typically carry genes responsible for antibiotic resistance. Through the production of a pilus, one bacterium can attach to another and share genetic material. This type of process is particularly significant in environments with high selective pressure because rapid dissemination of resistance traits becomes possible. The intricacies of the process of conjugation highlight the evolutionary advantage bestowed on bacteria capable of effectively transferring desirable genes. With the increasing complexity of microbial communities, understanding such mechanisms of genetic exchange is essential in formulating methods to overcome antibiotic resistance and improve public health outcomes (Milka et al., 2018).

5.4.3. Impact of Reproduction on Bacterial Evolution

The reproductive methods utilized by bacteria have a substantial impact on the evolutionary course of these microorganisms, and they are of vital importance in the adaptation and survival of the microbes. Prokaryotic reproduction mainly involves binary fission, which is a process of rapidly dividing cells to produce two genetically similar cells. This asexual form allows for the quick growth of populations and serves as a powerful method for the spread of beneficial characters in a population. However, the lack of genetic recombination with this type of reproduction can limit gene variety. In order to balance this limitation, many bacteria engage in horizontal gene transfer (HGT) so that new genetic information can be obtained from other organisms. This two-way system of reproduction not only facilitates the passing on of adaptive characteristics but also the development of new functions, thereby setting the evolutionary landscape within bacterial populations. Moreover, the relationship of reproductive processes with environmental stressors carries strong implications for bacterial evolution. In fluctuating environments, the ability of bacteria to reproduce asexually but also share genetic information through HGT allows for rapid adaptation to selective pressures. For example, studies have indicated that in the instance of staphylococcal pathogenicity islands (SaPIs), helper viruses develop rapidly to become immune to their satellite counterparts, an indication of a co-evolutionary arms race that promotes genetic innovation and responsiveness (Buckling et al., 2015). Such an interaction identifies that bacterial reproduction is more than mere survival; it is intricately related to ecological interaction and evolutionary pressure that can accelerate rapid genetic change. Thus, the action of reproduction on evolution must be viewed as an integrative dynamics between intrinsic biological mechanisms and environmental extrinsic forces. Second, the evolutionary path of bacterial reproduction must highlight the movement away from interspecies sharing of genetic materials towards individual vertical transmission. It is contended that early organisms had been relying heavily on HGT to develop a shared genetic environment where the traits would easily be traded among organisms.

Over time, selective pressures may have favored the evolution of more individuated reproduction approaches for greater stability and specialisation in bacterial lineages (Arnoldt et al., 2015). This transition marks an important juncture in microbial evolution because it provides a foundation for present-day bacterial diversity. In evolving to their environment, prokaryotes' reproduction approaches shape their short-term survival but also determine long-term evolutionary trajectories. Comprehending the intricacies of bacterial reproduction will ultimately shed light on microbial persistence and the constant, dynamic evolution of these microbes in an ever-evolving world (Figure 5.11).

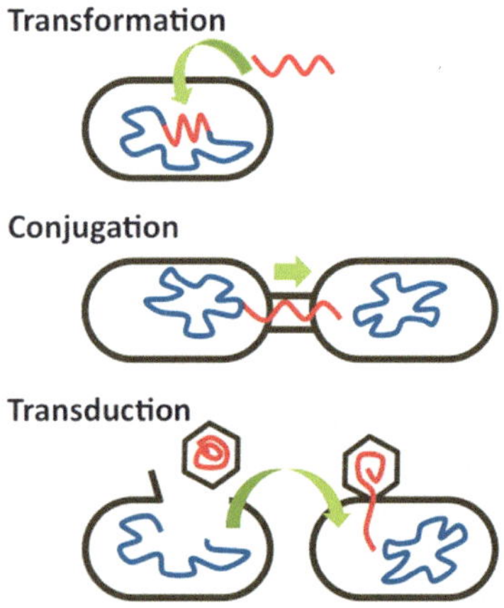

Figure 5.11. Mechanisms of bacterial horizontal gene transfer (HGT).

Source: https://www.researchgate.net/publication/280584808/figure/fig1/AS:324966294802456@1454489410517/Mechanisms-of-bacterial-horizontal-gene-transfer.png.

Test Your Knowledge

1. How does binary fission occur in bacteria, and what are the main stages involved in this process?
2. What are the different mechanisms of genetic exchange in bacteria, , such as transformation, transduction, and conjugation?

5.5. Gene Regulation in Bacteria

Learning Outcome

1. Describe operons and their function
2. Understand environmental factors influencing gene expression
3. Discuss the role of regulatory proteins in gene control

Gene expression in bacteria is a critical process that enables bacteria to adapt to fluctuating environmental conditions efficiently. Based on various systems , such as transcription factors, operons, and promoter regions, bacterial genes are regulated, allowing for the coordinated expression of a set of genes. An example is the lac operon. It regulates lactose metabolism in *Escherichia coli*. When lactose is present, it's attached to the repressor protein, allowing transcription of genes involved in lactose use. This flexibility shows the manner in which gene regulation is not only a means of biological regulation but also a response to changes in nutrient availability, demonstrating the evolutionary advantage offered by such mechanisms. Also, an understanding of these regulatory processes can provide information on more abstract principles of genetic adaptation, situating this fundamental concept within the context of bacterial structure and genetics. On a molecular level, bacterial gene regulation is shaped by many intrinsic and extrinsic factors that underlie the intricacy of gene expression. Experiments have shown that gene expression is susceptible to random fluctuation, causing variation in protein production among genetically similar organisms. The phenomenon, which has been termed "phenotypic noise," emphasizes the importance of regulation in ensuring gene expression stability. Significantly, variations may be caused by processes related to transcription and translation, with some regions of promoters playing a vital role in the level of noise. Experiments conducted in *E. coli* showed that essential genes and highly evolutionarily conserved genes possess promoters that maintain lower phenotypic noise, hence keeping essential cell functions under stable high performance. These findings suggest that natural selection can target gene expression noise, further solidifying the role of regulatory elements in the evolutionary trajectory of bacterial populations (Arkin et al., 2012). One of the intriguing aspects of bacterial regulation of genes is the dualistic nature of stability and adaptability as revealed through the scaling properties of their genome. The existing models, , such as the RAevol model, have begun to uncover the mechanisms of scaling of the genome and regulatory network complexities. These analyses suggest that scaling laws evident in the gene content of bacteria are not simply an expression of the divergent lifestyles but are more fundamentally connected to spontaneous rates of mutation and selective pressures for genome stability. During their movement through their habitats, scaling properties help us understand how modifications in the size and organization of the genome influence gene regulation. Therefore, a grasp of gene regulation's relationship to genome structure can illuminate the mechanisms of evolution by which bacteria thrive in disparate ecological niches, and also assist in the association between their structural genetics and regulatory systems (Adami et al., 2010).

5.5.1. Operons and Their Function

An operon is a fundamental concept in the regulation and expression of genes in prokaryotes, the hallmark of prokaryotic genetics. An operon refers to a cluster of genes that are transcribed together with the assistance of a shared promoter, which facilitates coordinated expression of functionally related genes. Such an organization is extremely cost-efficient for the bacteria since it permits coordinated protein production of proteins that belong to the same metabolic pathway or are activated by environmental signals. A good example is the *E. coli* lac operon, where genes for lactose metabolism are organized as a group in order to optimize resource utilization according to lactose concentration.

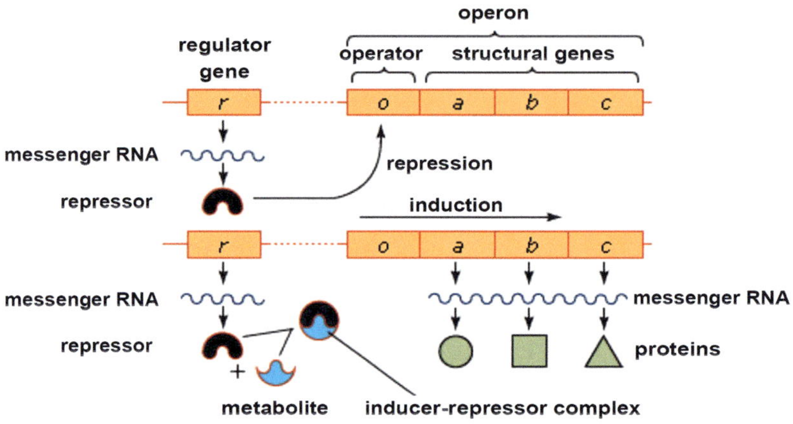

Figure 5.12. Model of the operon and its relation to the regulator gene.

Source: https://cdn.britannica.com/81/781-004-CA10795E/Model-operon-relation-regulator-gene.jpg?w=400&h=300&c=crop.

These systems show the flexibility of bacterial cells to rapidly adapt to changing environments without the need for intricate regulatory systems, thus demonstrating their efficiency in evolution. Operons are controlled by various mechanisms such that the genes are expressed only when the cell requires them. In the case of the lac operon, lactose availability leads to repression of a repressor protein, allowing RNA polymerase to bind and initiate transcription. But when there is no lactose, the repressor still occupies the operator site, inhibiting transcription. This toggle-like character indicates the operon's flexibility and thrift in resource utilization. Further, operon research has broad implications in bacterial adaptation and survival processes, as can be seen from experimental evolution studies. For instance, in *Pseudomonas* fluorescens, the formation of the Wrinkly Spreader mutant gives evidence regarding how alterations in the regulatory network mutational changes can enhance fitness through operon-like structure, whereby groups of genes work together to exploit new ecological niches and resources (Spiers et al., 2014). The genetic basis of operons also extends beyond regulation of transcription; it gives insight into evolutionary associations between bacteria.

Operons can have very long evolutionary histories, with conserved regions indicating common ancestry and functional homologies between different bacterial populations. The study of magnetotactic bacteria (MTB) provides an intriguing setting to study operon dynamics, particularly in the context of biomineralization. MTB possess specific operons that regulate the formation of magnetosomes, organelles that are pivotal in their magnetic navigation system (KOMEILI et al., 2020). By investigating the genetic architectures that control operon function in MTB, researchers gain profound insight into biochemical pathways and their evolutionary convergences, illuminating the intricate web of relationships between bacterial structure, genetics, and ecological success. The research into operons, therefore, not only expands our understanding of bacterial functions but also offers a vehicle through which the evolutionary processes of adaptation can be studied (Figure 5.12).

5.5.2. Environmental Factors Influencing Gene Expression

Environmental factors have a significant role in regulating the expression of genes in bacteria, a function that is central to their explanation of adaptability and survival. A number of external parameters, , such as temperature, pH, and availability of nutrients, can affect the processes of transcription and translation, leading to different phenotypic effects among genetically close organisms. This heterogeneity is crucial for the bacteria that are exposed to different environments. For instance, mutations within the promoter parts of some genes may give rise to different levels of protein synthesis, which sum up to so-called "phenotypic noise." Studies on *Escherichia coli* reveal that genes for vital functions have promoters with lower noise levels, and it is suggested that natural selection will favor stability in vital gene expression under environmental stress (Arkin et al., 2012). By gaining insight into how bacteria regulate their genetic responses to environmental cues, we can better understand their evolutionary strategies. Gene-environment interaction can also be viewed with the multifactorial disease paradigm of inflammatory bowel disease (IBD). While IBD has a dominant genetic component, host environmental factors, including diet and microbial exposure, interact with host genetic factors influencing susceptibility and disease progression. Current evidence is directed towards the contribution of specific genes, , such as NOD2/CARD15, which are not only implicated in genetic susceptibility but also mediate host responses to extrinsic environmental stimuli that can trigger IBD attacks. Because bacteria are a central element of gut environments, the way in which bacteria adapt the expression of their genes in response to genetic as well as extragenetic stimuli can tell us about disease and therapeutic processes (Fischer et al., 2006). The dual control of this indicates the necessity for adding environmental components to genetics research, especially that involving microbial pathogenesis. Further, environmental regulation of gene expression is not dissociable from the very principles of evolutionary biology. The ability of bacteria to change their environment through modulation of gene expression is a reflection of the interactive nature of genetics in response to external pressures. As external pressures exert their influence, bacteria may undergo epigenetic changes, allowing them to adjust quickly without altering the underlying genetic code. The capacity for environmental control of gene expression not only ensures survival in adverse conditions but also facilitates ecological diversification. Demonstration of this plasticity is provided by phenotypic variation between bacterial populations that are able to grow and survive in individualized environments by varying their genetic response to conformity. Hence, unraveling the mechanisms of environmental regulation of gene expression is central to comprehension of the complex interaction between bacterial architecture, genetics, and adaptation (Figure 5.13).

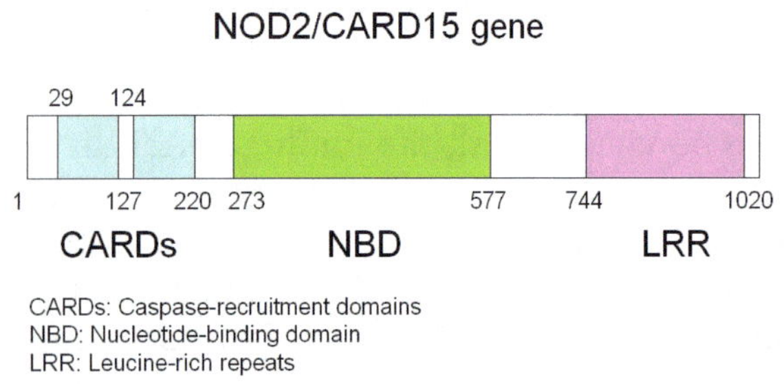

Figure 5.13. NOD2/CARD15 gene.

Source: https://upload.wikimedia.org/wikipedia/en/3/33/NOD2_CARD15.jpg.

5.5.3. Role of Regulatory Proteins in Gene Control

The complex processes of gene regulation in bacteria are primarily regulated by the activity of regulatory proteins, which are central in regulating the expression of genes for different physiological functions. These proteins, , such as transcription factors and repressors, react to environmental signals that enable bacteria to quickly adjust to changing environments. Effective regulation of gene expression is crucial to survival, particularly in dynamic environments where resources are limited or in stressed conditions. Regulatory proteins control promoter activity or act on the RNA polymerase to activate or suppress transcription and thereby regulate the production of proteins essential to growth and metabolism. This sophisticated regulatory system serves to emphasize the plasticity of bacterial systems, enabling them to adapt and succeed within their environments as they utilize many different niches. Post-transcriptional control as a means of gene expression is a significant factor within this regulatory environment. Proteins not only regulate at the transcriptional level but also become involved in the fine-tuning of mRNA stability and translation. For instance, small non-coding RNAs (sRNAs) can interact with messenger RNA to either regulate its degradation or the efficacy of translation, thereby being pivotal in gene expression regulation post-transcriptionally. Such interaction allows for rapid response to environmental stimuli without the need for novel transcription. Regulatory mechanisms using such sRNAs show an additional complexity to the regulation of bacterial gene expression, an instance of the multidimensional approaches through which bacteria regulate their gene expression machinery operationally. One of the best illustrations of regulatory protein regulation is in the regulation of *Salmonella enterica* pathogenicity island I (SPI-1) genes, vital to the bacteria's ability to invade epithelial cells. Expression of SPI-1 genes is tightly regulated and induced in controlled conditions, exhibiting a strategic adaptation mechanism. Experimental proof indicated that the silencing of SPI-1 gene expression during non-permissive conditions involves the CRP-cAMP complex. Significantly, the regulatory protein HilD, the invasion master regulator of Salmonella, is controlled by CRP-cAMP, indicating the determinant role of regulating networks in bacteria. This exchange shows the part that regulatory proteins have in the heavily regulated modulation of gene expression, which dictates bacterial activity and virulence and thereby makes regulatory proteins a necessity within bacterial architecture and genetics (Adami et al., 2010; Balsalobre et al., 2018).

Test Your Knowledge

1. What is an operon, and how does it regulate gene expression in bacteria?
2. What environmental factors can influence bacterial gene expression, and how do bacteria respond to these changes?
3. What roles do regulatory proteins , such as repressors and activators play in controlling bacterial genes?

5.6. Applications of Bacterial Genetics

Learning Outcome

1. Understand the use of bacteria in biotechnology
2. Explain the role of bacteria in medicine and antibiotic resistance
3. Discuss bacterial genetics in environmental science

Bacterial genetics has relevance in a number of applications beyond basic scientific research, having serious impacts on medicine, biotechnology, and the environment. Scientists can design genetically modified organisms (GMOs) to generate significant drugs , such as insulin and vaccines, through the manipulation of bacterial genes. These technologies are particularly worth their while in the context of escalating worldwide health demands, where standard drug development lead times become intolerable. By applying genetic engineering techniques like gene cloning and expression systems, microorganisms may be engineered to produce complex biological molecules more efficiently than could be otherwise accomplished by traditional methods. Thus, understanding bacterial genetics not only enhances our capability in medicine but also points to the significance of these microbes as a tool of innovation in the biotechnology sector (Seaman & Whitehouse, 2001). Moreover, advances in advanced genomic technologies have propelled bacterial genetics into areas of possibility heretofore unimaginable. Technologies , such as CRISPR/Cas9 have revolutionized the ability of scientists to edit genes with unprecedented precision, enabling opportunities for gene therapy and disease modeling. Bacterial systems have been particularly important for manipulating and assaying these genome editing tools, acting as platforms for the examination of genetic function and interactions. As researchers continue to fine-tune such methodologies, the potential for increasing agricultural sustainability and food security by genetically modifying bacteria becomes increasingly valid. Bacterial genetics knowledge lies at the heart of designing crops that are more resilient to environmental stress and insects and thus can protect sources of food as the population of the world continues to grow (Beccari et al., 2017). Aside from agriculture and medicine, bacterial genetics also has applications in environmental cleanup and biotechnology. Bacteria can be genetically modified to degrade contaminants and hence, are extremely valuable in bioremediation activities. The ability to engineer bacteria with favorable metabolic pathways allows scientists to harness them for the cleanup of oil spills, heavy metal contamination, and other hazardous wastes. Moreover, genetically modified microbes can be applied to enable sustainable use by recycling waste into biofuels or other useful substrates. On the one hand, the ongoing development of methods and knowledge in bacterial genetics not only facilitates ecological sustainability but also illustrates the interconnection between various scientific disciplines. Therefore, the uses of bacterial genetics highlight its critical significance in the resolution of some of the greatest challenges human society confronts today (Seaman & Whitehouse, 2001).

5.6.1. Use of Bacteria in Biotechnology

The use of bacteria in biotechnology is an outstanding intersection of microbiology with genetic engineering in which the natural ability of these microorganisms is exploited for biotechnological applications. Bacteria are focal points in this cutting-edge sector because of their ease, quick growth rates, and universality of environments for adaptation. Genetic manipulation methods make it possible for researchers to alter bacterial genomes to make them even more functional for biotechnological applications. For instance, techniques , such as CRISPR-Cas9 have enabled the insertion or excision of genetic material in ways previously unheard of, and genetically modified bacteria have been engineered that can produce essential compounds like insulin, growth hormones, and even biofuels. This vast potential renders bacteria valuable instruments for addressing global issues in the realms of health care and energy sustainability. Furthermore, bacterias function extends to medical and energy applications, serving beneficially in agricultural biotechnology. Genetic engineering of bacteria has led to the development of biofertilizers and biopesticides, which enhance sustainable agriculture at lower environmental costs and higher yields. Use of nitrogen-fixing bacteria or pesticide-degrading bacteria improves agriculture to be more environmentally friendly and cost-effective. Besides, biotechnology utilizes bacteria to produce primary nutrients, , such as vitamins and amino acids, that can be used directly to improve food security. This advancement of biotechnological strategies highlights the importance of studying bacterial genetics, particularly with the world facing growing food production challenges in the context of a growing population. The research on marine bacteria also further highlights the multiple applications of these bacteria to biotechnology. Recent studies have identified particular genetic features in marine bacteria that may lead to the generation of new compounds and enzymes of potential therapeutic use. The microorganisms not only have relevance with their functional implications to the functions of marine ecosystems, but are now also at the focus of biotechnological interest due to their ability to provide bioactive products of pharmaceutical value. As implied by recent surveys of research on marine biotechnology, making coordination among industry and academia easier can promote the transfer of this knowledge to applied situations, enabling the optimal potential of marine biodiversity to be realized in health and industrial applications (Seaman & Whitehouse, 2001; Toenniessen et al., 2001). Continuous focus on learning about bacterial structure and genetics will lead to such innovations, promising a future in which bacteria play a role in solving complex problems in technology and sustainability (Figure 5.14).

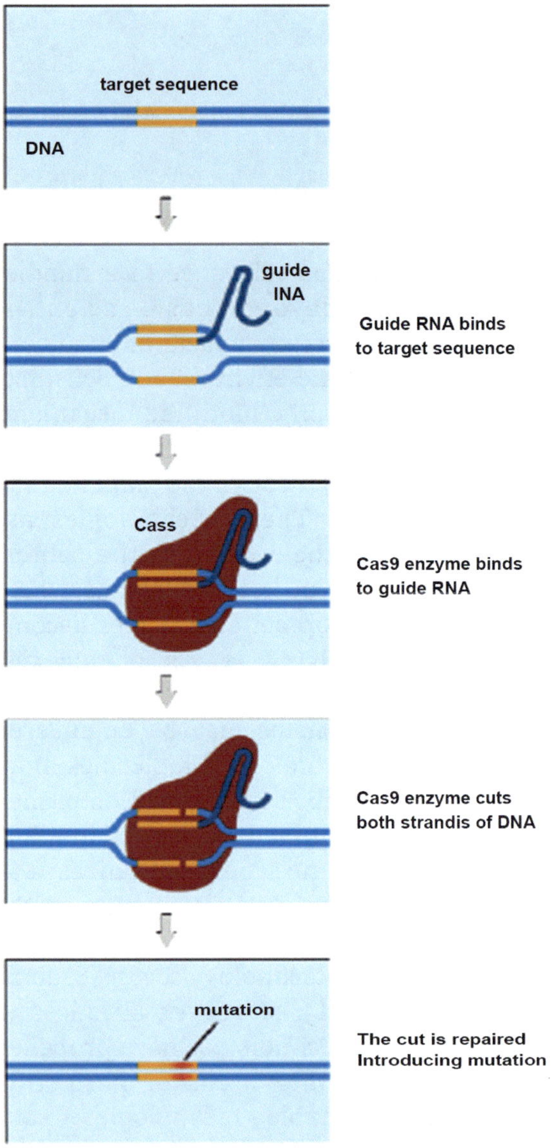

Figure 5.14. Diagram showing how the CRISPR-Cas9 editing tool works.

Source: https://www.yourgenome.org/wp-content/uploads/2023/12/1301-CRISPR-in-action-372x768.png.

5.6.2. Role of Bacteria in Medicine and Antibiotic Resistance

The increasing use of bacteria in medicine has gained significance with researchers exploring their possible utilization aside from pathology, in this instance, combating antibiotic resistance. Historically, antibiotics have been the pillar of contemporary medicine, effectively curing an assortment of bacterial infections. The development of antibiotic-resistant strains, however, has presented an enormous challenge and prompted a re-examination of how such microorganisms are conceptualized and utilized. As the disease has increasingly developed resistance, it has become possible to make new therapeutic strategies that attack not only the bacteria themselves but also the processes that cause them to be resistant. An understanding of bacterial structure and genetics has therefore become necessary, as it provides insight into how alterations in DNA can lead to resistance but also offers opportunities for the development of new therapies. In response to the antibiotic resistance crisis, researchers are investigating bacteriophages, viruses that infect and kill bacteria, as a potential new therapeutic. Bacteriophages are advantageous in being specific, which can minimize collateral damage done to useful microbiota, a significant problem with broad-spectrum antibiotics. That specificity is the product of the intricate genetics and phage and host bacterial architecture, testimony to the evolutionary race between the organisms. Contemporary interest in phage therapy also stems from the limitations of traditional antibiotics because much contemporary medicine has been made less effective due to ubiquitous resistance mechanisms. Dramatic expansion of our understanding of bacteriophage interactions with bacterial genetics is of prime importance in optimizing phage application, emphasizing the role of bacteria not only as causative agents of disease but as targets of study in designing new therapeutic medicine.

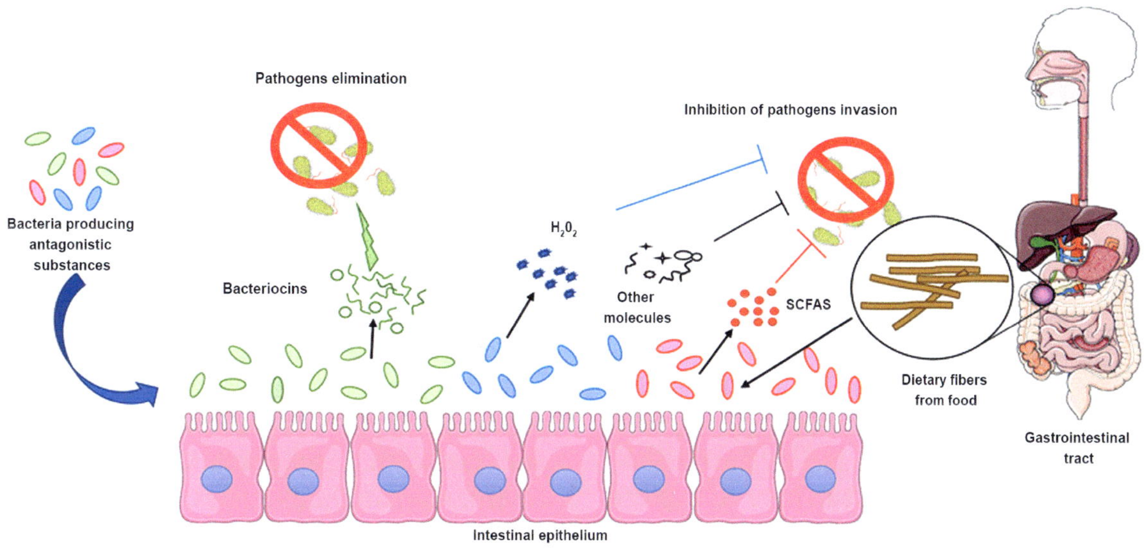

Figure 5.15. Protective effects and inhibitory actions of bacteria against pathogens in the gastrointestinal tract.

Source: https://www.researchgate.net/publication/354587584/figure/fig1/AS:1068170588721165@1631683122969/Protective-effects-and-inhibitory-actions-of-bacteria-against-pathogens-in-the.png.

Confronted with the evolving landscape of bacterial therapeutics, equally in the crosshairs are the legal and economic frameworks controlling the development of said therapies. The heavy investment in pharmaceutical research and development is likely to be based on strong patent protection. However, recent Supreme Court rulings have challenged the patentability of phage therapy, potentially stifling innovation in this area. As researchers urge phages to be effective alternatives to antibiotics, enabling frameworks need to be developed to ensure financial viability for corporations willing to invest in phage-based therapies. Without adequate protection, the therapeutic potential of bacteriophages, particularly against resistant bacterial infections, can be a lost potential. Developing an enabling environment for research and development, maybe through alternative regulatory channels or incentives, is therefore crucial to the future of medicine in the battle against antibiotic resistance (Todd et al., 2014, 2019) (Figure 5.15).

5.6.3. Bacterial Genetics in Environmental Science

The combination of bacterial genetics and environmental science is core to the comprehension of ecological dynamics and biogeochemical processes. Bacteria play crucial roles in processes of nutrient cycling, including the nitrogen and carbon cycles, and genetic diversity allows them to adapt to various environmental conditions. Advanced genetic techniques, , such as metagenomics and CRISPR-based methods, enable researchers to explore the metabolic potential of bacterial assemblages across various ecosystems. Through the examination of environmental bacteria's genetic composition, researchers are able to measure their functions in bioremediation, essentially maximizing their capacity to break down contaminants and restore the balance in the environment. This genetic information not only contributes to theoretical understanding but also has practical implications, indicating how bacterial genetics is crucial in resolving pressing environmental problems like climate change and environmental contamination and is therefore a significant area of multidisciplinary research under the broad umbrella of environmental science. In some settings, certain groups of bacteria have been of particular interest due to their distinctive genetic abilities that allow them to flourish in the environment. For instance, magnetotactic bacteria (MTB) have evolved specialized organelles known as magnetosomes, enabling them to orient according to magnetic fields in aquatic habitats. The genetic regulation of magnetosome formation reveals intricate pathways involving numerous genes that modulate biomineralization processes. This research not only enhances our knowledge of basic bacterial processes but also identifies potential biotechnological and environmental applications. Since the bacteria can survive in many conditions, from freshwater to marine, finding their genetics can potentially give insight into how microbial life adjusts and influences conditions within the environment and therefore advancing research in bacterial genetics concerning ecological function and sustainability (KOMEILI et al., 2020).

Also, the genetic variability within populations of the bacteria is a pool for traits beneficial for environmental adaptation. Horizontal gene transfer (HGT) plays a crucial role here, allowing the bacteria to gain beneficial genes from the organisms around them, thus facilitating rapid adaptation to evolving environmental conditions. Genetic transfer is particularly rampant in stressful conditions, , such as contaminated or harsh environments. Bacterial adaptability via HGT makes them more efficient in bioremediation processes, which further accelerates the degradation of toxic substances within contaminated environments. In addition, knowledge in bacterial genetics plays a crucial role in tracing and understanding antimicrobial resistance, a critical issue in environmental health and public safety. Consequently, identification of the genetic mechanisms of bacteria in the environment is essential, not only for research, but also for developing means to counteract environmental decline and human health protection (Seaman & Whitehouse, 2001).

Test Your Knowledge

1. How are genetically modified bacteria used in biotechnology?
2. Explain how bacterial genetics contributes to the development of new antibiotics or alternative therapies to combat resistant strains.
3. In what ways do bacteria genetically adapt to environmental pollutants, and how is this harnessed in bioremediation?

SUMMARY

In describing the intricate relationship between bacterial structure and genetics, each component of these systems is found to be dependent upon and crucial to the existence of bacteria. The structural characteristics of bacteria, , such as their solid cell walls and specialized membrane structures, make possible a variety of physiological functions governed by their genetic makeup. For instance, genetic blueprints in bacterial DNA regulate cellular functions, including how bacteria construct fundamental structures like pili and flagella. The former gives them mobility, while the latter confers adhesion functionality, and this illustrates how bacterial genetic structure is linked to structural function. Recognition of this interaction is not only expanding our foundation knowledge of microbiology but also highlighting potential applications in biotechnological avenues, where manipulation of these structures may lead to new answers in medicine and environmental science. The genealogical heterogeneity observed in the world of bacteria is phenomenal, which shows the evolutionary adaptability that has allowed the organisms to reproduce in the multiplicity of environments. Mechanisms , such as horizontal gene transfer, recombination, and mutation have contributed to this diversity and illustrate the heavy role of genetics in prokaryotic evolution and survival. Of particular interest is the role of DNA repair mechanisms, , such as recently discovered non-homologous end-joining pathways in prokaryotes, that shed light on prokaryotic adaptability to environmental stress and genomic stability. This heightened attention underscores the dynamic nature of bacterial genetics and its influence on structural integrity, further confirming the relevance of genetic study to the understanding of bacterial life cycles and phage interactions. These discoveries are seminal because they unlock the door to potential studies that can reveal new genetic mechanisms of manipulating bacterial behavior. The conclusion to this study of bacterial structure and genetics throws light on the interrelatedness and complexity that rule life at the microscopic level. The study of specialized bacterial structures like magnetosomes throws light on the excellent adaptations of microorganisms, as it gives an insight into their evolutionary past and ecological interactions. According to literature, the intricate processes of biomineralization and organelle formation are still the most developed sections in genetics, a very promising area for further breakthroughs (Komeili et al., 2020). Meanwhile, the development of DNA repair mechanisms testifies to the necessity for bacteria to maintain the stability of genes under broad environmental stress and mutation (Bowater et al., 2006). Together, these results not only enrich our understanding of the biology of bacteria but also frame essential debates about the implications of bacterial genetics in biotechnology, ecology, and medicine, demonstrating the persistent relevance of this work to the global scientific community.

Studies in bacterial structure and genetics give valuable insights into mechanisms controlling growth and cell division. Of the essential characteristics reported is the adder principle, to the effect that bacteria add a constant volume from birth to division with different amounts in genetically similar cells. This principle contradicts conventional paradigms of growth as pointing to stochastic control of the timing of cell division. A volume-proportionally expressed time-keeper protein in a cell volume might make this possible by regulating its expression in proportion to cell volume, further emphasizing the role of internal cellular regulators in homeostasis of size. The results from the experiment validate this model, where added volume between division events is constant despite newborn cell size fluctuations, thereby identifying a central mechanism that regulates bacterial growth dynamics (Ghusinga et al., 2015). Bacterial genetics also comprises the topic of genetic stability and transmissibility of information among bacteria. The structural component of the bacterial cell plays a decisive part in the exchange of genetics, particularly in terms of horizontal gene transfer. Given the various modes, e.g., transformation, transduction, and conjugation, in which bacteria operate, such genetic diversity plays a decisive influence on their adaptability and survival. The implications of the above processes are extended to the agricultural sector, related to the application of genetically modified organisms (GMOs), and this gives rise to crucial questions regarding their impact on organic agricultural practices. These discussions bring into perspective an in-depth knowledge of DNA's fate in various environmental conditions, , such as longevity in soil and spread through cattle feed (Clarke et al., 2001). Moreover, the interaction of bacterial structure and the regulation of genes is central to pathogenesis research and antibiotic resistance. Bacteria possess unique structural features, , such as peptidoglycan cell walls and heterogeneous membrane lipid composition, that not only serve as physical barriers but also as elements participating in signaling and gene expression. The structural components influence how bacteria respond to external stresses, including the development of antibiotic treatments. An understanding of these interactions is essential to the development of new strategies for fighting infections caused by bacteria and improving treatment outcomes. The exploration of genomic organization and regulatory systems enriches the bacterial genetics field, opening the door to future research focused on realizing such knowledge for biotechnology and therapeutic applications (Ghusinga et al., 2015).

KEY TERMS FROM THIS CHAPTER

Antibiotic resistance genes
Asexual reproduction
Bacterial DNA
Bacterial mobility
Binary fission
Biofilm development
Biomineralization
Antibiotic-resistant strains
Bacterial cell wall
Bacterial genomes
Bacterial morphology
Biochemical pathways
Biological systems
Biotechnology

CRITICAL THINKING QUESTIONS

1. **Which of the following structures is present in all bacterial cells?**
   a. Capsule
   b. Flagella
   c. Nucleoid
   d. Pili
2. **What distinguishes Gram-positive from gram-negative bacteria structurally?**
   a. Presence of outer membrane
   b. Absence of peptidoglycan
   c. Presence of nucleus
   d. Presence of endospores
3. **How do bacteria most commonly reproduce?**
   a. Mitosis
   b. Binary fission
   c. Budding
   d. Conjugation
4. **Which type of genetic material is usually found in bacteria?**
   a. Linear DNA in nucleus
   b. Single-stranded RNA in ribosomes
   c. Mitochondrial DNA
   d. Double-stranded circular DNA in nucleoid
5. **Which of the following is an example of gene regulation in bacteria?**
   a. Splicing of pre-mRNA
   b. Operon system
   c. Histone modification
   d. RNA interference

Short Answer Questions

1. What are the major structural components of a bacterial cell, and what is the function of each?
2. What are the key differences between cocci, bacilli, and spirilla bacterial shapes, and how do these relate to their classification?
3. Describe the structure and function of the bacterial chromosome and plasmids. How do they differ?
4. What is the role of plasmids in antibiotic resistance and horizontal gene transfer?
5. Explain the process of binary fission in bacteria. How does it differ from mitosis in eukaryotic cells?
6. What is an operon, and how does the lac operon function as an example of gene regulation in bacteria?

Answers to Critical Thinking Questions

1. (c) 2. (a) 3. (b) 4. (d) 5. (b)

REFERENCES

1. Adami, C., Balleza, E., Knibbe, C., Cases, I., Cordero, O. X., Parsons, D. P., Dittrich, P., et al. (2010). Scaling laws in bacterial genomes: A side-effect of selection of mutational robustness? https://core.ac.uk/download/148657306.pdf (accessed on 13th June 2025).
2. Ahern, H., & Habashi, J. (2020). *Cereus Fun: An Introduction to Microbiological Techniques*. https://core.ac.uk/download/395019283.pdf (accessed on 13th June 2025).
3. Anderson, J. G., Goudie, A. C., MacGregor, S. J., & Olateju, M. (2003). Inactivation of pathogens on food and contact surfaces using ozone as a biocidal agent. https://core.ac.uk/download/9020578.pdf (accessed on 13th June 2025).
4. McBurney, M. I., Davis, C., Fraser, C. M., Schneeman, B. O., Huttenhower, C., Verbeke, K., Walter, J., & Latulippe, M. E. (2019). Establishing What Constitutes a Healthy Human Gut Microbiome: State of the Science, Regulatory Considerations, and Future Directions. *The Journal of nutrition*, *149*(11), 1882–1895. https://doi.org/10.1093/jn/nxz154(accessed on 13th June 2025).
5. Arkin, A., Bar-Even, A., Lobner-Olesen, A., Raj, A., Zaslaver, A., Bishop, A. L., Zaslaver, A., et al. (2012). A genome-wide analysis of promoter-mediated phenotypic noise in *Escherichia coli*. https://core.ac.uk/download/4894249.pdf (accessed on 13th June 2025).
6. Arnoldt, H., Strogatz, S. H., & Timme, M. (2015). Simple model for the Darwinian transition in early evolution. http://arxiv.org/abs/1501.05073 (accessed on 13th June 2025).
7. Baldwin, I. T., Dorcheh, E. K., Li, R., Rameshkumar, A., et al. (2019). Antimicrobial peptide expression in a wild tobacco plant reveals the limits of host-microbe-manipulations in the field. https://core.ac.uk/download/225124661.pdf (accessed on 13th June 2025).
8. Balsalobre, C., El Mouali, Y., Gaviria-Cantin, T., Gilbert, S., et al. (2018). CRP-cAMP mediates silencing of *Salmonella* virulence at the post-transcriptional level. https://core.ac.uk/download/161254135.pdf (accessed on 13th June 2025).
9. Bandurski, R. S., & Singh, N. (1983). *The Alpha-Helix Concept: Innovative Utilization of the Space Station Program. A report to the National Aeronautical and Space Administration Requesting Establishment of a Sensory Physiology Laboratory on the Space Station*. Document ID
10. 19840012542, Acquisition Source, Legacy CDMS, Document Type Contractor Report (CR)
11. https://core.ac.uk/download/pdf/42849574.pdf (accessed on 13th June 2025).
12. Bankevich, A., Darling, A. E., Page, A. J., Kislyuk, A. O., Charlesworth, B., Buckee, C., et al. (2020). Bacterial microevolution and the pangenome. https://core.ac.uk/download/323058045.pdf (accessed on 13th June 2025).
13. Baumdicker, F., Hess, W. R., & Pfaffelhuber, P. (2010). The diversity of a distributed genome in bacterial populations. http://arxiv.org/abs/0907.2572 (accessed on 13th June 2025).
14. Beccari, T., Dundar, M., Gartland, J. S., Gartland, K., et al. (2017). Advances in biotechnology: Genomics and genome editing. https://core.ac.uk/download/293859551.pdf (accessed on 13th June 2025).
15. Bernardi, G., Calladine, C. R., Clay, O., Daniell, P. J., Holste, D., Gerton, J. L., Kong, A., et al. (2004). Spectral analysis of guanine and cytosine fluctuations of mouse genomic DNA. http://arxiv.org/abs/q-bio/0411017 (accessed on 13th June 2025).

16. Berry, A., Koukounari, A., Norton, A. J., Laird, A. R., Schelkle, B., Webster, B. L., Webster, B. L., et al. (2015). Hybridization in parasites: Consequences for adaptive evolution, pathogenesis and public health in a changing world. https://core.ac.uk/download/36778666.pdf (accessed on 13th June 2025).
17. Bois, A., Garcia-Roger, E. M., Hong, E., Hutzler, M., et al. (2019). Congenital anomalies from a physics perspective: The key role of "manufacturing" volatility. http://arxiv.org/abs/1905.04357 (accessed on 13th June 2025).
18. Boutry, S., Brisse, S., Bui Thi Ngoc, L., Gagnevin, L., et al. (2008). From local surveys to global surveillance: Three high-throughput genotyping methods for epidemiological monitoring of *Xanthomonas citri* pv. *citri* pathotypes. http://agritrop.cirad.fr/548014/1/document_548014.pdf (accessed on 13th June 2025).
19. Bowater, R., & Doherty, A. J. (2006). Making ends meet: Repairing breaks in bacterial DNA by non-homologous end-joining. https://core.ac.uk/download/2728184.pdf (accessed on 13th June 2025).
20. Buckling, A., Donderis, J., Elena, S. F., Frígols, B., et al. (2015). Virus satellites drive viral evolution and ecology. https://core.ac.uk/download/42366344.pdf (accessed on 13th June 2025).
21. Carroll, S., DeFrees, S., Georgiou, G., Johnson, K., et al. (2009). Expression of active human sialyltransferase ST6GalNAcI in *Escherichia coli*. https://core.ac.uk/download/211333360.pdf (accessed on 13th June 2025).
22. Clarke, B., Dale, P., Fontes, E., Martin, C., et al. (2001). A review of knowledge of the potential impacts of GMOs on organic agriculture. https://core.ac.uk/download/10923231.pdf (accessed on 13th June 2025).
23. Cockayne, A., Elias, A. F., Barbour, A. G., Hendrickx, A. P., Williams, A. W., Chi, B., Hu, B., et al. (2014). Initial characterization of the FlgE hook high molecular weight complex. https://core.ac.uk/download/78919273.pdf (accessed on 13th June 2025).
24. Draf, C., Fisch, K. M., Kurabi, A., Nasamran, C., et al. (2020). Single-cell transcriptomes reveal a complex cellular landscape in the middle ear and differential capacities for acute response to infection. https://core.ac.uk/download/323308745.pdf (accessed on 13th June 2025).
25. Fischer, S., Gál, I., Lakatos, L., Lakatos, G., et al. (2006). Current concept on the pathogenesis of inflammatory bowel disease: Crosstalk between genetic and microbial factors—Pathogenic bacteria and altered bacterial sensing or changes in mucosal integrity take "toll"? https://core.ac.uk/download/11855827.pdf (accessed on 13th June 2025).
26. Ghusinga, K. R., Singh, A., & Vargas-Garcia, C. A. (2015). A mechanistic first-passage time framework for bacterial cell-division timing. http://arxiv.org/abs/1512.07864 (accessed on 13th June 2025).
27. Haaber, J., Ingmer, H., & Penadés, J. R. (2017). Transfer of antibiotic resistance in *Staphylococcus aureus*. https://core.ac.uk/download/84148494.pdf (accessed on 13th June 2025).
28. Hofvander, P. (2004). Production of amylopectin and high-amylose starch in separate potato genotypes. https://core.ac.uk/download/11694800.pdf (accessed on 13th June 2025).
29. Emmett, K.J., Rabadan, R. (2014). Characterizing Scales of Genetic Recombination and Antibiotic Resistance in Pathogenic Bacteria Using Topological Data Analysis. In: Ślęzak, D., Tan, AH.,

Peters, J.F., Schwabe, L. (eds) Brain Informatics and Health. BIH 2014. Lecture Notes in Computer Science(), vol 8609. Springer, Cham. https://doi.org/10.1007/978-3-319-09891-3_49(accessed on 13th June 2025).

30. Horowitz, N. H., & Owen, R. D. (1954). *Physiological Aspects of Genetics.* https://core.ac.uk/download/4869317.pdf (accessed on 13th June 2025).

31. Jerdan, R., Lungin, O., Moshynets, O. V., Potters, G., et al. (2020). Extending an eco-evolutionary understanding of biofilm formation at the air-liquid interface to community biofilms. https://core.ac.uk/download/287584064.pdf (accessed on 13th June 2025).

32. Kaloshian, I., & Teixeira, M. (2019). Advances in plant-nematode interactions with emphasis on the notorious nematode genus *Meloidogyne.* https://core.ac.uk/download/305123985.pdf (accessed on 13th June 2025).

33. King, D. M. (2015). Evolutionary dynamics of speciation and extinction. https://core.ac.uk/download/217321608.pdf (accessed on 13th June 2025).

34. Komeili, A., & McCausland, H. (2020). Magnetic genes: Studying the genetics of biomineralization in magnetotactic bacteria. https://core.ac.uk/download/323080553.pdf (accessed on 13th June 2025).

35. Lagares, A., Pistorio, M., & Sanjuán Pinilla, J. (2014). The plasmid mobilome of the model plant-symbiont *Sinorhizobium meliloti*: Coming up with new questions and answers. https://core.ac.uk/download/159287717.pdf (accessed on 13th June 2025).

36. McGowan, T. L. (1996). *Construction of a Novel Fungal Gus Expression Plasmid, And Its Evaluation in Aspergillus nidulans: A Thesis Presented in Partial Fulfilment of The Requirements for The Degree of Master of Science in Genetics at Massey University.* https://core.ac.uk/download/148645080.pdf (accessed on 13th June 2025).

37. Milka, M. (2018). Role of horizontal gene transfer in bacteria. https://core.ac.uk/download/234687733.pdf (accessed on 13th June 2025).

38. Molineux, I. J., & Panja, D. (2010). Dynamics of bacteriophage genome ejection *in vitro* and *in vivo.* http://arxiv.org/abs/1012.0220 (accessed on 13th June 2025).

39. Parry, S. K. (1993). *Construction and Utilization of a Bidirectional Reporter Vector in The Analysis of Two Nod-Boxes in of Rhizobium loti: A Thesis Presented in Partial Fulfilment of The Requirements for The Degree of Master of Science in Molecular Genetics at Massey University.* https://core.ac.uk/download/222793743.pdf (accessed on 13th June 2025).

40. Seaman, W., & Whitehouse, J. H. (2001). *Florida Marine Biotechnology: Research, Development and Training Capabilities to Advance Science and Commerce.* Florida Sea Grant College Program University of Florida Sea Grant Technical Paper Number 110 March 2001 https://core.ac.uk/download/11016354.pdf (accessed on 13th June 2025).

41. Spiers, A. J. (2014). A mechanistic explanation linking adaptive mutation, niche change, and fitness advantage for the Wrinkly Spreader. https://core.ac.uk/download/228177282.pdf (accessed on 13th June 2025).

42. Taoka, A., Kaito, C., Nakane, D., Wada, H., Mori, H., Tulum, I., Shimabukuro, K., et al. (2020). Tree of motility–A proposed history of motility systems in the tree of life. https://core.ac.uk/download/327172571.pdf (accessed on 13th June 2025).

43. Todd, K. (2014). The promising viral threat to bacterial resistance: The uncertain patentability of phage therapeutics and the necessity of alternative incentives. https://core.ac.uk/download/213020895.pdf (accessed on 13th June 2025).
44. Toenniessen, G. H., O'Toole, J. C., Harris, R. R., Herdt, R. W., & Murashige, T. (2001). The Rockefeller Foundation's international program on rice biotechnology. https://core.ac.uk/download/71354545.pdf (accessed on 13th June 2025).
45. Wheeler, V. (2017). Preliminary analyses of the diversity of soil microbes on the campus of the University of the Incarnate Word. https://core.ac.uk/download/217400695.pdf (accessed on 13th June 2025).

GRAM-POSITIVE COCCI

6

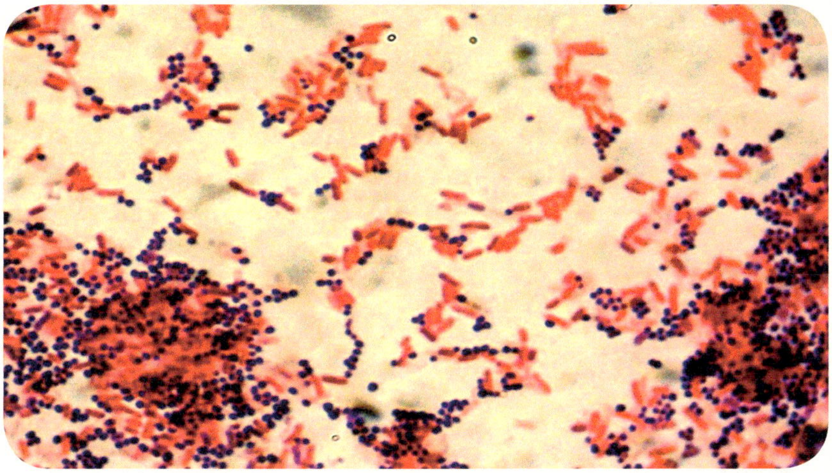

Introduction

In bacteria, the classification of bacteria as Gram-positive and gram-negative is fundamental, having implications both for laboratory diagnosis and clinical interventions. Gram-positive cocci form a subgroup of bacteria that retain the stain of crystal violet used in the Gram staining test and has significant implications in their interaction with infection. This chapter delves into the nature, pathogenicity, and clinical relevance of Gram-positive cocci that comprise salient genera, such as *Staphylococcus*, *Streptococcus*, and Enterococcus. Information regarding these microbes is significant since therapy regimens and management strategies for infections brought about by these microbes are significantly different from infection due to gram-negative microbes. Hence, a thorough research on Gram-positive cocci is not only significant for academic study but also crucial for the enhancement of patient care. Clinical significance of Gram-positive cocci is a reflection of clinical significance. These organisms have evolved so that most of them are resistant to traditional antibiotics and thus treatment

LEARNING OBJECTIVES

After studying this chapter, you will be able to:

1. Explain the characteristics of Gram-positive cocci
2. Describe the major types of Gram-positive cocci
3. Discuss pathogenicity and diseases
4. Understand laboratory identification of Gram-positive cocci
5. Focus on the treatment and management of infections caused by Gram-positive cocci
6. Deal with current research and developments

becomes challenging and requires continuous monitoring. Methicillin-resistant *Staphylococcus aureus* (MRSA) is a quintessential example of a Gram-positive species that poses some very serious issues in a clinical environment. Furthermore, the virulence determinants employed by these cocci, , such as the exotoxin production and adherence factors, contribute to their survival and virulence. The present study indicates the high rate of infection with these microbes, as the problems have come to such a critical juncture that the demand for effective infection control and antimicrobial stewardship has become indispensable. The specificity of Gram-positive coccis' interaction with the immune system of the host only amplifies the extent of their impact, rendering it the topic of ongoing debate in the scientific community on how to treat and prevent them. Emerging from biology, the knowledge derived from the ecology and microbiological processes of Gram-positive cocci depicts their complex interaction with the human being and the environment. For instance, studies have uncovered that infections associated with healthcare most often take root in the improper handling of biomedical waste, which can include pathogenic Gram-positive bacteria, thus exposing healthcare workers and patients to injury (Eyaufe et al., 2016). Beyond the clinical arena, the implications of these findings are to require increased standard operating procedures in how soiled materials are disposed of. Furthermore, understanding the environmental presence and resistance patterns of these organisms remains key in guiding public health intervention. Considering that more evidence now exists on the amenability of Gram-positive cocci to stress, the necessity of innovative treatment strategies becomes an exigency. The chapter aims to incorporate current research and clinical perspectives towards conceptualization of a uniform understanding of Gram-positive cocci and their significance in microbiology and infectious disease control.

Definition of Gram-positive Cocci

Gram-positive cocci are round-shaped bacteria with a peptidoglycan-thick cell wall that retains the crystal violet stain in Gram staining. This property makes them Gram-positive, not only due to their description but also because it suggests that they are sensitive to certain antibiotics. Gram-positive cocci also have significant roles in infectious disease as well as clinical microbiology due to the fact that they encompass several disease-causing species of *Staphylococcus*, *Streptococcus*, and Enterococcus. These groups are responsible for a wide range of infections from mild cutaneous disease to systemic severe illness, which emphasizes their clinical significance. It is necessary to know their biological and structural characteristics in order to make rational treatment choices and further the advancement of microbiological diagnostics. The pathogenicity is caused by the virulence factors of Gram-positive cocci, which can vary markedly between species. *Staphylococcus aureus* produces a number of toxins and enzymes, for instance, that help it evade the host immune system and induce diseases , such as pneumonia, sepsis, and skin infection. *Streptococcus* pyogenes, another significant Gram-positive cocci, is known to induce pharyngitis, scarlet fever, and rheumatic fever. To that effect, some Gram-positive cocci exhibit resistance to antibiotics, which complicate the process of treatment and present a public health issue. For example, the resistance level observed in skin organisms during blood contamination studies highlights the importance of constant surveillance for antimicrobial susceptibility, particularly in hospitals where patients are most vulnerable to infection (Malimu, 2012). The rise in antibiotic-resistant Gram-positive cocci emphasizes the necessity for constant research and development in the field of microbiology. Bacterial secondary infections have been found to complicate disease conditions, particularly when epidemic species like *Staphylococcus aureus* possess resistance to primary-line antibiotics (Pahlevan et al., 2013). This calls for a proper understanding of the epidemiology and mechanisms of resistance on the part of these microorganisms. Moreover, developing new therapeutic interventions, , such as new antibiotics or add-on therapy, is of utmost priority in Gram-positive coccus infection treatment. More studies on their clinical importance can allow healthcare providers to implement more effective interventions and combat the rising issue of antibiotic resistance, yielding better patient outcomes against these adaptive pathogens (Figure 6.1).

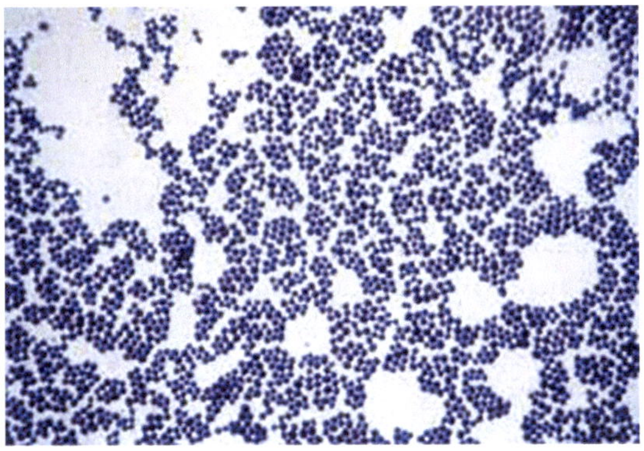

Figure 6.1. Gram-positive cocci in clusters.

Source: https://www.researchgate.net/publication/323977409/figure/fig3/AS:647032997957632@1531276096219/Gram-positive-cocci-in-clusters.png.

Importance in Microbiology and Medicine

Understanding the significance of Gram-positive cocci in medicine and microbiology reveals their pivotal role in disease pathology through infectious disease. Multiple species, , such as *Staphylococcus aureus* and *Streptococcus pneumoniae*, are normal pathogens responsible for numerous forms of illness ranging from skin infections to pneumonia and sepsis. By forming biofilm, evading the host immune system, and acquiring resistance to antibiotics, treatment becomes more effective. For instance, the emergence of methicillin-resistant *Staphylococcus aureus* (MRSA) indicates a sudden public health problem, demanding consistent investigation into effective management measures. Disruptions in the supply of effective antibiotics occasioned by such resistant microbes increased morbidity and mortality rates within hospitals and in the community, demanding that timely and knowledge clinical interventions be implemented to control infections caused by these virulent microorganisms.." Furthermore, the diagnostic significance of Gram-positive cocci should not be overemphasized. Proper identification and differentiation of these bacteria are of utmost importance, as they tend to present similar phenotypic features to each other, making misdiagnosis a possibility. A study pointed out the clinical and microbiological characteristics of *Staphylococcus* intermedius group (SIG) isolates from human samples, highlighting their potential to produce serious infections, especially in immunocompromised individuals (Burnham et al., 2018). Misidentification of such pathogens, perhaps due to their similarity to *Staphylococcus aureus*, can adversely affect therapy by encouraging delays in the implementation of appropriate therapy. Since such organisms are increasingly being identified as morbidity causative agents, clinical microbiologists and clinicians must set up strong parameters for correct identification and susceptibility testing to optimize patient management. At the clinical level, the significance of recognizing Gram-positive cocci extends beyond identification and treatment — it also extends to learning from newly acquired infections. An example of this is disseminated gonococcal infection (DGI), which illustrates how secondary complications can arise from primary infections, as in the case of atypical presentation leading to subcutaneous abscesses and pyomyositis (Boonyasiri et al., 2012). Such cases point out the interconnected nature of different pathogens and the need to have a broad concept of patient presentations. Gram-positive cocci microbiological investigations reveal such complex interactions and inform preventive measures in order to avoid severe complications. Ongoing research on the pathogens not only enhances diagnostic accuracy but also directs public health policy to retard the progress of infection spread and mitigate the impact of antibiotic resistance on healthcare.

6.1. Characteristics of Gram-positive Cocci

Learning Outcome

1. Understand the cell wall structure of Gram-positive cocci
2. Discuss staining properties and methods
3. Describe the morphological features of Gram-positive cocci

Gram-positive cocci group primarily on the basis of their typical cellular characteristics as well as biochemical properties. Microscopically, they appear as spherical, often clumped cells that absorb the crystal violet dye used in Gram staining tests. This is because they have a thick peptidoglycan layer present in the cell wall, which gives structural support and protection against adverse environmental conditions. Of the Gram-positive cocci, two large groups dominate: *Staphylococcus* and *Streptococcus*, both distinguished by their pattern of arrangement, biochemical activity, and disease-causing ability. For instance, while *Staphylococcus* species are generally found in irregular clusters with a grape-like arrangement, *Streptococcus* species are generally found in chains or pairs. These physical arrangements, in conjunction with some metabolic pathways, are used to identify them and serve as primary biomarkers for clinical diagnosis. Pathogenicity, Gram-positive cocci possess different virulence factors that allow them to cause disease. *Staphylococcus aureus*, for example, possesses several toxins, one of which is enterotoxin B, whose ingestion causes acute food poisoning. In investigative research, it is uncovered that most *Staphylococcus aureus* isolates from various sources have characteristics common to pathogenicity, , such as mannitol fermentation and coagulase production, along with their Gram-positive cocci morphology (Arifah et al., 2020). Another pathogen, *Streptococcus pneumoniae*, whose involvement in pneumonia and meningitis has been observed, contains a capsular polysaccharide responsible for evading host immune systems. The pathogenic potential of these bacteria highlights the necessity for proper identification and sensitivity testing, particularly in clinical microbiology laboratories. The prevalence of Gram-positive cocci in clinical specimens presents challenges as much as opportunities for microbiological practice. A study on corneal ulcers concluded that Gram-positive cocci made up the majority of the bacterial isolates, which emphasizes their significance in infections (Guramatunhu et al., 2001). This discovery is essential because it brings to the fore the necessity for efficient laboratory methodologies for identification and differentiation of these microorganisms. Gram staining, despite its shortcomings in some cases, is still a cornerstone in microbiology due to its speed and simplicity. Nevertheless, a multifaceted approach, including state-of-the-art methodologies like PCR and culture methods, is inevitable for successful pathogen identification. Sorting out the intricacies in Gram-positive cocci, as well as strict clinical assessment, will enhance infection care and therapeutic outcomes.

6.1.1. Cell Wall Structure and Composition

Cell wall structure of Gram-positive cocci is of cardinal significance in defining their physiological characteristics and potential pathogenicity. Essentially composed of a dense peptidoglycan layer, the cell wall provides rigidity and resistance to extraneous stresses. The matrix of this peptidoglycan is strongly cross-linked with teichoic acids, which are embedded in it and also impart overall stability to the cell wall itself. The presence of these teichoic acids not only contributes to the maintenance of cell integrity but also a significant role to play in the adhesion of bacteria to host tissues, hence facilitating infection. It is thus essential to learn the composition of the cell wall in order to comprehend the biology of Gram-positive cocci and their interactions with the host immune system. The morphological difference among various Gram-positive cocci is starkly evident if one considers the ultrastructure of their cell walls. For instance, it has been discovered through research that certain species , such as *Staphylococcus aureus,* possess a characteristic layered cell wall structure made up of two distinct layers. The surface layer, having resistance to lytic enzymes, is thought to consist predominantly of teichoic acid while the inner layer is amorphous in character and is enzymatically degradable.

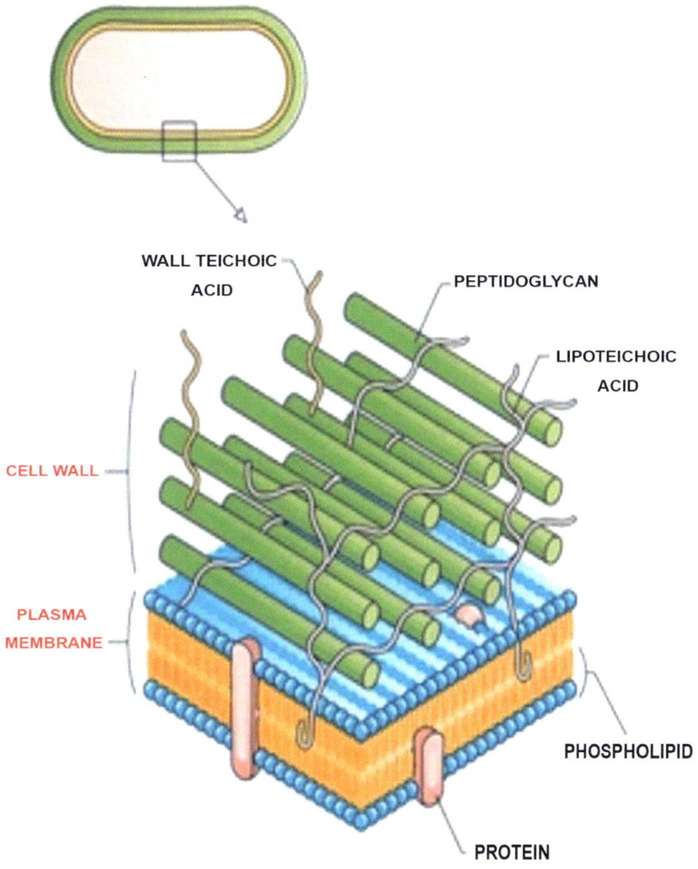

Figure 6.2. Cell wall structure of Gram-positive cocci.

Source: https://www.shutterstock.com/image-vector/Gram-positive-versus-negative-cell-600nw-2086382827.jpg.

This fine structure not only decides the mechanical properties of the cell wall but is also involved in pathogenicity and antibiotic resistance. By understanding these structural nuances, researchers can assess more precisely the behavior of Gram-positive cocci in various environmental and clinical conditions, which would assist in treatment for infections with these organisms (Kanemasa et al.,

1974). Additionally, the ecological versatility of Gram-positive cocci also arises due to their cell wall organization. For example, certain halophilic Gram-positive cocci have unique adaptations in cell wall composition that allow them to thrive in elevated salinity. Peptidoglycan composition variability and the presence of specific surface proteins allow these microorganisms to resist osmotic pressure and maintain cellular integrity. Phylogenetic analysis suggests that closely related genera , such as Salimicrobium, exhibit high genetic diversity, which is matched with environmental adaptations , such as the best growth conditions and salt tolerance. These findings put into question the central position of cell wall composition and environmental factors, their relevance to taxonomy and the evolutionary biology of Gram-positive cocci (Birbir et al., 2011) (Figure 6.2).

6.1.2. Staining Properties and Methods

Study of Gram-positive cocci using particular staining methods is an elementary technique of microbiology by which the bacteria are differentiated and identified. The Gram staining process, suggested by Hans Christian Gram in the 19th century, involves the sequential use of crystal violet and iodine, decolorization with alcohol or acetone, and ultimately, counterstaining with safranin. This response capitalizes on the structural diversity of the cell wall of Gram-positive bacteria, which possess a heavy peptidoglycan layer that retains the crystal violet dye, which the microscope sees as purple. Gram-negative bacteria possess thinner peptidoglycan and an outer membrane and fail to retain the crystal violet but absorb the safranin, which the microscope perceives as pink. Understanding of these staining features is significant as staining-based misidentification may lead to inadmissible treatment planning in the clinical laboratory. Aside from the usual Gram staining, additional staining methods further enable visualization and description of Gram-positive cocci. Such methods as the capsule stain, endospore stain, and acid-fast stain provide further details regarding morphological features and physiological capabilities of bacterial species. For example, capsule stain will be capable of identifying encapsulated Gram-positive cocci like *Streptococcus pneumoniae*, which will be beneficial to ascertain its pathogenesis. In the same way, the endospore stain will be capable of identifying the hardness of certain strains, like the genus Bacillus. Besides, the acid-fast stain technique can distinguish some Gram-positive bacteria, , such as those containing mycolic acid in their cell walls, , such as Mycobacterium species, demonstrating the diversity of this group.

Each one of these specialized tests gives valuable information that complements the fundamentals picked up from standard Gram staining. The use of staining properties in the diagnosis and treatment of infection by Gram-positive cocci cannot be overestimated. Clinicians typically use the result of Gram staining to decide on their choice of antibiotics, as most treatment protocols are based on the Gram reaction of the bacteria. For instance, detection of methicillin-resistant *Staphylococcus aureus* (MRSA) is problematic because it is resistant to β-lactam antibiotics and requires rapid detection using staining along with culture procedures. Recent studies indicate the antimicrobial possibility of lactic acid bacteria from conventional fermented foods that have been shown to repress both Gram-positive and Gram-negative pathogens to a significant degree (Widodo et al., 2021). In addition, endophytic bacterial studies have shown their capability to combat resistant strains, placing emphasis on alternative methods in antimicrobial therapy (Das et al., 2021). Understanding staining characteristics of Gram-positive cocci is not only critical in identification but also directs treatment strategies and consequently influences public health outcomes (Figure 6.3).

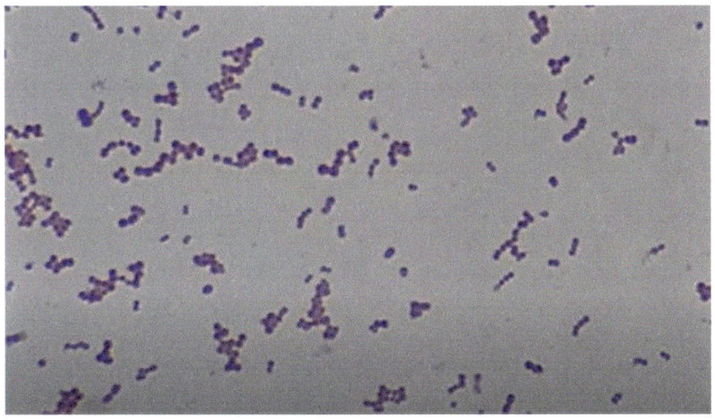

Figure 6.3. Gram-positive cocci in chains of *Streptococcus pyogenes* in Gram staining of culture.

Source: https://medicallabnotes.com/wp-content/uploads/2022/02/Gram-positive-cocci-in-chains-of-*Streptococcus*-pyogenes-in-Gram-staining-of-culture-1024x576.jpg.

6.1.3. Morphological Features

The morphological characteristics of the Gram-positive cocci are also important in their identification and for understanding their biological roles. These bacteria tend to be spherical and may exist in various arrangements , such as clusters, chains, or pairs, and they tell us a lot about their taxonomy. For instance, *Staphylococcus* exists in clusters that are irregular and grape-like, whereas *Streptococcus* exists in chains or pairs. These formations both reflect not only the pattern of bacterial cell division but also their pathogenicity and mode of interaction with the host environment. It would become more convenient to use corresponding laboratory methods of identification due to such formations, as holistic approaches under co-operational research projects , such as the Apollo-Soyuz Test Project suggest, where systematic identification of bacteria by formal laboratory procedures as presented in (Taylor et al.) is given top priority. Apart from shape and structure, the peptidoglycan structure of Gram-positive cocci is also important in their staining and resulting identification. The existence of a thicker peptidoglycan layer in Gram-positive bacteria holds on to crystal violet stain during Gram staining and produces well-defined results compared to Gram-negative bacteria.

This distinctive property is crucial in separating Gram-positive cocci into different genera, , such as Bacillus, Lactococcus, and enterococci species, among others. The rigidity of their cell walls also makes them resistant to environmental stresses, and this confers on them a survival benefit in various habitats. These morphological differences are crucial not only for laboratory identification but also for an understanding of how these organisms survive and interact with their environments and possible hosts, which further emphasizes the significance of a subtle understanding of their morphology in clinical microbiology. The study of morphological characteristics is more than just identification and tells us something about the probable biochemical characteristics and environmental roles of Gram-positive cocci. For example, studies on endophytic bacteria of the Micrococcus and Enterococcus genera not only reveal their morphological characteristics but also their excellent antimicrobial activity against pathogenic members , such as Salmonella. Additionally, the various colony morphologies that exist in fungal and bacterial endophytes propose an intense interaction with host plants that leads to the biosynthesis of useful metabolites. These intricate interactions prove the worth of the examination of morphological characters' in unraveling more extensive ecological mechanisms at play, as argued within the outcomes described in studies focused on endophytic endowments in plants, thereby affirming our knowledge of Gram-positive cocci not only as isolated microbes but also as integral components of complex biological processes (Das et al., 2021) (Figure 6.4).

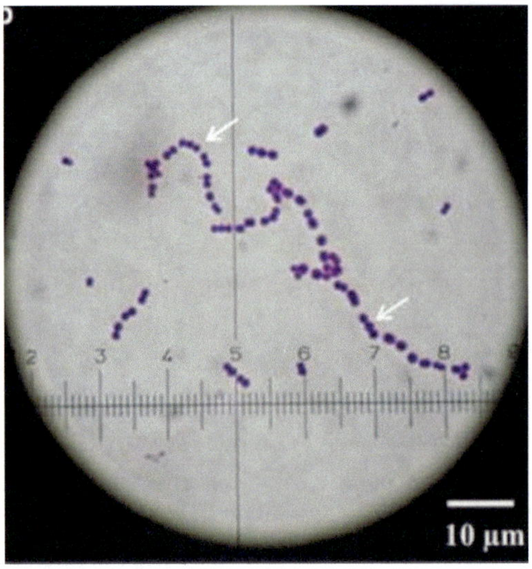

Figure 6.4. Gram-positive cocci arranged in chains, pairs or small groups; the chain lengths were highly variable. (Gram staining, bar = 10 µm).

Source: https://www.researchgate.net/publication/317660543/figure/fig3/AS:1182999710314508@1659060518547/Bacterial-morphology-a-Gram-positive-coccus-shaped-organisms-arranged-in-pairs-or.jpg.

Test Your Knowledge

1. What are the key structural components of the cell wall in Gram-positive cocci, and how do they contribute to its function?
2. Describe the typical morphology of Gram-positive cocci and how they are arranged microscopically.

6.2. Major Types of Gram-positive Cocci

Learning Outcome

1. Understand Staphylococcus species
2. Describe Streptococcus species
3. Describe the Enterococcus genus

The domain of Gram-positive cocci encompasses an array of bacterial genera characterized by distinctive features and pathogenic potential. *Staphylococcus* and *Streptococcus* are prominent among these, with their paramount significance in clinical microbiology attributed to their high incidence of presence in human infections. *Staphylococcus aureus*, for instance, is known to cause skin and soft tissue infections, pneumonia, and sepsis with broad implications for public health. Furthermore, the likelihood of certain strains becoming antibiotic resistant, namely methicillin-resistant *Staphylococcus aureus* (MRSA), complicates treatment protocols and prompts concerns regarding hospital infection control measures. The clinical relevance of such importance warrants ongoing monitoring and examination of the resistance and virulence factors of these pathogens. Familiarity with these Gram-positive cocci is central to effective diagnosis, treatment, and prevention practices in healthcare settings. Another familiar genus of the Gram-positive cocci is *Streptococcus*, which is itself further divided into several groups depending on their hemolytic capabilities and Lancefield group. Notably, *Streptococcus* pyogenes, Group A *Streptococcus*, is responsible for infections as benign as pharyngitis to as severe as life-threatening invasive disease , such as necrotizing fasciitis. *Streptococcus pneumoniae* is also a leading cause of pneumonia, meningitis, and otitis media, especially in children and elderly individuals. The pathogenicity of such bacteria can be attributed to some of the following virulence factors , such as toxins and the ability to evade the immune system. The recognition and discrimination of such *Streptococcus* species are of greater than theoretical significance; they have immediate clinical, vaccine, and public health implications for management of patients, development of vaccines, and outbreak control of streptococcal infections. Mounting evidence also suggests opportunistic potential for some Gram-positive cocci, particularly in immunocompromised individuals. For instance, Enterococcus species are normally found in the gastrointestinal tract and are a matter of concern only when they become translocated to other locations in the body or in the setting of underlying disease. *Enterococcus faecalis* and Enterococcus faecium are of greatest clinical significance and are frequently implicated in urinary tract infections, bacteremia, and endocarditis. The development of resistance among enterococci, especially to vancomycin, has made treatment more complex and necessitated a greater focus on antimicrobial stewardship and infection prevention practices. The presence of Gram-positive cocci in various clinical settings underscores not only their epidemiological significance but also the complex interdependency between microbial communities and host susceptibility that underlies the outcome of disease, as attested through studies of the bacterial flora in diseases , such as Buruli ulcer (Pahlevan et al., 2013).

6.2.1. Staphylococcus Species

The role of *Staphylococcus* species in the context of Gram-positive cocci cannot be underscored enough, particularly in clinical settings. The organisms are known for their ability to cause varied infections, with most significant among them being methicillin-resistant *Staphylococcus aureus* (MRSA) that presents a huge threat to healthcare systems. The prevalence of MRSA and other species of *Staphylococcus* in different infections, , such as diabetic foot ulcers, demonstrates their adaptive properties and capacity for antibiotic resistance acquisition. A study highlighted the isolation of MRSA as one of the most commonly present pathogens of infected diabetic foot ulcers, accounting for 19.4% of infections, highlighting the importance of effective empirical treatment regimens directed against these pathogens (Hayatshahi et al., 2012).

The emergence of resistance in non-*Staphylococcus* species not only complicates the treatment process but also demands continuous monitoring and the application of appropriate antimicrobial procedures. Apart from their clinical importance, the diversity of *Staphylococcus* species provides a fascinating aspect of microbial ecology. They are often found on human skin and mucous membranes, where they become commensals and are part of the normal flora. However, upon a breakdown of the cutaneous barrier or in immunocompromised individuals, these normally benign microorganisms can turn into opportunistic pathogens. For instance, in the management of chronic conditions like Buruli ulcer, *Staphylococcus aureus* is recovered as frequently as other pathogens, contributing to the treatment protocol complexities (Pahlevan et al., 2013). This phenomenon illustrates the delicate balance between microbial pathogenicity and host defense, which mirrors the necessity for full knowledge of *Staphylococcus* species in disease and health (Figure 6.5).

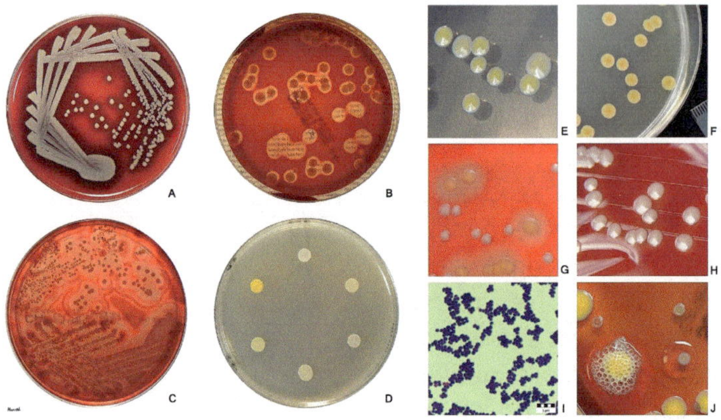

Figure 6.5. *Staphylococcus aureus* on basic cultivation media.

Source: https://upload.wikimedia.org/wikipedia/commons/thumb/0/08/*Staphylococcus*_aureus_appearance_on_agar_plates.jpg/1920px-*Staphylococcus*_aureus_appearance_on_agar_plates.jpg.

Staphylococcus species' role extends beyond the pathogenicity they have, as they are at the heart of arguments concerning antibiotic stewardship and the emergence of bacterial resistance. The increasing rate of antibiotic resistance, particularly in strains like MRSA, jeopardizes the efficacy of traditional treatment procedures. For example, *S. aureus* has demonstrated strong resistance to first-line antibiotics widely used in the majority of regions, as revealed in research on the bacterial flora of long-term infections (Pahlevan et al., 2013). This calls for ongoing research into alternative therapy protocols and developing new antimicrobial agents. Also, understanding the genetic mechanisms underlying the resistance observed in *Staphylococcus* species will inform clinical policies and guidelines that would arrest the virulence of such organisms in healthcare settings. There is thus a requirement for holistic methods to address the multifaceted issue that is *Staphylococcus* species both as a human skin commensal and virulent pathogen (Figure 6.6).

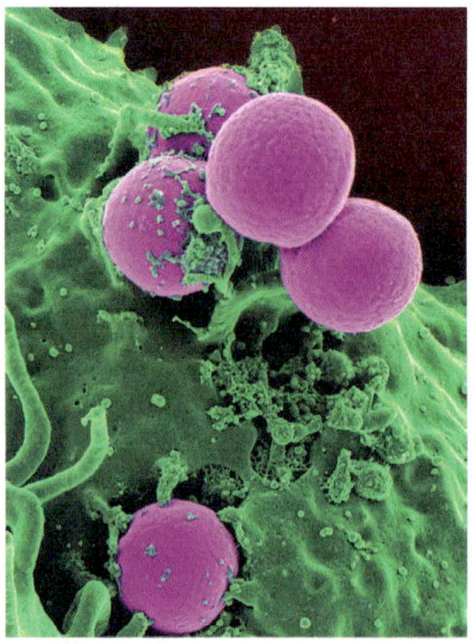

Figure 6.6. Colorized scanning electron micrograph of a human neutrophil ingesting methicillin-resistant *Staphylococcus aureus* (MRSA).

Source: https://upload.wikimedia.org/wikipedia/commons/thumb/0/01/Human_neutrophil_ingesting_MRSA.jpg/800px-Human_neutrophil_ingesting_MRSA.jpg.

6.2.2. Streptococcus Species

Streptococcus is a big genus of Gram-positive cocci with an extremely diverse group of pathogenic characteristics and clinical significations. They are round in shape and usually occur in chains or in pairs, a typical morphological characteristic. Streptococci belong to various groups based on the Lancefield classification, of which the most important medically significant streptococci belong to groups A (S. pyogenes), B (S. agalactiae), and others , such as *Streptococcus pneumoniae*. These groups are each linked with human diseases ranging from mild infections like pharyngitis and cutaneous infections to severe disease , such as rheumatic fever and pneumonia. Their virulence factors that include hemolysins, pyrogenic exotoxins, and biofilm-forming capability contribute to their pathogenicity. Information concerning these factors is thus crucial in effective clinical diagnosis and treatment in clinical microbiology.

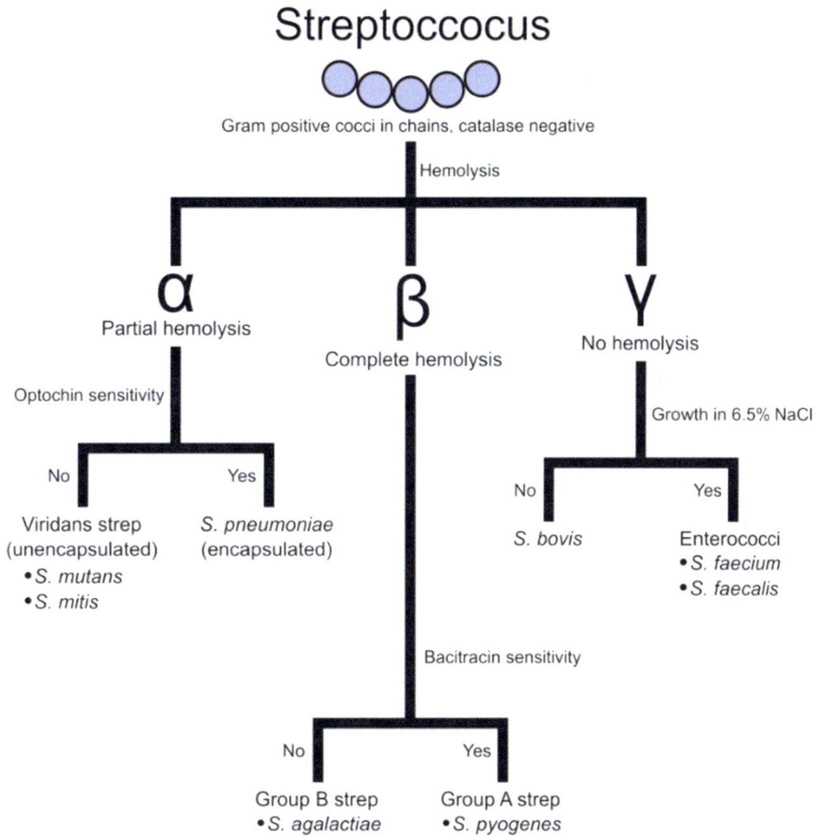

Figure 6.7. *Streptococcus.*

Source: https://upload.medbullets.com/topic/104175/images/*Streptococcus*%20classification%20-%20moises.jpg.

Another clinical importance of *Streptococcus* species comes in the form of involvement in polymicrobial infection, particularly involving gram-negative bacteria. The research on cervico-facial sepsis, for instance, indicates the complexity of infection where mixed bacterial flora are usually recovered. In a survey at Tygerberg Academic Hospital, it was observed that patients who reported with cervico-facial sepsis did not have gram-negative organisms cultured despite the presence of Gram stains for such bacteria, indicating predominance of Gram-positive cocci in such infections (Barnard, 2019). It raises questions regarding the interaction of streptococci with other bacterial populations and what that means for antibiotic treatment regimens. Survival of such microbes in polymicrobial environments indicates the need for directed therapeutic interventions against both Gram-positive and Gram-negative microbes on an equal basis. Analysis of epidemiology and resistance patterns of *Streptococcus* species is important due to their changing nature and impact on public health. The emergence of antibiotic resistance in certain strains, particularly *S. pneumoniae*, necessitates ongoing surveillance and revision of therapeutic recommendations. Research into the prevalence of these organisms across various clinical environments has indicated that while a majority continue to remain susceptible to standard antibiotic therapy, increasing reports of resistant organisms are infiltrating the community and clinical environments. As seen in another study conducted at the same university, while gram-negative organisms have been indicated within cultures, streptococci often prevail within pathogenic environments, requiring careful planning when creating treatment regimens (Barnard, 2019). Familiarity with these dynamics is crucial for clinicians to ensure maximum patient outcomes and to effectively treat against the hazards presented by these Gram-positive cocci (Figure 6.7).

6.2.3. Enterococcus Species

The Enterococcus species, , such as opportunistic pathogens *Enterococcus faecalis* and Enterococcus faecium, play a vital role in disease as well as in human health. They are Gram-positive cocci that naturally inhabit the gastrointestinal tract of human beings as well as other mammals and have already demonstrated their role in maintaining the gut flora and facilitating digestion. Yet, their ability to infect especially in the immunocompromised patient or in the medical device bearer has established Enterococcus species as serious clinical pathogens. Their resistance to numerous environmental stresses combined with antibiotic resistance presents serious challenges in clinical environments. Their identification and monitoring are significant in avoiding infection control and treatment effectiveness, particularly with their capability to contaminate the health environment and, in turn, increase nosocomial infections, as indicated by recent research (Mthembu et al., 2017).

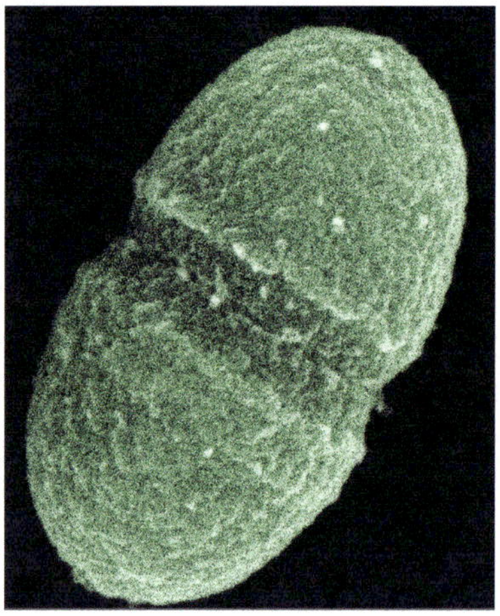

Figure 6.8. *Enterococcus faecalis.*

Source: https://upload.wikimedia.org/wikipedia/commons/thumb/4/4a/Enterococcus_faecalis20023-300.jpg/800px-Enterococcus_faecalis20023-300.jpg.

Increased Enterococcus species detection in clinical specimens in recent studies has led to concerns regarding their causative roles in producing wound infections and other critical complications. For instance, E. faecalis was identified as a significant isolate of diabetic ulcers in a study, and the organism's contribution to polymicrobial infections was highlighted (Mthembu et al., 2017). The importance of proper identification of Enterococcus species in clinical microbiology is highlighted in such instances. Identification using biochemical assays and molecular tools in patient samples becomes important in order to guide therapeutic interventions (Figure 6.8).

The extremely high rate of Enterococcus species among risk groups and chronic diseases warrants ongoing observation and research to understand their pathogenic mechanisms and patterns of susceptibility adequately. Further, the adaptability of Enterococcus species to different environments is unimaginable, as proved by their occurrence in unusual environments, even human breast milk. The characterization of breast milk commensal bacteria has yielded significant isolates, , such as E. *faecalis*, highlighting the complexity of microbiota involved in infant health. It highlights a two-faced role of Enterococcus species, they are crucial members of the microbiota and potential pathogens under certain circumstances. Additional studies and general investigations are required to clarify their role in disease and health, reiterating the significance of knowledge about these Gram-positive cocci to ensure better clinical outcomes and targeted therapeutic strategies (Figure 6.9).

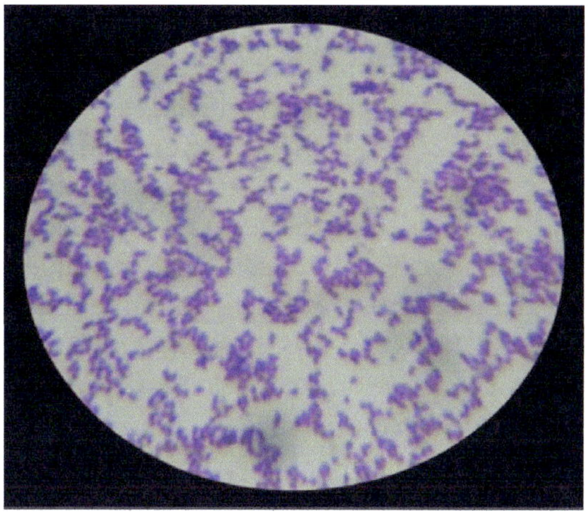

Figure 6.9. *Enterococcus faecalis* (microscopic view).

Source: https://www.researchgate.net/profile/Hardik-Patel 78/publication/353175503/figure/fig2/AS:1044656330649601@1626076886188/Enterococcus-faecalis-microscopic-view.png.

Test Your Knowledge

1. What are the main genera of Gram-positive cocci, and how are they typically classified?
2. What are the key characteristics and clinical significance of Staphylococcus aureus?

6.3. Pathogenicity and Diseases

Learning Outcome

1. Understand common infections caused by Gram-positive cocci
2. Describe mechanisms of virulence in Gram-positive cocci
2. Define antibiotic resistance issues

Pathogenicity of Gram-positive cocci entails a range of mechanisms through which these bacteria can infect and evade the host's immunity. One impressive case is that of *Staphylococcus aureus*, particularly methicillin-resistant *S. aureus* (MRSA), associated with catastrophic disease and high lethality. This bacterium has a number of virulence factors, including the exotoxin production and the enzymes that facilitate tissue invasion. MRSA prevalence is alarming and has reportedly been responsible for killing more individuals than AIDS in some regions, highlighting the need for proper treatment strategies and antibiotic stewardship. It is hence important to understand the underlying genetic and biochemical mechanisms behind the development of pathogenicity in order to design new therapies against these potent superbugs (Gillen et al., 2009). Another significant Gram-positive cocci of concern is *Streptococcus pneumoniae*, which is responsible for community-acquired pneumonia and meningitis. Its virulence relies on a number of factors, , such as the polysaccharide capsule that inhibits phagocytosis, hence enhancing bacterial survival in the host. Besides, pneumolysin, an exotoxin from *Streptococcus pneumoniae*, is able to cause cell lysis of host tissues and enhance disease progression.

The epidemiology of the pathogen has varied over time, mainly due to the use of vaccines against specific serotypes. Nevertheless, the emergence of vaccine-resistant strains remains a challenge. Thus, tracking such trends and an understanding of the mechanisms of serotype change are essential for public health programs that aim to regulate disease caused by this bacterium (Gall & Riely, 1965.). In addition to these direct pathogenic mechanisms, even the healthy mixed Gram-positive cocci flora can cause disease under certain circumstances, , such as immunocompromised conditions or disruption of the skin. As an example, such the presence of cocci in human skin colonially tends to exclude more virulent pathogens from colonizing. Disruption of the environment, however, can disrupt the above balance and cause opportunistic infection. The character of interaction with the habitat among skin microflora becomes extremely relevant in unique situations, , such as long-duration space exploration, where traditional microbial interaction would significantly change. Research into these areas can provide leads to the pathogenic potential under new conditions and stress the need to conduct more research on human-associated microbiomes (Gall & Riely, 1965).

6.3.1. Common Infections Caused by Gram-positive Cocci

The contribution of Gram-positive cocci to infectious diseases cannot be underestimated since they continue to be a major cause of many clinically relevant infections. Of these, *Staphylococcus aureus* is a well-known pathogen responsible for a wide range of conditions, ranging from innocuous skin infections to life-threatening conditions , such as pneumonia, endocarditis, and sepsis. This pathogenic versatility is, in turn, due to its ability to produce a variety of virulence factors like toxins and nutrient-acquisition enzymes that help the bacteria to obtain nutrients and evade the immune system. Besides, the emergence of methicillin-resistant *Staphylococcus aureus* (MRSA) has contributed to the burden that falls on healthcare systems, rendering routine treatment regimens ineffective and requiring new management methods (Pieniążek et al., 2024). The ongoing researches on the epidemiology and treatment of MRSA still highlight the importance of strict surveillance of infections of Gram-positive cocci in the community and in hospitals. Another major genus among Gram-positive cocci is *Streptococcus*, with several species bearing varied clinical importance. *Streptococcus* pyogenes is responsible for infections , such as pharyngitis, impetigo, and rheumatic fever, for example. Its propensity to cause very serious complications renders it of interest in the public health discourse. *Streptococcus pneumoniae*, on the other hand, is notoriously known for causing infections in the respiratory system, particularly pneumonia, meningitis, and otitis media. *S. pneumoniae* vaccination campaigns have evolved over time, although antibiotic resistance complicates therapy. Evidence indicates the effectiveness of antibiotic prophylaxis varies considerably, necessitating specific therapy patterns depending on the individual strains seen in clinical practice (Bryant et al., 2017). The wide clinical presentation and stable resistance patterns of these streptococcal infections necessitate ongoing research to maximize treatment regimens. Enterococcus species, particularly *Enterococcus faecalis* and *Enterococcus faecium*, are emerging pathogens in the field of Gram-positive cocci. Historically a component of the normal gut microbiota, they are capable of causing nosocomial infection, particularly in immunocompromised patients. Enterococci are naturally resistant to many antibiotics, making treatment challenging. They are perhaps best known for their role in urinary tract infection, bacteremia, and endocarditis, particularly in patients with underlying disease.

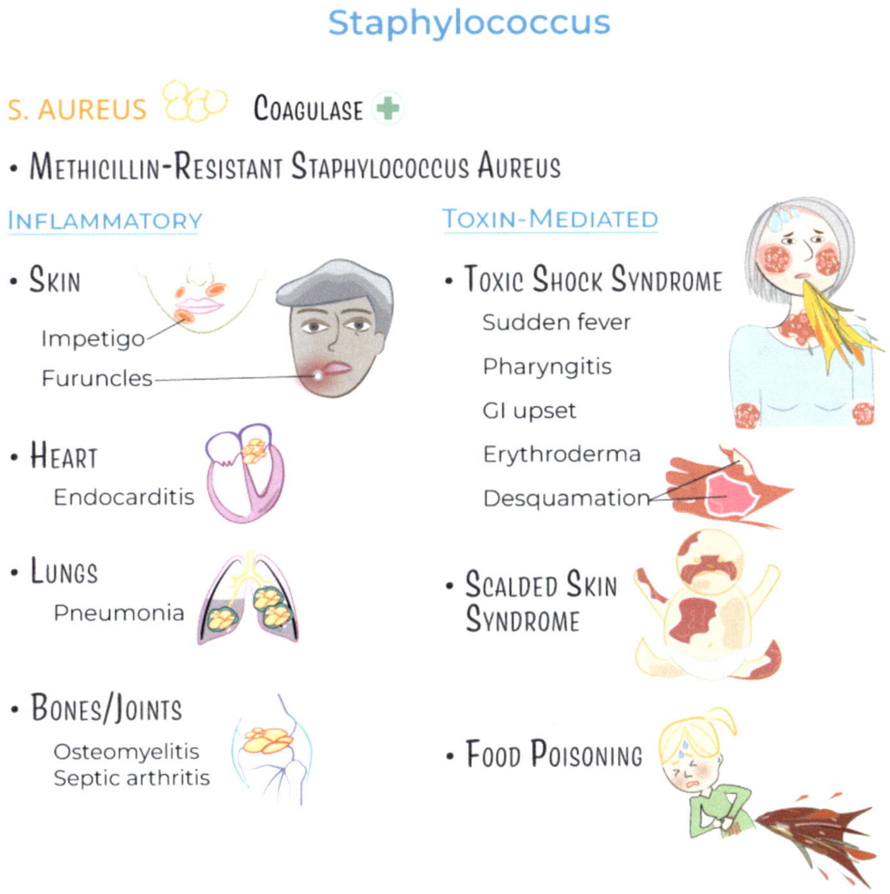

Figure 6.10. *Staphylococcus* infection.

Source: https://d1j63owfs0b5j3.cloudfront.net/term/images/Gram-positive-cocci-4718.png.

The emergence of vancomycin-resistant enterococci (VRE) once again points to the challenge of these bacteria as VRE infection is associated with increased morbidity and healthcare costs. Continuous surveillance and research into enterococcal infection are required to promote the outcome of treatment and map out effective measures of prevention, thus emphasizing the supreme importance of clinical awareness and antimicrobial stewardship in the treatment of Gram-positive cocci infection (Bryant et al., 2017; Pieniążek et al., 2024) (Figure 6.10).

6.3.2. Mechanisms of Virulence

The virulence processes of Gram-positive cocci are multifaceted and involve the production of numerous factors that promote colonization, survival, and evasion of host defenses. Biofilm formation is one of the most significant determinants of pathogenicity among these factors. Gram-positive cocci , such as *Staphylococcus aureus* are capable of adhering to host tissue and medical devices and forming biofilms that protect them against both the immune system and antibiotic treatment. This characteristic is most problematic in chronic wound infections, where strains that produce biofilm have been implicated in delayed healing and antibiotic resistance. Research has shown that 80% of bacterial strains from chronic wound isolates exhibit biofilm production, highlighting its position as an essential virulence factor that allows such pathogens to persist more effectively (Bordignon et al., 2017).

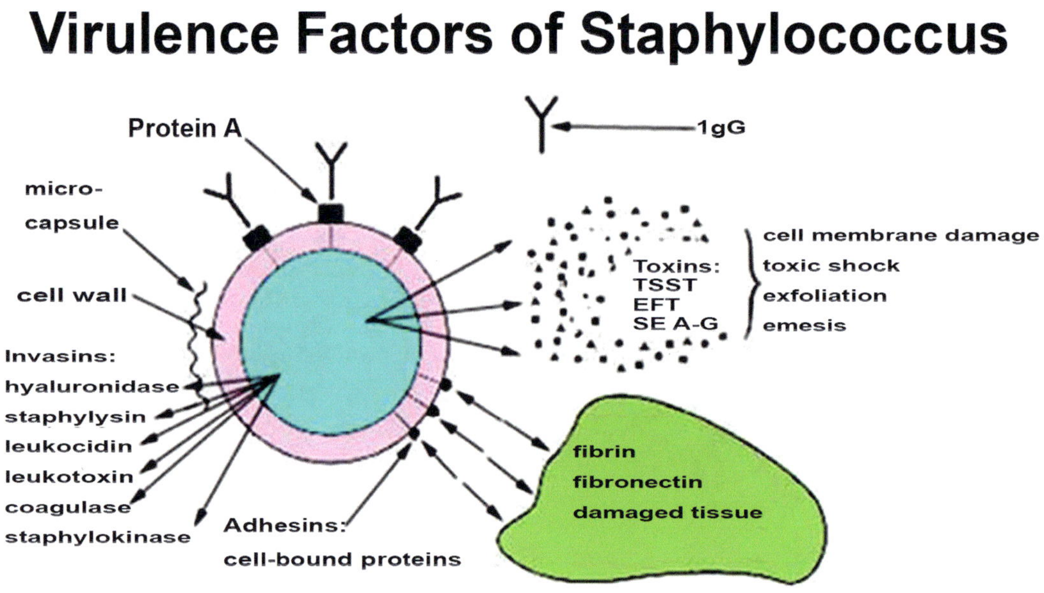

Figure 6.11. Virulence factors of *Staphylococcus*.

Source: https://microbiologyinfo.com/wp-content/uploads/2016/01/Virulence-Factors-of-*Staphylococcus*.jpg.

Therefore, treating infections associated with biofilm poses a challenging problem in clinical microbiology. The second essential virulence strategy in Gram-positive cocci is in the gene transfer process, whereby the transfer of antibiotic resistance and virulence factors between populations of bacteria occurs. Horizontal gene transfer can occur via processes, such as transformation, transduction, and conjugation that enable bacteria to acquire genes that contribute to their survival as well as versatility within hostile environments. For instance, under conditions, such as the gastrointestinal tract and oral cavity, Gram-positive bacteria can exchange genes encoding virulence factors, thereby increasing their virulence. The exchange is worst when under antibiotic stress, where resistant bacteria multiply and disseminate resistant genes to previously susceptible organisms

(Mullany et al., 2000). When these pathogenic strains proliferate, they underscore the need for continued research on mechanisms of gene transfer and their importance to public health. In addition to biofilm formation and gene transfer, the production of specific virulence factors, , such as exotoxins and surface proteins, are central to Gram-positive coccid pathogenicity. For instance, *Staphylococcus aureus* secretes enterotoxins that can cause severe gastrointestinal disease, and toxins like hemolysins that can damage host tissues, facilitating the entry and spread of the bacteria. Surface proteins like clumping factor and protein A, besides augmenting adhesion to the host tissue, also suppress the immune system by preventing opsonization and phagocytosis. The coordinated action of these pathways produces a firm virulence plan that allows Gram-positive cocci to effectively infect and colonize hosts. Knowledge of such pathways is essential for the design of targeted therapeutic strategies against fighting infections caused by these resilient pathogens (Figure 6.11).

6.3.3. Antibiotic Resistance Issues

Antibiotic resistance has emerged as a matter of utmost public health concern, particularly in Gram-positive cocci , such as *Staphylococcus aureus* and Enterococcus. These organisms possess the intriguing ability to acquire resistance genes, most commonly through horizontal gene transfer, and thereby thrive under antibiotic conditions. This lack of predictability not only complicates the treatment plan but also enhances the nosocomial infection risk and that of epidemic community infection. Methicillin-resistant *Staphylococcus aureus* (MRSA), for instance, has become endemic in various settings, leading to increased morbidity and mortality. Hence, it is essential to discern the processes by which these bacteria become resistant to antibiotics so that one can implement efficient therapeutic practices and public health strategies aimed at the control of transmission of resistant bacteria. Experiments have established that the use of antibiotics in agricultural practice has a core contribution to the emergence of resistant bacterial species, both human and non-human. For instance, the application of antibiotics in pig farming has long-term effects, as it promotes the development of multidrug-resistant Enterococcus and other coagulase-negative staphylococci. Evidence indicates that 98% of the isolates gained from the air within the concentrated swine feeding operations were resistant to multiple antibiotics that are usually used in their treatment (Chapin et al., 2004). This stark evidence of antibiotic resistance in farm environments reveals an immediate need for stricter controls on the use of antibiotics in farm animals. Lacking such reform of these farming practices, the ecological reservoirs of antibiotic-resistant bacteria can continue to threaten human health, aggravating the challenge of treatment of uncomplicated infections that were once easily curable. Secondary infections complicating diseases like Buruli ulcer also reveal the complexity of antibiotic resistance in healthcare. Buruli ulcer patients also experience infections from resistant bacterial strains, most prominent among them being *Staphylococcus aureus* and *Pseudomonas aeruginosa*, which make them more difficult to treat (Pahlevan et al., 2013). The evidence of over 60% of Buruli ulcers with resistant pathogens highlights a critical shortfall in curing such infections effectively. Such a long-standing issue not only prolongs the healing period but also health expenditure and chances of subsequent complications. Combining antibiotic resistance in the case of disease like Buruli ulcer entails a multi-faceted approach that comprises improving the surveillance of bacterial infections, improving infection control, and antibiotic stewardship programs. As bacteria become increasingly prevalent with resistance, the health system should adapt in due time to ensure patient outcomes are safeguarded.

Test Your Knowledge

1. What common infections are caused by Staphylococcus aureus, and what makes it a particularly dangerous Gram-positive cocci?
2. What are the main virulence factors of Streptococcus pneumoniae, and how do they contribute to its pathogenicity?

6.4. Laboratory Identification

Learning Outcome

1. Describe culture techniques and media
2. Explain how biochemical tests play a crucial role in identifying Gram-positive cocci
3. Understand molecular methods for the detection of Gram-positive cocci

Laboratory identification of Gram-positive cocci is an important feature in microbiology due to their clinical significance in various infections. Gram-positive cocci are identified by a thick peptidoglycan cell wall that retains the crystal violet stain used in Gram staining and thus presents a purple color when examined under a microscope. These are typically found under genera like *Staphylococcus*, *Streptococcus*, and Enterococcus, which have numerous species under each that need to be identified using specific methods. Laboratory workup most often begins with the collection and culturing of the clinical specimens, i.e., blood, pus, or throat swabs. The different biochemical tests, like the catalase test for distinguishing Streptococci from Staphylococci, following culturing assist in initial identification. Laboratory identification is important because it decides the treatment and patient outcome in cases of infection caused by these organisms. After preliminary testing, more sophisticated identification techniques may be employed to come to a definitive diagnosis. For instance, selective media, , such as mannitol salt agar to culture *Staphylococcus aureus*, allow isolation on the basis of specific growth factors. Further testing, such as hemolysis on blood agar, separates *Streptococcus* species. In addition to biochemical tests, molecular methods, , such as PCR, have emerged at the forefront of identifying and characterizing Gram-positive cocci with accuracy. The methods are more specific and sensitive than traditional culture approaches. Additionally, (Taylor et al.) outlines systematic laboratory procedures that involve immunological methods, which can complement biochemical testing and provide a reliable identification system. By applying a combination of these techniques, laboratories can facilitate correct identification of pathogenic strains. Ultimately, effects of laboratory identification of Gram-positive cocci are greater than classification because they have an impact on public health and infection control strategies. Identification of the specific strain of a pathogen enables clinicians to manage antibiotic therapy correctly, thereby minimizing antimicrobial resistance and patient cure rates. Besides, awareness of the virulence factors of each species informs surveillance and control of infections. The synergy between traditional microbiologic methods and advanced molecular diagnostics provides the basis for effective laboratory practice in this area. Proper identification of Gram-positive cocci is thus not a classification issue; it is an essential step in the control of bacterial infections and the avoidance of public health crises from misdiagnosis or late treatment. To this end, (Bizzini et al., 2013) supports the contention that effective laboratory identification is a key component of disease control as it allows doctors to properly react to the complexities of microbial infections.

6.4.1. Culture Techniques and Media

Gram-positive cocci in clinical settings require special culture techniques and a proper medium for identification and subsequent investigation. In clinical lab settings, most conventional techniques, like blood agar and mannitol salt agar, are utilized by most institutions in growing Gram-positive cocci. Blood agar provides an enriched medium to encourage the growth of a wide variety of bacteria, with hemolytic patterns seen that can be used to differentiate species within the *Streptococcus* and *Staphylococcus* genera. Mannitol salt agar, on the other hand, enriches for *Staphylococcus* species and differentiates *Staphylococcus aureus* from other coagulase-negative staphylococci. These differential culture techniques enable clinicians to rapidly identify pathogens, ultimately leading to effective treatment regimens in the era of rising antibiotic resistance and a need for more advanced diagnostics (Golia et al., 2018). In addition to traditional culturing methods, automated platforms have emerged in their role of minimizing the risk of human error and accelerating the process of Gram-positive cocci identification. For instance, automated blood culture systems, , such as Bact/Alert, allow early identification of microorganisms in sepsis resulting from bloodstream infection, a very clinical issue because of their association with high morbidity and mortality. Automated processing of samples in such systems reduces specimen-to-species time, which is critical to patient outcome. Aside from automation, technologies like Vitek II enable streamlined drug susceptibility testing that helps clinicians make informed decisions regarding antibiotic therapy. Combined, these technologies not only improve diagnostic accuracy but also enable ongoing surveillance of resistant strains that could complicate treatment regimens (Durfee et al.). Lastly, the relationship between culture methodology and microbiological media serves as the foundation of the underlying principles in microbiology, most especially the clinical relevance of Gram-positive cocci. Continual monitoring through such systems is important since Gram-positive bacteria can be differently susceptible to drugs. For instance, the pervasiveness of coagulase-negative staphylococci in bacteremia depicts the need for tailored culture techniques to identify multiple pathogens simultaneously and ascertain their antimicrobial resistance profiles. Enhanced diagnostic regimens are essential not only for infection management but also for eradicating resistant organisms from healthcare environments. With technology advancement, integrating traditional methods with new technologies will enhance clinical microbiology's role in combating infectious diseases effectively (Golia et al., 2018).

6.4.2. Biochemical Tests for Identification

Biochemical tests are necessary for the identification of Gram-positive cocci, which include significant pathogens , such as *Staphylococcus*, *Streptococcus*, and Enterococcus species. The first step involves Gram staining, distinguishing these bacteria based on the cell wall component. The following biochemical tests involve catalase testing and coagulase testing. For instance, *Staphylococcus aureus* is catalase positive and coagulase positive, in contrast to coagulase-negative staphylococci. This initial classification is rudimentary, as it allows microbiologists to limit the scope of possible pathogenic agents effectively, so therapeutic interventions are appropriately done. These diagnostic processes are vital with the increasing incidence of antibiotic resistance among Gram-positive cocci, which further proves the significance of proper identification (Purushottam et al., 2025).

Further biochemical tests are required to narrow down the identification of Gram-positive cocci. Carbohydrate fermentation tests can provide additional information, particularly for the *Streptococcus* species, which can be categorized based on their ability to ferment various sugars. For example, *Streptococcus pneumoniae* ferments maltose and glucose but not lactose, and *Streptococcus* pyogenes also prefers the same.

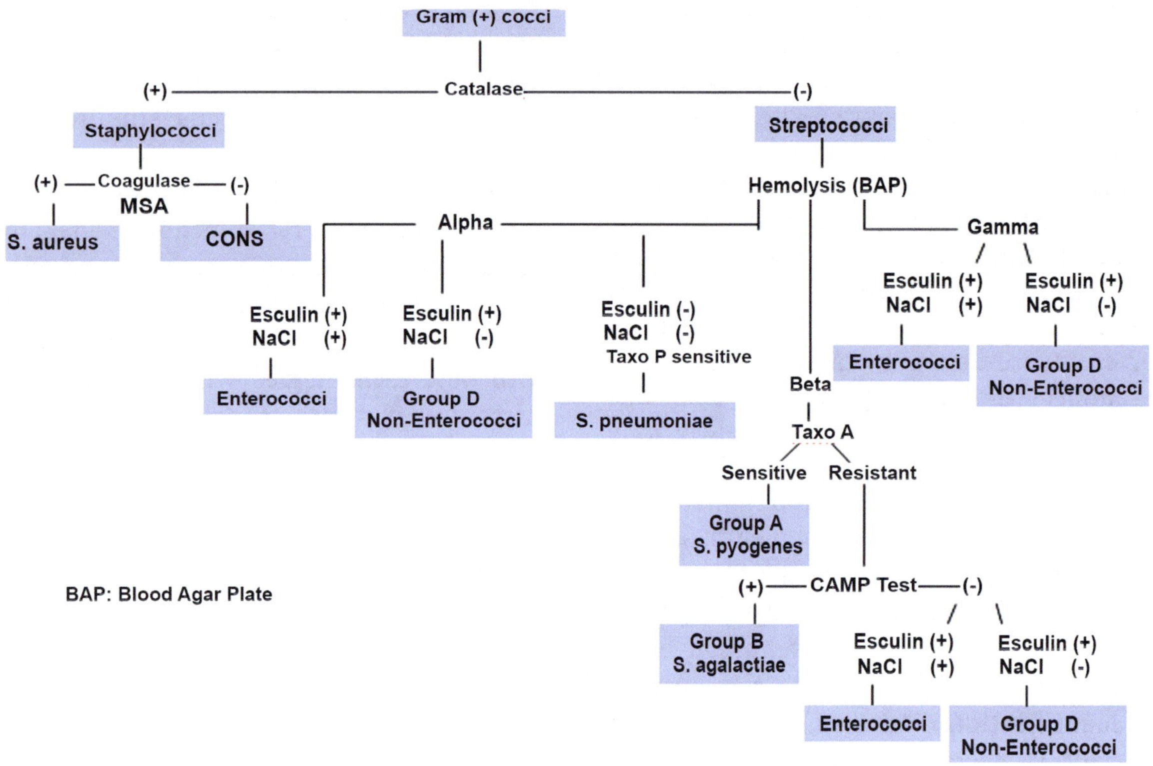

Figure 6.12. Biochemical tests for differentiating Gram-positive cocci.

Source: https://i0.wp.com/microbeonline.com/wp-content/uploads/2013/05/Biochemical-tests-for-differentiating-Gram-positive-cocci.png?w=686&ssl=1.

Further, the presence of the Lancefield system of classification is an added possibility for differentiation among beta-hemolytic streptococci, which helps clinicians identify specific strains responsible for outbreak syndromes. Understanding these biochemical characteristics is important in that they guide the effect of treatment options and interventions, particularly in clinical settings that may be delayed from appropriate therapy due to misidentification (Eyaufe et al., 2016).

Ultimately, the integrated method of biochemical analysis not only serves the specific identification of Gram-positive cocci but also guides wider community health initiatives. Monitoring pathogenic strains, particularly multi-drug resistant strains, is necessary for the prevention and control of infection. For instance, as recently identified, the emergence of Methicillin-resistant *Staphylococcus aureus* (MRSA) poses a threat to the healthcare systems worldwide and needs to be monitored continuously for its biochemical markers. The integration of new testing technologies, i.e., multiplex PCR with the traditional biochemical tests, can be beneficial in the enhancement of the accuracy and speed of identification. Therefore, a sound understanding of biochemical testing is priceless for clinical microbiologists, ultimately resulting in improved patient outcomes and interventions in public health following emerging bacterial threats (Purushottam et al., 2025) (Figure 6.12).

6.4.3. Molecular Methods for Detection

The evolution of molecular methods of detection has transformed the diagnostic process in Gram-positive cocci, particularly in the identification of clinically significant pathogens , such as *Staphylococcus* and *Streptococcus* species. Some of the methods that allow rapid amplification of specific genetic sequences of these cocci include polymerase chain reaction (PCR) and real-time PCR. The specificity decreases the possibilities of false positives or false negatives, which enhances the process of identification of pathogens. Use of molecular diagnostics not only enhances detection sensitivity but also allows for the early initiation of optimal treatment regimens, an essential consideration in managing infections caused by such pathogens. In addition, molecular methods could detect antibiotic resistance genes, thereby informing healthcare workers about the appropriate treatment options on time, which could be important with the rising antimicrobial resistance (Bizzini et al., 2013). Also, multiplex PCR has emerged as a prime candidate for simultaneous detection of several pathogens, thereby being greatly useful in clinical settings where co-infections are prone to occur. This method allows concurrent identification of various Gram-positive cocci and other pathogens from the same sample, hence saving time and resource utilization involved in laboratory diagnosis. For instance, discrimination between pathogenic and non-pathogenic strains of *Streptococcus pneumoniae* improves clinical management. Moreover, techniques , such as whole-genome sequencing can provide total data regarding the genetic makeup of Gram-positive cocci, hence allowing epidemiological and outbreak investigation. The integration of these molecular techniques into routine microbiological practices is an imperative for the advancement of public health policy, as well as patient welfare in infectious diseases (Malimu, 2012).

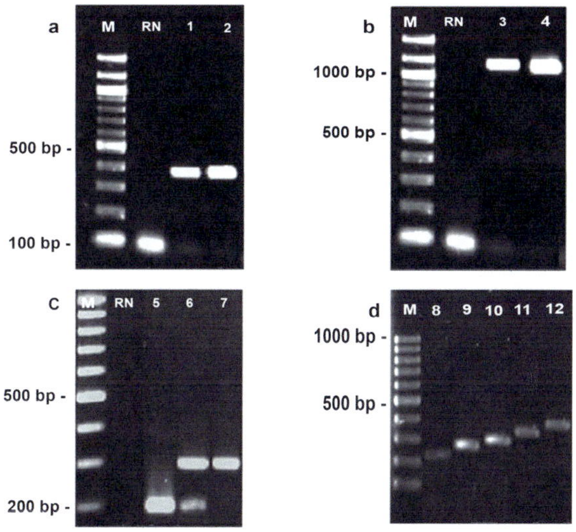

Figure 6.13. Agarose (1.5%) gel electrophoresis of *Staphylococcus aureus* PCR products of virulence factor genes. M = molecular weight standard; RN = negative reaction; (a) 1 = icaD-positive isolate (381 bp), 2 = control reaction; (b) 3 = icaA-positive isolate (1,315 bp), 4 = control reaction; (c) 5 = hla-positive isolate (210 bp), 6 = positive isolate for both genes (hla and hlb), 7 = hlb-positive isolate (300 bp); (d) 8 = spaA-positive isolate (polymorphic region; 220 bp), 9 = spaA-positive isolate (250 bp), 10 = spaA-positive isolate (280 bp), 11 = spaA-positive isolate (300 bp); and 12 = spaA-positive isolate (315 bp).

Source: https://www.researchgate.net/profile/Miliane-Souza/publication/51244861/figure/fig1/AS:305924746039300@1449949551517/Agarose-15-gel-electrophoresis-of-*Staphylococcus*-aureus-PCR-products-of-virulence.png.

Within the broader scope of clinical microbiology, the application of molecular methods in identifying Gram-positive cocci emphasizes the necessity of continuous development of, as well as validation for, molecular assays. With improvement in diagnostic technologies, quality control processes and standardization processes are most important to ensure consistency in settings. Advances in sample collection and preparation techniques are equally important to improve the ability of molecular detection methods to reach their optimal capacity. It is important that health facilities are updated with the generation of new technologies and apply processes that meet existing standards in order to optimize detection capacity. With an increase in understanding of microbial pathogenesis, molecular techniques will increasingly significantly influence the diagnosis and treatment of Gram-positive cocci infection, ultimately leading to improved health (Bizzini et al., 2013) (Figure 6.13).

Test Your Knowledge

1. What type of culture media is commonly used to isolate Gram-positive cocci?
2. Which biochemical test is used to distinguish Staphylococcus aureus from other Staphylococcus species, and what is the expected result?

6.5. Treatment and Management

Learning Outcome

1. Understand the antibiotic landscape for treating infections caused by Gram-positive cocci
2. Discuss about challenges in the treatment of infections caused by Gram-positive cocci
3. Explain the role of vaccines in preventing infections

Management and treatment of Gram-positive coccus infections require a multi-modal strategy because these pathogens present unique challenges due to their intrinsic resistance and variability in susceptibility patterns. Effective management starts with accurate identification of the causative pathogen because therapeutic action can differ significantly depending on the pathogen. For instance, *Staphylococcus aureus*, particularly its methicillin-resistant strains (MRSA), requires focused antibiotics , such as vancomycin or linezolid. Similarly, *Streptococcus pneumoniae* infection typically requires targeted therapy based on susceptibility testing since resistance trends may vary geographically. Emergence of drug-resistant strains necessitates ongoing monitoring and evolution of treatment regimens to provide effective patient outcomes with minimal risk for additional development of resistance. In addition to antibiotic therapy, supportive therapy is also a key in the treatment of Gram-positive coccus infections, especially in severe cases. For example, Enterococcus infections tend to develop high morbidity when they present as polymicrobial infections. Combination therapy could enhance therapeutic efficacy and also prevent resistance development. On top of this, resolution of contributing conditions, , such as diabetes or immunocompromised state, may also enable more efficient healing and reduce the risk of chronic infection. Utilization of multidisciplinary approaches, , such as the integration of infectious disease specialists, can also optimize management plans, providing maximized patient care through personalized treatments based on up-to-date clinical guidelines. The growing issue with bacterial biofilm production is one of the biggest obstacles in the successful treatment of chronic Gram-positive coccus infections, particularly those involving implanted medical devices or chronic wounds. Studies have shown that biofilm-producing strains , such as methicillin-resistant *Staphylococcus aureus* (MRSA) result in wound healing defects and increased resistance against regular antibiotic regimens. These biofilms are recalcitrant and need not only pharmacologic therapy but mechanical removal procedures where appropriate. As is evident from recent reports, eradication of these biofilm-related infections requires a synergistic strategy combining debridement with high-level antibiotics individually tailored to the biofilms pattern of susceptibility. Hence, discovering solutions for the problems of biofilm-based infections in treatment mode is very important for attaining optimal outcomes for patients affected with Gram-positive cocci infection (Malimu, 2012; Bordignon et al., 2017).

6.5.1. Antibiotic Options and Effectiveness

The antibiotic context for the therapy of Gram-positive cocci infections is complex, particularly due to the rising trend of antibiotic resistance. Methicillin-resistant *Staphylococcus aureus* (MRSA) ranks among the most common and dangerous pathogens of Gram-positive cocci. Effective control demands a careful manner in choosing antibiotics, , such as vancomycin, which remains the drug of choice for treating MRSA infections. The existence of vancomycin-resistant organisms necessitates searching for alternative therapies. Daptomycin and linezolid are established effective agents, offering new therapeutic alternatives. Yet their clinical usefulness may vary, necessitating susceptibility testing to guide appropriate therapy. The physician has the dilemma of balancing the efficacy of existing antibiotics in light of the growing threat of microbial resistance, highlighting the urgent need to pursue research and development of novel antimicrobial agents to counter this menace. In the context of antibiotic therapy, biofilm and resistance in Gram-positive cocci have clinical relevance. Such strains complicate treatment regimes, as they are more resistant to standard antibiotics. For instance, research indicates that nearly all methicillin-resistant *Staphylococcus aureus* (MRSA) strains were identified to produce moderate to high biofilm levels, which complicates eradicating them from chronic infections and wounds. The fact that clinical isolates have such a high rate of biofilm production accounts for their importance as a virulence factor, which strongly determines the result of treatment. This is particularly alarming because biofilms facilitate chronic infection, often necessitating long antibiotic courses or surgery to ultimately lead to resolution. Hence, understanding biofilm dynamics and its implications for antibiotic effectiveness is the crux for devising targeted approaches against these recalcitrant infections, particularly in chronically ill patient groups. There is increasing evidence supporting the rethinking of antibiotic protocols to include the new paradigm of resistance and biofilm-based infections in the context of Gram-positive cocci. The Surgical Infection Societys model of intra-abdominal infections (IAI) illustrates this response to shifts in resistance patterns, highlighting the need for updated recommendations regarding antimicrobial therapy selection and treatment duration. Employing a systematic, evidence-based approach allows healthcare providers to apply the most current available data to make clinical decisions, ultimately leading to improved patient outcomes. As underscored in recent guidelines, knowledge of the risk factors, source control interventions, and individualized antibiotic protocols is still critical to the prevention of IAI from Gram-positive cocci. This is one trend in infectious disease management where antibiotic stewardship and continued resiliency in adapting to resistance patterns are essential to maximize successful treatment as well as prevent deleterious outcomes because of emerging antibiotic resistance and biofilm (Bordignon et al., 2017; Chang et al., 2017) (Figure 6.14).

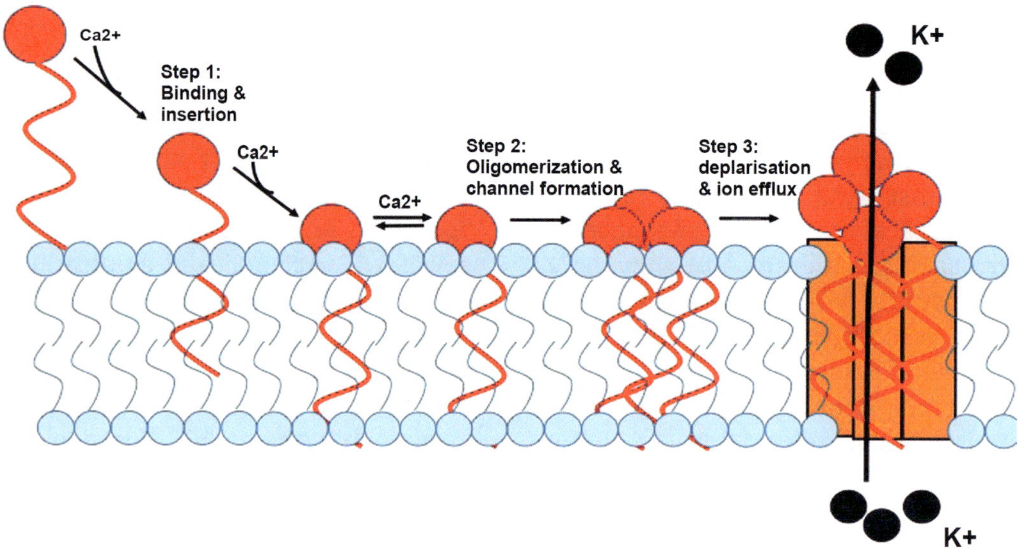

Figure 6.14. Mechanism of daptomycin action. (1) Daptomycin binds and inserts into the cell membrane; (2) aggregates the cell membrane; and (3) alters the shape of the cell membrane to form a hole in the cell, allowing ions in and out of the cell easily.

Source: https://upload.wikimedia.org/wikipedia/commons/1/12/Mechanism_of_Daptomycin_Action.jpg.

6.5.2. Challenges in Treatment

Gram-positive coccus infection management is faced with significant challenges that must be addressed with care. One of the greatest challenges is the escalating antibiotic resistance rates, particularly among methicillin-resistant *Staphylococcus aureus* (MRSA). MRSA infections are very difficult to manage due to their beta-lactam resistance and are likely to necessitate options that are more expensive or less potent. Furthermore, the employment of broad-spectrum antibiotics can compromise the healthy microbiota and the ability of other pathogens to proliferate and develop a complex therapeutic situation. This interaction results in antibiotic resistance and difficult-to-control infections constituting a vicious cycle, which is an important barrier to favorable treatment in clinics, especially in risk groups , such as neonates and the elderly. Other than resistance to antibiotics, variability of responses between patients to treatment also further complicates infection control by Gram-positive cocci more complicated. Age variability, comorbidities, and immune status all play a crucial role in determining the effectiveness of antimicrobial agents. Neonates, for instance, are placed at higher risk due to their immature immune systems and thus treated with mupirocin to decolonize MRSA, which will minimize the risk of associated infections (Bryant et al., 2017). Introduction of such interventions comes with risks because the risks of adverse effects and the emergence of new pathogens have to be weighed considerably against the benefits. Therefore, individualized treatment courses based on patient profiles and consideration of these factors still challenge health professionals. Furthermore, the limited range of available agents makes the process of treating Gram-positive coccus infections difficult. Most of the existing treatment regimens are based on traditional antibiotics, but the emergence of resistant strains warrants ongoing research and discovery of new agents. While mupirocin has been effective at preventing MRSA infections, its limited activity spectrum requires complementary measures for the prevention of other Gram-positive infections (Pieniążek et al., 2024). The urgency for new solutions requires increased collaboration among scientists, clinicians, and industry stakeholders to develop more potent antimicrobial drugs and prophylactics. Thus, the conquest of the therapy conundrum of Gram-positive cocci not only relies on the development of existing therapies but also highlights the importance of preemptive research and education in the battle against bacterial infections.

6.5.3. Role of Vaccines in Prevention

Vaccination is an important means of preventing disease caused by Gram-positive cocci, including such familiar pathogens as *Streptococcus pneumoniae* and *Staphylococcus aureus*. The development and deployment of vaccines have had a major impact on limiting morbidity and mortality due to infections caused by these microbes.

For instance, the pneumococcal vaccine has exhibited a remarkable efficacy in the prevention of invasive pneumococcal disease, particularly among vulnerable populations like the aged and immunocompromised individuals. Through the immunization of the immune system to recognize and respond rapidly to the polysaccharide capsules of *Streptococcus pneumoniae*, not only do vaccines mitigate the severity of infection, but also limit the spread of antibiotic resistance by eliminating cases that would require intensive treatments, thus supporting public health interventions in limiting bacterial infection. Furthermore, the vaccine field has grown due to the discovery of novel antimicrobial strategies that employ vaccine technology. For example, research has shown that vaccines directed against pathogens, which are most often associated with catheter-related urinary tract infections and which prominently feature Gram-positive cocci secondary infections, lead to improved patient outcomes.

The integration of vaccines with preventive measures, , such as the use of anti-infective urinary catheters, is a multifaceted patient care modality. These catheters have been constructed in such a way that they exhibit antiinfective surface activity, thereby reducing the risk of complications and infections that would otherwise give rise to severe medical conditions, showing how vaccination, as a healthcare development, can collaborate with other medical innovations to facilitate infection control within health care settings (Maki et al., 2001). Additionally, vaccines are included in veterinary practice, particularly in calf diarrhea, in which multifactorial pathogens like Gram-positive cocci contribute to disease incidence. Immunization of pregnant calves and cows against specific pathogens was successful in reducing the incidence of diarrhea episodes, which form a critical factor contributing to rates of neonatal morbidity and mortality. Arguments for vaccination as a protective measure in livestock highlight the broader context of immunization strategies throughout the medical disciplines, cementing their protective function against disease. In the face of continued threats of evolving pathogen strains along with increasing antibiotic resistance, the protective function of vaccines becomes increasingly critical in safeguarding human and animal health, ultimately supporting an integrated approach to epidemiological control (Blanchard et al., 2012) (Figure 6.15).

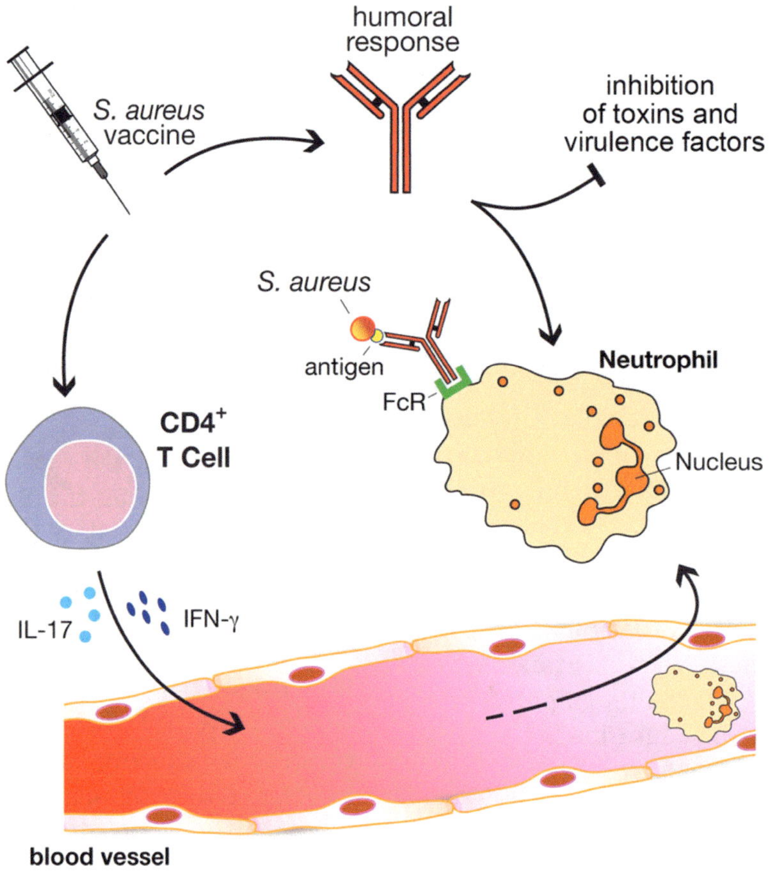

Figure 6.15. A model to generate protective immunity against *S. aureus* infections through vaccination. Protective vaccines should be able to elicit three major immune responses: (i) antibodies to directly inhibit bacterial viability and/or toxicity; (ii) antibodies to mediate opsonophagocytosis; and (iii) cell-mediated immunity to stimulate recruitment of phagocytes (e.g., neutrophils) at the site of the infection.

Source: https://www.researchgate.net/publication/230736119/figure/fig1/AS:11431281238590593@1713997231457/A-model-to-generate-protective-immunity-against-S-aureus-infections-through-vaccination.tif.

Test Your Knowledge

1. What are the first-line antibiotic treatments for infections caused by methicillin-sensitive Staphylococcus aureus (MSSA)?
2. Which antibiotics are commonly used to treat Streptococcus pneumoniae infections?

6.6. Current Research and Developments

Learning Outcome

1. Understand the advances in understanding pathogenic mechanisms
2. Describe advances in diagnostic techniques for Gram-positive cocci
3. Focus on emerging treatments and therapies

Recent advances in technologies for rapid identification have greatly revolutionized the way health practitioners approach the diagnosis and treatment of Gram-positive coccus infections. Perhaps one of the biggest breakthroughs is the use of matrix-assisted laser desorption/ionization time-of-flight (MALDI-TOF) mass spectrometry, which has made it possible to quickly identify pathogens from positive blood culture. A recent study indicated the effectiveness of a direct method that makes it possible to identify Gram-positive cocci within 30 minutes. This method demonstrated a 90% concordance level with traditional MALDI-TOF procedures performed on isolated bacteria, which had established its viability in clinical settings (Lupetti et al., 2015). The potential to accelerate antimicrobial therapy in septic patients significantly enhances treatment conditions and stresses the necessity for further investigation into the best methods of diagnostic techniques for Gram-positive infections. In addition to better identification methods, computer-assisted image analysis in clinical microbiology is a promising development for the identification of Gram-positive cocci. Classical classical methods based on manual microscopy are unimaginable for efficiency and standardization. A breakthrough research paper introduced a digital image analysis program to identify Gram-stained microorganisms with high levels of accuracy. Initial tests indicated sensitivity of 66% to 99% and 78% to 99% specificity, which characterized the ability of this technology to augment traditional methods (Hauser et al., 2011). Because the program demonstrated an accuracy rate of 94% across multiple trials after further training, it suggests that computer aids can yield consistent, quantifiable results and streamline laboratory protocols for identifying Gram-positive cocci, eventually contributing towards improved clinical decision-making. Continual improvement in diagnostic instruments and methods puts researchers and clinicians better equipped to manage infections of Gram-positive cocci. The application of sophisticated technology, including MALDI-TOF and digital image analysis, not only simplifies the identification process but also increases the overall efficiency of patient care. Future studies need to strive to further develop such methodologies with an aim to further enhance their utility in various clinical settings and increase their ability to differentiate between closely related bacterial species. With each new volume of information and growth in the sophistication of these technologies, enormous potential for improved surveillance and regulation of Gram-positive cocci exists. This is all the more relevant with growing antimicrobial resistance, underscoring the imperative for continued innovation on both the diagnostic and therapeutic avenues in microbiology.

6.6.1. Advances in Understanding Pathogenic Mechanisms

Improved knowledge of pathogenic mechanisms of Gram-positive cocci has revealed complex mechanisms used by these organisms to cause infections. Increasing research has centered on host-pathogen interactions that enable the virulence of pathogens like *Staphylococcus aureus* and *Streptococcus pneumoniae*. Scientists have identified the genetic determinants for their pathogenicity using advanced tools like transcriptomic profiling and genomic sequencing. For instance, the ability of these bacteria to form biofilm not only assists their survival in host environments but also aids resistance to antibiotics. This increasing knowledge of pathogenic mechanisms becomes an imperative for specific therapeutic interventions that can block these interactions, ultimately bringing about more successful management of infections caused by Gram-positive cocci. Implications of this research have implications within clinical settings, where a greater understanding can determine better treatment and diagnosis policies. Furthermore, exploration of mechanisms of pathogenicity has drawn attention to immune evasion strategies adopted by Gram-positive cocci. As a case in point, the secretion of a number of surface proteins interfering with complement activation is a remarkable strategy in evading host immune attacks. Proteins with LPXTG motifs have been demonstrated to anchor virulence factors onto the bacterial cell wall, increasing the survival and infectivity of pathogens. These findings support the idea that it is critical to understand the mechanisms of anchoring for better knowledge of the biology of the pathogens and the generation of new vaccines and therapeutic compounds. With further research through groundbreaking studies that continue to identify and define these surface proteins, it opens new avenues for the research of Gram-positive pathogenic processes, , such as their relevance to clinical microbiology (Hoick et al., 1999). Research on the role of the microbiome in Gram-positive cocci pathogenicity also exhibits that there is a complex interaction between the host's innate flora and the pathogenic microbe. Recent evidence has shown that the architecture of skin and mucosal microbiota can significantly influence susceptibility to such infections. The co-action between commensal bacteria and putative pathogens can enhance the host defense mechanisms or encourage pathogen development. For instance, the dynamics of skin microfloras under controlled conditions, i.e., space mission simulation, have demonstrated how microbial communities are influenced and affected by external stimuli and play a mediating role in opportunistic infections (Gall et al.). This knowledge contributes to improved understanding of disease mechanisms and presents a potential for microbiota modulation as an infection prevention of Gram-positive cocci, thus opening a new frontier in clinical and translational microbiology.

6.6.2. New Diagnostic Techniques

Advancements in diagnostic techniques for Gram-positive cocci have transformed microbiological tests, particularly the identification of pathogenic strains. Traditional culturing protocols, though the cornerstone, are wanting in specificity for accurate identification of coagulase-negative staphylococci and other Gram-positive bacteria. Novel molecular techniques, , such as polymerase chain reaction (PCR) and nucleic acid amplification tests (NAATs), are now essential tools that enable speedy detection and identification of bacteria on a genetic level. These methods not only raise the incidence of diagnosis but also improve accuracy by minimizing contamination risk inherent with traditional techniques. Ongoing knowledge of bacterial epidemiology necessitates such an improvement with a critical impact in clinical decision-making, where prompt intervention is crucial to patient outcome. Another hopeful diagnostic method is the application of pulsed field gel electrophoresis (PFGE) to define DNA patterns for coagulase-negative staphylococci, an organism that is most often implicated in catheter-related bloodstream infection. The PFGE technique provides a good basis for tracing and identifying bacterial strains, which indicates that most of the cases attributed to such organisms are not properly diagnosed without prejudice. This deployment of the methods enlightens the epidemiology of Gram-positive cocci infection by revealing sources and modes of transmission of the infections. Where at most 33 different strains can be present, phenotypic alone can be inaccurate in a clinical setting, thus the necessity to integrate genealogical approaches into standard diagnostic processes (Dobbins et al., 2002). Such advances allow clinicians to tailor their therapeutic approaches, thereby optimizing patient care. Moreover, the application of genetic engineering techniques for the production of bacterial proteins has created new opportunities for diagnostics, particularly in surface display systems. Anchoring of proteins to the bacterial cell surface of, e.g., lactic acid bacteria (LAB) is a novel method that enhances the display of chimeric proteins for use in diagnostics and therapy. The LPXTG box anchoring motif, widely utilized, can be used to covalently anchor proteins to the cell wall and thus usher in the possibilities of vaccine technologies and enhanced enzyme immobilization (Hoick et al., 1999). As further research ensues, the potential of such techniques to enhance diagnostic processes also becomes clearer, mirroring the new reality of precision medicine. By applying advances in genetic engineering and molecular biology, the field of microbiology is able to develop reliable, rapid diagnostic systems that yield improved outcomes for infected patients caused by Gram-positive cocci (Figure 6.16).

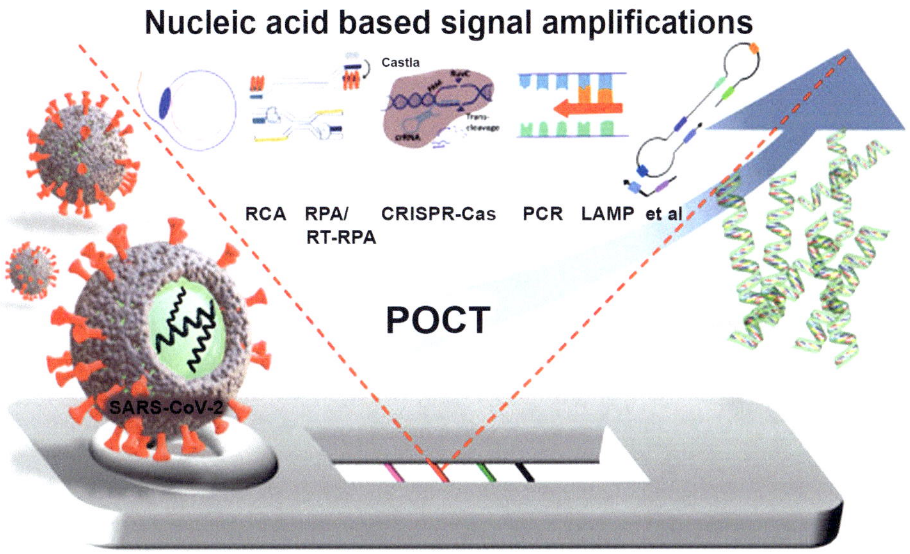

Figure 6.16. Nucleic acid-based amplification tests.

Source: https://ars.els-cdn.com/content/image/1-s2.0-S095656632200149X-gr1.jpg.

6.6.3. Emerging Treatments and Therapies

The emergence of multi-antibiotic resistant Gram-positive cocci presents critical challenges to clinical practice. With organisms like Methicillin-resistant *Staphylococcus aureus* (MRSA), Vancomycin-resistant Enterococcus (VRE), and resistant streptococci still replicating, the effectiveness of traditional antimicrobial therapy is grossly compromised. The introduction of novel drugs like linezolid and daptomycin is a paradigm shift in therapeutic regimes. These drugs introduce new modes of action, enhancing efficacy in resistant populations. In addition, by targeting pharmacokinetic and pharmacodynamic properties, clinicians can optimise dosing schemes with the aim of optimizing patient outcomes. A way of dealing with such infections is being aware of the epidemiological trends and clinical relevance associated with these resistant pathogens, as presented in recent literature, highlighting the utmost necessity of continuing research into novel treatments with promise to control these difficult pathogens (MANFREDI et al., 2006). Chronic infections by Gram-positive cocci, particularly in wounds, complicate treatment strategies. Chronic wounds like pressure sores and diabetic foot sores are prone to harbor populations of resistant bacteria, leading to persistent inflammation that complicates healing mechanisms. Infections may significantly impair quality of life, calling for cutting-edge therapeutic interventions outside the purview of traditional antibiotics. Working on the development of therapies , such as bioengineered dressings and antimicrobial topicals to manage bacterial burden and aid healing is ongoing. Clarifying the intricate host-microbe interaction in chronic wound microenvironments may assist in designing such therapies. Furthermore, approaches that employ knowledge of microbial interaction function to generate synergistic effect on infection control and wound healing, paving the way for improved patient outcome and reduced surgery if other treatments are unsuccessful (Alhede et al., 2016). As Gram-positive climate continues to change, the incorporation of good surveillance and research on novel therapies is essential. Surveillance for patterns of resistance to antibiotics and for the effectiveness of new therapeutic agents has lessons for clinicians. Careful evaluation of new drugs, , such as quinupristin-dalfopristin and tigecycline, alongside proven regimens are essential for guiding clinical decisions. Recent clinical trials establishing safety and effectiveness of these newer treatments promise to fortify our arsenal against resistant bacteria. Furthermore, interdisciplinary approaches that integrate drug development ingenuity with profound understanding of microbiology and mechanisms can achieve care are crucial. A multi-departmental solution is necessary to not only arrest the flow of multi-drug resistant Gram-positive cocci but also to maximize treatment models that are sensitive to the evolving danger of antibiotic resistance (Manfredi et al., 2006).

Test Your Knowledge

1. What recent discoveries have been made about the virulence factors of Staphylococcus aureus?
2. What is the current status of vaccine development against Streptococcus pneumoniae and other Gram-positive cocci, and what novel antigen targets are being explored?

SUMMARY

In explaining the complex dynamics of Gram-positive cocci, it is evident that such microbes play a significant role in human disease and health. Their prevalence in infection necessitates a comprehensive understanding of their characteristics, identification, and control. The chapter has outlined the important implications of Gram-positive cocci in hospitals, emphasizing the need for accurate microbiological diagnosis. The findings of various studies indicate that despite the presence of gram-negative organisms in some cases, clinical presentation in most cases is caused by Gram-positive strains, which underscores their relevance to infection control (Barnard, 2019). Health practitioners thus have to stay up to date with the virulence factors of Gram-positive cocci for the purposes of improving treatment outcomes. Furthermore, the vulnerability of Gram-positive cocci to antimicrobial treatment provides yet another complication to their therapeutic manipulation. Resistance in these bacteria, , such as the establishment of biofilm and the acquisition of antibiotic-resistant genes, complicates traditional methods of therapy. As testified by recent research, the establishment of resistant strains provides a impetus for ongoing surveillance and new treatment approaches. In particular, concerns around empirical versus directed therapy are pertinent, especially where gram-negative bacteria are suspected from Gram stain results (Barnard, 2019). This highlights the importance of an integrated approach bringing together both laboratory testing and clinical expertise in individualizing patient management strategies. Lastly, infection treatment caused by Gram-positive cocci needs to be founded on a multi-dimensional strategy combining the most recent research information and clinical experience. By constantly updating the knowledge related to the pathogenicity, antibiotic resistance, and treatment efficacy, healthcare workers can enhance patient outcomes. Coordination among microbiologists, clinicians, and pharmacists is also as important in the battle against the potential growing menace posed by these bacteria. Follow-up studies on prevention measures and other therapies will be critical in the treatment of the public health problems presented by Gram-positive infections. A well-rounded understanding and strategy, thus, are essential for maximizing these bacteria's treatment in optimal terms in order to secure better patient outcomes in various groups.

In summarizing the key points regarding Gram-positive cocci, their clinical significance and the diverse genera that fall under this classification must be noted. Gram-positive cocci encompass some of the important pathogens like *Staphylococcus* and *Streptococcus* species, which cause a series of infections from infection of the skin to life-threatening diseases. *Staphylococcus aureus*, notorious for producing skin infections and toxic shock syndrome, possesses the peculiarity of exhibiting antibiotic resistance, thus compromising treatment. Furthermore, *Streptococcus pneumoniae*, being a prime etiologic agent of pneumonia, highlights the prevention of infection due to such agents by vaccination. The ability of the cocci to cause significant morbidity and even mortality indicates the importance of sustaining research effort and judicious clinical management. A second important element concerns pathogenicity mechanisms of Gram-positive cocci. Their virulence factors, , such as toxins, adhesins, and immune evasion mechanisms, all contribute to their pathogenic capacity. For example, enterotoxin production by *Staphylococcus aureus* leads to food poisoning, demonstrating its outbreak capacity. Further, *Streptococcus* pyogenes, the etiologic agent of infections like pharyngitis and rheumatic fever, can produce streptolysins that cause red blood cells and white blood cells to lyse. This knowledge is not only necessary for diagnosis and treatment but also for the prevention of these diseases effectively. Research on such virulence factors is ongoing, and it can result in the development of targeted treatments and vaccines and thus improve patient outcomes. Furthermore, Gram-positive cocci co-occurrence with polymicrobial infection is most difficult to clinically treat. The presence of such pathogens as *Staphylococcus aureus* and *Pseudomonas aeruginosa* together in infections, particularly infections , such as Buruli ulcer, is most difficult to treat therapeutically. Secondary Buruli ulcers showed high rates of isolation of *Staphylococcus aureus*, and these tend to be resistant to the most common drugs used for treatment, thus the necessity of close monitoring and particular antibiotic treatment. It is also a cause for worry regarding the influence of hygiene practices and microbiological balance of the cutaneous flora. Analysis of such interactions shows the importance of understanding the ecological dynamics of microbial populations in relation to Gram-positive cocci, which ultimately brings about more effective infection control measures in clinical settings (Whitmore et al., 1965; Pahlevan et al., 2013).

KEY TERMS FROM THIS CHAPTER

- Adaptive pathogens
- Antibiotic resistance
- Antibiotic treatment regimens
- Antimicrobial therapy
- Biochemical mechanisms
- Buruli ulcer
- Community-acquired pneumonia
- Antibiotic prophylaxis
- Antibiotic stress
- Antimicrobial stewardship
- Bacterial species
- Biofilm production
- Cervico-facial sepsis
- Diagnostic accuracy

CRITICAL THINKING QUESTIONS

1. **Which of the following is a catalase-positive Gram-positive coccus?**
   a. *Streptococcus* pyogenes
   b. *Enterococcus faecalis*
   c. *Staphylococcus aureus*
   d. *Streptococcus pneumoniae*
2. **What is the most common cause of bacterial endocarditis among Gram-positive cocci?**
   a. *Streptococcus* pyogenes
   b. *Staphylococcus* epidermidis
   c. *Enterococcus faecalis*
   d. Viridans group streptococci
3. ***Streptococcus pneumoniae* is best differentiated from other alpha-hemolytic streptococci by:**
   a. Catalase test
   b. Coagulase test
   c. Optochin sensitivity
   d. Bacitracin sensitivity
4. **Which Gram-positive cocci is most commonly associated with urinary tract infections?**
   a. *Staphylococcus saprophyticus*
   b. *Staphylococcus aureus*
   c. *Streptococcus agalactiae*
   d. *Streptococcus pyogenes*
5. **The Lancefield classification is primarily used for:**
   a. Differentiating types of *Staphylococcus*
   b. Classifying beta-hemolytic streptococci
   c. Identifying Gram-negative bacilli
   d. Distinguishing Enterococcus species

Short Answer Questions

1. What are the major genera of Gram-positive cocci and how are they classified based on their morphology and arrangement?
2. How can you differentiate *Staphylococcus aureus* from other staphylococci in the lab?
3. What virulence factors are associated with *Streptococcus* pyogenes (Group A *Streptococcus*)?
4. What laboratory test differentiates *Streptococcus pneumoniae* from other alpha-hemolytic streptococci?
5. Which Gram-positive cocci are common causes of hospital-acquired infections?
6. What is the clinical significance of Enterococcus species, and how are they identified?
7. What are the distinguishing features of *Staphylococcus* saprophyticus in urinary tract infections?
8. How does hemolysis on blood agar help differentiate Streptococcal species?

Answers to Critical Thinking Questions

1. (c) 2. (d) 3. (c) 4. (a) 5. (b)

REFERENCES

1. Abdul Rahim, R., Hassan, Z., Mat Isa, N., Mustafa, N., et al. (2016). Identification, characterization and phylogenetic analysis of commensal bacteria isolated from human breast milk in Malaysia. https://core.ac.uk/download/153810919.pdf (accessed on 13th June 2025).
2. Alhede, M., Baltzis, D., Barbour, A., Berezow, A., Bi, L., Borges, A., Brossard, K., et al. (2016). Micro-management: Curbing chronic wound infection. https://core.ac.uk/download/77287389.pdf (accessed on 13th June 2025).
3. Pieniążek, J. M., Padkowska, A., Dobosz, M., Arciszewska, K., Buczkowski, J., Miazga, M., ... Mataczyńska, A. (2024). Overview Of The Main Bacterial Infections In Humans. *Quality in Sport, 23*, 54786. https://doi.org/10.12775/QS.2024.23.54786 (accessed on 13th June 2025).
4. Arifah, S., Effendi, M. H., & Sektiari, B. (2020). Encoding gene identification in *Staphylococcus aureus* enterotoxin B from nasal mucosa of the dog. https://core.ac.uk/download/328104122.pdf (accessed on 13th June 2025).
5. Barnard, N. (2019). Prevalence of gram-negative infections in cervical-facial sepsis. https://core.ac.uk/download/289120735.pdf (accessed on 13th June 2025).
6. Birbir, M., Ruiz de la Haba, R., Sánchez-Porro, Á., Ventosa, U., et al. (2011). *Salimicrobium salexigens* sp. nov., a moderately halophilic bacterium from salted hides. https://core.ac.uk/download/51387441.pdf (accessed on 13th June 2025).
7. Bizzini, A., Fajardo, A., Gardner, A., Rahman, A., Vickers, A. A., Marshall, B. M., Benagli, C., et al. (2013). Could public restrooms be an environment for bacterial resisters? https://core.ac.uk/download/30696462.pdf (accessed on 13th June 2025).
8. Blanchard, P. C. (2012). Diagnostics of dairy and beef cattle diarrhea. https://core.ac.uk/download/323069372.pdf (accessed on 13th June 2025).
9. Boonyasiri, A., Jitmuang, A., Keurueangkul, N., Leelaporn, A., et al. (2012). Gonococcal subcutaneous abscess and pyomyositis: A case report. https://core.ac.uk/download/156738799.pdf (accessed on 13th June 2025).
10. Bordignon, V., Cavallo, I., Cilli, L., De Santis, C., et al. (2017). Biofilm is a major virulence determinant in bacterial colonization of chronic skin ulcers independently from the multidrug resistant phenotype. https://core.ac.uk/download/188832167.pdf (accessed on 13th June 2025).
11. Bryant, K., Elward, A., Lessler, J., Milstone, A., et al. (2017). Bacterial infections in neonates following mupirocin-based MRSA decolonization: A multicenter cohort study. https://core.ac.uk/download/84911302.pdf (accessed on 13th June 2025).
12. Burnham, C. A. D., Lainhart, W., & Yarbrough, M. L. (2018). Epidemiology, clinical characteristics, and antimicrobial susceptibility profiles of human clinical isolates of *Staphylococcus intermedius* group. https://core.ac.uk/download/212860634.pdf (accessed on 13th June 2025).
13. Chang, P. K., Diaz, J. J., Jr., & Huston, J. M., et al. (2017). The Surgical Infection Society revised guidelines on the management of intra-abdominal infection. https://core.ac.uk/download/74358329.pdf (accessed on 13th June 2025).
14. Chapin, A., Rule, A., Jensen, L. B., Schwab, K., Gibson, K., Mackiewicz, B., Buckley, T., et al. (2004). Airborne multidrug-resistant bacteria isolated from a concentrated swine feeding

operation. https://core.ac.uk/download/pdf/3797183.pdf (accessed on 13th June 2025).

15. Das, S., Gowthami, G. A., Karthik, Y., Manjula, K., et al. (2021). Study of antibacterial, anti-proliferative and pro-apoptotic potential of the cell extracts of endophytic fungi and bacteria isolated from *Pajanelia longifolia* (Willd.) K. Schuman. https://core.ac.uk/download/490618308.pdf (accessed on 13th June 2025).

16. Dobbins, B. M., Kindon, A., Kite, P., McMahon, M., et al. (2002). DNA fingerprinting analysis of coagulase-negative staphylococci implicated in catheter-related bloodstream infections. https://core.ac.uk/download/59668.pdf (accessed on 13th June 2025).

17. Whitmore, F. C., Durfee, R. L., Spurlock, J. M., (2025). Evaluation of proposed Skylab and SSP soap products. Document ID 19730011416, Acquisition Source, Legacy CDMS, Document Type, Contractor Report (CR)

18. https://core.ac.uk/download/pdf/80641742.pdf (accessed on 13th June 2025).

19. Eyaufe, A. A., Ireye, F., & Osagie, R. N. (2016). Microbial analysis of biomedical wastes from selected health facilities in parts of Edo South and its public health implication. https://core.ac.uk/download/480549410.pdf (accessed on 13th June 2025).

20. Gall, L. S., & Riely, P. E. (1965). Effect of diet and atmosphere on intestinal and skin flora. Volume II–Literature survey. Document ID, 19660023332 Acquisition Source, Legacy CDMS, Document Type Contractor Report (CR)

21. https://core.ac.uk/download/pdf/85249155.pdf (accessed on 13th June 2025).

22. Gillen, A. L. (2009). The genesis of methicillin-resistant *Staphylococcus aureus*: A modern-day leprosy and hospital menace. https://core.ac.uk/download/227056809.pdf (accessed on 13th June 2025).

23. Golia, S., Swamy, M. A., & Varania, N. (2018). Spectrum of aerobic bacteria and their antimicrobial pattern in bloodstream infections of hospitalized patients: A retrospective study. https://core.ac.uk/download/539913600.pdf (accessed on 13th June 2025).

24. Guramatunhu, S., Mkangamwi, N. A., & Wani, M. G. (2001). Prevalence of causative organisms in corneal ulcers seen at Sekuru Kaguvi Eye Unit, Harare, Zimbabwe. https://core.ac.uk/download/286042264.pdf (accessed on 13th June 2025).

25. Hauser, R. G. (2011). Digital image analysis of Gram-stained culture specimens. https://core.ac.uk/download/232768842.pdf (accessed on 13th June 2025).

26. Hayatshahi, A., Heshmat, R., Nikoo, M. K., Qorbani, M., et al. (2012). Clinical microbiology study of diabetic foot ulcer in Iran; pathogens and antibacterial susceptibility. https://core.ac.uk/download/84432172.pdf (accessed on 13th June 2025).

27. Hoick, A., Mercenier, A., Robert, A., Strauss, A., Strauss, A., Haandrikman, A. J., Pugsley, A. P., et al. (1999). Anchoring of proteins to lactic acid bacteria. https://core.ac.uk/download/pdf/12905226.pdf (accessed on 13th June 2025).

28. Kanemasa, Y., & Tomochika, K. (1974). Freeze-etch studies on the bacterial cell surfaces: Action of the cell wall lytic enzymes on the Gram-positive cocci. https://core.ac.uk/download/12547174.pdf (accessed on 13th June 2025).

29. Kannapiran, E., Muraleedharan, H., & Kalaigandhi, V. (2009). Microfouling of manganese-oxidizing microorganisms in Rameswaram coastal waters. https://core.ac.uk/download/pdf/288822.pdf (accessed on 13th June 2025).

30. Lupetti, A., Ghelardi, E., Morici, P., Barnini, S., & Brucculeri, V. (2015). Rapid and reliable identification of Gram-negative bacteria and Gram-positive cocci by deposition of bacteria harvested from blood cultures onto the MALDI-TOF plate. https://core.ac.uk/download/pdf/81273900.pdf (accessed on 13th June 2025).

31. Maki, D. G., & Tambyah, P. A. (2001). Engineering out the risk for infection with urinary catheters. https://core.ac.uk/download/pdf/8251600.pdf (accessed on 13th June 2025).

32. Malimu, E. Z. (2012). The prevalence of bacterial contamination in donated blood in Dar es Salaam, Tanzania. https://core.ac.uk/download/pdf/16666702.pdf (accessed on 13th June 2025).

33. Manfredi, R. (2006). Update on the appropriate use of linezolid in clinical practice. https://core.ac.uk/download/226361801.pdf (accessed on 13th June 2025).

34. Mthembu, Wendy & Penduka, Dambudzo & Mosa, Rebamang & Shoba, Bonginkosi & Zobolo, A & Opoku, A. (2017). The bacteria profiles of wounds in diabetic patients hospitalized in northern Kwazulu-Natal, South Africa. African Journal of Clinical and Experimental Microbiology. 18. 186. 10.4314/ajcem.v18i4.2. (accessed on 13th June 2025).

35. Mullany, P. (2000). Gene transfer in the GI tract and oral cavity. https://core.ac.uk/download/1707214.pdf (accessed on 13th June 2025).

36. Pahlevan, A. A., Wysocki, A. B., Paintsil, A., Shittu, A. O., Shittu, A. O., Bauer, A. W., Anku, B., et al. (2013). Secondary bacterial infections of Buruli ulcer lesions before and after chemotherapy with streptomycin and rifampicin. https://core.ac.uk/download/18261879.pdf (accessed on 13th June 2025).

37. Purushottam, D., Padmaja, N., & Ganja, S. (2025). Infections caused by Gram-positive cocci and their microbiological pattern in a tertiary care hospital. https://core.ac.uk/download/647975798.pdf (accessed on 13th June 2025).

38. Taylor, G. R., & Zaloguev, S. N. (2025). Methods for microbiological and immunological studies of space flight crews. https://core.ac.uk/download/pdf/42873204.pdf (accessed on 13th June 2025).

39. Widodo, Y. R., & Wirawati, C. U. (2021). Assessment of antimicrobial and proteolytic activity of lactic acid bacteria isolated from *dadih*: Naturally fermented buffalo milk from West Sumatra, Indonesia. https://core.ac.uk/download/483682919.pdf (accessed on 13th June 2025).

GRAM-NEGATIVE COCCI

7

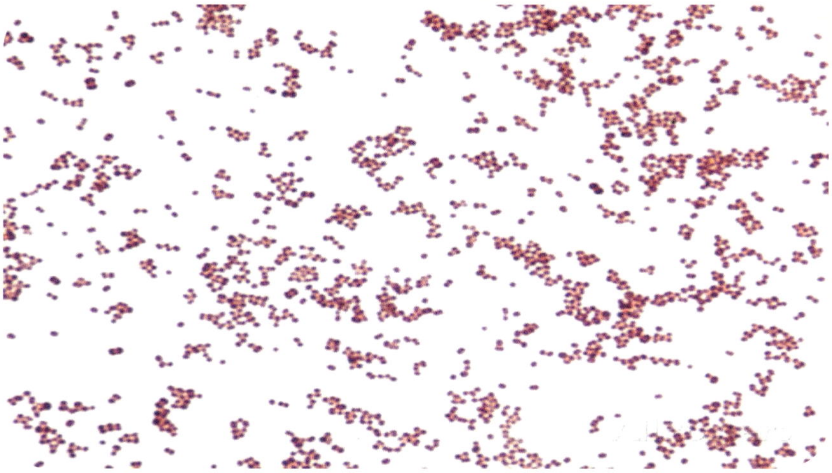

LEARNING OBJECTIVES

After studying this chapter, you will be able to:

1. Understand the characteristics of gram-negative cocci
2. Explain the major types of gram-negative cocci
3. Discuss pathogenicity and diseases
4. Describe laboratory identification techniques
5. Focus on treatment and antibiotic resistance
6. Deal with prevention and control measures

Introduction

Classification of bacteria as Gram-positive or gram-negative is the backbone of microbiology, especially in the therapeutic management of infections. Gram-negative cocci constitute a special group of bacteria with a specific cell wall structure affecting their pathogenicity and response to antibiotics. This section is intended as an introduction to lay the groundwork for the significance of gram-negative cocci in clinical microbiology based on their roles in various infectious processes. The structural differences in their membranes render gram-negative bacteria inherently more resistant to certain antibiotics, complicating treatment regimens for patients infected with these organisms. Knowledge of such characteristics is important for health professionals to effectively manage infections and prevent bacterial resistance. Gram-negative cocci, especially from the Neisseria and Moraxella genera, have been known to be linked with a wide range of medical conditions ranging from minor infections to serious disease like meningitis. The pathogenic capability in these bacteria is normally maximized in compromised hosts, emphasizing the importance of rapid detection and correct treatment regimes. As demonstrated in clinical settings, co-infections involving other species of bacteria make the clinical scenario more difficult and therefore require observation and examination of bacterial spread in infections. This complexity is perhaps best demonstrated by the isolation of several pathogenic organisms, , such as in diabetic wound infections where gram-negative bacilli were the dominant flora with other species, leading to polymicrobial infections (Mthembu et al., 2017). Such findings only serve to underscore the necessity of extensive diagnostic procedures in treating infections. In addition to the problems created by antibiotic resistance, socioeconomic impacts of gram-negative coccid infection warrant serious attention. These infections occur largely in high-risk populations and accompanying morbidity and health care expenditures are major. Studies have also shown that chronic infections, like those in the case of Buruli ulcer disease, can be aggravated by secondary infection by the causative agents like Pseudomonas aeruginosa and Staphylococcus aureus, which can significantly influence healing processes (Pahlevan et al., 2013). An appreciation of these connections illuminates the complicated nature of gram-negative coccid illness and highlights the importance of interdisciplinary approaches to clinical and public health realms. Conquering such hurdles is crucial for effective management and prevention methods that can minimize the impact of such pathogens on patient health and community well-being.

Definition of Gram-Negative Cocci

Gram-negative cocci are another category of bacteria that are rounded, and they possess a specific cell wall structure with an outer membrane made of lipopolysaccharides. Their unique cellular arrangement accounts for their resistance to certain antibiotics, and they are therefore of clinical importance as causative agents of infections. Genera within this group of species include Neisseria and Moraxella, which are significant in producing human clinical disease. Neisseria meningitidis, for example, initiates bacterial meningitis, while Neisseria gonorrhoeae leads to gonorrhea. Knowledge of gram-negative cocci is essential in diagnostic microbiology because their identification dictates the treatment strategy and public health measures based on their importance in both medical and environmental fields. The pathogenicity of gram-negative cocci can be attributed to various virulence factors enhancing their survival and infectivity. For instance, pili in Neisseria strains are helpful for attachment to host tissues, while their immune evasion mechanisms are the reason for the long-term infection. Additionally, the beta-lactamase enzyme production by certain isolates is a demonstration of how some bacteria become resistant to certain antibiotics , such as penicillin.

This adaptability underscores the need for continuous surveillance and study of antimicrobial resistance patterns of these pathogens, as attested by studies that indicate a shift in susceptibility, where some of the species are more resistant to first-line antibiotics (Malimu, 2012). These findings underscore the need to understand the epidemiology of gram-negative cocci in the clinical setup and the need to apply effective infection control practices. Finally, the definition and terminology of gram-negative cocci include not only their structural character but also their clinical importance, therapeutic challenges, and their impact on public health. With the evolving face of microbial infection, particularly in the framework of emergent antimicrobial resistance, more work on the dynamics of gram-negative cocci is necessary. Impact of these microbes on patient outcomes and the healthcare system ensures that their action in various environments should be familiar, like in the case of secondary infection complicating the primary condition, such as in Buruli ulcers patients (Pahlevan et al., 2013). An in-depth knowledge of gram-negative cocci is therefore essential to clinicians and researchers, creating platforms towards improved therapeutic interventions and public health practice (Figure 7.1).

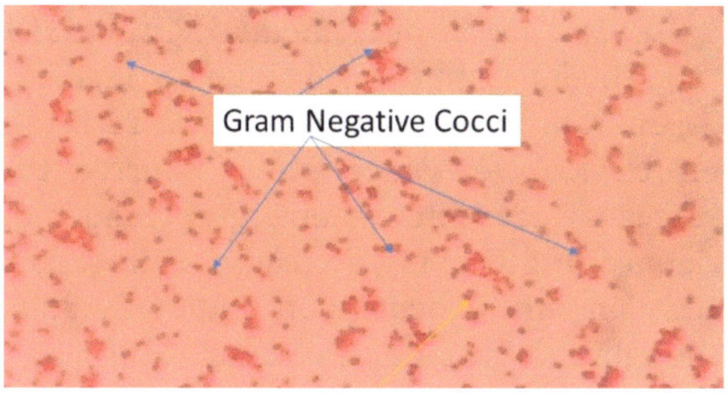

Figure 7.1. Gram-negative cocci.

Source: https://universe84a.com/wp-content/uploads/2019/06/Gram-negative-diplococci.jpg.

Importance in Microbiology and Medicine

The contribution of Gram-negative cocci to medicine and microbiology cannot be overstated since they have several pathogenic roles and present challenges in clinical practice. Gram-negative cocci, especially Neisseria species , such as Neisseria gonorrhoeae and Neisseria meningitidis, are responsible for deadly infections , such as gonorrhea and bacterial meningitis. Their complex outer membrane architecture not only enables them to endure unfavorable conditions but also renders them resistant to antibiotics. Reports have indicated a worrisome increase in antimicrobial resistance among these microorganisms, making them hard to cure and posing public health hazards. These traits emphasize the need for ongoing surveillance and innovative approaches in prevention and infection control by Gram-negative cocci, as they form a critical point of concern for health care systems around the world. In medical diagnosis, identification and detection of Gram-negative cocci are very important in the understanding and management of infectious diseases. Techniques, such as culture methods and biochemical tests, as the targets of current research, help differentiate between pathogenic microorganisms and non-pathogenic flora among the human microbiome. Bacterial infection of blood transfusion facilities, for instance, identified Gram-negative bacteria as a serious patient safety risk, with rates of contamination revealing an overall infection control issue in clinical procedures. Identification of these pathogens enables the delivery of timely and sufficient therapeutic measures, thereby reducing morbidity and mortality due to bacterial infections.

As observed by (Malimu, 2012), strategies employed in antimicrobial resistance pattern determination can inform treatment, which can make patient management more effective. Their pathogenicity and environmental stability also enhance their relevance in microbiology and public health. These microorganisms tend to live in other ecological niches, for example, clinical settings, and are able to survive under dirty biomedical waste, as shown through studies on microbial characterization of the said waste. Bacterial pathogens like *Staphylococcus aureus* and *Escherichia coli* in biomedical waste pose serious health risks to healthcare workers and members of the public, highlighting the need for stringent waste management procedures (Eyaufe et al., 2016). The understanding of their epidemiology, mechanisms of resistance, and public health importance is critical to the development of effective interventions. With respect to the growing antibiotic resistance anxiety and despite the rising trend in antibiotic resistance, curing the threat of Gram-negative cocci is not only a clinical issue but a imperative public health priority.

7.1. Characteristics of Gram-Negative Cocci

Learning Outcome

1. Understand wall structure and composition of gram-negative cocci
2. Describe staining properties and identification
3. Explain metabolic and growth characteristics of gram-negative cocci

The microbiological landscape of Gram-negative cocci is characterized by specific cell structures that distinguish them from Gram-positive equivalents. One of the most distinguishing features of Gram-negative cocci is their characteristic outer membrane, which has a distinctive lipopolysaccharide (LPS) component. This structure not only serves as a barrier to certain antibiotics and detergents but also plays a central part in causation of infection through inducing strong host defense responses. The denser peptidoglycan layer in Gram-negative cocci also leads to loss of violet color on Gram staining, which provides them with the characteristic pink color. This differential structure is essential in clinical diagnosis as it determines the treatment protocol through the determination of antibiotic resistance and sensitivity mechanisms, which are increasingly becoming essential in infection management caused by these microorganisms. Clinical practice in identification of Gram-negative cocci is primarily achieved by observing their biochemical characteristics and pathogenicity. Well-studied groups , such as Neisseria are thoroughly researched for their clinical significance, particularly in meningitis and sexually transmitted illness. Their virulence is augmented by their ability to form biofilms and resist host immune mechanisms. Their virulence factors, pili and other adhesins, allow them to bind to mucosal surfaces and cause infection in human hosts. For instance, Neisseria gonorrhoeae has been observed to have sophisticated mechanisms for enhancing its survival in the host, including genetic diversity and antimicrobial agent resistance, which emphasizes the importance of correct identification and selective antibiotherapy in the management of infections by these Gram-negative cocci. The increasing recognition of Gram-negative cocci, particularly members of the *Staphylococcus* intermedius group (SIG), as significant pathogens in human medicine has generated considerable interest regarding their clinical relevance. It is reported that research has identified an emerging trend in the incidence of SIG being the cause of infections, mainly in immunocompromised individuals. Although they are similar to *Staphylococcus aureus*, the misleading characterization of SIG can lead to erroneous therapy, hence making it important to have proper diagnostic methods. The emergence of methicillin resistance in SIG isolates is another challenge with great public health and infection control significance. A high percentage of SIG isolates exhibited differences in susceptibility to commonly used antibiotics in research, reiterating the need for microbiologic caution and targeted therapeutic approaches in managing infections caused by Gram-negative bacteria (Au et al.; Burnham et al., 2018).

7.1.1. Cell Wall Structure and Composition

One of the most important features of gram-negative cocci is the typical cell wall structure and composition, which plays a significant role in their physiology and virulence. Unlike the thick peptidoglycan layer found in Gram-positive bacteria, gram-negative cocci possess a more differentiated cell wall structure with a thin peptidoglycan layer sandwiched between two lipid membranes. Their outer membrane contains lipopolysaccharides (LPS), which not only contribute to structural stability but also initiate host immunity. The LPS is an endotoxin, and they are classified as virulent pathogenic gram-negative cocci due to this. This combination of a thin peptidoglycan layer with an outer membrane defines their vulnerability to antibiotics and other antimicrobial drugs, necessitating specific therapeutic measures. The gram-negative coccus peptidoglycan wall is also uneven in thickness but again too fragile to withstand the physical forces of invading the host. Cell wall composition is dynamic, and therefore, there is flexibility to exist in any habitat. The outer cell wall layer also consists of complex polysaccharides and proteins that may be implicated in bacterial virulence by adhering to host tissues or evading the immune system. These structural components are key to an understanding of the interaction of gram-negative cocci with their host organism. An analysis of the structure and organization of molecules within cell walls of such organisms can give insights into pathogenic mechanisms and design of drugs against such pathogens in the future.

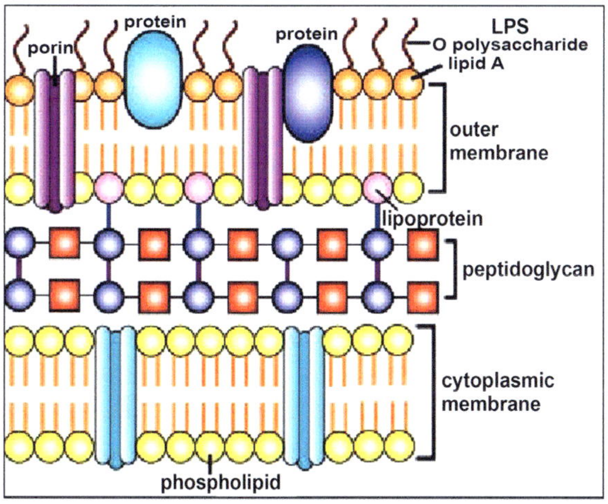

Figure 7.2. The structure of a gram-negative cocci cell wall.

Source: https://www.researchgate.net/profile/La-Fletcher/publication/228499811/figure/fig1/AS:301911971516419@1448992831636/The-structure-of-a-gram-negative-cell-wall.png.

Research on individual components of gram-negative cocci cell walls also established the presence of distinguishing structural components that set these bacteria apart from their closely related Gram-positive relatives. For example, it has been confirmed through research that differences in cell wall architecture among certain gram-negative species impact their classification and pathogenesis research. For example, the cell wall structure in gram-negative cocci demonstrates a characteristic binding of lipoproteins to the peptidoglycan, which adds strength and contributes to the stability of the cell envelope as a whole. These findings are meant to emphasize the importance of specialized analyses in ascertaining the structure and functional importance of various cell wall components, contributing to taxonomic inconsistency as well as clinical significance in treating infections caused by these bacteria (Kanemasa et al., 1974) (Jones et al., 2012) (Figure 7.2).

7.1.2. Staining Properties and Identification

The gram-negative cocci are distinguished mainly on the basis of their staining properties, which practically differentiate them from the Gram-positive ones. The Gram staining technique is essential in this case, since it exploits the structural differences between bacterial cell walls. Gram-negative bacteria contain a thin layer of peptidoglycan that is covered by an outer membrane with lipopolysaccharides that hold on to the counterstain, usually safranin, during decoloration. Thus, gram-negative cocci turn pink on the microscope, and these vital visual cues help microbiologists throughout the identification process. Such staining features not only help in initial classification but also dictate the additional biochemical testing and isolation methods used in the laboratory. Such methods, like selective medium, allow us to narrow down the specific type of gram-negative cocci involved, gaining further information on their pathogenicity and ecological habitats.

After Gram staining of gram-negative cocci, the morphological analysis is of vital importance for identification. Various techniques can be used to analyze colony morphology and cell pattern, , such as microscopy and streak plating. Neisseria species with their typical diplococci arrangement, for instance, can be distinguished from other gram-negative cocci based on morphology as well as on growth on selective media like chocolate agar. Current methods, such as the API 20NE test are an affordable pathway for phenotypic characterization, integrating multiple biochemical tests on one platform. Most importantly, integration of both traditional and current methods gives a comprehensive examination of the bacterias biochemical capabilities, allowing directed therapy in clinical practice. Morphological identification thus has a key role to play in a sequence of diagnostic methods aimed at precise characterization of these pathogens. In addition to this, discrimination among gram-negative coccid species is more complex than mere staining and morphological techniques; it's typically a combination of immunological, genetic, and specialized biochemical techniques. Phage typing and antimicrobial susceptibility testing, not only assist in the identification of specific strains of bacteria but also provide information regarding their resistance patterns, which is indispensable for proper treatment. For the instance, information on the phenotype of potential pathogens , such as Neisseria gonorrhoeae by testing influences major intervention strategies in public health. The scientific approach towards identification of gram-negative cocci through the use of newer researches and characterizations points to their antimicrobial capability and proteolytic nature, as in research with lactic acid bacteria, , such as those found in conventional fermented foods, with appreciable antimicrobial activity against both Gram-positive and gram-negative bacteria (Taylor et al.; Widodo et al., 2021). This multidisciplinary strategy offers precise identification and efficient control of gram-negative coccus-induced infections in clinical and environmental contexts (Figure 7.3).

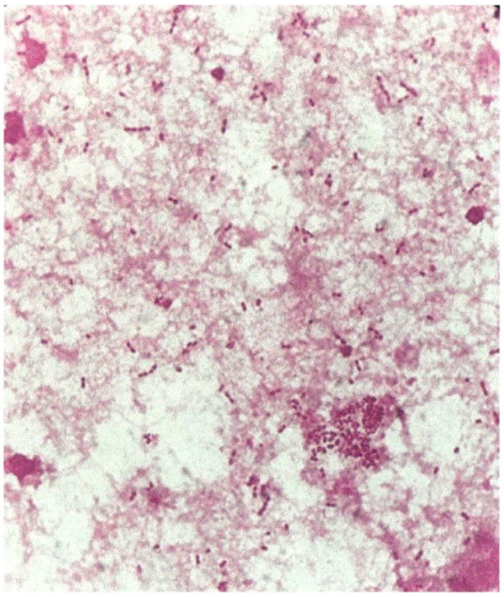

Figure 7.3. Gram staining of the blood culture isolated displayed gram-negative coccobacilli.

Source: https://www.researchgate.net/publication/331057317/figure/fig2/AS:725684502675459@1550028076797/Gram-staining-of-the-blood-culture-isolated-displayed-Gram-negative-coccobacilli.png.

7.1.3. Metabolic and Growth Characteristics

The metabolism and growth characteristics of Gram-negative cocci are of key importance to the understanding of their ecological roles and significance to human health. The bacteria typically have a diverse range of metabolic processes that enable them to survive in varying conditions available in the environment. For instance, some species can ferment carbohydrates for the production of organic acids and gases, facilitating their cultivation in anaerobic environments. The Gram-negative coccoid metabolism is generally linked with fermentative processes by which energy can be generated in the absence of oxygen. Also, their ability to metabolize different substrates, , such as sugars, is a demonstration of the versatility of these bacteria and their capability to thrive in different ecological niches, , such as the human digestive tract and other biological systems. A very good example of such metabolic flexibility in their own species has been reported in strain Cello (Akkermans et al., 2003), which demonstrates the capacity to degrade cellobiose and grow on a range of different sugars. Such a distinct metabolic fingerprint of such strains demonstrates the function of some sugars in supporting bacterial growth, with glucose functioning best because it degrades into byproducts like acetate and hydrogen. These byproducts of metabolism not only reflect the supply of energy to the bacterium but also identify its environmental potential for interaction, especially with other bacteria in syntrophic interactions that can utilize such byproducts. The significance of this metabolic flexibility extends beyond ecological competitiveness; it reflects aspects of microbial community dynamics, including their potential role in bioconversion and association with host organisms. In addition to their metabolic flexibility, Gram-negative cocci possess some requirements for growth that can either increase or influence their virulence and survival mechanisms. The majority of these bacteria need specific temperature and pH conditions in order to grow, which tend to closely represent the conditions under which they thrive in nature, e.g., inside the human body. For instance, bacteria can have growth adaptation mechanisms in which they are able to survive and grow at temperatures around 37 degrees Celsius, for instance, with various cocci. Moreover, the ability to form biofilms confers a competitive advantage in natural and clinical environments, offering protection against antimicrobial agents and the immune system of the host. This biofilm production is the most significant of the determinants of pathogenicity of certain Gram-negative cocci, emphasizing how valuable it is to be aware of their growth tendencies not only for basic microbiological facts but also for specific therapeutic strategy design (Krastanov et al., 2018).

Test Your Knowledge

1. What are the key structural components of the cell wall in Gram-negative cocci, and how do they differ from Gram-positive bacteria?
2. How do Gram-negative cocci appear after Gram staining, and what accounts for this staining pattern?

7.2. Major Types of Gram-Negative Cocci

Learning Outcome

1. Describe Neisseria species
2. Understand Moraxella species

The most significant groups of gram-negative cocci are essentially represented by the genera Moraxella and Neisseria. The genus Neisseria is possibly more famous by its pathogenic species Neisseria meningitidis and Neisseria gonorrhoeae. Neisseria is a significant genus in human health because these bacteria are responsible for sexually transmitted disease and bacterial meningitis, respectively. Their ability to live on mucosal membranes as well as their transmission modes show their significance in public health. Moreover, virulence factors expressed by the bacteria , such as pili and endotoxins assist in adhesion to host cells and in inflammatory processes. Understanding of these mechanisms is crucial in order to develop successful therapy and prophylactic treatment against Neisseria spp. infection, which mirrors the importance of continued research and clinical microbiology surveillance. Moraxella catarrhalis is another notable example of gram-negative cocci, and it is primarily known to be an opportunistic pathogen. The bacterium is often found to colonize the upper respiratory system and is most often implicated in respiratory infections, particularly in children and patients with serious medical conditions , such as COPD.

Moraxella catarrhalis is also able to colonize the upper respiratory system and result in otitis media and sinusitis, and resistance to beta-lactam antibiotics is a possible challenge in treatment. Its resistance to the host's immune system, combined with its potential to affect susceptible populations, highlights the importance of information about resistance profiles and epidemiology. This type of information has the potential to influence clinical practice and inform the use of antibiotic stewardship in an effort to treat Moraxella catarrhalis infections. Geographical prevalence and distribution of gram-negative cocci in various niches show their ecological adaptability and public health importance. They have been found through studies to be predominantly isolated from clinical specimens, and also from environmental samples, proving that they are versatile. For instance, in studies on bacteriological characterization of food processing environments, there have been established strong correlations of some gram-negative cocci with food contamination episodes. Such cases as are noted in the Cochin area underscore the need for ongoing monitoring to monitor populations of bacteria within food production systems because some strains can serve as carriers for pathogenic strains. Through understanding , such associations and their implications, scientists and public health workers are best able to assess risk and implement proper control measures, ultimately bettering public health and food safety (Taylor et al.; Iyer et al., 1971).

7.2.1. Neisseria Species

The Neisseria genus contains a variety of Gram-negative cocci that are mostly famous for their application in human health and disease. Neisseria gonorrhoeae and Neisseria meningitidis are two of the most well-known species, where the former causes sexually transmitted disease and the latter causes bacterial meningitis. The organisms thrive in the mucosal surfaces of the human host since their growth is facilitated by the nutrient-rich habitat of the host. Their evasion of the host immune response is aided by a number of virulence factors, including pili and outer membrane proteins, that increase host tissue adherence and invasion. The highly specialized nature of their metabolic requirements is also a source of difficulty in their diagnosis, which entails specialized methods of culture and media for their recovery and identification within clinical samples. Phylogenetic relationships in the Neisseria genus have been explored in recent studies and the diversity and evolutionary significance of new species determined. For instance, a polyphasic strategy with a group of isolates led to the taxonomic designation of a new species, Neisseria oralis, on the basis of distinctive genetic and phenotypic features. This organism had a high-level similarity to Neisseria lactamica, indicating the need for further studies to understand the complexity of Neisseria taxonomy and its implications in clinical microbiology. The isolates presented an unprecedented 99.7–100% identity in their 16S rRNA gene sequences, indicating their genetic similarity but morphologically and functionally distinct characteristics. These investigations contribute to the understanding of Neisseria diversity and the necessity of accurate identification within the clinical setting to prevent misdiagnosis and improve patient management strategies (Carpenter et al., 2013).

In addition to their clinical relevance, the Neisseria species provide some unique challenges in lab diagnosis and identification. Traditional culture methods, despite their effectiveness, consist of specialized requirements which are sometimes not attainable within the average laboratory.

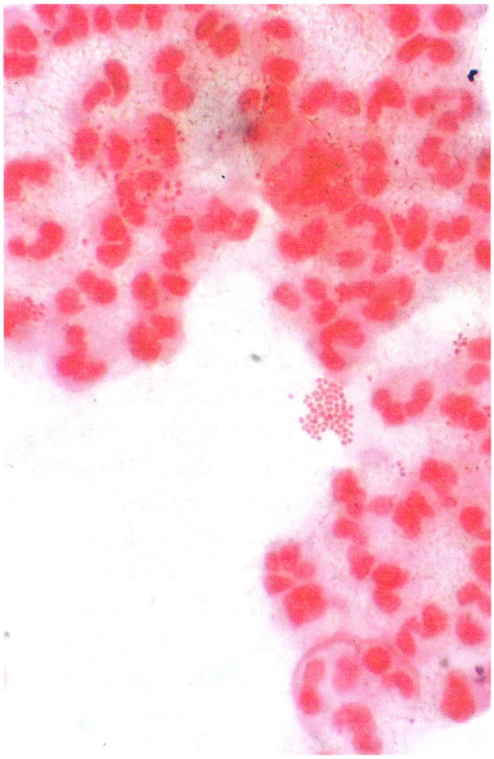

Figure 7.4. Neisseria gonorrhoeae with pus cells, Gram-stain.

Source: https://upload.wikimedia.org/wikipedia/commons/thumb/f/ff/Neisseria_gonorrhoeae_with_pus_cells.jpg/800px-Neisseria_gonorrhoeae_with_pus_cells.jpg.

As in systematic laboratory schemes that have developed as a result of collaborative microbiological research, compatible strategies for the identification of Neisseria and other Gram-negative cocci have been refined to ensure maximum accuracy and reliability (Taylor et al.). These strategies utilize routine biochemical tests along with advanced molecular methods that facilitate the rapid identification of bacterial species. The ongoing evolution of identification systems is in reaction to the complexities present in Neisseria species, which their pathogenicity necessitates to be solved by immediate and precise laboratory response to infections. Hence, complete knowledge about both the biological characteristics of Neisseria and the methods applied for their analysis is needed for public health management (Figure 7.4).

7.2.2. Moraxella Species

The Moraxella genus, comprising several species of Gram-negative cocci, plays a role in human health and disease. Perhaps most notably, Moraxella catarrhalis is an opportunistic organism commonly involved in respiratory infections, particularly in pediatric and in some underlying medical patients. Its ability to colonize the upper respiratory tract without causing harm in normal conditions seems to transform into pathogenic status in conditions of immunocompromised or viral infiltration, , such as influenza. Also, Moraxella species exhibit resistance to numerous antibiotics, and this has caused concern over treatment efficacy and public health interest. Studies have shown that Moraxella organisms contain β-lactamase enzymes, which are part of their resistance factor, and make infection management due to Moraxella organisms challenging (Barnard, 2019). Thus, understanding the pathogenic activity and antibiotic resistance of Moraxella species will be crucial in the formulation of effective therapeutic interventions as well as checking their impact on susceptible populations. The epidemiology of Moraxella species also supports their position as hospital pathogens. M. catarrhalis was identified as a rare isolate in patients with otitis media and sinusitis, two conditions prevalent among children. Such infection often results in chronic pain and can result in further complications when not addressed. Aside from respiratory tract infection, Moraxella species are implicated in infections of the middle ear and sinuses, which are extremely problematic due to their recurrence and association with bacterial resistance

(Barnard, 2019). The presence of Moraxella in such infections underscores the need for a comprehensive diagnostic strategy to identify this pathogen since standard culture methods will fail to detect it. Continued investigations into epidemic patterns of Moraxella species provide insight into their role in infectious diseases and inform clinical practice regarding diagnosis and treatment. In addition to their medical relevance, the challenge of treating Moraxella species serves as a reminder for ongoing research. The establishment of antibiotic-resistant Moraxella strains necessitates reconsideration of current treatment approaches and the discovery of new treatment modalities. New vaccine candidates, for instance, are being explored to augment immune response to Moraxella infection with the aim of reducing disease incidence in high-risk populations. Further, sustained collaborative work between infectious disease and clinical microbiology experts is needed to monitor resistance trends and optimize antibiotic stewardship (Barnard, 2019). In this way, by considering Moraxella species as not only commensals but also important drivers of pathogenesis of many infections, the medical profession can optimize prevention strategies and further enhance patient outcomes. Ultimately, deeper insights into the biology and ecology of Moraxella will be reflected in better control measures in the face of growing antibiotic resistance problems (Figure 7.5).

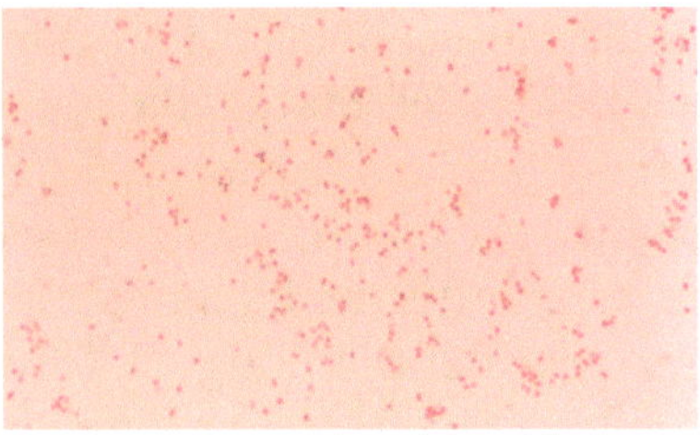

Figure 7.5. Pictorial representation of diplococcuus formation in *M. catarrhalis.*

Source: https://upload.wikimedia.org/wikipedia/commons/4/48/Moraxella_Catarrhalis.png.

7.2.3. Other Notable Genera

Among the wide variety of Gram-negative cocci, a number of prominent genera play important roles in understanding their ecological and pathogenic significance. *Pseudomonas* stands out with its impressively wide range of habitats, surviving in a wide variety of environments , such as soil and aquatic systems. Its opportunistic nature is most feared in immunocompromised patients, where it is capable of inducing infections ranging from pneumonia to bacteremia. Of most significance is that *Pseudomonas aeruginosa*, the most common isolate from chronic wound biofilms, highlights its importance in the capacity to maintain infection through biofilm formation and antibiotic resistance. Understanding *Pseudomonas*' behavior in the biofilm environment is important as such environments typically encompass multi-dimensional bacterial communities that complicate diagnosis and treatment. Enterobacter is also a significant genus, for which it is most well known due to its role in hospital-acquired infections and its development as a clinical pathogen. Species like Enterobacter cloacae are frequently the cause of urinary tract and wound infections, particularly in the hospital environment. The genus is highly adaptable and prone to developing resistance to many different antibiotics, causing huge treatment issues. Studies have proven that the Enterobacter species will synergistically interact with other bacteria within chronic wound biofilms to form a more stable pathogenic population. This synergy points to the need for new therapeutic approaches aimed at these complex interactions in biofilms to achieve improved healing in patients. Stenotrophomonas is another genus of note, with Stenotrophomonas maltophilia emerging as a serious opportunistic pathogen in cystic fibrosis patients and in patients receiving extended courses of antibiotic therapy. Environmental resilience allows it to survive well in a broad spectrum of environments, contributing to its reluctance to be eradicated from clinical settings. Current research has indicated S. maltophilias capacity to form biofilms on health care devices, a key factor towards sustaining infection. Of concern, this genus is also naturally resistant to many of the most commonly used antibiotics, and thus alternative therapy options need to be explored. Lastly, the study of these major genera of the Gram-negative cocci universe not only identifies and assists in the discovery of their unique pathogenic mechanisms but also works to indicate the imperative of ongoing research into combating the challenges posed by multi-species biofilm infections and their therapeutic implications (Kannapiran et al., 2009; Dowd et al., 2008) (Figure 7.6).

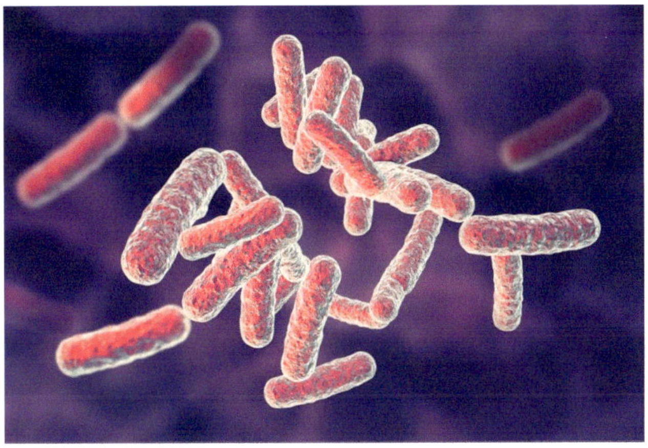

Figure 7.6. *Pseudomonas* is a type of bacteria that can cause infections.

Source: https://www.medicalnewstoday.com/articles/322386#causes.

Test Your Knowledge

1. What are the key differences between Neisseria gonorrhoeae and Neisseria meningitidis in terms of disease?
2. What clinical conditions are associated with Moraxella catarrhalis, and how is it identified in the lab?

7.3. Pathogenicity and Diseases

Learning Outcome

1. Understand common infections caused by gram-negative cocci
2. Discuss the mechanisms of pathogenicity in gram-negative cocci
3. Describe risk factors for infection involving gram-negative cocci

Pathogenicity of Gram-negative cocci is an extremely crucial element in identifying their role in a host of diseases. Gram-negative cocci contain a more intricate outer membrane that serves as not just a defense shield against the external environment but also a virulence factor reservoir necessary for causing an infection. For instance, structural composition of lipopolysaccharides can provoke virulent immune responses that can, in turn, induce septic shock under extreme conditions. Their ability to evade host defense mechanisms is supplemented by the exoenzyme and other factors that enable them to colonize and persist in human tissues. The intricate relationship between the host and the bacterial pathogens is the basis of disease processes of Gram-negative cocci, hence the need for thorough studies on their biology and pathogenicity. A significant characteristic of Gram-negative coccus pathogenicity is their involvement in polymicrobial infection, particularly in oral and systemic environments. Research has shown that these bacteria, including species within the Bacteroides and Fusobacterium genera, tend to co-occur with other pathogens in complex infections.

Their presence in oral infections has been documented extensively, where they are involved in periodontal disease and other oral pathologies, thus showing their role in both localized and systemic infections. The capacity of these cocci to form biofilms enhances their strength, thus proving them to be difficult to treat and often leading to chronic infections. Research has shown that ecological processes in microbial communities can affect the pathogenicity of Gram-negative cocci since they interact with host tissues and coexisting microorganisms, which ultimately play a role in disease severity and progress. Antibiotic resistance in Gram-negative cocci is becoming a major concern in clinical environments, as it restricts treatment for infected patients.

The transfer of resistance genes, often mediated through plasmids, significantly impedes the treatment of infections produced by such organisms. For example, Bacteroides fragilis group isolates have been shown to harbor plasmids that contain resistances to multiple classes of antibiotics, which poses dire challenges in the treatment of infections. In addition, oral isolates' differences in antibiotic susceptibility, as highlighted by recent studies, show that the environment and selective pressures are significant determinants of resistance patterns. It addresses the antibiotic resistance and pathogenicity of Gram-negative cocci in a multidisciplinary manner that combines microbiological studies with clinical techniques of resisting infections, identifying the pressing need for emerging therapeutic regimens and prevention measures to counter the threats of these pathogens (Gall & Riely, 1965; Mooney et al., 1987).

7.3.1. Common Infections Caused by Gram-Negative Cocci

Gram-negative cocci are significant pathogens of many human infections, especially in the healthcare setting where they impart a lot of morbidity and mortality. Of specific interest are the Neisseria species, Neisseria meningitidis and Neisseria gonorrhoeae. N. meningitidis is responsible for meningitis and septicemia, mostly in adolescents and young adults, while N. gonorrhoeae causes gonorrhea, a prevalent sexually transmitted infection. Understanding of the epidemiology of these infections is important, with the possibility of occurring abruptly in highly populated settings making a swift response from public health and vaccination imperative. In addition to these classic infections, the emerging resistance of gram-negative cocci poses the risk of more failures at the therapeutic level, with constant surveillance and study of therapeutic agents an imperative.

The clinical manifestations of gram-negative coccus infections are varied, depending on the involved organism and patient population. For instance, in neonatal intensive care units, gram-negative coccus infections, including various strains of *Pseudomonas aeruginosa*, are on the rise. These organisms not only infect the localized area but also produce systemic infections, which impair the tenuous health status of neonates. Colonization with gram-negative bacteria in such vulnerable populations has been seen to result in increased risks of nosocomial infection with significant causes of healthcare problems (Figure 7.7).

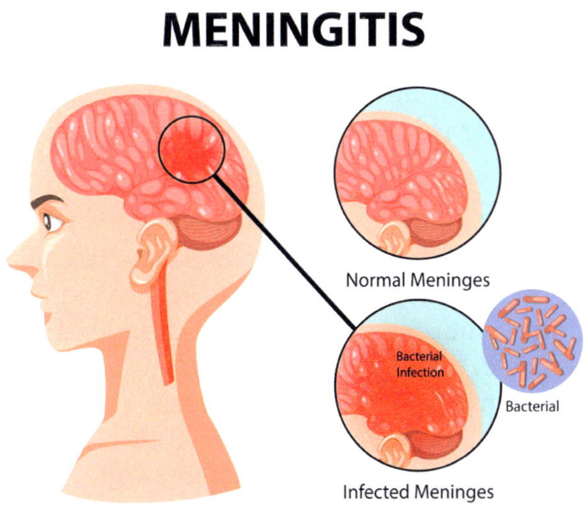

Figure 7.7. Meningitis.

Source: https://www.fortishealthcare.com/drupal-data/2024-08/y5zj_iwgh_220217.jpg.

As exemplified in current efforts, while treatments with mupirocin strategies can effectively minimize the risk for Gram-positive infections, they yield insignificant results on the incidence of gram-negative species infections, reinforcing the complexity of controlling such infections and the need for combined antimicrobial stewardship efforts (Bryant et al., 2017). Moreover, gram-negative cocci are frequently isolated in secondary infections, particularly among patients with underlying medical conditions or those on treatment for other infections. For example, patients with Buruli ulcers or chronic wounds are susceptible to co-infection by gram-negative organisms like Proteus mirabilis and *Pseudomonas aeruginosa*. Their presence complicates the clinical picture since they are resistant to multiple antibiotics, thereby limiting the treatment options. A high incidence of antimicrobial resistance among these organisms is demonstrated by research, which can lead to delayed healing of wounds and unfavorable patient outcomes (Pahlevan et al., 2013). It is therefore important to determine the role of gram-negative cocci in primary and secondary infections so that the clinical establishment of effective therapeutic treatment protocols and patient outcomes can be derived (Figure 7.8).

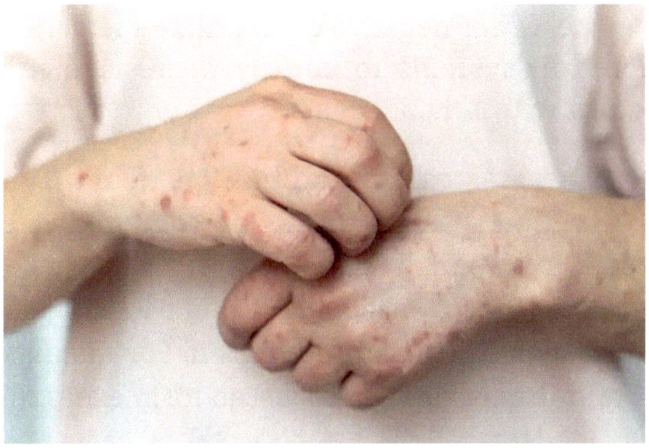

Figure 7.8. Septicemia.

Source: https://www.metropolisindia.com/upgrade/blog/upload/25/02/septicemia-recognizing-the-signs-of-blood-poisoning1739965327.webp.

7.3.2. Mechanisms of Pathogenicity

The pathogenic processes in Gram-negative cocci involve a multiplicity of mechanisms and encompass interaction between virulence factors enabling them to colonize, resist the host's defense, and cause disease. An important element of pathogenicity is having certain surface appendages , such as pili and fimbriae that enhance adhesion to host tissues. These organisms enable Gram-negative cocci to cause infections by binding to mucosal surfaces and thereby circumvent the hosts mechanical defense barriers. Moreover, these bacteria possess lipopolysaccharides (LPS) in their outer membrane, which not only play an important function in immune evasion by acting as a barrier to antimicrobial agents but also cause inflammatory reactions after interacting with the immune cells of the host. Strategic manipulation of these factors renders Gram-negative cocci particularly well adapted to survival in hostile environments, such as those presented by the human immune system, thereby increasing their pathogenic potential. Another major mechanism of pathogenicity is through the secretion of a variety of toxins, which have the capacity to disrupt host cell processes and cause tissue damage. Gram-negative cocci utilize specialized secretion systems to convey these virulence factors within host cells.

These systems, including Type III and Type IV secretion systems, enable bacteria to deliver proteins responsible for controlling host cell processes that contribute to immune evasion and bacterial survival and replication. For instance, certain Gram-negative cocci can form exotoxins that lead to cell lysis while others can cause cell signaling disruption, ultimately interfering with the host's immune response. The ability to actively compromise host cell integrity not only enhances the bacterias possibility of proliferation but also complicates treatment due to the huge range of virulence factors employed, which are constantly challenging the host defense system. The antibiotic resistance factor has a major effect on the pathogenicity of Gram-negative cocci and presents a significant challenge in the clinical context. Studies have indicated that the majority of strains harbor plasmids with multi-antibiotic resistance, which later renders it difficult to treat. During infections, mechanisms of resistance , such as production of beta-lactamases will deactivate the antibiotics, rendering them useless against certain pathogens. The genes of resistance are typically on mobile genetic elements, which enable them to be disseminated from one group of bacteria to another, resulting in widespread resistance among Gram-negative cocci in various environments. For example, research on oral infection isolates established differential antibiotic susceptibility patterns and illustrated that while certain strains were sensitive to traditional drugs, others exhibited high levels of astounding resistance through plasmid acquisition (Mooney et al., 1987). Not only does this exhibit the capacity for adaptation in pathogenic Gram-negative cocci, but it also highlights the importance of ongoing monitoring and setting new therapeutic strategies to counteract resistant infections effectively.

7.3.3. Risk Factors for Infection

Risk factors for gram-negative coccus infection are numerous and can significantly impact clinical courses. In hospitalized individuals, particularly intensive care unit populations, compromised immune function secondary to underlying conditions, such as diabetes, malignancies, and immunosuppressive therapy, predisposes individuals to infection. Furthermore, invasive medical devices , such as catheters and ventilators offer sites of entry for pathogens, , such as gram-negative cocci, to obtain entry into the bloodstream or other sterile sites. This is even more so in neonatal intensive care units (NICUs), where immature immune systems render neonates extremely vulnerable to such infections. More recent research indicates decolonization interventions, including the use of mupirocin among MRSA-colonized neonates, decrease successfully the incidence of Gram-positive infections but appear to have no discernible effect on subsequent gram-negative infections, further indicating the need for targeted infection control interventions (Bryant et al., 2017). Second, the presence of antibiotic-resistant strains among gram-negative cocci is a major risk factor for infection. Multi-drug resistant organisms can flourish in hospitals, primarily due to excessive and inappropriate use of antibiotics. This results in limited treatment options and higher probabilities of treatment failure, complicating patient management. For instance, transfusion patients can be infected by contaminated blood products if they contain resistant gram-negative cocci. A study of bacterial contamination in blood bags revealed substantial proof of coagulase-negative staphylococci, which, although are commonly referred to as skin flora and are generally contaminants, also possess antimicrobial resistance genes. Therefore, the risk of infection with blood transfusions could be significantly elevated if such organisms find their way into the circulatory system of a patient (Malimu, 2012). Preventive care against gram-negative cocci infections is possible with a multi-factorial approach of improved hygiene measures, careful use of antimicrobials, and vigilance of invasive devices. Surveillance for resistant organism outbreaks should be implemented in healthcare institutions to curb possible infections from spreading. Besides, education of healthcare personnel in the practice of strict aseptic techniques during procedures, , such as catheterization or transfusions, can help minimize risk. Emphasis on protocols of regular screening and utilization of effective decolonization methods in risk patients—particularly pediatrics and immunocompromised—is an integral part of overall risk management planning. Synthesis of these with ongoing studies on the pathophysiology and resistance of gram-negative cocci is essential to reducing rates of infection among high-risk patients (Figure 7.9).

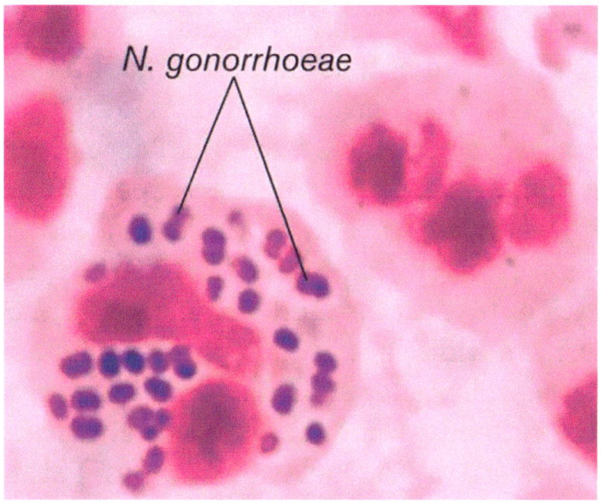

Figure 7.9. Neisseria gonorrhoeae (Gram-negative diplococci).

Source: https://i0.wp.com/microbeonline.com/wp-content/uploads/2013/06/Neisseria-gonorrhoeae.png.

Test Your Knowledge

1. What are the most common infections caused by Gram-negative cocci, particularly Neisseria and Moraxella species?
2. What are the primary mechanisms of pathogenicity in Neisseria gonorrhoeae?

7.4. Laboratory Identification Techniques

Learning Outcome

1. Understand culture methods and media
2. Discuss about biochemical tests for identification of gram-negative cocci
3. Describe molecular techniques for detection of gram-negative cocci

Efficient laboratory identification techniques are crucial for the accurate diagnosis of gram-negative coccus infections. These bacteria, which typically comprise Neisseria meningitidis and Neisseria gonorrhoeae strains, require specific techniques for effective identification. Serological tests are equally essential, especially in the identification of bacterial antigens. The enzyme-linked immunosorbent assay (ELISA) is widely employed to detect these antigens during rapid diagnosis while informing effective treatment interventions. Moreover, molecular techniques , such as polymerase chain reaction (PCR) are sensitive and specific and can identify genetic material of such bacteria even during low bacterial loads. Such advancements in the diagnostic techniques enhance our potential in controlling and treating gram-negative coccus infections and ultimately improve the outcomes in patients. Apart from serological and molecular techniques, traditional culture methods remain core to gram-negative coccus identification in the laboratory. They involve inoculation of special growth medium that supports proliferation of target organisms but inhibits others. For instance, selective media , such as Thayer-Martin agar supports growth of Neisseria species due to its high nutrient levels and addition of antibiotics to suppress contaminant flora. Apart from isolation, further biochemical analysis enables discrimination between species based on metabolic characteristics. Standard tests involve oxidase testing that facilitates identification of Neisseria by its positive test for oxidase. Such techniques, although being cumbersome compared to molecular techniques, are of great value to confirm diagnostics and differentiate epidemiologic trends associated with gram-negative coccid infections. Another significant part of laboratory identification techniques involves antimicrobial susceptibility testing. This is a vital step towards the management of the increasing problem of antibiotic resistance among gram-negative cocci, especially within clinical practice. The Kirby-Bauer disk diffusion method is widely used, whereby bacterial isolates are subjected to antibiotic-impregnated disks on an agar plate. The inhibition zones are read to determine susceptibility levels, and this aids clinicians in choosing the right therapeutic approach. Especially, since resistance patterns change with the passage of time, regular follow-up through these testing protocols guarantees evidence-based treatment protocols. Scientific research has established, for instance, that while some gram-negative cocci are amenable to conventional antibiotics, others exhibit scary resistance profiles, necessitating continuous research and adaptation in lab protocols to yield effective control of such microorganisms (Malimu, 2012). Therefore, an integrated approach blending both traditional and modern methods of identification is crucial in gram-negative coccus infection control.

7.4.1. Culture Methods and Media

The cultivation of gram-negative cocci is special and involves special culture procedures and media that take into consideration the distinctive requirements for growth of these organisms. Culture media , such as chocolate agar and MacConkey agar provide required nutrients as well as inhibit competing flora growth. Chocolate agar favors the growth of demanding bacteria by supplementing with hemoglobin and other additives, whereas MacConkey agar differentiates gram-negative bacteria based on lactose fermentation, and thus pathogenic species , such as Neisseria gonorrhoeae can be isolated and differentiated by clinicians. Furthermore, specialized media may incorporate selective agents to favor the isolation of particular gram-negative cocci through inhibiting non-target microbes. Thus, the selection of media plays a central role in the successful culturing and identification of gram-negative cocci in clinical microbiology. Apart from selecting appropriate media, culturing gram-negative cocci involves accurate laboratory procedures in accordance with accepted protocols. Procedures may involve streak plating and broth cultures that enhance growth of target organisms without encouraging contamination. The main techniques employed in culturing bacteria can significantly affect the outcomes, including the number and viability of gram-negative cocci species. The systematic laboratory procedures scheduled during the Apollo-Soyuz Test Project, as presented in literature, represent an excellent model for these techniques, demonstrating the value of rigid adherence to protocol in obtaining good results. By explaining the efficacy of these methods, the lab can offer accurate identification and typing of gram-negative cocci, thereby resulting in effective clinical management and treatment (Taylor et al.). Additionally, the use of immunological and biochemical approaches also enhances the capacity to diagnose infections caused by gram-negative cocci. These methods can complement traditional culture techniques by providing rapid identification of the causative agents. Antibiotic susceptibility testing, for instance, is particularly critical in the treatment of Neisseria species infections because resistance patterns can be complex and diverse. Media formulation and reagent preparation in the laboratory are critical steps in this context, directly influencing the result of susceptibility testing. These stringent requirements are reflected in standards for enriched media preparation, through which gram-negative cocci can be cultured and examined to optimal standards. Finally, the integration of culture methods, media preparation, and immunological tests is a multidisciplinary approach to the investigation and management of infections caused by gram-negative cocci, and it reflects the sophisticated nature of contemporary microbiological practice (Bizzini et al., 2013) (Figure 7.10).

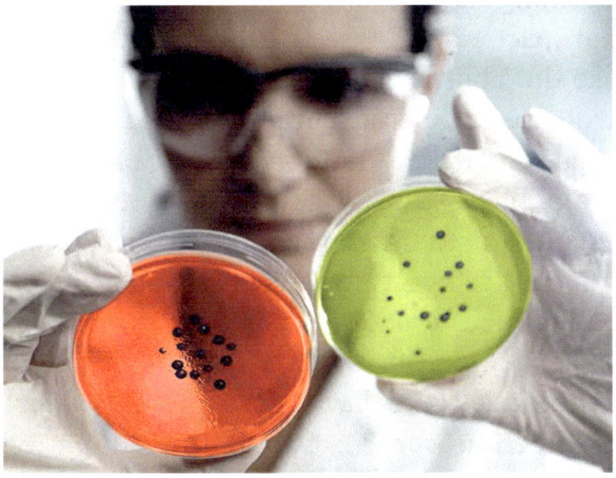

Figure 7.10. Culture methods and media.

Source: https://media.post.rvohealth.io/wp-content/uploads/sites/3/2022/09/Gram-positive-negative-bacteria-thumb.jpg.

7.4.2. Biochemical Tests for Identification

Gram-negative cocci identification is often reliant on a mixture of biochemical testing that identifies their metabolic processes and enzymatic properties. They are required to differentiate species within genera , such as Neisseria and Moraxella, whose analogous clinical features do not map to analogous biochemical patterns. Catalase and oxidase are common tests for the detection of the enzymes that play very crucial roles in detecting certain organisms. For instance, Neisseria are oxidase-positive, an important feature that is utilized to differentiate them from other bacteria. Application of such tests not only streamlines laboratory procedures but also enhances the precision of diagnosis, therefore enabling targeted treatment for infections caused by such microbes. In addition to routine enzymatic tests, additional sophisticated biochemical tests also aid in the typing of Gram-negative cocci. Fermentation tests, which test the ability of an organism to catabolize different carbohydrates, provide valuable information regarding its biochemical pathways. This is particularly relevant in the separation of pathogenic Neisseria species from non-pathogenic species. Additionally, tests , such as the API 20NE system allow for a systems approach where one can study a number of biochemical parameters in combination. These combination test strategies have proved effective in clinical microbiology laboratories as well, enabling early detection and an enhanced understanding of the pathogen's pathogenicity and resistance pattern, which are required for effective treatment (Dr. Purushottam et al., 2025).

Apart from mere detection, biochemical tests also play a significant role in tracking the antimicrobial resistance patterns of Gram-negative cocci. Emergence of multidrug-resistant strains necessitates continuous monitoring, which biochemical analysis addresses through susceptibility determination to various antibiotics. In clinical sample research, e.g., samples collected from healthcare facilities, the prevalence of resistant strains of bacteria takes center stage as requiring immediate improved infection control measures (Eyaufe et al., 2016).

Through the integration of biochemical test results with epidemiological data, healthcare professionals are able to conduct more effective strategies of combat against Gram-negative coccus infections, thus safeguarding the general population and informing therapy (Figure 7.11).

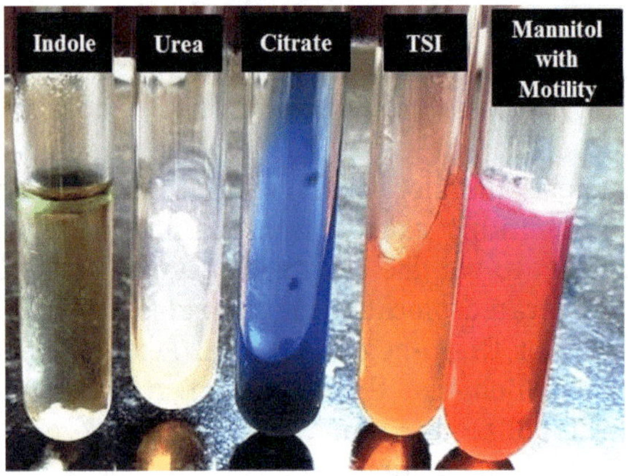

Figure 7.11. Various biochemical reactions for identification of gram-negative cocci.

Source: https://www.researchgate.net/profile/Prasanna-Sarangan-2/publication/310314206/figure/fig2/AS:432189646086145@1480053449895/arious-biochemical-reactions-for-identification-of-non-fermentative-gram-negative-bacilli.png.

7.4.3. Molecular Techniques for Detection

Application of molecular techniques in the identification of Gram-negative cocci has significantly enhanced our understanding and management of these bacteria. Microbiological culture was employed previously for the detection of pathogens, and this was challenging because of time-consuming growth and contamination. However, with the introduction of molecular technology , such as polymerase chain reaction (PCR), real-time PCR, and next-generation sequencing, diagnosis has changed for the better. These methods are based on the amplification of unique DNA sequences so that organisms can be rapidly identified and characterized. For example, PCR is used to detect the occurrence of pathogens even at low levels, and hence it remains an incredibly useful tool to identify drug-resistant strains that may impact cure. Besides, molecular tests can be constructed to identify genes involved in virulence determinants or resistance to antibiotics and therefore provide the clinician with useful information for the proper therapeutic strategy.

Another notable characteristic of molecular detection techniques is that they can quantify biofilm formation by Gram-negative cocci. Biofilms, which are aggregates of bacteria surrounded by an extracellular matrix that protects them, represent important issues in both the clinical and environmental contexts. Molecular methods , such as quantitative PCR can quantify biofilm-associated genes, thereby providing data regarding the pathogenicity of some bacterial strains. It has been demonstrated that the ability to form biofilms is related to virulence and persistence of chronic infection. In particular, the development of high levels of biofilms has been described in multidrug-resistant organisms (MDROs), which makes it more difficult to treat. By using these molecular approaches, clinicians are able to properly identify biofilm producers versus non-producers to have more targeted efforts in infection control and improved patient outcome. Beyond identification only, molecular detection plays a further role in surveillance and epidemiological monitoring of Gram-negative cocci. With increasing antibiotic resistance, timely and precise detection is instrumental in reducing the transmission of these organisms.

Molecular techniques facilitate fast characterisation of the resistance genes and immediate intervention measures. For example, identification of some plasmid-borne resistance genes by molecular typing techniques can be utilized to direct public health intervention to prevent further transmission of resistant strains.

In addition, studies indicate that the healthcare facility biofilm-forming bacteria cause complex infections, and molecular techniques are crucial when interpreting interactions (Bizzini et al., 2013). With the addition of molecular detection techniques, healthcare workers can enhance their ability to combat the growing menace of Gram-negative cocci and treat patients more effectively (Bizzini et al., 2013).

Test Your Knowledge

1. What culture media are commonly used for isolating pathogenic Neisseria species, and why are they preferred?
2. What biochemical tests are used to differentiate Neisseria gonorrhoeae, Neisseria meningitidis, and Moraxella catarrhalis?

7.5. Treatment and Antibiotic Resistance

Learning Outcome

1. Understand common antibiotics used against gram-negative cocci
2. Discuss the mechanisms of antibiotic resistance
3. Focus on strategies to combat resistance

The treatment of Gram-negative coccus infections continues to be a significant problem in today's medicine, particularly due to the fear of rising antibiotic resistance. The bacteria, typically associated with fatal infections, possess inherent mechanisms of resistance to most common and popular antibiotics. One of the critical issues in combating these infections is proper monitoring of antibiotic susceptibility patterns among the Gram-negative isolates. With targeted treatments by susceptibility testing, professionals can choose to make informed decisions regarding how best to preserve antibiotic efficacy while decreasing the selection pressure that creates further resistance. A targeted approach, especially in neonatal intensive care, has demonstrated that strategic use of antibiotics, such as mupirocin is easily able to decrease the risk of infection from specific Gram-positive pathogens, but the role for Gram-negative therapy is not well understood (Bryant et al., 2017). In the context of modern treatment protocols, the role of newer antibiotics and other treatment modalities becomes increasingly significant. Multidrug-resistant forms of Gram-negative cocci have necessitated taking combination therapies and adjunctive treatments as a form of maximizing microbial susceptibility and limiting virulence. Innovative approaches, including the use of bacteriophage therapy and immunomodulatory drugs, have shown promise in the treatment of resistant infections either by directly acting on the bacteria or boosting the host's immune system. In addition, strict infection control measures, , such as increased hygiene measures and focused screening processes, play a key role in averting the spread of resistant strains in the clinical setting (Barnard, 2019). Investigation of the genetic mechanisms of resistance could potentially offer novel therapeutic targets. Secondly, education of physicians and the community on responsible use of antibiotics is also critical in the battle against antibiotic resistance. These include the importance of good prescribing practices and promotion of patient compliance to prescribed regimens. Their improper use not only fails to treat infections but also plays a part in the overall issue of resistance among Gram-negative cocci. Health promotion efforts to educate the public can decrease infection occurrence and enhance patient outcomes by making the current antibiotics' use more conservative. In tandem, these measures underscore the necessity for an all-encompassing approach to prevention and treatment, as it has been realized that the battle against antibiotic resistance is not only a healthcare issue but a social phenomenon necessitating concerted effort at various levels of healthcare (Bryant et al., 2017).

7.5.1. Common Antibiotics Used Against Gram-Negative Cocci

In the management of Gram-negative coccus infections, various groups of antibiotics are generally employed to achieve effective therapeutic outcomes. Selecting the appropriate antibiotics would depend on the specific bacterial species and their sensitivity. The penicillins and the cephalosporins are examples of the beta-lactam antibiotics that have been long-standing cornerstones in combating such infections. Aminopenicillins, for instance, , such as ampicillin are quite effective against certain Neisseria meningitidis strains, while third-generation cephalosporins , such as ceftriaxone are most commonly applied in the treatment of cases with severe infections. The pharmacological properties of these drugs as well as their ability to penetrate the bacterial cell walls greatly enhance their therapeutic effectiveness, making them indispensable tools when treating Gram-negative cocci infections. Another critical class of antibiotics effective against Gram-negative cocci are aminoglycosides, , such as gentamicin and tobramycin. They exert their effect by binding to the bacterial ribosomes, ultimately stopping protein synthesis, which is crucial for bacterial growth and division. Aminoglycosides are particularly effective against enteric Gram-negative cocci, , such as certain strains of *Escherichia coli* and Klebsiella pneumoniae. Studies have indicated that combined use of aminoglycosides with other agents has synergistic action and, therefore, the overall response against resistant organisms is improved. Additionally, with the increased prevalence of multidrug-resistant organisms, surveillance for resistance patterns needs to be carried out from time to time so that the effective therapeutic management remains available, especially in serious infection involving Gram-negative cocci. Besides this, fluoroquinolones and carbapenems are both important members of the antibiotic arsenal against these microorganisms. Fluoroquinolones, such as ciprofloxacin and levofloxacin, are particularly very effective at their wide range of action and penetration into most tissues.

They are widely used in circumstances where resistance would render other antibiotics ineffective. Concurrently, carbapenems like imipenem and meropenem are used as last-resort treatments due to their immense potency against the majority of Gram-negative bacteria. Nevertheless, the emergence of carbapenem-resistant Gram-negative cocci is a significant public health issue, hence the critical need for sustained research and development of antibiotic treatment. Both (Malimu, 2012) and (Bordignon et al., 2017) present essential details of the dynamics of antibiotic resistance and susceptibility patterns, as well as emphasize the demand for particular antibiotic strategies in clinical practice (Figure 7.12).

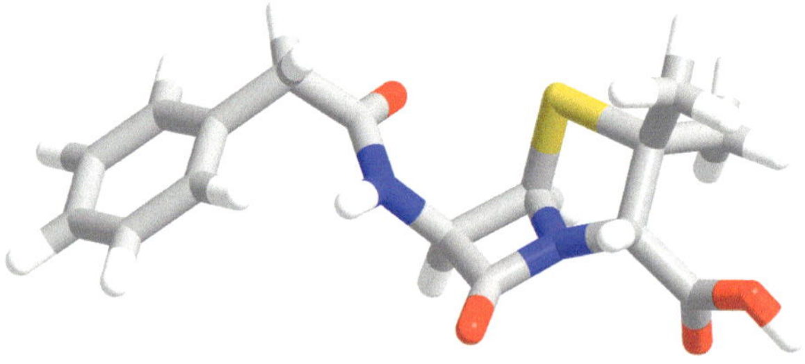

Figure 7.12. Chemical structure of *Penicillin* G.

Source: https://upload.wikimedia.org/wikipedia/commons/thumb/4/42/Penicillin-G_3D.png/1920px-Penicillin-G_3D.png.

7.5.2. Mechanisms of Antibiotic Resistance

Antibiotic resistance in gram-negative cocci is a developing clinical microbiology problem to a large extent as a function of their complex cell wall architecture. The outer membrane of gram-negative bacteria is both a primary defense against the penetration of antibiotics. This complex architecture, characterized by lipopolysaccharides, impairs entry by hydrophilic agents and renders many antibiotics ineffective. Adding to the complexity of treatment is the fact that many of these species possess efflux pumps that actively export antibiotic substances from the cell. This process allows bacteria to become resistant to a broad spectrum of antibiotics, including β-lactams and fluoroquinolones, hence treatment becomes difficult. Moreover, the horizontal transfer of the resistance genes allows the pathogens to become more adept in varying environments. Subsequently, understanding of these processes is critical in the development of novel therapeutic approaches to combating antibiotic-resistant gram-negative cocci and ensuring patient safety within the hospital environment. Biofilm formation is another critical mechanism of the antibiotic resistance of gram-negative cocci.

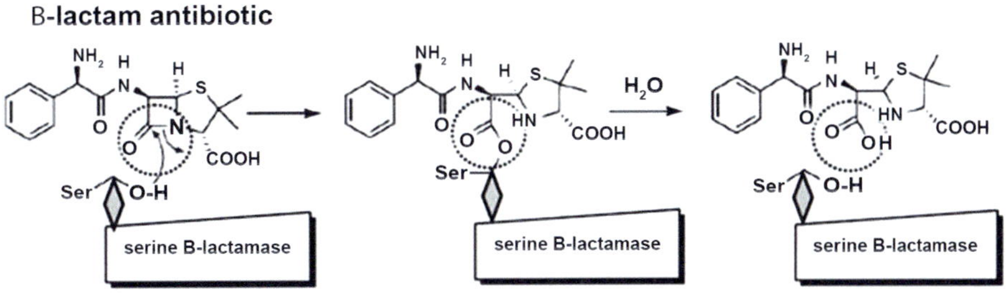

Figure 7.13. Mechanism of the hydrolysis of β-lactam antibiotics through serine-β-lactamases.

Source: https://www.researchgate.net/publication/307818439/figure/fig1/AS:404605822357505@1473476953975/Mechanism-of-the-hydrolysis-of-b-lactam-antibiotics-through-serine-b-lactamases.png.

Biofilms are complex groups of microbes that are enclosed within a protective extracellular matrix that is a sanctuary for bacteria against host defense mechanisms as well as against antimicrobial compounds. Studies have shown that drug-resistant pathogens (MDROs), such as *Pseudomonas aeruginosa*, have high biofilm yields, thus predisposing treatment in chronic infection to be difficult. Of particular concern were 80% of chronic wound patient clinical isolates that had the capacity to produce biofilms, noting the association of biofilm production with successful clinical persistence of these pathogens. The occurrence of biofilm producers in chronic infections indicates that this is a key virulence factor because bacteria can survive harsh conditions and lower the effectiveness of antibiotic treatment. It is essential to comprehend the dynamics of biofilms in order to devise methods for degrading such resistant structures and increasing drug effectiveness. Further, the role of enzyme production in the development of antibiotic resistance cannot be disregarded, particularly in gram-negative cocci. Enzyme-mediated resistance results primarily because of the production of β-lactamases that hydrolyze β-lactam antibiotics and inactivate them. The emergence of extended-spectrum β-lactamases (ESBLs) in gram-negative bacteria like Klebsiella pneumoniae and *Escherichia coli* has added to the challenges for healthcare professionals. Although ESBL production may lead to multidrug resistance, the presence of a correlation between biofilm production and resistance patterns among these organisms is also an observed fact. While 80% of *Pseudomonas aeruginosa* MDR isolates were high to moderate biofilm producers, an inconsistent subpopulation of other species produced less prevalent biofilm characteristics (Bizzini et al., 2013). This demonstrates the complex nature of resistance mechanisms calling for comprehensive approaches targeting both enzymatic neutralization and biofilm-based resistance to adequately manage infections with gram-negative cocci (Bizzini et al., 2013) (Figure 7.13).

7.5.3. Strategies to Combat Resistance

The increasing prevalence of resistance in gram-negative cocci necessitates assessing alternative approaches to deal with this chronic issue. Traditional antibacterial agents are not usually effective towards adamant strains, and therefore scientists seek alternative modes of therapy. A promising avenue of study focuses on improving existing antibiotics with the aim of enhancing effectiveness against resistant phenotypes. For instance, the delineation of the resistance mechanisms provides the basis for developing drug combinations that take advantage of specific vulnerabilities in bacterial pathogens. Additionally, on top of pharmacogenomics, it is possible to tailor antimicrobials to combat explicit genetic profiles of resistant organisms, maximizing therapeutic effect with minimal toxicity. These developments are important since they provide a multi-dimensional platform to tackle the complexities associated with gram-negative cocci infection treatment, with the ultimate aim of reducing morbidity and mortality rates due to these recalcitrant pathogens. Apart from modifying antibiotic regimens, the use of non-antibiotic adjunct therapies is another important strategy towards combating resistance among gram-negative cocci. Studies have shown that the addition of agents , such as antimicrobial peptides and bacteriophage therapy can restore sensitivity in resistant bacteria by degrading biofilms or enhancing the natural immune response against infection. These combination therapies not only add firepower against such pathogens but also lower selective pressure that contributes to the development of resistance. For example, the establishment of biofilms, a critical virulence factor, might be inhibited by application of green tea extracts, i.e., Epigallocatechin Gallate-Stearate (EGCG-S), which exhibit antimicrobial potency against various resistant isolates (Aponte et al., 2018). The new perspective points towards possibilities for synergies through integrative combination of alternative remedies and standard antibiotics, thereby opening new avenues to successful therapy. Efforts directed towards antibiotic stewardship and control of infection support the development of new therapies and adjunctive treatments against the struggle for resistance in gram-negative cocci. Stringent infection prevention measures put in practice can reduce infections due to resistant organisms by a significant extent. Furthermore, promoting appropriate prescribing of antibiotics by clinicians restricts unnecessary exposures to cause the development of resistance. Education and training of health care professionals on the effects of antibiotic misuse are at the heart of the establishment of a drug-use culture of responsibility. The necessity for embracing prevention measures is emphasized by the high rates of resistance among clinical isolates (Napolitano et al., 2005). Collectively, these measures point towards a general strategy to the management of resistance which enables gram-negative cocci to be treated effectively while preserving the efficacy of current and future antimicrobial medications.

Test Your Knowledge

1. What are the first-line antibiotics used to treat infections caused by Neisseria gonorrhoeae and Neisseria meningitidis?
2. What antibiotics are commonly used to treat Moraxella catarrhalis infections, and why is penicillin alone often ineffective?

7.6. Prevention and Control Measures

Learning Outcome

1. Understand vaccination strategies for controlling infections caused by gram-negative cocci
2. Deal with infection control practices in healthcare settings
3. Explain how public health initiatives play a crucial role in mitigating the impact of infectious diseases

Effective prevention and control measures are part of the management of Gram-negative coccus infections, particularly due to their emergent patterns of resistance. Implementation of strict sterilization protocols in health institutions can significantly lower the risk of transmission. This includes regular disinfection of equipment and surfaces and implementation of asepsis measures during procedures. Additionally, strict screening of blood donations is also crucial to prevent bacterial contamination. A study at the Eastern Zone Blood Transfusion Services confirmed that bacterial contamination rates of blood products are frequently startling, where a 2.8% frequency of Gram-positive cocci was recognized as the highest priority concern, underlining the need for increased testing and surveillance practice in blood banks (Malimu, 2012). By placing these practices at the highest level of priority, healthcare centers can minimize the risk of administering Gram-negative cocci to vulnerable patient populations, consequently enhancing overall patient safety. In addition to regular disinfection procedures, educational courses for healthcare workers and members of the general public are crucial in controlling Gram-negative cocci infection. Training programs on hygiene practices, , such as correct hand-washing techniques and adequate attention while donating blood, are essential. Public awareness campaigns can also contribute to increased awareness of the risks of bacterial infections and timely diagnosis and treatment. The multidimensional prevention is particularly necessary because, as research states, environmental factors play a gigantic role in the prevalence of such pathogens (Klaas et al., 2017). Through establishing an environment centered on education and awareness, health agencies can successfully empower individuals towards engaging in preventive measures that reduce the spread of Gram-negative cocci. In addition, vaccine and other therapeutic modality development is important for the long-term control of Gram-negative coccid infections. Although advances in vaccine research are promising, implementation is constrained, especially against frequently misclassified Gram-positive organisms. Preventive control of environmental risks, , such as those posed by mastitis pathogens in dairy cattle, requires a requirement to address both mechanisms of bacterial transmission and healthcare implications of causing such pathogens (Klaas et al., 2017). Improving vaccine development and advancing its application along with antimicrobial stewardship initiatives can be a solid platform for prevention and control. In the end, an integrated strategy that includes education, environmental management, and the use of vaccines will be crucial in combating the challenges caused by Gram-negative cocci in all environments.

7.6.1. Vaccination Strategies

With regard to infectious diseases, vaccination strategies form a significant component of public health interventions for the control of infections due to gram-negative cocci. Vaccines are employed to stimulate the immune system, leading to the development of immunity against specific pathogens. To illustrate this, in the case of Neisseria meningitidis—another predominant gram-negative cocci, which is responsible for causing meningococcal disease—vaccination strategies have made great progress. A number of conjugate vaccines are being engineered to provide immunity against more than one serogroup, demonstrating the worth of continued innovation in vaccine design to capture up-and-coming strains as they appear. Success of vaccination programs depends equally on the formula of the vaccine itself as on the acceptance and use of vaccination regimens by the public, so strong education campaigns are needed to describe the benefits of immunization to risk groups. particularly in farm settings, vaccination strategies for zoonotic gram-negative cocci , such as those addressed to livestock must be carefully considered to prevent risks of transmission to humans. Environmental mastitis, common in dairy farms, illustrates the amount of complexity surrounding the control of gram-negative bacteria , such as *Escherichia coli* and Klebsiella pneumoniae. To properly control environmental mastitis involves the execution of complete vaccination programs, of which only coliform mastitis is currently the focus. Current advancements in vaccine development against other Gram-positive agents of mastitis lag behind, creating a gap which requires further study and innovation. Moreover, the integration of vaccines with other control measures—i.e., environment alteration and host immunity enhancement—has the potential to present a multidisciplinary approach to the reduction of infection incidence, highlighting the necessity of adopting a comprehensive strategy in addressing vaccine efficacy in livestock health management (Klaas et al., 2017). The use of vaccination strategies against gram-negative cocci demands ongoing scrutiny and reformulation to changing epidemiologic situations, particularly in the face of emerging antibiotic resistance. Not only is vaccination a means of prevention, but it also helps reduce reliance on antimicrobials, as implied by calls for sustainable practice within human as well as veterinary medicine. Studies indicate that the incorporation of innovative biotechnological tools, for example, exogenous enzymes supplemented in poultry feed, is likely to improve the overall effectiveness of vaccines by stimulating gut health and influencing microbial communities during infection (Clack et al., 2007). Such integrative approaches could significantly enhance the effectiveness of vaccination programs and contribute to the development of a more sustainable agricultural system. With increasing social demands for limiting the usage of antimicrobials, ongoing development and deployment of effective vaccination approaches remain significant to safeguard both public health and agricultural ecosystems (Figure 7.14).

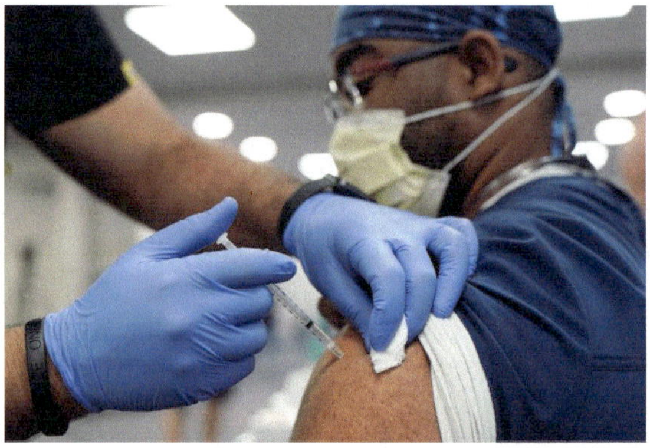

Figure 7.14. Vaccination strategies.

Source: https://images.wsj.net/im-425247?width=700&height=466.

7.6.2. Infection Control Practices in Healthcare Settings

Healthcare facility infection control is important in preventing the spread of pathogenic microorganisms, like Gram-negative cocci, that pose significant clinical risks. These pathogens, which are often found in various infections, can lead to serious complications when not prevented. Universal measures like hand hygiene, use of personal protective equipment (PPE), and a sterile environment are of paramount importance in infection prevention. Implementation of these practices is not merely a matter of procedure; education and sensitivity on the part of healthcare workers to following protocol need to be continual. The use of antimicrobial therapy, particularly infection therapy, also needs to be carefully controlled so as not to allow resistance to develop, which can often follow exposure to a given pathogen in the clinical setting and make further treatment more and more difficult. Decolonization methods have been shown to be a vital component of infection prevention, particularly for patients colonized with Methicillin-resistant *Staphylococcus aureus* (MRSA) and Gram-negative organisms. Research has confirmed the efficacy of mupirocin, a decolonizing antibiotic, in preventing recurrent infection caused by some Gram-positive pathogens, as demonstrated in a multicenter cohort of MRSA-colonized newborns (Bryant et al., 2017). However, mupirocin's action appears weaker against Gram-negative infection, implying the necessity for targeted approaches when planning decolonization treatment in healthcare settings. The challenge lies in balancing treatment efficacy with preventing resistance development in bacterial populations, which translates into continuous assessment and adjustment of infection control to respond to emerging information. In addition, use of smartphones in clinical environments is also a source of concern regarding their role as reservoirs of bacterial pathogens. Such a study on phones of healthcare workers indicated a high rate of bacterial colonization with a high percentage of these bacteria possessing multidrug resistance (Bhat et al., 2011). This means there is a need for strict policies regulating the use and hygiene of personal devices in clinical environments. To effectively manage Gram-negative cocci and other nosocomial infections, hospitals must have detailed guidelines that include regular disinfection of movable equipment and promoting a culture of hygiene among personnel. Hospitals can enhance patient safety and reduce the rate of infection transmission by both traditional infection control measures and future challenges.

7.6.3. Public Health Initiatives

Public health interventions play a critical role in restraining the impact of infectious illnesses caused by gram-negative cocci , such as Neisseria gonorrhoeae and Neisseria meningitidis. Through frequent checks and follow-up, public health agencies are capable of identifying outbreaks as well as promptly responding to contain transmission of these microorganisms. Identification in the early stage becomes possible with interventions that promote routine screening and vaccinations, which ensure significantly reducing morbidity and mortality caused by infections. Through the implementation of evidence-based interventions, , such as education campaigns for the prevention of sexually transmitted diseases, public health programs empower communities to adopt safer behavior, which ultimately lowers infection levels. The interventions not only deal with current outbreaks but also prevent future infections, thereby contributing to a healthier population overall. Moreover, the incorporation of antimicrobial stewardship programs is vital in public health initiatives against the growing threat of antibiotic resistance, particularly among gram-negative cocci. The programs ensure responsible use of antibiotics and, therefore, their effectiveness against resistant organisms. The adoption of such initiatives can be encouraged by public health organizations through the encouragement of appropriate antibiotic prescription and sensitization by healthcare providers on patterns of resistance. For instance, use of potential dietary feed additives (pDFA) with antibacterial activity has shown great promise in animal production, impacting human health indirectly by preventing the use of traditional antibiotics in farm animals (Bruggeman et al., 2019). Through the reduction of the use of antibiotics in agriculture, these measures work to reduce the likelihood of the development of resistance, which may cross-over into human populations. In addition, public health activities in research and development are the key to the battle against gram-negative cocci. Assistance and funding for continuous research aimed at new vaccines and treatment must continue to counter the developing threats from these organisms. Collaboration between government and non-governmental organizations can stimulate innovation in vaccine technology in conjunction with addressing the social determinants of disease spread. For example, the meta-analysis of potential dietary feed additives displays how new approaches can lead to improved results for animals, mirroring the appeal for revolutionary trends among human health (Bruggeman et al., 2019). Grasping research as a priority, public campaigns for health can aid in instilling more efficient ways of avoiding infections and increasing the general public's resistance to gram-negative cocci.

Test Your Knowledge

1. What vaccines are available for the prevention of Neisseria meningitidis infection, and which populations are targeted?
2. What infection control practices are essential in healthcare settings to prevent the spread of Gram-negative coccal infection?

SUMMARY

The microbiology of gram-negative cocci reveals complex interactions within microbiological dynamics, primarily within clinical contexts in which such pathogens participate in infections. The characterization of the complexity of their pathogenicity has significant significance for diagnosis and therapy. For example, in cervico-facial sepsis, the most frequent staining of gram-negative bacteria is observed; nonetheless, the correlation between staining and real presence of the bacteria is not so definitive. The research by Tygerberg Academic Hospital and Tygerberg Oral Health Centre provides evidence that while the majority of pus swabs produce gram-negative stains, very few of them culture gram-negative organisms effectively, potentially reflecting a gap in diagnostic competence (Barnard, 2019). The findings support the urgency for continued investigation into the validity of the application of Gram staining as a diagnostic tool for therapeutic intervention. Moreover, the study on gram-negative cocci reveals the imperative need for innovation in microbiological methods. The disparity between Gram stain results and culture positivity hints towards the participation of anaerobes that favor evading standard laboratory detection. The study data here are inspiring in that only two out of 90 pus samples cultured grew gram-negative organisms, despite a considerable number of specimens being gram-negative for staining (Barnard, 2019). This is a concerning finding that underestimates their presence, making it challenging to determine their contribution to infection. With improved laboratory techniques and the implementation of a multimodal diagnosis strategy, health professionals are better placed to diagnose and treat gram-negative cocci infections, ultimately improving patient care. In the end, research on gram-negative cocci is far from over and needs more intensive research that completes gaps in our current knowledge base. Tygerbergs findings indicate that the outcomes of their investigations raise a key issue: sole diagnostic dependence on Gram staining could be inadequate to establish accurate diagnosis of pathogens causing infection. As we continue to advance our microbiological methodology, the incorporation of new technologies and approaches will be imperative. By embracing these developments and expanding our understanding of gram-negative cocci, the medical community can assist in facilitating increased protocols that enable proper identification and treatment of infections, leading to improved healthcare responses and patient safety. Thus, ongoing researches and clinical vigilance remain invaluable in the fight against bacterial infections.

In their investigation of the nature and clinical importance of gram-negative cocci, their biological and pathogenic characteristics must be known. They are distinguished by a distinct structure with a thin peptidoglycan layer covered by a complicated outer membrane. It acts as a defense system of these bacteria against certain antibiotics, thus making them more difficult to treat. Furthermore, the ability of such organisms to develop genetic variation is accountable for their virulence and treatment resistance. Research on the mechanisms of resistance has indicated that such gram-negative organisms can infect extensive populations in host tissues, , such as in Buruli ulcer, where secondary infection is common, making clinical presentation and sustaining the disease complicated (Pahlevan et al., 2013). Clinical manifestations of gram-negative coccid infections extend beyond simple pathogenicity. Isolation and identification of the bacteria from clinical specimens are crucial for successful therapy, particularly because they are often conjugated with other pathogens at the time of infection. For example, in Buruli ulcers, over 60% of the lesions were co-infected with other bacteria , such as *Staphylococcus aureus*, which considerably affects healing. Implications of such findings underscore the necessity of empirical knowledge in the administration of routine antibiotic regimens, as secondary infection can lead to very prolonged treatment durations and increased healthcare costs. The emergence of drug-resistant strains, particularly *S. aureus*, underscores the need to monitor and manage resistance patterns, in order to improve patient outcomes and direct future therapeutic guidelines (Pahlevan et al., 2013). Developments in gram-negative coccus research also reveal their genetic backgrounds, and the mechanisms of evolution guide their comprehension. Especially, SaPIs research shows that horizontal gene transfer plays a key role in adaptive potential among these bacteria. The discovery of similar PICI factors in various genera puts forward a convergent evolution approach as proof of a highly successful and promiscuous lifestyle among gram-negative cocci. This information increases the horizon of the field of bacterial genetics, ushering in the prospect of new therapeutic techniques and prevention. Through the study of these complicated interactions, the medical community can better predict complications created by these resilient pathogens within the clinical setting, finally leading to more efficient strategies in the battle against infection created by gram-negative cocci.

KEY TERMS FROM THIS CHAPTER

- Alternative therapy
- Antibiotic efficacy
- Antibiotic-resistant strains
- Antimicrobial resistance patterns
- Bacterial contamination
- Bacterial ribosomes
- Bacteriophage therapy
- Aminoglycosides
- Antibiotic susceptibility
- Antimicrobial medications
- Antimicrobials
- Bacterial meningitis
- Bacterial spread
- Biofilm-based resistance

CRITICAL THINKING QUESTIONS

1. **Which of the following is a characteristic feature of Gram-negative cocci?**
   a. They retain crystal violet stain and appear purple under a microscope
   b. They have a thick peptidoglycan layer in their cell wall
   c. They appear pink or red after Gram staining due to a thin peptidoglycan layer
   d. They are typically acid-fast bacteria
2. **Which of the following genera are examples of Gram-negative cocci commonly implicated in human infections?**
   a. *Staphylococcus* and *Streptococcus*
   b. Neisseria and Moraxella
   c. *Clostridium* and Bacillus
   d. Listeria and Corynebacterium
3. **The most common disease caused by Neisseria gonorrhoeae is:**
   a. Meningitis
   b. Gonorrhea
   c. Tuberculosis
   d. Pneumonia
4. **Which laboratory test is typically used to identify Neisseria species?**
   a. Catalase and oxidase tests
   b. Acid-fast staining
   c. Coagulase test
   d. Endospore staining
5. **Which of the following is true regarding antibiotic resistance in Neisseria gonorrhoeae?**
   a. It is universally sensitive to penicillin
   b. It is resistant only to macrolides but sensitive to all beta-lactams
   c. Antibiotic resistance is not a concern in Neisseria species
   d. It has developed resistance to multiple antibiotics , including penicillin and tetracycline

Short Answer Questions

1. What are the general characteristics of Gram-negative cocci, and how do they differ from Gram-positive cocci in terms of structure and staining?
2. What are the major genera and species classified as Gram-negative cocci, and how are they taxonomically categorized?
3. Which diseases are commonly caused by Gram-negative cocci , such as Neisseria gonorrhoeae and Neisseria meningitidis, and what are their primary pathogenic mechanisms?
4. How does the immune system respond to infections caused by Gram-negative cocci, and what virulence factors contribute to their ability to evade host defenses?
5. What laboratory techniques are used to identify Gram-negative cocci, including culture methods, staining, and molecular diagnostics?

Answers to Critical Thinking Questions

1. (c) 2. (b) 3. (b) 4. (a) 5. (d)

REFERENCES

1. Akkermans, A. D. L., Plugge, C. M., de Vos, W. M., et al. (2003). *Victivallis vadensis* gen. nov., sp. nov., a sugar-fermenting anaerobe from human faces. https://core.ac.uk/download/pdf/29294961.pdf (accessed on 13th June 2025).
2. Aponte, T. R. (2018). Green tea polyphenol EGCG-S as an antimicrobial agent. https://core.ac.uk/download/234620901.pdf (accessed on 13th June 2025).
3. Au, F., Bollen, W. B., & Byers, K. M. (2025). Systematic description and key to isolates from Atacama Desert, Chile. https://core.ac.uk/download/pdf/85244762.pdf (accessed on 13th June 2025).
4. Barnard, N. (2019). Prevalence of Gram-negative infections in cervical-facial sepsis. https://core.ac.uk/download/289120726.pdf (accessed on 13th June 2025).
5. Bhat, S. S., Hegde, S. K., & Salian, S. (2011). Potential of mobile phones to serve as a reservoir in spread of nosocomial pathogens. https://core.ac.uk/download/pdf/13598633.pdf (accessed on 13th June 2025).
6. Bizzini, A., Fajardo, A., Gardner, A., Rahman, A., Vickers, A. A., Marshall, B. M., Benagli, C., et al. (2013). Could public restrooms be an environment for bacterial resisters? https://core.ac.uk/download/30696462.pdf (accessed on 13th June 2025).
7. Bolotin, A., Chopin, A., Ruzin, A., Frígols, B., Duerkop, B. A., Ubeda, C., Ubeda, C., et al. (2016). Phage inducible islands in the Gram-positive cocci. https://core.ac.uk/download/46558936.pdf (accessed on 13th June 2025).
8. Bordignon, V., Cavallo, I., Cilli, L., De Santis, R., et al. (2017). Biofilm is a major virulence determinant in bacterial colonization of chronic skin ulcers independently from the multidrug resistant phenotype. https://core.ac.uk/download/188832167.pdf (accessed on 13th June 2025).
9. Bruggeman, G., Dewulf, J., Papadopoulos, D., Sarrazin, L., et al. (2019). Potential dietary feed additives with antibacterial effects and their impact on performance of weaned piglets: A meta-analysis. https://core.ac.uk/download/227040221.pdf; https://core.ac.uk/download/225124686.pdf (accessed on 13th June 2025).
10. Bryant, K., Elward, A., Lessler, J., Milstone, A. M., et al. (2017). Bacterial infections in neonates following mupirocin-based MRSA decolonization: A multicenter cohort study. https://core.ac.uk/download/84911302.pdf (accessed on 13th June 2025).
11. Burnham, C. A. D., Lainhart, W., & Yarbrough, M. L. (2018). Epidemiology, clinical characteristics, and antimicrobial susceptibility profiles of human clinical isolates of *Staphylococcus intermedius* group. https://core.ac.uk/download/212860634.pdf (accessed on 13th June 2025).
12. Carpenter, A. N., Cole, J., Coorevits, A., Dewhirst, F., et al. (2013). *Neisseria oralis* sp. nov., isolated from healthy gingival plaque and clinical samples. https://core.ac.uk/download/286364429.pdf (accessed on 13th June 2025).
13. Clack, B. A., Clemente-Hernandez, S., Kettunen, H., Makivuokko, H., et al. (2007). Enzymes as feed additive to aid in responses against *Eimeria* species in coccidia-vaccinated broilers fed corn-soybean meal diets with different protein levels. https://core.ac.uk/download/286641567.pdf (accessed on 13th June 2025).

14. Dowd, S. E., James, G. A., Rhoads, D. D., Secor, P. R., et al. (2008). Survey of bacterial diversity in chronic wounds using pyrosequencing, DGGE, and full ribosome shotgun sequencing. https://core.ac.uk/download/pdf/7970332.pdf (accessed on 13th June 2025).

15. Eyaufe, A. A. (Aidevbo), Ireye, F. (Faith), & Osagie, R. N. (Rachael). (2016). Microbial analysis of biomedical wastes from selected health facilities in parts of Edo South and its public health implication. https://core.ac.uk/download/480549410.pdf (accessed on 13th June 2025).

16. Gall, L. S., & Riely, P. E. (2025). Effect of diet and atmosphere on intestinal and skin flora. *Volume II–Literature Survey.* https://core.ac.uk/download/pdf/85249155.pdf (accessed on 13th June 2025).

17. Jones, A. L., Sutcliffe, I. C., & Goodfellow, M. (2013). Prescottia equi gen. nov., comb. nov.: a new home for an old pathogen. *Antonie van Leeuwenhoek*, *103*(3), 655–671. https://doi.org/10.1007/s10482-012-9850-8(accessed on 13th June 2025).

18. Iyer, K. M., & Nambiar, V. N. (1971). Bacteriological investigations of prawn canneries 1. Incidence of aerobic spore formers. https://core.ac.uk/download/33721349.pdf (accessed on 13th June 2025).

19. Kanemasa, Y., & Tomochika, K. (1974). Freeze-etch studies on the bacterial cell surfaces: Action of the cell wall lytic enzymes on the Gram-positive cocci. https://core.ac.uk/download/12547174.pdf (accessed on 13th June 2025).

20. Kannapiran, E., Muraleedharan, H., & Kalaigandhi, V. (2009). Microfouling of manganese-oxidizing microorganisms in Rameswaram coastal waters. https://core.ac.uk/download/pdf/288822.pdf (accessed on 13th June 2025).

21. Klaas, I. C., & Zadoks, R. N. (2017). An update on environmental mastitis: Challenging perceptions. https://core.ac.uk/download/132211360.pdf (accessed on 13th June 2025).

22. Krastanov, A., Lante, A., & Tumbarski, Y. (2018). Immobilization of bacteriocins from lactic acid bacteria and possibilities for application in food bio preservation. https://core.ac.uk/download/154331336.pdf (accessed on 13th June 2025).

23. Malimu, E. Z. (2012). The prevalence of bacterial contamination in donated blood in Dar es Salaam, Tanzania. https://core.ac.uk/download/pdf/16666702.pdf (accessed on 13th June 2025).

24. Mooney, C. A. (1987). The antibiotic sensitivity patterns and plasmid DNA content of gram-negative anaerobic bacteria isolated in Palmerston North, New Zealand: A thesis presented in partial fulfilment of the requirements for the degree of Masters in Science at Massey University. https://core.ac.uk/download/187503948.pdf (accessed on 13th June 2025).

25. Mthembu, Wendy & Penduka, Dambudzo & Mosa, Rebamang & Shoba, Bonginkosi & Zobolo, A & Opoku, A. (2017). The bacteria profiles of wounds in diabetic patients hospitalized in northern Kwazulu-Natal, South Africa. African Journal of Clinical and Experimental Microbiology. 18. 186. 10.4314/ajcem.v18i4.2. (accessed on 13th June 2025).

26. Napolitano, L. M. (2005). Emerging issues in the diagnosis and management of infections caused by multi-drug-resistant, Gram-positive cocci. https://deepblue.lib.umich.edu/bitstream/2027.42/63395/1/sur.2005.6.s2-5.pdf (accessed on 13th June 2025).

27. Pahlevan, A. A., Wysocki, A. B., Paintsil, A., Shittu, A. O., Shittu, A. O., Bauer, A. W., Anku, B., et al. (2013). Secondary bacterial infections of Buruli ulcer lesions before and after

chemotherapy with streptomycin and rifampicin. https://core.ac.uk/download/18261879.pdf (accessed on 13th June 2025).

28. Purushottam, D. M., Padmaja, N., & Ganja, S. (2025). Infections caused by Gram-positive cocci and their microbiological pattern in a tertiary care hospital. https://core.ac.uk/download/647975798.pdf (accessed on 13th June 2025).

29. Taylor, G. R., & Zaloguev, S. N. (2025). Methods for microbiological and immunological studies of space flight crews. https://core.ac.uk/download/pdf/42873204.pdf (accessed on 13th June 2025).

30. Widodo, Y. R., & Wirawati, C. U. (2021). Assessment of antimicrobial and proteolytic activity of lactic acid bacteria isolated from dudhi: Naturally fermented buffalo milk from West Sumatra, Indonesia. https://core.ac.uk/download/483682919.pdf (accessed on 13th June 2025).

GRAM-POSITIVE BACILLI

8

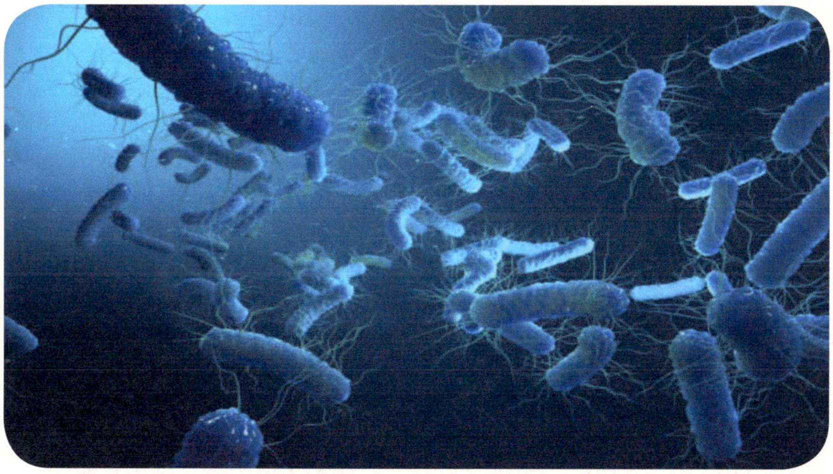

LEARNING OBJECTIVES

After studying this chapter, you will be able to:

1. Understand the characteristics of Gram-positive bacilli
2. Describe major types of Gram-positive bacilli
3. Focus on pathogenicity and diseases
4. Describe laboratory identification techniques
5. Deal with treatment and management of infections

Introduction

Gram-positive bacilli are a significant research area in the field of microbiology due to their significant roles in clinical and environmental environments. These bacteria, depending on whether or not they will retain the crystal violet dye when subjected to Gram staining, possess different potentials for pathogenicity which need to be detected with great caution. Understanding the identification, classification, and effects of these bacteria is important to defeat various health illnesses, including infectious diseases which impact a significant percentage of the population. This introduction lays the groundwork for a comprehensive study of the diverse group of Gram-positive bacilli, their importance in microbial ecology as well as human health. Gram-positive bacilli are traditionally linked with opportunistic infections in clinical practice, particularly in immunocompromised patients. The ability to recognize these organisms accurately can be a determining factor in infection control, allowing for the selection of successful antimicrobial therapy. Traditional identification methods are being complemented by newer methodologies , such as Matrix-Assisted Laser Desorption/Ionization Time-of-Flight mass spectrometry (MALDI-TOF MS), which further enhance precision in discriminating between close relatives. As noted in recent studies, the hierarchical structure of microbial identification needs to be integrated within machine learning algorithms to automate diagnosis and improve patient outcomes (Vervier et al., 2015). This scholarly exploration of Gram-positive bacilli will therefore emphasize traditional and modern approaches towards their identification and characterization. Besides, it is essential to recognize the prevalence and distribution of Gram-positive bacilli in various environments, including clinical settings. For example, in diabetic wound infections, it has been found that there is an extremely complicated interaction between the bacteria and host response, where proper and timely identification is important to the success of therapy (Mthembu et al., 2017). The presence of Gram-positive bacilli with other pathogens is likely to yield polymicrobial infections that complicate therapeutic interventions. This introduction thus seeks to establish a foundation for reasoning through the wide-ranging implications of Gram-positive bacilli in medicine, ultimately correlating their microbiological characteristics to broader health concerns faced in todays era.

Definition of Gram-positive Bacilli

The Gram-positive bacilli are primarily identified based on the type of their cell wall composition that retains the crystal violet used in the Gram staining process. This is due to the thick peptidoglycan layer present in their cell wall that separates these bacteria from the Gram-negative group. Gram-positive bacilli are a large group of rod-shaped bacteria and consist of such genera as Bacillus, *Clostridium*, and Listeria. Understanding their morphological features is significant because these aspects not only aid in identification but also contribute to pathogenicity and the role in the environment. Understanding Gram-positive bacilli is critical to understanding their ecological impact and the infections they can cause, from food poisoning to more lethal infections in immunocompromised individuals. From the clinical significance of Gram-positive bacilli, it can be seen that they serve a dual role as both beneficial and pathogenic microorganisms. For instance, beneficial species , such as Lacto*Bacillus* are critical for food fermentation and the health of humans, forming gut microbiota. Conversely, pathogenic species , such as *Clostridium* tetani, responsible for tetanus, are serious health hazards. Besides, some Gram-positive bacilli are capable of producing biofilms, which will enhance their survival in various environments and contribute to recurrent infections. A study revealed that biofilm production is common among multidrug-resistant pathogens, highlighting the involvement of Gram-positive bacilli in chronic wound infections, as they can hinder healing and induce complications (Bordignon et al., 2017). This Gram-positive *Bacillus* duality explains the necessity of ongoing research on the interaction between Gram-positive bacilli and human beings and their ecological habitats. Along with that, study in Gram-positive bacilli encompasses areas , such as antibiotic resistance patterns, which are now significant public health concerns. Microorganisms , such as *Staphylococcus aureus* and *Bacillus* cereus possess various degrees of antimicrobial resistance, rendering treatment of infections due to them complex. For instance, the prevalence of methicillin-resistant *Staphylococcus aureus* (MRSA) within Gram-positive bacilli highlights the critical need for effective antibiotic resistance measures. It has also been evidenced through studies that there is a high prevalence of Gram-positive bacilli in transfused blood products, showing chronic problems of contamination associated with the process of transfusion (Malimu, 2012). These findings not only inform clinical practice but, significantly, emphasize the importance of strict screening processes to ensure transfusion safety and demonstrate the essential interfacing of Gram-positive bacilli research and public health initiatives (Figure 8.1).

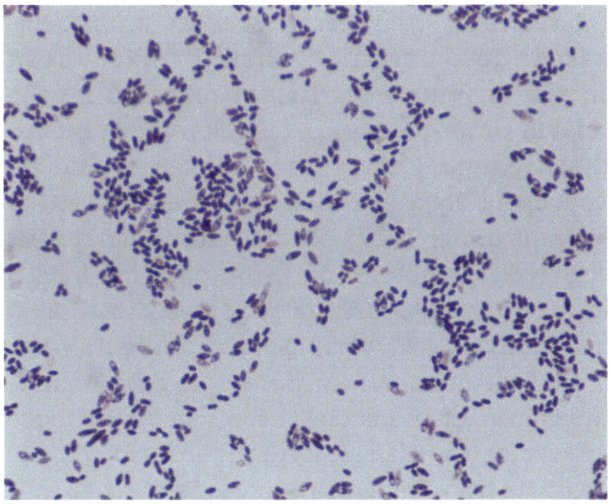

Figure 8.1. Gram-positive bacilli with subterminal spores are visible.

Source: https://www.researchgate.net/publication/47675814/figure/fig2/AS:11431281221193740@1706709169261/Gram-stained-smear-showing-R-peoriensis-Gram-positive-bacilli-with-subterminal-spores.jpeg.

Importance in Microbiology

In microbiology, Gram-positive bacilli are of great concern to research because they impact human disease and health. They are also important for the study of pathogenic mechanisms because some of them produce infectious diseases that are very dangerous. *Bacillus anthracis*, which is the anthrax bacterium, demonstrates the virulence of infection that may be caused by Gram-positive bacilli. The treatment of these infections not only requires acquaintance with the pathogens themselves, but also an acute sense of their pattern of antibiotic resistance, which has been ominously rising in recent years. As highlighted in current studies, the occurrence of antimicrobial-resistant Gram-positive cocci and bacilli requires innovative approaches in the clinical setting to address these new threats (Anjaneya Swamy & Andhale, 2021). Hence, it is important to know the nature and resistance mechanisms of these bacilli if a public health response has to be effective. Gram-positive bacilli are significant, not only for their disease potential, but also for their beneficial roles in most ecological niches. They recycle nutrients, particularly in decomposing organic matter and in symbiosis within human flora. For instance, there are some species that serve as a foundation for the production of fermented foods and probiotics, which maintain a healthy gut. However, the interaction between their positive and negative roles emphasizes the need for extensive microbiological studies to determine the dynamics of their interaction. As physicians are encountering an increasing number of patients suffering from infections caused by these bacilli, an appreciation of their dual roles is found to be necessary. The microflora and the importance of Gram-positive bacilli in disease and health bring out the importance of ongoing research and monitoring (Barnard, 2019).

In addition, the clinical relevance of Gram-positive bacilli has been increased with the emergence of antibiotic resistance patterns complicating treatment options. The patterns of resistance in clinical isolates underscore the necessity for medical practitioners to adapt strategies in the use of antibiotics, as evident in recent retrospective studies that gave an overview of the susceptibility of various pathogens. The high level of resistance among Gram-positive pathogens calls for the formulation of localized antimicrobial policies and guidelines for optimizing effective therapy. Clinically significant Gram-positive bacilli, ranging from those responsible for common infections to those responsible for severe outcomes, highlight the vulnerabilities in our health care systems. Microbiological research must continue to advance and overcome these shortcomings so that microbiologists and clinicians can work hand-in-hand to limit the impact of resistant pathogens on public health (Anjaneya Swamy & Andhale, 2021).

8.1. Characteristics of Gram-positive Bacilli

Learning Outcome

1. Understand the cell wall structure of Gram-positive bacilli
2. Describe staining properties and identification
3. Discuss about metabolic characteristics of Gram-positive bacilli

Gram-positive bacilli are a heterogeneous group of bacteria distinguished by the presence of a thick peptidoglycan cell wall. This is a characteristic that differentiates them from gram-negative bacilli. Besides giving firmness and shape to the cells, this characteristic plays a great role in their ability to hold the crystal violet stain employed during Gram staining. Gram-positive bacilli are mostly divided into two categories: spore-forming and non-spore-forming. Genera like *Bacillus* and *Clostridium* represent the spore-forming group, distinguished by their ability to withstand severe environmental conditions through sporulation. Other adaptive features of non-spore-forming genera like Listeria and Corynebacterium include unique metabolic pathways and the ability to cause disease. Structural differences and classifications of these bacilli show how adaptable and significant they are, particularly in clinical microbiology and infectious disease control. Pathogenicity in the Gram-positive bacilli is extremely variable between the different genera, and the majority of the species are harmful to human health. For instance, anthrax-producing *Bacillus anthracis* and *Clostridium perfringens* which induce gas gangrene, demonstrate the severe consequences of infection with these organisms. *Listeria monocytogenes* has also emerged as a leading foodborne pathogen that is fatal in immunocompromised persons and pregnant women. Recognition of the virulence determinants of such pathogens, such as toxins and adhesins, is necessary in order to develop effective treatment regimens and prophylaxis. Interestingly, treatments, such as mupirocin-based decolonization therapy have been shown to reduce the risk of infection by the related Gram-positive pathogens, which means that treatment of such pathogens should be appropriately controlled in a clinical setting (Bryant et al., 2017). Furthermore, the special cell wall structure of Gram-positive bacilli influences not just pathogenicity but also interaction with various environments, e.g., biological membranes. Based on new results, the character of bacteria seems to play a more important role than hitherto with respect to their ability to transfer across porous membranes, e.g., in filtration techniques used in microbiological processes. This is particularly important in the implication of why Gram-positive and gram-negative bacteria respond differently to environmental stress. For instance, the flexibility of cell wall structure can cause uncontrolled transfers through filters, hence complicating the sterility assurance in laboratory environments (Aimar et al., 2009). Thus, recognition of the characteristics of Gram-positive bacilli is important in clinical microbiology and scientific investigation, determining how these bacteria are handled in various industrial environments and medical contexts.

8.1.1. Cell Wall Structure and Composition

The cell wall composition of Gram-positive bacilli is a fundamental part of their biology and determines both their viability and infectivity. Mostly consisting of high peptidoglycan layers, the cell walls give the bacteria their structural strength and osmotic resistance. This peptidoglycan is a polymer chain consisting of sugar chains cross-linked by peptide chains, which give them stability and protection from stress factors in the environment. In Gram-positive bacteria, such a layer can represent as much as 90% of the structure of the cell walls, a distant cry from Gram-negative bacteria, whose peptidoglycan layers are considerably thinner and include an outer membrane. Not only does the unique structure of the Gram-positive cell wall make it possible for retention of crystal violet stain in Gram staining, but it also aids the bacteria in resisting a wide range of antibiotics, influencing cell wall synthesis. Thus, the cell wall is a fundamental structure that is responsible for determining the identity and susceptibility of these microbes. In addition to peptidoglycan, the cell walls of Gram-positive bacilli are often found to contain some teichoic acids, which are concerned with cell wall structural integrity and function. These acids, , such as lipoteichoic acid (LTA) and wall teichoic acid (WTA), are found within the peptidoglycan layer to provide additional structural rigidity as well as a phosphate reservoir necessary for cell metabolic processes. These teichoic acids also contribute to the interaction between Gram-positive bacteria and their environment, in the ability to bind to host tissues and prevent immune response. In addition, their structural components are highlighted by host immune responses, sometimes as virulence factors inducing inflammation. Therefore, the intricate composition of the Gram-positive *Bacillis* cell wall significantly enhances their infective potential, as well as offering a target for therapeutic approaches attempting to disrupt cell wall integrity. Moreover, recent studies highlight the evolutionary significance of prokaryotic cell wall structures, traceable back to old protection and environmental adaptation mechanisms. For instance, recurring crystalline surface layers (S-layers) are among the most old forms of cell wall structures found in numerous prokaryotic species, , such as Gram-positive bacilli. These S-layers, composed of glycoprotein lattices, have diverse architectural patterns that all serve the overall stability of the cell wall. They not only bestow protective coverings against physical and biological stresses but also have evolved multifunctional roles, including molecular sieves, sites for enzyme attachment, and virulence factors. As they become integrated into the broader context of cellular function, understanding these intricate details of cell wall composition is crucial for developing targeted antibacterial therapies that exploit the vulnerabilities inherent in Gram-positive bacilli's architecture (Figure 8.2).

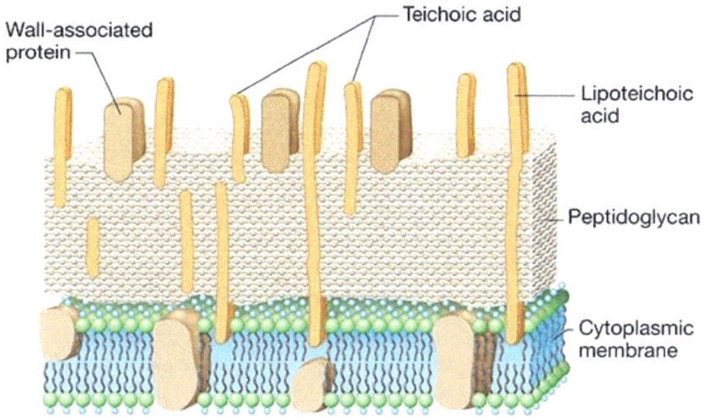

Figure 8.2. Gram-positive bacilli cell wall.

Source: https://microbenotes.com/wp-content/uploads/2018/04/Gram-positive-cell-wall.jpg.

8.1.2. Staining Properties and Identification

In the identification of Gram-positive bacilli, the characteristics of staining play a pivotal role in it, especially in the process of Gram staining. The process identifies bacteria based on the cell wall content, where Gram-positive bacteria are stained purple as a result of the retention of crystal violet. This is owing mainly to the thick peptidoglycan layer of the cell wall for Gram-positive bacilli, which contributes to extra structural strength. For instance, species , such as *Bacillus* subtilis have this property evidently, hence can be easily identified in routine microbiological examinations. Second, the precision of this staining process has made it an indispensable tool for clinical labs, permitting direct discrimination of pathogenic Gram-positive bacilli from other bacteria and thereby making early and correct treatment decisions possible. In addition to the Gram stain, other biochemical tests also support the identification process of Gram-positive bacilli. Such tests as the catalase test, which identifies the presence of the enzyme catalase, can distinguish between genera within the Gram-positive group. For instance, while *Staphylococci* spp. test positive for the catalase test, *Streptococci* spp. test negative, hence confirming their classification. Furthermore, newer techniques, like API (Analytical Profile Index) testing and 16S rDNA sequencing, provide precise profiles of bacterial isolates with proper identification independent of morphology and staining characteristics. These methods are particularly significant in clinical settings, where accurate identification is critical to the treatment of infection, most notably that involving diabetic wounds, as identified in studies on the significance of monitoring pathogen distribution and antibiotic resistance (Mthembu et al., 2017). The significance of staining features also applies to the discipline of clinical microbiology, where the identification of strains with potential probiotic properties becomes increasingly pertinent (Figure 8.3).

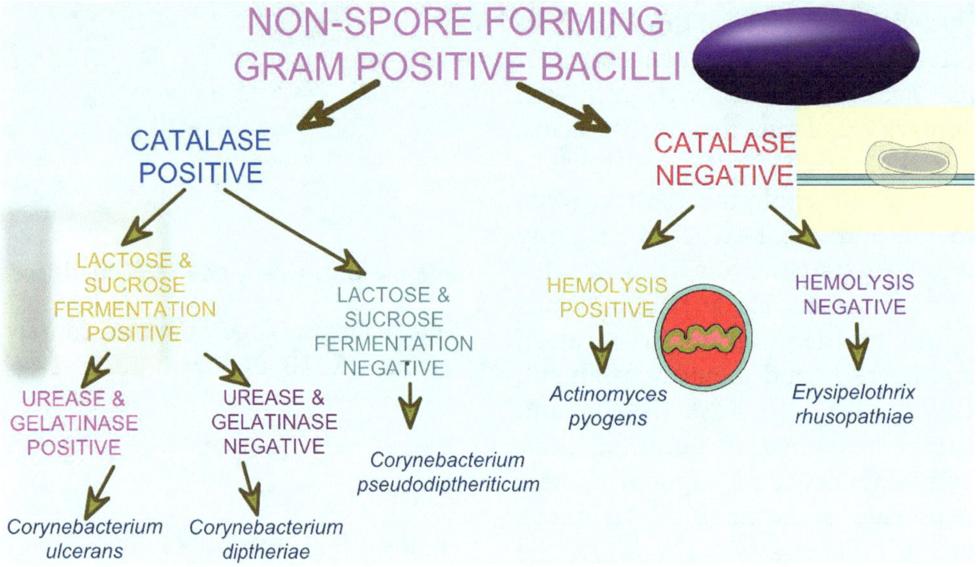

Figure 8.3. Flowchart of bacterial tests: Gram-positive bacilli.

Source: https://i.ytimg.com/vi/2xV-HkB1iWA/maxresdefault.jpg.

Studies have established that certain strains of *Bacillus* possess better surface properties , such as hydrophobicity, which are critical for their application as probiotics in animal nutrition. The identification of such strains through rigorous staining and testing protocols has been crucial in determining their viability for further research and application. For example, studies separated *Bacillus* subtilis strains and examined their beneficial qualities like biosurfactant production and pathogen inhibition, further confirming the importance of proper identification methods in enhancing the development of probiotics (Maldonado et al., 2015). With advancing science, the correlation between staining characteristics and subsequent identification protocols will definitely dictate the fate of microbial probiotics and therapeutic applications (Figure 8.4).

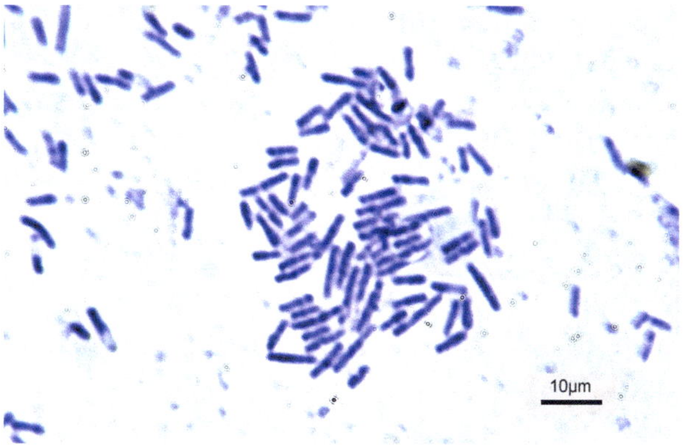

Figure 8.4. *Bacillus* subtilis (Gram stain).

Source: https://upload.wikimedia.org/wikipedia/commons/thumb/5/52/Bacillus_subtilis_2.jpg/1280px-Bacillus_subtilis_2.jpg.

8.1.3. Metabolic Characteristics

The metabolic characteristics of Gram-positive bacilli are key to their ecological environment and virulence. Primarily, the bacteria exist as heterotrophic in their metabolism, obtaining energy and their carbon source from organic molecules. This characteristic allows them to inhabit an extensive array of environments, ranging from soil and water to host organisms. For instance, certain species like *Bacillus* and Listeria are perfectly adapted to nutrient-rich substrates where they can catabolize carbohydrates, proteins, and lipids. In addition, their ability to respire both aerobically and anaerobically contributes significantly to their survival under various conditions. This metabolic flexibility not only enhances their adaptability but also facilitates competition with other microbial populations, thus controlling the overall microbial dynamics of their environments. Additionally, Gram-positive bacilli frequently employ fermentation pathways, which yield energy without oxygen. For instance, bacteria , such as Lacto*Bacillus* play a key role in food production, especially in fermenting dairy products. In this case, their ability to ferment lactose to lactic acid not only serves to preserve food but also creates favorable flavors and textures. In the same way, some pathogenic Gram-positive bacilli, for example, *Clostridium* species, exhibit special fermentative mechanisms that can result in different metabolites, like butyric acid and acetone. These metabolic byproducts can be useful to the bacteria and toxic to their hosts, and lead to spoilage of food or disease. These bifunctional metabolic activities underlie the duality of Gram-positive bacilli as useful and disease-causing organisms, depending on their location. The study of metabolic characteristics extends beyond energy production to encompass the genetic and regulatory systems that control these activities. Advances in molecular biology have significantly enriched the understanding of metabolism and gene expression in Gram-positive bacilli. Techniques , such as transcriptomics have shown intricate networks of metabolic genes that are regulated by environmental cues, the availability of nutrients, and stress. Understanding such pathways is significant not only for theoretical microbiology but also for applied reasons , such as industrial fermentation and pathogenicity control. For example, identification of genes that promote enhancement of spoilage processes in *Bacillus* species may guide better preservation procedures in the food industry (Aarts et al., 2015). Likewise, knowing metabolic strategies applied by pathogenic Gram-positive bacilli may guide treatment procedures against infections (Altschul et al., 2013).

Test Your Knowledge

1. What key components distinguish the cell wall structure of Gram-positive bacilli from Gram-negative bacteria?
2. How does the thick peptidoglycan layer in Gram-positive bacilli affect their staining properties during Gram staining?

8.2. Major Types of Gram-positive Bacilli

Learning Outcome

1. Describe Bacillus species
2. Understand Clostridium species
3. Discuss Listeria monocytogenes

Classification of Gram-positive bacilli is of prime importance in microbiology, particularly the identification of mechanisms of pathogenicity and methods of treatment of the infection. Gram-positive bacilli are broadly classified into spore-producing and non-spore-producing ones. Under the spore-producers, the *Bacillus* genus includes both pathogenic and asepathogenic species, of which the most dreaded *Bacillus anthracis* causes anthrax. In contrast, the non-spore-forming bacilli, , such as Listeria and Corynebacterium, are likewise crucial in disease in humans. For instance, *Listeria monocytogenes* is a virulent pathogen that induces listeriosis, which may cause complicated secondary infections in the highly vulnerable group of pregnant females and immunocompromised individuals. Understanding these differences is vital for effective diagnosis and treatment protocols in the hospital environment. A summary of the clinical significance of various Gram-positive bacilli illustrates their multifarious function in health and disease in man. *Streptococcus* species, including *Streptococcus pneumoniae* and *Streptococcus pyogenes*, are strongly implicated in respiratory and cutaneous infections, respectively. The pathogenicity of these organisms is further augmented by their ability to evade host immunity and develop antibiotic resistance. Moreover, the occurrence of multidrug-resistant pathogens (MDRO) among Gram-positive bacilli, especially in diseases like prosthetic joint infections, has grave implications for treatment. Interestingly, a study noted that infection in the early postoperative time period was predominantly by virulent *S. aureus* isolates and polymicrobial infections, and stressed the importance of prudent antimicrobial stewardship to combat the emergence of MDROs in clinical environments (Cardenal et al., 2019; Toro López, 2019). Besides, Gram-positive bacilli possess more than a mere role as pathogens; the majority of them are engaged in beneficial processes in their habitats. Some species of the *Bacillus* genus, for example, are applied in industrial microbiology as a result of their enzymatic synthesis. Other probiotics like Lacto*Bacillus* and Bifidobacterium, which belong to the groups of more general collections of bacilli, have a very critical function in enhancing intestinal health and activating the immune system. This Gram-positive bacilli dualism of being pathogenic and beneficial brings them into the focus of ongoing research. Improved comprehension of their resistance mechanisms and metabolic processes is the key to future therapeutic interventions, particularly in a day and age where antibiotic resistance is increasing. Their intricacy necessitates a thorough examination of both their detrimental and benevolent impact on the health of human beings.

8.2.1. Bacillus Species

Of the heterogeneous group of Gram-positive bacilli, the *Bacillus* species are specifically fascinating because of their unique characteristics and widespread presence in most environments. The group is comprised of a diverse range of motile, spore-producing bacteria with the ability to thrive in various ecological niches like soil, water, and living organisms. It is noteworthy that *Bacillus anthracis*, the causative agent of anthrax, is unique owing to its importance in public health as well as biosafety (Figure 8.5).

Bacillus cereus, another member of this genus, is also often implicated in food poisoning and is pathogenic and non-pathogenic in nature, indicating the complex nature of microbial community interactions. Being soil bacteria, the members of the *Bacillus* genus can also contribute significantly to nutrient turnover, increasing soil fertility and overall health, and this therefore indicates their ecological significance aside from their impacts on human health. The survival mechanisms of *Bacillus* species are largely due to their ability to form endospores, a property that allows them to survive extreme environmental conditions like heat, drying, and starvation. Such resting forms are crucial to survival and can persist for several years under adverse conditions, but germinate only to vegetative cells that divide actively upon exposure to supportive conditions. Endosporulation is not merely a survival mechanism but also makes it possible for the transfer of these organisms from one environment to another. Thus, the *Bacillus* species can quickly colonize new environments, something that may have implications for agriculture and food safety.

The spores' resistance also makes them important in microbial spoilage studies, particularly in the food industry, where certain strains cause product contamination leading to serious economic losses and health hazards among consumers, as seen through the increasing focus on foodborne pathogen management. Moreover, the functional diversity of *Bacillus* species is also utilized in biotechnological applications, including their utilization for fermentation technologies and enzymes and other bioactive molecules. For example, *Bacillus* subtilis is widely utilized in the food and agriculture sectors due to the capability of this organism to secrete enzymes that help in animal feed digestibility and increase crop yields. The industrial importance of the *Bacillus* species is also illustrated by their potential as biocontrol agents against pests and plant diseases in agriculture. As improvements become public about their genomic and metabolic capabilities, the potential for the utilization of these Gram-positive bacilli in diverse applications increases. This understanding of *Bacillus* species use in different environments has to be interdisciplinary, bringing in microbiology, ecology, and applied sciences to use their full potential with a reduction in the accompanying risk, particularly in applications of food safety (Bevilacqua et al., 2015; López et al., 2019) (Figure 8.6).

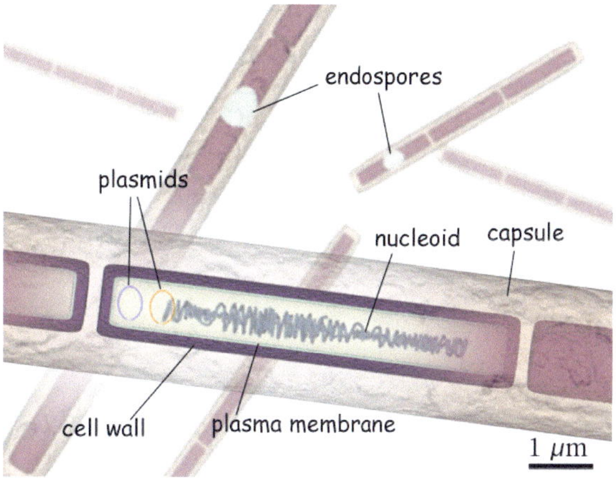

Figure 8.5. Structure of *B. anthracis.*

Source: https://upload.wikimedia.org/wikipedia/commons/3/30/B_anthracis_diagram_en.png.

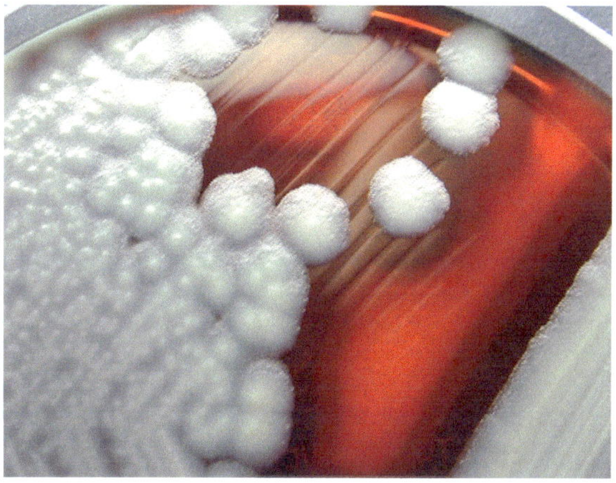

Figure 8.6. *Bacillus* cereus showing hemolysis on sheep blood agar.

Source: https://upload.wikimedia.org/wikipedia/commons/0/02/Bacillus_cereus_01.png.

8.2.2. Clostridium Species

Amongst the diverse genera of Gram-positive bacilli, *Clostridium* species are significant due to their unique characteristics and pathogenicity. These bacteria are best known for the spores they produce, which render them resistant to a range of environmental stress conditions and thus favor their existence even under unfavorable environments. The group includes several medically significant species, a few of which include *Clostridium* tetani, the etiologic agent of tetanus; *Clostridium* botulinum, the etiologic agent of botulism; and *Clostridium* difficile, the agent of antibiotic-associated diarrhea.

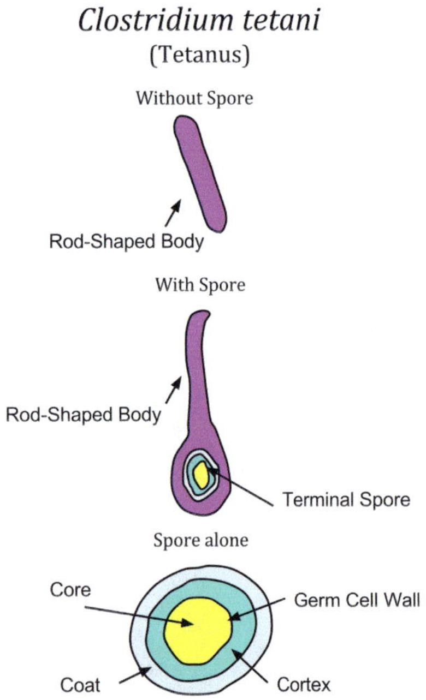

Figure 8.7. A diagram of *C. tetani* showing the bacterium alone, with a spore being produced, and the spore alone.

Source: https://upload.wikimedia.org/wikipedia/commons/thumb/f/f2/*Clostridium*_Tetani.svg/800px-*Clostridium*_Tetani.svg.png.

The pathogenic activities employed by *Clostridium* members frequently involve the production of highly potent exotoxins that disrupt physiological functions, resulting in disease that is typically profound. The prevalence of these infections poses notable challenges to public health systems, which need heightened awareness and effective control measures in order to work against their impacts (Ajani et al., 2010). The epidemiology of the *Clostridium* species is such that it is based on reliance on certain environments and risk factors. For instance, *C. difficile* infections are usually linked with antibiotic exposure and health care facilities, in which disruption of normal gut flora allows for the overgrowth of this pathogen. *C. botulinum* is also naturally linked with improperly handled food, pointing to the risks in food handling techniques. Traumatic injury or surgery can introduce *C. tetani* into vulnerable hosts, leading to potentially fatal complications. It is vital to comprehend these epidemiological patterns in order to impose preventative measures to curb infection rates (Figure 8.7).

Surveillance systems monitoring *Clostridium* species epidemics can inform public health action and improve treatment protocols, with appropriate care being delivered to infected individuals (Ajani et al., 2010). The clinical relevance of *Clostridium* species infection underscores the need for ongoing research in this field. Advances in microbiological techniques and immunology have allowed us to gain knowledge on how the organisms interact within host systems. Recent studies have revealed potential therapeutic approaches to reverse the effects of *Clostridium* toxins and ensure improved patient recovery. A good example is the development of monoclonal antibodies to neutralize *C. botulinum* toxins, which offers a promising approach to therapy. In addition, more advanced diagnosis is required for the effective fast detection of *Clostridium* species to allow for timely intervention during severe disease outbreaks. Continued research into the *Clostridium* pathogenicity and resistance mechanisms will be critical to establishing a proper treatment and total control measures against these formidable Gram-positive bacilli (Figure 8.8).

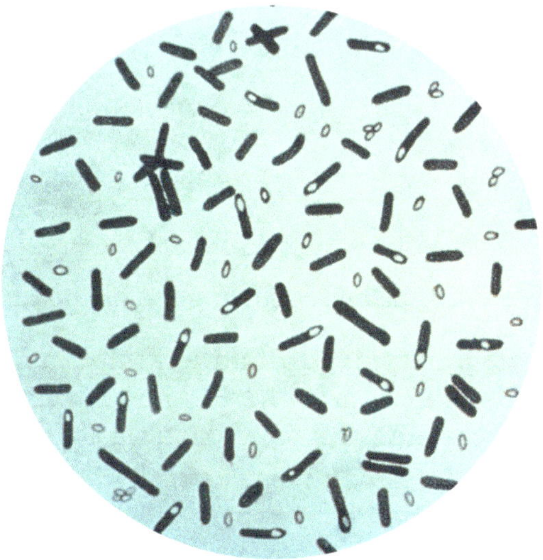

Figure 8.8. A photomicrograph of *Clostridium botulinum* bacteria.

Source: https://upload.wikimedia.org/wikipedia/commons/5/58/*Clostridium_*botulinum_01.png.

8.2.3. Listeria Species

Listeria species, and particularly *Listeria monocytogenes*, are a significant problem in the category of Gram-positive bacilli since they are disease-causing and can result in serious clinical presentations. On the basis of its ability to grow at refrigeration temperatures, *L. monocytogenes* is of particular significance in food safety since it tends to infect dairy products, meats, and ready-to-eat foods. The pathogenicity of the organism can be largely attributed to its unique virulence factors, which allow it to survive and multiply within the host cells. The ability of the pathogen to evade the immune mechanisms of the host, along with its intracellular existence, leads to pathologies , such as listeriosis, which can have serious manifestations in different vulnerable populations of individuals, including the aged, pregnant women, and immunocompromised hosts. Understanding these factors in Listeria species is crucial to successful public health interventions and strengthening food safety measures (Figure 8.9).

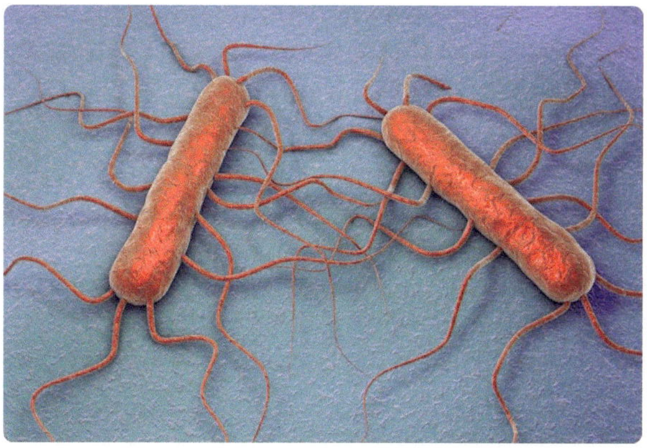

Figure 8.9. Listeria.

Source: https://www.news-medical.net/image-handler/ts/20210928105416/ri/673/picture/2021/9/shutterstock_400088737.jpg.

Insights into specific outbreaks provide valuable information regarding the epidemiological patterns of Listeria infection. A prominent study documented an outbreak of neurological disease in red-legged partridges, demonstrating how *L. monocytogenes* is capable of infecting avian hosts. Clinical manifestations , such as torticollis and head tilt were observed among the infected birds, and microbiological examination certified encephalitis caused by *Listeria monocytogenes*. The outbreak was caused by the introduction of day-old chicks infected with the disease, highlighting the pathogens' transmission pathways and ecological adaptability. Such results make it imperative to track Listeria not only in the sources of human food but also in animal husbandry facilities, where detection can be devastating to the health and productivity of animals and agriculture (Lopez, 2019). The pathogenicity of Listeria species is closely tied to how it interacts with the immune system of the host. As a pathogen, *L. monocytogenes* employs multiple mechanisms to evade the host cell functions and immune response. The microorganism employs bacterial exotoxins in intracellular migration and dissemination and thereby increasing pathogenicity and causation of disease (Elmanama et al., 2007).

Secondly, the character of the host-parasite association highlights the necessity of ongoing research on the host immune response as a vehicle of pursuing an understanding of listeriosis pathogenesis. This data may pave the way for new treatments and vaccines, supporting public health measures to avert Listeria infections. As research continues to untangle the intricacies of these correlations, it is increasingly clear that Listeria species are an attractive model for the exploration of pathogenicity in Gram-positive bacilli (Figure 8.10).

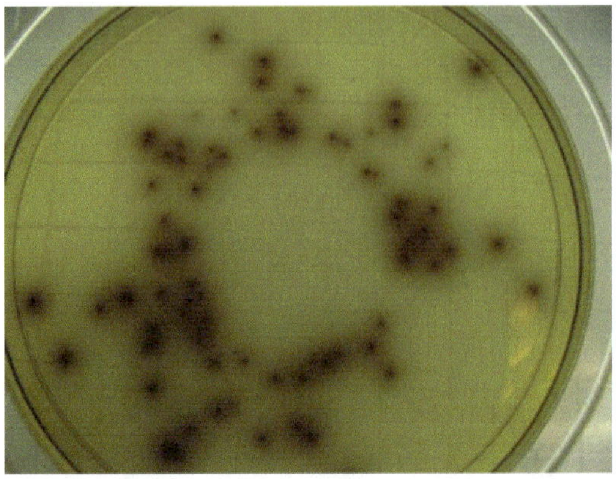

Figure 8.10. Listeria grown on agar medium.

Source: https://upload.wikimedia.org/wikipedia/commons/7/7c/Listeria_monocytogenes_grown_on_Listeria_Selective_Agar.jpg.

Test Your Knowledge

1. What are the key distinguishing characteristics of Bacillus species compared to Clostridium species?
2. What are the common species of Listeria that are pathogenic to humans, and which species is the most clinically significant?
3. What are the typical environmental sources and transmission routes for Listeria monocytogenes infections in humans?

8.3. Pathogenicity and Diseases

Learning Outcome

1. Understand infections caused by Bacillus anthracis
2. Describe clostridial infections and their implications
3. Focus on Listeriosis and its impact on public health

The pathogenicity of the Gram-positive bacilli, and particularly the genera *Bacillus* and Listeria, is used to highlight their far-reaching implication on human diseases worldwide. *Bacillus anthracis*, through its reputation for causing anthrax, under optimum environmental conditions, can produce spores that play an essential role in its persistence and dissemination. Infection is established through a variety of routes of invasion, cutaneous, inhalational, and gastrointestinal, each having a corresponding clinical challenge and expression. Its pathogenicity is to blame for its capsule and very toxic exotoxins produced, which are to blame for systemic symptoms and high mortality rates in case of failure to treat. An understanding of these mechanisms is important in the development of effective prevention and therapeutic strategies, with a focus on research in disease control and public health intervention (Gall & Riely, 1965). Other than *Bacillus* species, *Listeria monocytogenes* is a particular problem, particularly among pregnant females and immunocompromised individuals, where it can cause fatal meningitis and septicemia. *L. monocytogenes*' virulence comes from its intracellular growth and dissemination mechanisms to invade host cells and evade immunity, respectively. This adaptability allows the infection to pass through the placenta, resulting in adverse outcomes , such as fetal loss or neonatal infection. Moreover, the pathogen's association with contaminated food products adds to its public health interest, necessitating stringent food safety measures. Effective Listeria outbreak management is reliant on having good knowledge of its ecology, transmission routes, and related risk factors accountable for its intensified effects on disease (Alippi et al., 2011). Recent studies on interactions between Gram-positive bacilli and their habitats reinforce the complex dynamics accountable for their pathogenicity. It has also been evidenced through study that bacterial strains, , such as those obtained from insect cuticles, can be antagonistic towards pathogenic fungi , such as Beauveria bassiana and thus suggest a more sophisticated role in ecological systems. Being harbored by beneficial bacteria like *Bacillus* thuringiensis suggests the potential for biocontrol mechanisms that might limit pest populations while addressing disease vectors in agricultural management. This brings to the fore the holistic vision of pathogenicity, in which microbial ecosystem knowledge may be utilized to guide interventions for reducing disease burdens due to Gram-positive bacilli. This knowledge is pivotal in the creation of novel prevention and treatment strategies, eventually contributing to enhanced public health (Gall & Riely, 1965) (Alippi et al., 2011).

8.3.1. Infections Caused by Bacillus anthracis

Bacillus anthracis infection is a critical concern in the clinical discipline of microbiology and public health due to the zoonotic transmission potential of the organisms. As a Gram-positive bacillus, B. anthracis is defined by the development of anthrax, which can occur in the form of cutaneous, gastrointestinal, inhalational, and, on rare occasions, meningitis. The cutaneous type accounts for approximately 95% of infections in humans, which commonly follow direct exposure to infected animal products. Gastrointestinal anthrax, although less common, includes severe complications following the consumption of raw, infected meat of animals, reiterating the public health risk in places where the disease remains endemic. This requires heightened vigilance and ongoing education regarding the identification and management of anthrax infection, particularly among communities that may be brought into close contact with animals or animal products, as illustrated by the finding of atypical cases due to food contamination (Arjmand et al., 2006). The pathogenicity of *Bacillus anthracis* is largely due to its capacity to form spores and toxins, enabling it to survive in a variety of settings and withstand the host immune system. Infection is possible through a number of different routes, with inhalation anthrax posing the highest risk of mortality due to its rapid onset. This type is found when spores are inhaled, resulting in serious respiratory disease that will rapidly progress to systemic infection. The pathways through which the bacterium pathogenically acts include both biochemical and cellular processes and account for its designation as a serious biothreat agent. Additionally, the novel pathogenesis of B. anthracis emphasizes the importance of innovative diagnostic methods and efficient treatment measures to reduce the burden of such infections on public health systems (Ajani et al., 2010).

Considering the complexities posed by infections caused by *Bacillus anthracis*, there is a critical need for integrated strategies aimed at prevention and control. Vaccination remains the primary means of defense against anthrax, particularly for those at higher risk, such as animal handlers and laboratory personnel. Public health initiatives that create awareness of the dynamics of the disease transmission are vital in reducing its occurrence. Further, research that endeavors to determine the ecological behaviors of B. anthracis and its interaction with animal populations is essential for the detection of outbreaks and timely intervention. Continued efforts in augmenting the surveillance, diagnosis, and treatment of anthrax will be significant in mitigating the public health risk posed by this powerful Gram-positive *Bacillus* to anticipate future events (Arjmand et al., 2006; Ajani et al., 2010) (Figure 8.11).

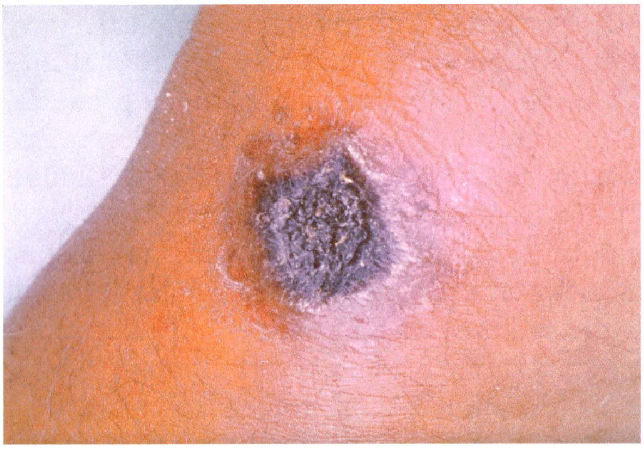

Figure 8.11. Anthrax: an infection caused by the bacterium *Bacillus anthracis*.

Source: https://upload.wikimedia.org/wikipedia/commons/thumb/5/5f/Anthrax_PHIL_2033.png/1280px-Anthrax_PHIL_2033.png.

8.3.2. Clostridial Infections and Their Implications

Clostridial infections, which are mostly caused by members of the genus *Clostridium*, constitute a serious public health problem because of their potential for fast progression and very high mortality. Of the clinically significant species, *Clostridium sordelli* and *Clostridium perfringens* have been of great interest because of their involvement in toxic shock syndromes. Such infections are of serious concern when found in obstetric settings, wherein *C. sordellii* carries a greater than 90% case-fatality rate. The challenge of early diagnosis contributes to the risk, with the rapid development of severe symptoms overloading clinical centers and emphasizing the urgent need for creative diagnostic approaches. Advances, such as the development of duplex PCR-based microsphere assays offer promising methodologies for early detection of these microorganisms from formalin-fixed, paraffin-embedded tissue, making identification easier and potentially improving patient outcomes (Antoniadou et al., 2012). The implications of clostridial infections extend to indirect health consequences, significantly impacting clinical management protocols and patient care standards. For instance, the unrelenting unpredictability of *C. sordellii* and *C. perfringens* infections renders them critically dependent on vigilance in obstetric and surgical cohorts, whose invasive treatment increases the risk of exposure to such pathogens. The causation of toxic shock associated with these pathogens does call for extensive education of healthcare providers in the recognition of signs and symptoms of infection to save the patient from the life-and-death distinction of early treatment. By raising the level of awareness of such infections, health care providers can impart preventive practices and induce early referral to specialists in the event of suspected high-risk exposure. The presence of rapid, sensitive diagnostic tests is set to transform the management of clostridial infections and allow more rational clinical choices, and enhance mortality rates related to the disease (Antoniadou et al., 2012). In addition, fighting clostridial infections needs an understanding of the microbiological environment at large and the role played by antibiotic usage in clinical management. The emergence of antibiotic resistance in clostridial organisms introduces an added level of complexity, impacting the effectiveness of treatment and complicating treatment. Of concern is the excessive use of antibiotics, which will disrupt the natural microbial environment, leading to a habitat where clostridia can thrive. This becomes a strong indicator of the importance of prudent antibiotic stewardship and the introduction of treatment regimens oriented around the prevention of infection. Further research is needed to elucidate clostridia's mechanisms of resistance, and to construct viable vaccines that will eventually stem the tide of such infections. Through efforts to tackle the complicated nature of clostridial infections, from diagnosis and treatment to prevention, the health industry can greatly reduce its impact on public health (Figure 8.12).

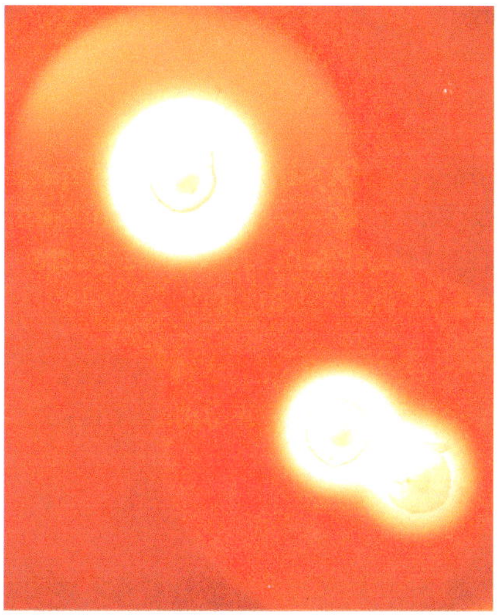

Figure 8.12. *Clostridium* perfringens: *Clostridium perfringens* bacteria from an infected human gall bladder.

Source: https://www.britannica.com/science/clostridial-infection.

8.3.3. Listeriosis and Its Impact on Public Health

Of the myriad of public health issues caused by bacterial infection, listeriosis, which is an infection by the Gram-positive *Bacillus Listeria monocytogenes*, is of critical concern, particularly to vulnerable groups , such as the elderly, pregnant women, and immunocompromised individuals. The illness is also characterized by the high rates of morbidity and mortality it results in, up to 25-30% among affected individuals, which signifies severe consequences of listeriosis outbreaks. Its prevalence in most settings, including food products, makes the control and prevention efforts particularly challenging for public health officials. This is the reason why enforcement of food safety through regulation and public education campaigns to reduce the risk of contamination, as well as ensure the vulnerable groups are informed of safe consumption practices, is paramount. The prevalence of *Listeria monocytogenes* in food products contributes to the complexity of its challenge to public health. There has also been proof to demonstrate that raw and not treated properly foods have high levels of this bacterium, and hence there has been an investigation of a variety of food matrices, including dairy. In the Maseru district of Lesotho, for instance, it was demonstrated through a study that there were startling rates of bacterial contamination in raw and pasteurized milk, with Listeria species isolated solely from raw samples. The findings, which indicate high total aerobic plate count and high coliform levels, prove that food safety precautions are not being adhered to strictly, and as such, a major public health risk is being created. Additionally, the presence of *Listeria monocytogenes* in milk products demonstrates the need for frequent monitoring of food hygiene levels, particularly in regions where food safety knowledge may be lacking (Lopez, 2019). Direct response to the increasing prevalence of listeriosis has instigated new strategies for enhancing food safety through controlling Listeria in food chains under research. There is evidence from science for the potential usefulness of bacteriocins, such as nisin, and specific essential oils in combating *Listeria monocytogenes* in model food systems and in vitro systems. This combination of antimicrobial chemicals has been shown to significantly increase the lag phase for Listeria development, reducing cell counts in testing conditions efficiently. Such advancements have the potential to improve food safety initiatives, but effective implementation is subject to a collaborative effort from food producers, regulators, and health agencies. As awareness for listeriosis increases, integration of these scientific findings within public health policy can help abate the impact of this possible devastating pathogen on society (Cotter et al., 2015) (Figure 8.13).

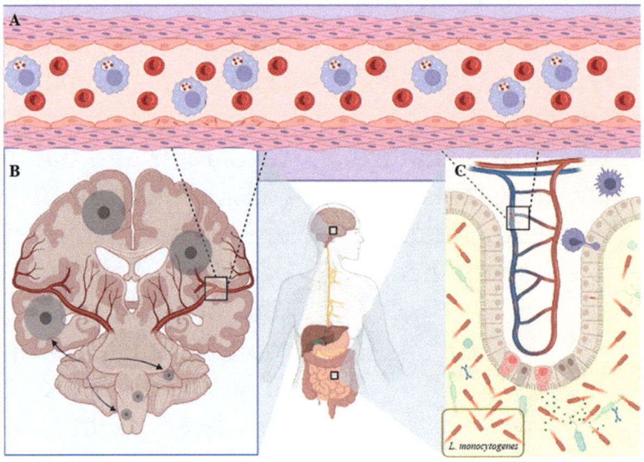

Figure 8.13. Most frequent clinical manifestations of listeriosis. (A) Blood dissemination of *L. monocytogenes* inside the macrophages; (B) neurolisteriosis. The arrows show the ring-enhancing lesions affecting the encephalon and rhombencephalon; and (C) gastroenteritis. The bacteria affect intracellularly and provoke the release of cytokines intro the intestinal lumen.

Source: https://www.researchgate.net/publication/361556630/figure/fig2/AS:11431281115281291@1674828624508/Most-frequent-clinical-manifestations-of-listeriosis-A-Blood-dissemination-of-L.png.

Test Your Knowledge

1. What are the key virulence factors of Bacillus anthracis that contribute to its pathogenicity in causing anthrax?
2. What are the major types of infections caused by Clostridium species, and how do their toxins affect human tissues?
3. What is listeriosis, which populations are most at risk, and why is it considered a significant public health concern?

8.4. Laboratory Identification Techniques

Learning Outcome

1. Describe microscopy and staining methods for identification of Gram-positive bacilli
2. Understand culture techniques and media
3. Discuss molecular methods for identification

In microbiology, Gram-positive bacilli identification plays a vital role in the diagnosis of infections caused by various bacteria. Laboratory methods of identification include both phenotypic characterization, biochemical testing, and newer molecular methods. Traditional techniques , such as Gram staining, microscopy, and growth on selective media, are useful in preliminary identification of these microorganisms. The Gram staining procedure highlights some morphological characteristics by which microbiologists are able to differentiate Gram-positive bacilli from other bacterial forms. Further, after preliminary identification, other biochemical tests , such as catalase and urease activity, are performed to make it species-specific. Such processes, being effective, normally require subsequent verification by molecular methods to ascertain species-specificity and reliability for clinical applications. The advent of molecular techniques has revolutionized laboratory detection of Gram-positive bacilli, enabling rapid and accurate diagnosis. Polymerase Chain Reaction (PCR) and sequencing technology are the defining milestones that enhance the understanding of genetic material in pathogens. PCR allows the identification of target organisms even from traces by amplifying particular DNA sequences. Sequencing provides useful information regarding genetic variation and phylogenetic evolution of different bacilli species. This integration of molecular methods in laboratory analysis not only increases accuracy but also simplifies the identification of antibiotic resistance genes, a growing concern in clinical microbiology. Laboratories are thus better equipped to tackle emerging infections and modify treatment strategies accordingly. Despite the high advantage contributed by molecular techniques, traditional methods remain essential, particularly in resource-limited settings. The economic and logistics constraints normally faced in clinical laboratories necessitate a cost-benefit strategy in microbial identification. Structured machine learning platforms have emerged as an option of preference to enhance identification processes via the use of hierarchical species data and existing laboratory practices, as observed in recent research. While a few of these structured methods have demonstrated accuracy in identification improvement, conventional methods are useful in providing context when separating highly similar species. Thus, a comprehensive strategy involving both conventional and new laboratory identification systems can enhance the overall effectiveness of Gram-positive bacilli diagnosis in clinical microbiology (Vervier et al., 2015).

8.4.1. Microscopy and Staining Methods

Gram-positive bacilli need a proper understanding of microscopy and staining methods, as these are the most crucial methods to be employed for observing and identifying such microorganisms. Gram staining, a rudimentary method in microbiology, allows bacteria to be identified on the basis of the properties of their cell walls. This is a multi-step process in which a heat-fixed bacterial smear is first stained with crystal violet and then iodine is added to form a complex that remains in the thick peptidoglycan layer of Gram-positive bacteria. The decolorizing process with alcohol or acetone that follows is important because the dye gets removed from Gram-negative bacteria but not from Gram-positive bacteria. Finally, a counterstain, typically safranin, is added, enhancing the contrast and showing a greater differentiation on the microscope. This ability to separate Gram-positive bacilli from other forms of bacteria is invaluable in clinical diagnosis and therapy. Furthermore, advanced microscopy techniques are able to significantly enhance the description of Gram-positive bacilli. Techniques , such as phase-contrast microscopy and fluorescence microscopy provide additional planes of detail not open to ordinary light microscopy. Phase-contrast microscopy uses variations in cellular structures' refractive index and is capable of optically analyzing living bacteria without staining or fixation, preserving their original morphology. Fluorescence microscopy, on the other hand, uses fluorescent dyes that bind to specific cell structures, leading to details relevant to the thriving and shape of such microorganisms becoming highlighted. The integration of these methods into microbiological research enhances resolution and even allows bacterial behavior and interaction to be visualized within complex environments. These advances pinpoint the contribution of high-technology microscopy in microbiological research, particularly for organisms like Gram-positive bacilli. Apart from microscopy, the advancement of staining procedures has also enhanced further understanding Gram-positive bacilli. Current techniques, including immunofluorescence and molecular staining, allow specific identification based on discrete antigens or genes. Immunofluorescence, for instance, applies fluorescently labeled antibodies to bind in a specific manner to antigens on the cell surface of bacteria for precise identification of complex microbial suspensions. The technique finds application in isolating specific Gram-positive bacilli from clinical specimens and will allow targeted treatment regimens. Furthermore, molecular stains, for example, nucleic acid-binding-based, may be employed to obtain information regarding the genetic composition of such microbes and hence enabling inference about their pathogenicity mechanism as well as resistance pattern. The integration of these newer staining methods with traditional microscopy gives an even higher degree of analysis in the study of Gram-positive bacilli, and this creates new avenues for further microbiological investigation and clinical diagnostics (Cardozo et al., 2015; Ahern et al., 2018) (Figure 8.14).

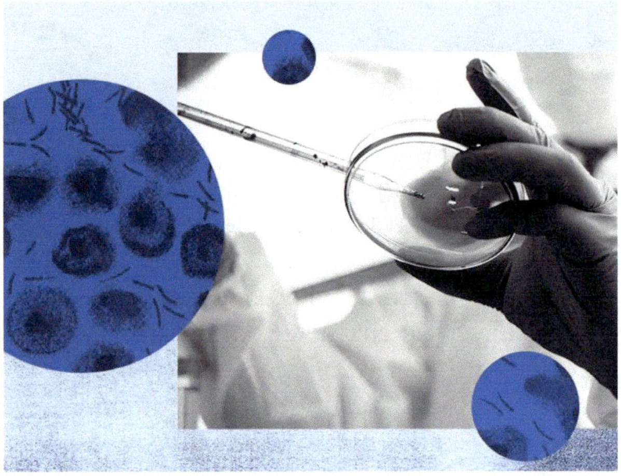

Figure 8.14. Microscopy and staining methods.

Source: https://media.post.rvohealth.io/wp-content/uploads/sites/3/2022/09/gram_positive_bacteria_collage_732x549_thumb-732x549.jpg.

8.4.2. Culture Techniques and Media

The examination of culture methods and media is part of the study of the growth habits and traits of Gram-positive bacilli. Such bacteria, which encompass key pathogens , such as *Listeria monocytogenes*, need special growth conditions to allow them to be isolated and experimented on. Techniques , such as the preparation of selective media play a critical role in separating several bacterial species; for example, utilizing MacConkey agar can purify Listeria from mixed bacterial samples due to its nutritional characteristics. The selectivity in selecting the medium not only impacts the growth but also the viability of the bacilli, hence giving information regarding their dynamics as well as resistance patterns towards antimicrobials. The identification of the best methods for culture is central to the correct diagnosis of infection and epidemiological patterns in Gram-positive bacilli, especially considering that they have the potential to bring about severe health problems in man and animals. Besides selective media, various enrichment cultures can help with improved identification of Gram-positive bacilli. For instance, incubation in the nutrient broth before plating on solid media offers the possibility to double the number of some of the bacterial populations, thus increasing the possibility of recovery of low-abundance pathogens. It is particularly useful in the clinical setting where samples may have a mixture of microbial communities. Also, specific temperature and atmospheric controls, i.e., anaerobias or elevated CO2 levels, may significantly increase the viability of specific Gram-positive bacilli during the culturing process. An understanding of such enrichment methods is not only crucial to good laboratory technique but also to the clinical interpretation of the organism recovered. The prevalence of antibiotic resistance in such isolated bacilli, as evidenced in research in the case of blood transfusion settings, again indicates strict culture techniques (Malimid et al., 2012). The detection of Gram-positive bacilli by culture techniques also involves determining their pathogenicity and antibiotic sensitivity. Sufficient antimicrobial susceptibility testing methods, , such as the Kirby-Bauer disk diffusion method, are applied following culture to determine the effective antibiotics against isolated bacteria. The distinction between the susceptibility patterns of Gram-positive bacilli species implies a demand for targeted therapeutic approaches in treating infections on a clinical basis. These facts also gain further significance in consideration of contaminant commonality as observed in blood transfusion procedures. By strictly following culture techniques that consider environmental aspects, scientists can better delineate the microbiological environment and draw well-informed strategies against bacterial infections caused by Gram-positive bacilli. This wider perspective emphasizes the need for advanced culture techniques and media not only in scientific research, but also in maintaining public health (Figure 8.15).

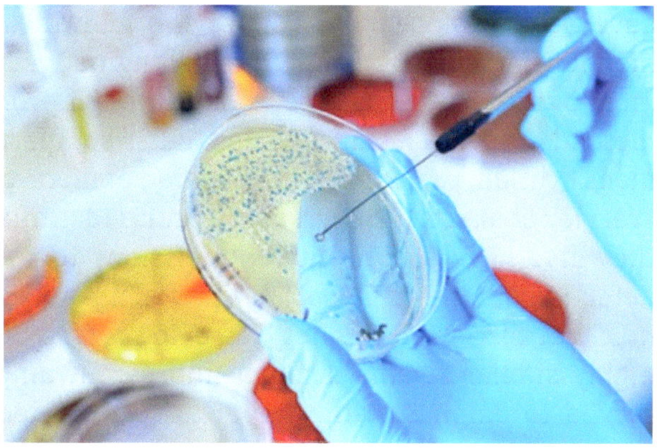

Figure 8.15. Culture techniques and media.

Source: https://www.shutterstock.com/image-photo/petri-dish-microbiological-laboratory-mold-260nw-1122280157.jpg.

8.4.3. Molecular Methods for Identification

The application of molecular methods in the identification of Gram-positive bacilli has extensively transformed microbiology, particularly in therapy and diagnosis. Techniques , such as polymerase chain reaction (PCR) and ribosomal RNA sequencing allow the identification of bacterial species with a high degree of accuracy by targeting special genetic sequences. Such techniques not only enhance the specificity of microbial identification but also speed up the process involved in the diagnosis of infection. Traditional phenotypic identification is sometimes slow and subject to misidentification on the basis of shared features in very closely related species. By incorporating molecular techniques, as noted in contemporary studies, the validity of identification procedures has been strengthened, allowing efficient treatment regimens to be initiated in time to prevent the spread of infectious diseases. Another significant technological breakthrough in the area of molecular identification is the use of Matrix-Assisted Laser Desorption/Ionization Time-of-Flight mass spectrometry (MALDI-TOF MS), which has emerged as a valuable tool in microbiological studies. MALDI-TOF MS allows for rapid profiling of bacterial proteins with a simple method of organism identification based on their unique protein spectra. Current research indicates that even though machine learning models with a structured methodology have been explored to optimize the identification process, the traditional methods have a very high level of accuracy in distinguishing between closely related species. The challenge here is that most of these advanced methods, although promising, are not necessarily superior to conventional methods in every instance, as in studies comparing various machine learning strategies for microbial identification, e.g., the new application of hierarchical architectures in learning protocols described in (Vervier et al., 2015). Correct molecular identification implications reach beyond simple diagnostics; they also have significant repercussions for public health and disease control. For instance, the detection of *Listeria monocytogenes* using molecular methods has significance not only in the clinical field but also in food safety, as evidenced by outbreak studies in animal herds. The detection of highly similar strains through fluorescent amplified fragment length polymorphism (fAFLP) has served to emphasize the importance of understanding the transmission dynamics of pathogens able to cause severe neurological disease. These molecular techniques enhance monitoring and are capable of tracking public health risks back to their origins. Thus, by employing advanced molecular techniques for the identification of Gram-positive bacilli, a critical role is played in the overall system of infectious disease control and prevention and, ultimately, human and animal health protection, as indicated in (Vervier et al., 2015) (Figure 8.16).

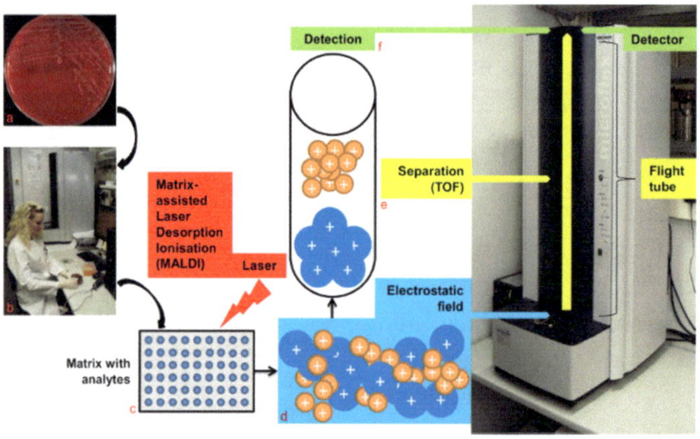

Figure 8.16. Analysis procedure using MALDI-TOF MS for identification of clinically relevant bacteria.

Source: https://www.researchgate.net/profile/Wolfram-Rudolph/publication/305219120/figure/fig2/AS:383299043250177@1468397021342/Analysis-procedure-using-MALDI-TOF-MS-for-identification-of-clinically-relevant-bacteria.png.

Test Your Knowledge

1. What are the key differences in the staining characteristics of Gram-positive bacilli when using the Gram stain versus the acid-fast stain?
2. How can spore staining be used to identify specific genera of Gram-positive bacilli, and which species commonly produce endospores?

8.5. Treatment and Management of Infections

Learning Outcome

1. Understand the phenomenon of antibiotic resistance among Gram-positive bacilli
2. Describe vaccination strategies for prevention
3. Explain the importance of supportive care in managing the clinical manifestations associated with infections caused by Gram-positive bacilli

The diagnosis and treatment of Gram-positive bacilli infection focus on the early diagnosis and successful antibiotic treatment. Clinically important species , such as *Bacillus* and Listeria are involved. They usually require measures that enhance their natural resistance patterns. Antibiotic susceptibility testing is important because the majority of Gram-positive bacilli have high resistance to commonly available antibiotics, e.g., methicillin. Information regarding the specific bacterial microbiota during infection is critical to the efficacy of treatment; for instance, evidence shows that 5.5% of blood culture isolates in adult patients had Gram-positive bacteria and exhibited high resistance to key antibiotics like imipenem and methicillin (Kante et al., 2017). Similarly, intervention in septic conditions at an early stage can significantly reduce mortality, setting the tone for the life-saving potential of accurate laboratory diagnosis combined with efficient empirical therapies. For the management of infections caused by Gram-positive bacilli, the variety of clinical approaches is wider than just antibiotics and supportive care and adjunctive therapy. A multi-dimensional approach is most evident in sepsis or septic shock, when prompt recognition of pathogens and timely administration of broad-spectrum antibiotics are paramount. For example, although gram-negative bacteria are mostly attributed with cervico-facial sepsis, evidence indicates that a considerable percentage of Gram-positive bacteria are also culpable for the infection, which affects treatment protocols (Barnard, 2019). Not only is treatment done with antibiotic modification in line with susceptibility patterns but also hydration, hemodynamic stabilization, and possibly surgical procedures in the event of abscess or other conditions. A full understanding of the Gram-positive bacilli situation in infections, therefore, forms a foundation for effective clinical management. Moreover, rising rates of antibiotic resistance among Gram-positive bacilli necessitate that health workers always be vigilant and responsive in their treatments. This pattern calls for ongoing education and research into new therapeutic agents with efficacy against resistant organisms. Surveillance data indicate that Gram-positivesome Gram-positive bacilli are resistant to neither vancomycin nor to erythromycin, but the prevalence of the rest of the remaining resistant strains poses severe obstacles to efficient treatment (Kante et al., 2017). Public health recommendations, thus, should be paramount in stewardship programs that promote responsible prescribing of antibiotics and contemplation of alternative therapy options, , such as bacteriophage therapy or immunomodulatory therapies. Through the promotion of a dynamic and educated perspective regarding the treatment and management of Gram-positive bacilli infection, healthcare practitioners are empowered to enhance patient outcomes and reduce the strain of antibiotic resistance.

8.5.1. Antibiotic Susceptibility and Resistance

The process of antibiotic resistance in Gram-positive bacilli is increasingly becoming a cause for concern, especially considering that the microorganisms are known to cause serious infections within clinical environments. The resistance patterns depict substantial difficulty in treating infections due to these microorganisms. Cases of high resistance have been reported, for example, against the use of tetracycline, penicillin, and erythromycin, which are frequently utilized antibiotics. Infections that classically would be amenable to such agents are increasingly becoming resistant, and treatment regimens must be adjusted. Up-to-date evidence underscores the importance of ongoing surveillance and assessment of regional antibiotic resistance, as this is critical in guiding empirical treatment and enabling optimal patient management in light of emergent bacterial resistance (Abdelaziz et al., 2022). Compounding the problem of antibiotic resistance is the fact of the methicillin-resistant *Staphylococcus aureus* (MRSA), a revered Gram-positive *Bacillus* that poses formidable therapeutic challenges. This organism is a classic demonstration of the remarkable potential for gaining resistance genes, undermining the efficacy of beta-lactam antibiotics and causing outbreaks of infection that would otherwise have been under successful control. Furthermore, a study also finds that while gram-negative bacilli predominate in bloodstream infections, Gram-positive cocci also continue to be a major problem, with their growing resistance to simple antibiotics. Facts show that monitoring resistant strains is not just a matter of scholastic concern but also a matter of immediate public health measure to prevent making infections untreatable (Anjaneya Swamy & Andhale, 2021). These forces together play to highlight the imperative of establishing robust antibiotic stewardship programs focused on Gram-positive bacilli. These programs must be coordinated among healthcare providers in order to ensure that antimicrobial choice is effective and guided by the most recent resistance information. An active response through continuous education of clinicians, investment in rapid diagnostic methods, and stringent adherence to updated clinical guidelines will provide effective management of the crisis of resistance. Lastly, addressing the problem of antibiotic susceptibility and resistance in Gram-positive bacilli becomes important to achieve patient outcomes and ascertain the continuity of effective antibiotic therapy in the future (Figure 8.17).

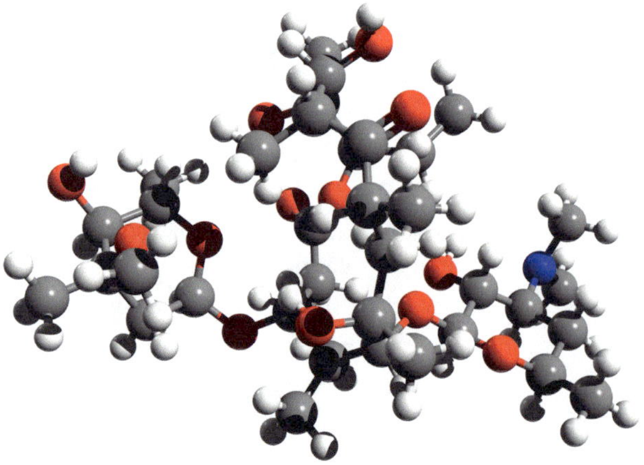

Figure 8.17. Erythromycin structure.

Source: https://upload.wikimedia.org/wikipedia/commons/d/d5/Erythromycin_3d_structure.png.

8.5.2. Vaccination Strategies for Prevention

The vaccine strategies are significantly complemented in avoiding diseases caused by Gram-positive bacilli. These bacteria, with notable pathogens among them being *Bacillus anthracis* and *Listeria monocytogenes*, pose tremendous threat to human health and agricultural production. Vaccination is a critical first-line defense, especially as the threat of antibiotic resistance continues to grow. Pre-exposure vaccination not only stimulates immunity in susceptible groups but also limits disease transmission. Countries implementing rigorous vaccination campaigns have seen a decrease in the frequency of disease events, emphasizing the worth of vaccine integration in public health initiatives aimed at controlling Gram-positive bacilli. Moreover, planned vaccination activities should consider the specific characteristics of different groups. For instance, the immunocompromised, like those who are transplanted with the liver, require specific vaccination schedules due to heightened vulnerability. It is revealed through studies that time matters; optimal vaccination would be before transplantation and initiation of the disease process to elicit the best immunity response (2011 Group AST et al., 2013). Medical professionals are hence recommended to utilize personalized vaccine regimens by patient status to offer the utmost protection against Gram-positive bacilli. Timing of vaccine administrations and the type of vaccines utilized can significantly complement preventive interventions in this high-risk group. The type of vaccines utilized, other than timing, is essential in the prevention of infection from Gram-positive bacilli. Inactivated vaccines are the preferred preoperative recommendation based on their safety profile, whereas live attenuated vaccines are contraindicated in post-transplant care (2011 Group AST et al., 2013). Public health interventions must also seek to address education among healthcare professionals and the populace at large on the necessity of vaccination for disease avoidance from such pathogens. The banning of antibiotic growth promoters in animal husbandry has provoked wake-up calls on the detriments of antibiotic resistance, compelling consideration of vaccination interventions as a means of countering the commonality of resistant organisms. Lastly, production and promotion of combined vaccination strategies along with regulatory measures can take far and bring down the role of Gram-positive bacilli in public health.

8.5.3. Supportive Care and Management of Symptoms

Supportive care is of central importance in the management of the clinical presentation of Gram-positive bacillary infections. In particular, muscle spasms and respiratory distress, the characteristic of tetanus infection, require urgent and adequate management. Tetanospasmin, the powerful neurotoxin produced by *Clostridium* tetani, induces severe muscle rigidity and spasmodic pain, significantly impairing the quality of life of patients. Supportive care interventions involve meticulous observation of vital parameters, maintenance of airway patency, and administration of antitoxins and antibiotics, as the key to early intervention. The application of all these therapeutic modalities in conjunction with appropriate supportive care can dramatically change patient outcomes as well as avert potentially lethal complications. Thus, the knowledge of early signs of tetanus and supportive treatment becomes very important in the provision of effective care to victims of this disease, and this emphasizes the need for balance between knowledge and early medical intervention (Sunilkumar et al., 2014). Treatment of infected patients due to Gram-positive bacilli also needs to be supplemented with consideration of total supportive care for patients with solid tumors. Risk factors for infection among such patients are more than one and usually involve drug treatment complications, which make symptomatic treatment more difficult. For example, an extreme neutropenia, which may be produced as a consequence of chemotherapy, can lead to increased susceptibility to infections, particularly within compartments , such as the bloodstream and skin. Supportive care is critical in the management of such symptomatology, where interventions like antibiotic therapy, fluid and electrolyte replacement, and careful monitoring of vitals are important. Importantly, conservative treatment continues to be effective in most cases, but can be complemented by surgery when indicated, particularly where deep abscesses are present or removal of infected prostheses becomes necessary (Rolston, 2017). Also, infection prevention and control strategies remain an integral part of the supportive care model for infection control by Gram-positive bacilli. These infections also tend to manifest in overlapping clinical syndromes, and thus, diagnosis and treatment initiation may be challenging. Thus, effective symptom control must be followed by stringent infection control measures and antimicrobial stewardship to control the tidal wave of resistant organisms that are increasingly becoming widespread. The recognition of these infections as multifactorial and the prioritization of preventative care can greatly improve patient outcomes. Through the clinician's journey in supportive care, the integration of strategies addressing both immediate symptoms and long-term prevention is required for full patient management. Through judicious assessment and symptom-oriented management, healthcare providers can simplify treatment protocols and improve the quality of life of patients afflicted with Gram-positive bacilli (Rolston, 2017).

Test Your Knowledge

1. What are the common antibiotic resistance mechanisms found in Listeria monocytogenes and Bacillus cereus?
2. What vaccines are currently available for the prevention of infections caused by Gram-positive bacilli?

SUMMARY

In conclusion to studying Gram-positive bacilli, it is clear that such bacteria are important in both human health and disease. The diverse genus of Gram-positive bacilli, , such as Bacillus, *Clostridium*, and Listeria, has different functions, from being probiotics in certain settings to causing disease in most infections. Knowledge about their biology, mechanisms of pathogenesis, and environmental niches where they have been found to grow will facilitate the planning of proper therapeutic approaches and prevention strategies. This overall understanding enables improved clinical management and underscores the need for further research in microbiology. The clinical significance of Gram-positive bacilli cannot be underscored enough, particularly in relation to their role in public health. Infections caused by such pathogens, e.g., those in cervico-facial sepsis, have shown foreboding trends in their presence and identification in clinical practice. Evidence suggests that gram-negative bacteria are prevalent in staining but infrequently isolated in culture, suggesting a disruption in diagnostics that may impact patient outcomes (Barnard, 2019). These findings highlight the importance of proper microbiological protocols and the need for healthcare practitioners to be vigilant for the identification and treatment of Gram-positive bacilli infection. In addition, the fact that Gram-positive bacilli have become resistant to antibiotics further complicates clinical microbiology.

The emergence of resistant organisms calls for reassessment of existing treatment protocols and increased emphasis on antimicrobial stewardship. As noted by a number of studies, overuse or misuse of antibiotics results in increased resistance levels, making infections harder to manage for Gram-positive bacilli-related infections (Barnard, 2019). It is therefore critical to develop a synergistic interaction between clinicians, researchers, and public health experts to resist these emerging infections and deliver enhanced health benefits to the affected patients. The intricate nature of Gram-positive bacilli necessitates ongoing effort and initiative on the part of the healthcare community. In analyzing the traits and clinical relevance of Gram-positive bacilli, it is crucial to identify their varied genera and the pathogenic potential they possess. *Bacillus* and Listeria are among those, with the former having a significant influence on human health. *Bacillus* species, with special mention of *Bacillus anthracis*, is considered to be responsible for anthrax, and thus, knowledge and awareness of its transmission are critical to public health programs. In addition, *Listeria monocytogenes* is also a causative factor due to its ability to cause severe systemic infection, particularly in pregnant women and immunocompromised individuals. Information about virulence factors of these bacteria and their infection mechanisms adds to the development of preventive strategies, which also underscores the significance of Gram-positive bacilli in clinical microbiology and epidemiology. Lastly, the industrial significance of Gram-positive bacilli cannot be overemphasized. These microorganisms have a crucial role to play in numerous biotechnological applications, from food production to environmental cleanup. For instance, some members of the *Bacillus* species are used in the production of enzymes, probiotics, and fermented foods, which are key components of the food industry. The biocontrol potential of *Bacillus* thuringiensis to control pests is an indicator of the ecological significance of these bacteria. Understanding the biochemical processes and metabolic characteristics of Gram-positive bacilli opens doors to new uses in food science and sustainable processes, hence their applicability beyond clinical environments. With every development in the study of microbiology, knowing the interactions between Gram-positive bacilli and the environment becomes increasingly vital. Current research aims toward understanding how they react when exposed to varying environments, which may influence food product contamination. Although gram-negative bacteria are the focus of immense attention due to their role in food spoilage, research indicates that some Gram-positive species also contribute significantly to food spoilage (Mohareb et al., 2015). In addition, the capacity of the bacteria to adapt to modified environmental stresses holds implications for both food industry operations and clinical treatments. Understanding genetic expressions of the strains under different conditions is not only important for comprehending the mechanism of spoilage but also assists in the formulation of targeted strategies for controlling bacterial food product contamination, ultimately serving the cause of public health (Altschul et al., 2013).

KEY TERMS FROM THIS CHAPTER

- Antibiotic exposure
- Antibiotic resistance patterns
- Antibiotic-associated diarrhea
- Bacteriocins
- Biological membranes
- Butyric acid
- Cell wall integrity
- Cell wall synthesis
- Clostridial infections
- Corynebacterium
- Disease transmission
- Disease-causing organisms
- Endosporulation
- Energy production
- Epidemiological patterns
- Flight mass spectrometry
- Gastrointestinal anthrax
- Gram-positive bacilli
- Gram-positive bacteria
- Gram-positive pathogens calls

CRITICAL THINKING QUESTIONS

1. **Which of the following is a typical characteristic of Gram-positive bacilli?**
   a. Thin peptidoglycan layer and outer membrane presence
   b. Presence of thick peptidoglycan layer and no outer membrane
   c. Lack of peptidoglycan and presence of lipopolysaccharide
   d. Ability to form spores and are always anaerobic
2. **Which of the following bacteria is NOT classified as a Gram-positive bacillus?**
   a. *Bacillus anthracis*
   b. *Listeria monocytogenes*
   c. *Clostridium* difficile
   d. *Escherichia coli*
3. **Which disease is caused by** *Clostridium* **tetani, a Gram-positive bacillus?**
   a. Tetanus
   b. Tuberculosis
   c. Botulism
   d. Diphtheria
4. **Which laboratory technique is most commonly used to confirm the presence of Gram-positive bacilli?**
   a. Acid-fast staining
   b. Gram staining
   c. India ink staining
   d. Capsule staining
5. **Which virulence factor is primarily responsible for the pathogenicity of** *Bacillus anthracis***?**
   a. Endotoxin
   b. Capsule
   c. Exotoxin
   d. Lipopolysaccharide

Short Answer Questions

1. What are the defining morphological and biochemical characteristics that distinguish Gram-positive bacilli from other bacterial groups?
2. What are the major genera of medically important Gram-positive bacilli, and what are the key differences in their pathogenic potential?
3. Which diseases are commonly caused by *Listeria monocytogenes*, *Bacillus anthracis*, and Corynebacterium diphtheriae, and what are the main virulence factors involved?
4. How do the toxins produced by Corynebacterium diphtheriae and *Bacillus anthracis* contribute to the clinical manifestations of diphtheria and anthrax, respectively?
5. What staining methods and culture media are typically used to identify *Listeria monocytogenes* and *Bacillus* species in the laboratory?
6. How do molecular methods , such as PCR and sequencing improve the accuracy of identifying Gram-positive bacilli compared to traditional culture techniques?

Answers to Critical Thinking Questions

1. (b) 2. (d) 3. (a) 4. (b) 5. (c)

REFERENCES

1. Mohareb et al. (2015). Identification of meat spoilage gene biomarkers in *Pseudomonas putida* using gene profiling. https://core.ac.uk/download/74410385.pdf (accessed on 13th June 2025).
2. Abdelaziz, M., Bashir, T., Hamadalnil, Y., Abdelkhalig, M., et al. (2022). Bloodstream infection in cancer patients; susceptibility profiles of the isolated pathogens, at Khartoum Oncology Hospital, Sudan. https://core.ac.uk/download/552647155.pdf (accessed on 13th June 2025).
3. Abdelkader, A. A. J. (2018). Isolation and characterization of phenol degrading bacterium strain *Bacillus thuringiensis* J20 from olive waste in Palestine. https://core.ac.uk/download/287331564.pdf (accessed on 13th June 2025).
4. Ahern, H. (2018). *Microbiology: A Laboratory Experience*. https://core.ac.uk/download/234027666.pdf (accessed on 13th June 2025).
5. Aimar, P., Causserand, C., Lebleu, N., Roques, C., et al. (2009). Role of the cell-wall structure in the retention of bacteria by microfiltration membranes. https://core.ac.uk/download/12043328.pdf (accessed on 13th June 2025).
6. Ajani, O. O., & Nwinyi, O. (2010). Identification and clinical relevance of Gram–positive spore formers. https://core.ac.uk/download/32224855.pdf (accessed on 13th June 2025).
7. Akça, E., Claus, H., Debaerdemaeker, T., Declercq, E., et al. (2005). Molecular organization of selected prokaryotic S-layer proteins. http://orbi.ulg.ac.be/bitstream/2268/57472/1/Claus05-CanJMicrobiolPP.pdf (accessed on 13th June 2025).
8. Alippi, A. M., de Remes Lenicov, A. M. M., & Toledo, A. V. (2011). Growth inhibition of *Beauveria bassiana* by bacteria isolated from the cuticular surface of the corn leafhopper, *Dalbulus maidis* and the planthopper, *Delphacodes kuscheli*, two important vectors of maize pathogens. https://core.ac.uk/download/323211016.pdf (accessed on 13th June 2025).
9. Anjaneya Swamy, M., & Andhale, J. D. (2021). Profile of pathogens isolated from different clinical samples and their antimicrobial pattern: a retrospective study. *International Journal of Research in Medical Sciences*, *9*(11), 3324–3329. https://doi.org/10.18203/2320-6012.ijrms20214075 (accessed on 13th June 2025).
10. Antoniadou, Z. A., Bandyopadhyay, K., Bhatnagar, J., DeLeon-Carnes, M., et al. (2012). Rapid, simultaneous detection of *Clostridium sordellii*and *Clostridium perfringens* in archived tissues by a novel PCR-based microsphere assay: Diagnostic implications for pregnancy-associated toxic shock syndrome cases. https://core.ac.uk/download/pdf/8706759.pdf (accessed on 13th June 2025).
11. Anzai, M. C., Gompertz, O. F., & Machado, A. P. (2010). *Bacillus subtilis* induces morphological changes in *Fonsecaea pedrosoi in vitro* resulting in more resistant fungal forms *in vivo*. https://core.ac.uk/download/37708865.pdf (accessed on 13th June 2025).
12. Ariza Cardenal, J., Bahamonde, A., Baraia Etxaburu, J., Benito Hernández, R., et al. (2019). The different microbial etiology of prosthetic joint infections according to route of acquisition and time after prosthesis implantation, including the role of multidrug-resistant organisms. https://core.ac.uk/download/344893862.pdf (accessed on 13th June 2025).
13. Artale, B. (2014). Developing genetic tools for *Geobacillus*. https://core.ac.uk/download/72048095.pdf (accessed on 13th June 2025).

14. Ascione, T., Bassetti, M., Bonnet, E., Bouza, E., et al. (2018). Hot topics in necrotizing skin and soft tissue infections. https://core.ac.uk/download/188186147.pdf (accessed on 13th June 2025).

15. Babamahmoodi, F., Aghabarari, F., Arjmand, A., & Ashrafi, G. H. (2006). Three rare cases of anthrax arising from the same source. *Journal of Infection, 53*(4), e175–e179. https://doi.org/10.1016/j.jinf.2005.12.018 (accessed on 13th June 2025).

16. Barnard, N. (2019). Prevalence of gram-negative infections in cervical-facial sepsis. https://core.ac.uk/download/289120726.pdf (accessed on 13th June 2025).

17. Barnes, H. J., Basher, H. A., Fonnesbech Vogel, B., Gitter, M., Ivanics, E., Lucas, A., McDiarmid, A., et al. (2015). Outbreak of encephalitic listeriosis in red-legged partridges (*Alectoris rufa*). https://core.ac.uk/download/36778157.pdf (accessed on 13th June 2025).

18. Beresford, T., Cotter, P. D., Fenelon, M., Gopal, P., et al. (2015). The prevalence and control of *Bacillus* and related spore-forming bacteria in the dairy industry. https://core.ac.uk/download/45656804.pdf (accessed on 13th June 2025).

19. Bevilacqua, A., Ciuffreda, E., Corbo, M. R., Mischitelli, M., et al. (2015). Genotypic and phenotypic heterogeneity in *Alicyclobacillus acidoterrestris*: A contribution to species characterization. https://core.ac.uk/download/54524234.pdf (accessed on 13th June 2025).

20. Bordignon, V., Cavallo, I., Cilli, L., De Santis, R., et al. (2017). Biofilm is a major virulence determinant in bacterial colonization of chronic skin ulcers independently from the multidrug resistant phenotype. https://core.ac.uk/download/188832167.pdf (accessed on 13th June 2025).

21. Bryant, K., Elward, A., Lessler, J., Milstone, A. M., et al. (2017). Bacterial infections in neonates following mupirocin-based MRSA decolonization: A multicenter cohort study. https://core.ac.uk/download/84911302.pdf (accessed on 13th June 2025).

22. Cardozo, M. G., Carrascal, A. K., Daza, C. E., et al. (2015). Tratamiento de agua residual de microbiología usando películas delgadas de TiO_2. https://core.ac.uk/download/511515063.pdf (accessed on 13th June 2025).

23. Cotter, P. D., Daly, K. M., Field, D., et al. (2015). Efficacy of nisin A and nisin V semi-purified preparations alone and in combination with plant essential oils to control *Listeria monocytogenes*. https://core.ac.uk/download/45656539.pdf (accessed on 13th June 2025).

24. Elmanama, A. A. (2007). *Diagnostic Medical Microbiology*. https://core.ac.uk/download/385924572.pdf (accessed on 13th June 2025).

25. Gall, L. S., & Riely, P. E. (2025). *Effect of Diet and Atmosphere on Intestinal and Skin Flora. Volume II – Literature Survey*. https://core.ac.uk/download/pdf/85249155.pdf (accessed on 13th June 2025).

26. Hafez, H. M. (2011). *Enteric Diseases of Poultry with Special Attention to Clostridium perfringens*. https://core.ac.uk/download/199415510.pdf (accessed on 13th June 2025).

27. Kante, M., Muni Lakshmi, P., & Sreenivasulu Reddy, P. (2017). Bacterial profile of bloodstream infections and their antibiograms. https://core.ac.uk/download/539910262.pdf (accessed on 13th June 2025).

28. Kleerebezem, M., Kuipers, O. P., et al. (1997). Expression systems for industrial Gram-positive bacteria with low guanine and cytosine content. https://core.ac.uk/download/pdf/12904458.pdf (accessed on 13th June 2025).

29. Leo, B. F., López-Heras, M., Porter, A. E., et al. (2015). Towards understanding the antibacterial activity of Ag nanoparticles: Electron microscopy in the analysis of the materials-biology interface in the lung. https://core.ac.uk/download/77002723.pdf (accessed on 13th June 2025).

30. Vervier, K., et al. (2015). Benchmark of structured machine learning methods for microbial identification from mass-spectrometry data. http://arxiv.org/abs/1506.07251 (accessed on 13th June 2025).

31. Maldonado, N. C., Nader, M. E. F., & Silva de Ruíz, C. (2015). "*In vitro*" evaluation of some properties in spore former bacteria isolated from calves' faces. https://core.ac.uk/download/159301332.pdf (accessed on 13th June 2025).

32. Malimu, E. Z. (2012). The prevalence of bacterial contamination in donated blood in Dar es Salaam, Tanzania. https://core.ac.uk/download/pdf/16666702.pdf (accessed on 13th June 2025).

33. Menon Narayanankutty, S., & Vadakut Krishnan, P. (2014). Tetanus trismus in a 2-year-old child: Case report. https://core.ac.uk/download/pdf/27205248.pdf (accessed on 13th June 2025).

34. Mthembu, Wendy & Penduka, Dambudzo & Mosa, Rebamang & Shoba, Bonginkosi & Zobolo, A & Opoku, A. (2017). The bacteria profiles of wounds in diabetic patients hospitalized in northern Kwazulu-Natal, South Africa. African Journal of Clinical and Experimental Microbiology. 18. 186. 10.4314/ajcem.v18i4.2. (accessed on 13th June 2025).

35. Moshoeshoe, S. L. (2025). Incidence of *Listeria monocytogenes* in milk from producers in the Maseru area. https://core.ac.uk/download/222966397.pdf (accessed on 13th June 2025).

36. Rolston, K. V. I. (2017). Infections in cancer patients with solid tumors: A review. https://core.ac.uk/download/pdf/81700368.pdf (accessed on 13th June 2025).

37. Sridhar, M. (1998). *Probiotics in Mariculture–Applications and Future Prospects.* https://core.ac.uk/download/33018681.pdf (accessed on 13th June 2025).

38. Stabler, R. A., Larsson, J. T., Al-Jaberi, S., Nielsen, E. M., Kay, E., Tam, C. C., Higgins, C. D., Rodrigues, L. C., Richardson, J. F., O'Brien, S. J., & Wren, B. W. (2013). Characterization of water and wildlife strains as a subgroup of *Campylobacter jejuni* using DNA microarrays. *Environmental Microbiology, 15*(8), 2371–2383. https://doi.org/10.1111/1462-2920.12111 (accessed on 13th June 2025).

39. Toro López, M. D. del. (2019). The different microbial etiology of prosthetic joint infections according to route of acquisition and time after prosthesis implantation, including the role of multidrug-resistant organisms. https://core.ac.uk/download/231995576.pdf (accessed on 13th June 2025).

GRAM-NEGATIVE BACILLI

9

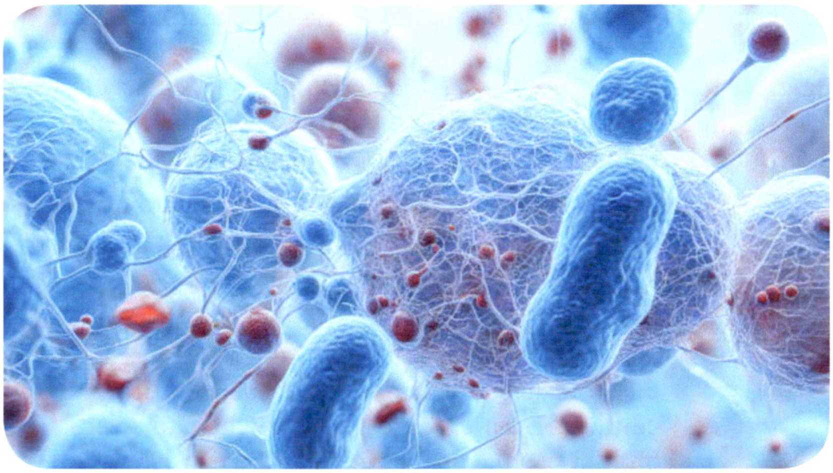

LEARNING OBJECTIVES

After studying this chapter, you will be able to:

1. Understand the characteristics of gram-negative bacilli
2. Describe major types of gram-negative bacilli
3. Explain the pathogenicity and disease associations
4. Discuss laboratory identification techniques
5. Deal with the treatment and management of infections
6. Focus on current research and developments

Introduction

It is essential to investigate gram-negative bacilli to determine their role in numerous infectious diseases. That gram-negative bacilli possess a unique cell wall structure that renders them resistant to most antibiotics used clinically makes them an issue of concern within the clinical field. Their resistance is primarily due to their outer membrane, which makes the microorganisms resistant to destructive agents and hence challenging to attack by antibiotics. The awe-inspiring variety of gram-negative bacilli, among them notorious ones like Pseudomonas aeruginosa and Escherichia coli, warrants appreciation of their clinical importance. As these bacteria are encountered by healthcare professionals in a range of infections, , such as urinary tract infection and sepsis, an intimate understanding of their biology, pathogenicity, and ecological niches becomes imperative. The importance of gram-negative bacilli extends beyond their mere identification; they are paramount in the epidemiology of infection. Recent studies have illustrated that a high proportion of causative organisms of cervico-facial sepsis are of gram-negative type. Research within Tygerberg Academic Hospital and Tygerberg Oral Health Centre suggests this prevalence, adding that while the majority of anaerobes are in fact present, the correlation between staining and culture may not be as predicted. Specifically, it has been resolved that while Gram-negative organisms will generally be found in Gram stains, fewer are identified using culture methods. This contrast reflects greater complexities in microbiological diagnosis and management, echoing the demand for a general infection control approach to clinical practice (Barnard, 2019; Barnard, 2019). Furthermore, Gram-negative bacilli reveal their evolving process of resistance and its public health consequences. Since resistance among these microbes is perpetually on the rise, it is endangering treatment efficacy and patient outcome severely. Detection of causes of resistance, suh as horizontal gene transfer and selective pressure due to the use of antibiotics, is essential for planning effective infection-fighting measures. Due to the rise in multi-drug-resistant Gram-negative bacilli, health organizations are emphasizing the importance of surveillance, stewardship, and new therapeutic approaches. With the changing epidemiology of infectious diseases, continued research into the behavior and nature of Gram-negative bacilli becomes increasingly important for maximizing clinical management and maintaining public health.

Definition of Gram-negative Bacilli

Gram-negative bacilli represent a heterogeneous and diverse group of bacteria characterized by their unique cell wall structure, significantly influencing their drug resistance and pathogenicity. They are characterized by the presence of a thin peptidoglycan wall overlaid with an outer membrane composed of lipopolysaccharides. Gram-negative bacteria are more drug-resistant than Gram-positive bacteria in general. This resistance is due in part to the outer protective membrane that can hinder the entrance of antimicrobial drugs and other molecules. Gram-negative bacilli include a number of genera, including *Escherichia*, Klebsiella, and *Pseudomonas*, each with distinctive biological characteristics and clinical importance. The ability to form biofilms is common in these bacteria and contributes to long-term infections, complicating treatment in hospitals, where the need for ongoing research on effective care is clear. The occurrence of Gram-negative bacilli in numerous infections highlights their relevance in clinical microbiology. Such organisms are frequently the cause of healthcare-associated infections, particularly in immunocompromised hosts, and their virulence factors may lead to severe clinical outcomes.

For instance, evidence has shown that Gram-negative bacilli, most notably multidrug-resistant bacteria (MDROs), are prevalent in chronic wounds and produce delayed healing and persistent infection. In one recent study, 80% of various Gram-negative bacterial strains cultured from chronic ulcers of the skin were biofilm producers, confirming the contribution of biofilm in bacterial persistence and virulence (Bordignon et al., 2017). That these bacteria thrive very well in polymicrobial environments aggravates the treatment situation further, necessitating profound understanding of their biological behavior and the development of innovative therapeutic interventions. Furthermore, understanding the antimicrobial resistance patterns of Gram-negative bacilli is essential to effective clinical practice.

The emergence of multidrug resistance poses serious challenges since many strains exhibit decreased susceptibility to the regular antibiotics, rendering treatment regimens difficult. The level of bacterial contamination of blood transfusions was demonstrated through a cross-sectional study where Gram-negative bacilli were among the reported isolates, thus raising an alarm about their impact on transfusion safety (Malimu, 2012). As the prevalence of these organisms goes up, it is even more critical for health care providers to monitor patterns of resistance and implement focused antibiotic stewardship programs. Not only will this enhance patient outcomes, but it will also help curb the spread of resistant Gram-negative bacilli among the health care and community environments, reminding again the pressing need for ongoing studies and collaborative effort in addressing this public health threat (Figure 9.1).

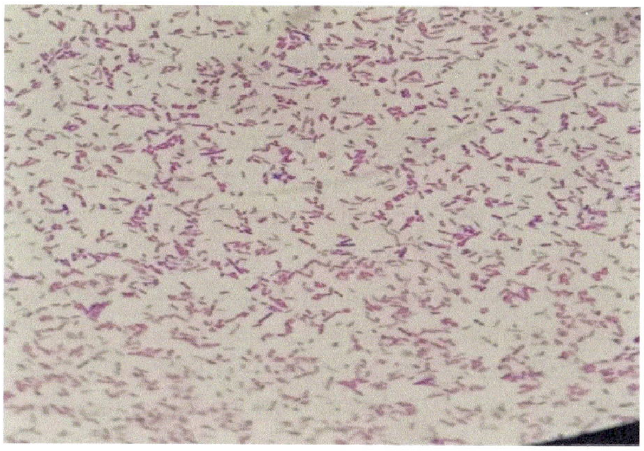

Figure 9.1. Gram-negative bacilli with bipolar staining.

Source: https://www.researchgate.net/profile/Maanasa-Bhaskar/publication/373747760/figure/fig3/AS:11431281187127328@1694138507930/Gram-negative-bacilli-with-bipolar-staining.png.

Importance in Microbiology and Medicine

The significance of Gram-negative bacilli to medicine and microbiology cannot be overstated, particularly in view of their roles in infectious diseases. Not only are they widespread in the environment but also in human flora, where they can change from non-pathogenic to pathogenic based on the environment. The ability of Gram-negative bacilli, , such as *Escherichia coli* and Klebsiella pneumoniae, to adapt to unfavorable environments and express resistance to a range of antibiotics is of utmost concern within the clinical setting. Furthermore, the increase in the incidence of antibiotic-resistant strains necessitates continuous monitoring and research, as these pathogens are more likely to cause severe healthcare-related infections, including urinary tract infections and sepsis. Their widespread nature gives rise to the importance of developing effective surveillance systems and antibiotic stewardship programs to mitigate their role in public health. In transfusion medicine, the importance of Gram-negative bacilli is increased by considering the potential for contamination of blood cultures.

A study conducted at the Eastern Zone Blood Transfusion Services revealed a high 2.8% rate of bacterial contamination of donated blood that was primarily caused by Gram-positive cocci, but did point towards some of the skin contaminant-related issues, including Gram-negative species. The contamination has far-reaching implications for the safety of patients since it can lead to transfusion-related infections and complicate the management of patients who have received transfusions. Understanding of the organisms and their nature assists in creating donor collection and screening guidelines to reduce rates of contamination.

The adaptable nature of the bacteria also warrants performing rigorous antibiotic susceptibility testing to ensure safe and effective blood products for transfusion (Malimu, 2012). Application of newer microbiological methods is necessary in the identification of Gram-negative bacilli within a short duration, particularly in urine specimens, which are responsible for urinary tract infections. Investigations on new chromogenic media, , such as chromID CPS Elite, have indicated a sharp reduction in time consumed for the identification of organisms compared to conventional tests with 82% recovery of pathogens. This expedited analysis is essential within the clinic, where delayed detection can impede treatment and increase morbidity within affected patients. Also, the reduction in consumable use and hand time with these newer methodologies demonstrates their value in optimizing lab efficiency, a key component of high-patient flow healthcare institutions. In conclusion, prompt identification of Gram-negative bacilli not only avails proper management but also gives the support of enhanced stewardship of antibiotic use, thus addressing the fiery issue of antimicrobial resistance (Burnham et al., 2016).

9.1. Characteristics of Gram-negative Bacilli

Learning Outcome

1. Understand cell wall structure of Gram-negative bacilli
2. Describe staining properties and identification
3. Focus on metabolic and growth characteristics

The characteristics of Gram-negative bacilli are central to understanding their biological activity and impact on human health. They are notable for their unusual cell wall structure, a characteristic not present in Gram-positive bacteria. The outer membrane of these bacteria has lipopolysaccharides (LPS) in it, and they contribute to the bacterias virulence and serve as an endotoxin if and when they are released upon bacterial lysis. The distinctive structure not only contributes to the permeability of substances into the cell but also imparts a resistance against most antibiotics, rendering Gram-negative bacilli unusually resistant in the clinical setting. Greater structural complexity requires special antibacterial strategies when working with infections caused by these organisms, necessitating ongoing research into microbial resistance mechanisms and therapy. In addition to their structural characteristics, Gram-negative bacilli are also highly metabolically diverse, which allows them to adapt to survive under various conditions. For instance, they can employ diverse substrates, thus playing a crucial role in ecological processes, , such as nutrient cycling and organic matter decomposition. Some of the species, for instance, *Pseudomonas* fluorescens, can survive under extreme environments with high temperatures, an aspect that proves their versatility (Decicco et al.). The diversity of their metabolic pathways not only ensures their survival in different milieus but also is invariably linked with their virulence. Certain Gram-negative bacilli, for example, possess particular virulence factors that enhance their pathogenicity, , such as their ability to obtain nutrients from tissue within a host and resist the body's immune mechanisms. Clinical significance must not be overlooked when looking at the character of Gram-negative bacilli. These pathogens include notorious culprit, such as *Escherichia coli* and Klebsiella pneumoniae, which are responsible for all types of infection ranging from urinary tract infection to fatal pneumonia. The emergence of multidrug-resistant strains in such organisms represents a serious public health concern that calls for novel therapeutic approaches and an understanding of their resistance mechanisms (Gall & Riely, 1965). In addition to this feature, the understanding of their genetic and environmental elements of pathogenicity is a prerequisite for the development of effective prevention and treatment measures. As more research is conducted, it is significant to study their evolution and adaptation to both environmental pressure and medical treatments, so that there can be a preventive measure towards preventing and controlling subsequent outbreaks.

9.1.1. Cell Wall Structure and Composition

Gram-negative bacilli's cell wall structure is a significant aspect of their biology, giving both form and integrity and acting as a major defense against environmental stress. Gram-negative cell walls possess a thin peptidoglycan layer between the inner and outer membranes compared to the thicker peptidoglycan found in Gram-positive bacteria. This unique architecture affords many physiological advantages, including selective permeability that dictates the entry and exit of molecules, thus enhancing metabolic efficiency. Additionally, the presence of lipopolysaccharides (LPS) on the outer membrane not only serves to ensure structural integrity but also plays pivotal functions in immune evasion, which points to the close correlation between cellular structure and pathogenicity, particularly for increasing bacterial infections in the pulmonary system (Leo et al., 2015). In contrast to the other prokaryotic morphologies, however, Gram-negative bacilli have a heterogeneous cell wall that is adapted to environmental changes. The outer membrane consists primarily of lipids, proteins, and lipopolysaccharides, and is responsible for the bacterias interaction with its environment. S-layers, for instance, periodic crystalline surface layers, are universal among the organisms and employed as protective coats. These structures not only contribute to physical protection but have also evolved to act as molecular sieves and binding sites for extracellular enzymes that catalyze various metabolic processes (Akça et al., 2005). The genetic heterogeneity among the various Gram-negative species has led to a number of adaptations, which have allowed for a more precise response to environmental deprivations and enhanced their overall survival and pathogenicity. The presence of specific proteins in the cell wall of Gram-negative bacilli also highlights the complexity and functionality of their structure. The proteins are part of important processes like the transportation of nutrients, cellular signaling, and interaction with host tissue, thus contributing to the general pathogenicity of such bacteria. For example, adherence factors in the cell wall can facilitate colonization and aggression against host immune responses. Furthermore, the dynamicity of the cell wall allows such microorganisms to respond promptly to changes in their environment, which is most basically essential in the hospital environment, where antibiotic resistance is increasing. As the increasing wealth of information regarding these structural and compositional aspects unfolds, it is worth noting their impact on developing effective therapeutic strategies against Gram-negative infections (Figure 9.2).

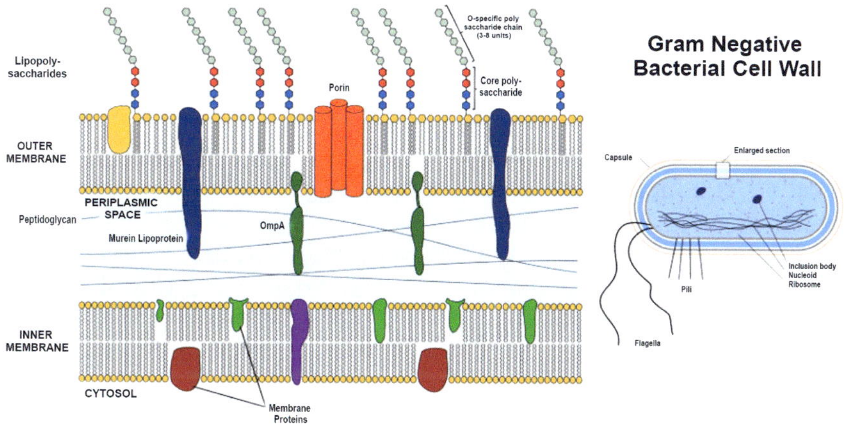

Figure 9.2. Gram-negative (LPS-diderm) cell wall structure.

Source: https://upload.wikimedia.org/wikipedia/commons/thumb/8/8b/Gram_negative_cell_wall.svg/960px-Gram_negative_cell_wall.svg.png.

9.1.2. Staining Properties and Identification

Staining typical of Gram-negative bacilli is a unifying factor in their identification in clinical and environmental microbiology. The underlying technique employed is the Gram stain, in which bacteria are differentiated according to cell wall composition. Gram-negative bacilli possess a thinner peptidoglycan layer and an outer lipopolysaccharide-containing membrane in such a way that they keep the counterstain, typically safranin, pink under the microscope. This identifying characteristic is crucial in laboratories to rapidly identify infection-causing bacteria, especially in opportunistic infections like those in wounds of diabetics. The rapid visualization of such bacteria enables early medical intervention and effective antibiotic therapy, which are crucial in the successful treatment of infections. Biochemical characteristics of Gram-negative bacilli also help with further identification. Following presumptive identification using Gram staining, additional biochemical tests like catalase and oxidase tests aid in identification confirmation of such microorganisms. For instance, the reactions related to the fermentation of certain sugars or the activity of certain enzymes could be suggestive of the presence of organisms like *Escherichia coli* or *Salmonella* spp. Additionally, the advent of molecular techniques, , such as 16S rDNA sequencing, has revolutionized the process of bacterial identification. This molecular method, as identified in studies involving the isolation of bacterial strains from clinical specimens, allows for a high degree of accuracy so that proper antibiotic sensitivity patterns can be determined for successful therapy, particularly in the event of complicated polymicrobial infections with the predominance of Gram-negative bacilli (Mthembu et al., 2017). Understanding staining features and consequent identification of Gram-negative bacilli is not entirely a laboratory practice; it has an important bearing on clinical outcomes. Accuracy in the diagnosis of such bacteria has direct implications for treatment approaches, as incorrect identification may lead to ineffective treatment procedures that may further aggravate the patient's outcome. Complementing this knowledge is the growing evidence that aims to find the probiotic value of certain Gram-negative bacteria, , such as *Bacillus* subtilis (Maldonado et al., 2015). This twin focus on pathogenicity and potential probiotic use demonstrates the intertwined nature of Gram-negative bacilli, an indicator of the need for effective identification tools taking into account both their harmful and beneficial traits within the microbiome and health care facilities (Figure 9.3).

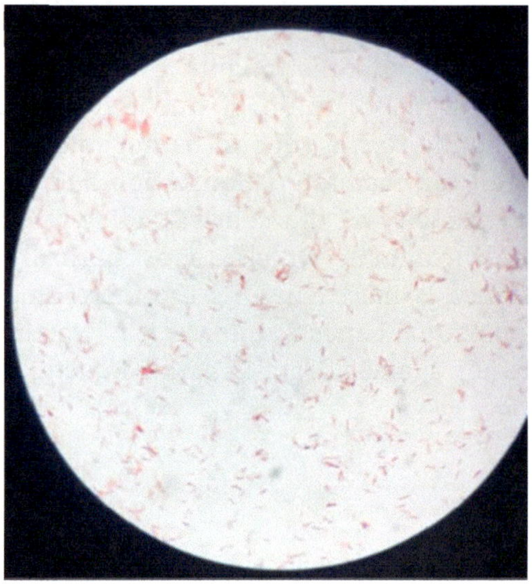

Figure 9.3. Gram staining: Gram-negative bacillus.

Source: https://www.researchgate.net/publication/373388841/figure/fig3/AS:11431281183724989@1692977037664/Gram-staining-A-Gram-negative-bacillus-and-B-Gram-positive-bacillus.png.

9.1.3. Metabolic and Growth Characteristics

The metabolic and growth characteristics of Gram-negative bacilli are the key to their pathogenicity and ecological competitiveness. These bacteria are extremely versatile, and they can live in different milieus, for example, soil, water, and host organisms. Gram-negative bacilli, for example, *Pseudomonas* species, are metabolically extremely varied, and they can utilize numerous different organic compounds as a source of energy. This adaptability is further enhanced by their ability to grow in aerobic and anaerobic conditions; indeed, *Pseudomonas* strains have been shown to grow vigorously in cold temperatures, causing spoilage of meat under aerobic condition. Using a comparison of *Pseudomonas* putida KT2440 gene expression across temperatures, researchers have discovered enormous variation in metabolic functions, indicating the ability of the organism to adapt to a range of environmental stresses, a necessary requirement for its survival under varying conditions (Aarts et al., 2015). Other Gram-negative bacilli, however, , such as Campylobacter jejuni, possess specialized growth requirements that dictate their metabolic characteristics. Being one of the most widespread causes of bacterial gastroenteritis in the world, the development of C. jejunis is closely connected with niche adaptation, most notably its preference for microaerophilic conditions. The organism possesses a multifaceted metabolic network by which it is capable of thriving in bird and mammal gastrointestinal tracts. Genome analysis has revealed distinct genetic distinctions among different strains of C. jejuni, with clonal complexes being correlated with livestock dominating specific clusters. Furthermore, more recent research utilizing multilocus sequence typing (MLST) has proven how these new genetic accommodations contribute to the organism's overall pathogenicity and enable it to exploit alternative environments and hosts (Altschul et al., 2013). The biochemical and growth characteristics of Gram-negative bacilli possess importance that extends beyond mere microbial ecology; they are a key to understanding food safety and public health. For instance, the susceptibility to spoilage of *Pseudomonas* in meat foods influences not merely quality but also carries economic and impacts consumer confidence in meat. Identification of differentially expressed genes in *Pseudomonas* at varying storage conditions provides insights into how these bacteria respond to stressors relevant to food preservation. Similarly, traceability of *C. jejuni* strains from either wildlife or livestock sources emphasizes the importance of understanding these organisms' growth needs, directing control of their presence in food systems and minimizing the risk of foodborne disease (Aarts et al., 2015).

Test Your Knowledge

1. What are the key structural components of the cell wall in Gram-negative bacilli, and how do they differ from Gram-positive bacteria?
2. Why do Gram-negative bacilli appear pink or red after Gram staining, and what does this indicate about their cell wall?

9.2. Major Types of Gram-negative Bacilli

Learning Outcome

1. Understand the Enterobacteriaceae family
2. Describe Pseudomonas species
3. Explain Vibrio

In Gram-negative bacilli, one of the most significant of these groups is Enterobacteriaceae, a family that contains numerous clinically significant pathogens. Among these species, some are very well known to cause community-acquired as well as healthcare-associated infections, , such as *Escherichia coli* and Klebsiella pneumoniae. *E. coli*, for instance, is a leading cause of urinary tract infection and may present in more severe forms , such as sepsis. Simultaneously, Klebsiella pneumoniae has also been associated with pneumonia, sepsis, and is a cause of multidrug resistance. The epidemiology of these microorganisms is characterized by an alarming trend in the development of antibiotic resistance, which poses serious obstacles to treatment protocols. Moreover, the virulence factors these microorganisms possess, , such as exotoxins and adherence, enhance their pathogenicity, complicating both prevention and therapeutic interventions in clinical situations. Another of the significant Gram-negative bacilli is the *Pseudomonas* genus, namely *Pseudomonas aeruginosa*. This organism is notorious for its environmental adaptability and is typically responsible for opportunistic infections in immunocompromised patients and patients who have underlying respiratory disease , such as cystic fibrosis. Due to its intrinsic resistance to a broad range of antibiotics, *P. aeruginosa* is exceedingly difficult to treat, commonly necessitating combination antibiotic therapy. The ability of the organism to form biofilms complicates treatment, resulting in reduced efficacy of standard antimicrobial agents. Based on existing research, *Pseudomonas* species infections have been exacerbated by the emergence of multidrug-resistant pathogens that have largely impacted the morbidity and mortality of patients in hospital settings, thereby perpetuating the need for empirical treatment recommendations that address the evolving nature of such pathogens (Toro López et al., 2019). Some of the other significant Gram-negative bacilli include Haemophilus influenzae and Neisseria species, which are clinically and of public health significance. Although H. influenzae has been supplanted to secondary pathogen status by effective vaccination, it is still able to cause severe infection, particularly in a population without this protection, i.e., children and the elderly. Neisseria meningitidis, for instance, is notorious for its causation of meningococcal disease, an acute life-threatening condition that mandates prompt diagnosis and treatment. The endemicity of these microorganisms also emphasizes the need for surveillance since trends in infection and resistance rates affect vaccination policy and treatment regimens. With multi-modal treatment regimens of the infections from these Gram-negative bacilli being developed, there is an increasing need to know their particular epidemiological and pathogenic characteristics to optimize patient outcomes (Cardenal et al., 2019).

9.2.1. Enterobacteriaceae Family

The family Enterobacteriaceae is a large group in the kingdom of Gram-negative bacilli, characterized by their diverse metabolic potential and ecological roles. The family includes the well-known genera *Escherichia*, Salmonella, and *Shigella* that occur as common environmental organisms and human pathogens. The versatility of Enterobacteriaceae is evident in their capability to survive under different environments from soil and water to the human and animal gut flora. This adaptability of Enterobacteriaceae pinpoints the function of the family in microbiological research as well as in public health due to their connection with diseases from gastroenteritis to severe systemic infection. Their capacity to become antibiotic-resistant also makes their study relevant through the challenge posed by proper treatment procedures in the clinical field. Proteus, which is among the well-known genera of Enterobacteriaceae, is a vivid example of these species as opportunistic pathogens and commensals. These can be readily distinguished by their role in urinary tract infection (UTI) and their ability to swarm, aiding in colonization and biofilm formation. They are multifactorial, with virulence factors, such as fimbriae, flagella, and a variety of enzymes, including urease, which helps in the development of urinary calculi. Opportunistic pathogens exploit certain conditions to cause infections, particularly in immunocompromised hosts. The significance of Proteus within the Enterobacteriaceae family indicates the severe need for comprehensive knowledge and monitoring of these microorganisms, especially keeping in view their implication in healthcare-associated infections (Drzewiecka et al., 2013). Moreover, the Enterobacteriaceae family is gaining relevance in environmental health, particularly water pollution. Thermotolerant coliforms are members of this family and are monitored most often in drinking water reservoirs because their presence will indicate fecal contamination and risk of waterborne disease. Experiments have established that the occurrence of these coliforms in drinking water may be due to various sources, and therefore, it becomes necessary to maintain strict water quality testing protocols to ensure public health (Camargo et al., 2024). Enterobacteriaceae that include thermotolerant coliforms are capable of thriving under diverse conditions, thereby making it difficult for water quality control. Therefore, an understanding of their environmental dynamics is important in order to create effective monitoring strategies and interventions for safeguarding human health in the context of rising antimicrobial resistance and environmental degradation (Figure 9.4).

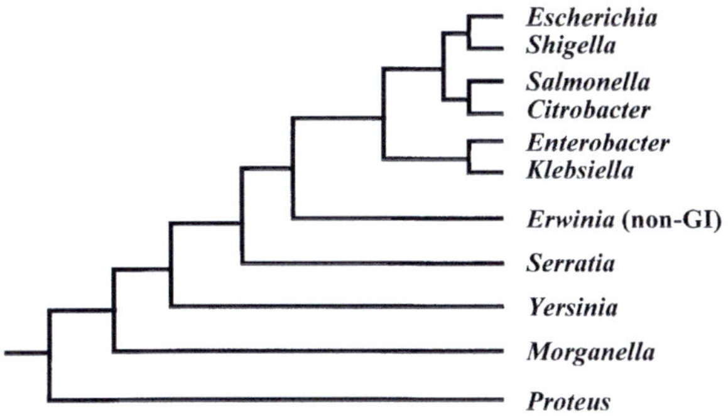

Figure 9.4. Relatedness among the family Enterobacteriaceae.

Source: https://www.researchgate.net/profile/Alan-Wolfe-2/publication/14164979/figure/fig3/AS:667801199075330@1536227621265/Relatedness-among-the-family-Enterobacteriaceae-7-All-genera-are-associated-with-the.png.

9.2.2. Pseudomonas Species

Pseudomonas is a key genus among the Gram-negative bacilli, with which most remarkable metabolic versatility underlies ecological ubiquity. *Pseudomonas* species live in widely diverse habitats that range from soil and water to several man-made habitats , such as hospital settings and laboratory settings. *Pseudomonas aeruginosa* is by far the best-studied species and is extremely high in significance due to opportunistic pathogenicity in immunocompromised hosts. The ability of the organism to metabolize diverse carbon substrates and to withstand adverse conditions, including heat and the introduction of antibiotics, qualifies it as a formidable opponent in hospital settings. Its adaptability mechanisms are essential in comprehending its environmental durability as well as its virulence determinants involved in its pathogenicity, particularly in nosocomial infections. The virulence of *Pseudomonas* species is particularly influenced by the production of virulence factors, which enhance their infectivity in host tissues and ability to resist immune response. These factors include an array of extracellular enzymes and exotoxins that impair the host cell functions and facilitate colonization by the bacteria. Studies involving *Pseudomonas* fluorescens mutants revealed significant information about how alterations in metabolic processes, , such as heat resistance, could affect virulence attributes (Gall & Riely, 1965). These experiments demonstrate the intricate relationship between genetic traits and environmental resistance, revealing how such bacteria are able to thrive under hostile conditions but still pose health risks to humans.

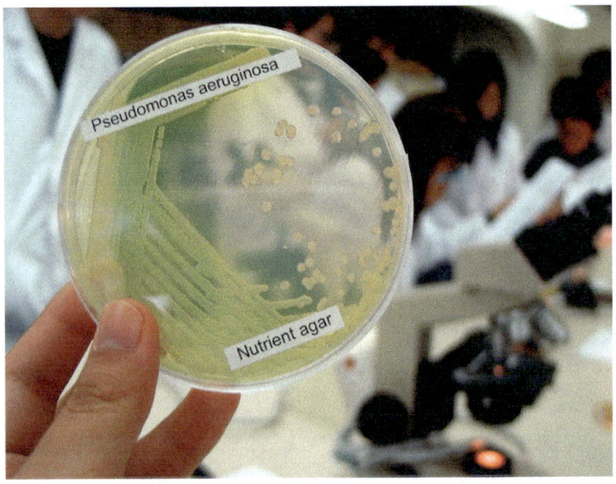

Figure 9.5. *Pseudomonas aeruginosa* in a Petri dish.

Source: https://upload.wikimedia.org/wikipedia/commons/6/6a/*Pseudomonas*_Aeruginosa.jpg.

Understanding how these interactions are utilized is significant in designing the appropriate therapeutic strategies against infections by *Pseudomonas* species. Apart from their virulence determinants, *Pseudomonas* species are also fascinating because they make significant contributions to the human microbiome, particularly in specialized niches , such as compact spaces. Research on human microflora has also shown that *Pseudomonas,* at times, makes contributions towards skin and respiratory microbiomes as a protective agent and also as an opportunistic pathogen (Gall & Riely, 1965). The dualism hinders the treatment of infections, particularly in patients who might have compromised microbial communities because of exposure to antibiotics. The ecological dynamics of *Pseudomonas* in various environments, coupled with their ability to evolve and cause disease, underscore the imperative for continued investigation and surveillance. A greater understanding of their biology could guide clinical practice and inform efforts to mitigate their impact on public health (Figure 9.5).

9.2.3. Vibrio Species

Vibrio species, a large group under the family Vibrionaceae, are characterized as Gram-negative bacilli that primarily inhabit aquatic environments. Their ecological flexibility allows them to exist in marine as well as freshwater environments.

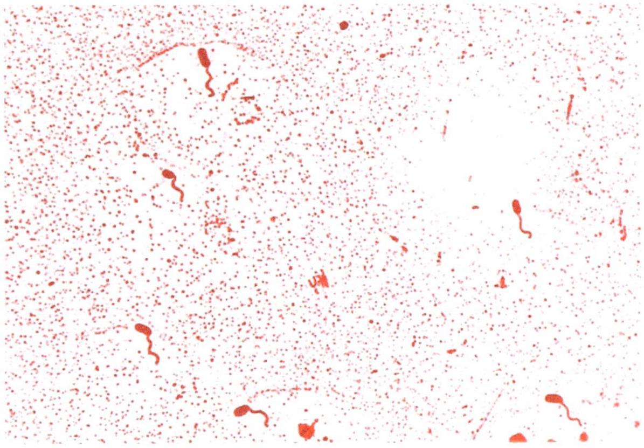

Figure 9.6. *Vibrio cholerae.*

Source: https://upload.wikimedia.org/wikipedia/commons/thumb/d/db/Vibrio_cholerae_01.jpg/1280px-Vibrio_cholerae_01.jpg.

Vibrio bacteria are of pivotal importance in nutrient cycling and serve as a source of food for enormous populations of marine animals. However, numerous Vibrio species, , such as *Vibrio cholerae* and Vibrio parahaemolyticus, are similarly reported as human pathogens, causing a range of diseases from gastroenteritis to fatal cholera. Vibrio species have been reported to be pathogenic as they possess multiple virulence factors, , such as the excretion of exotoxins that enable them to endure host habitats, which demonstrates their dual significance in ecological as well as clinical situations (Elmanama et al., 2007).

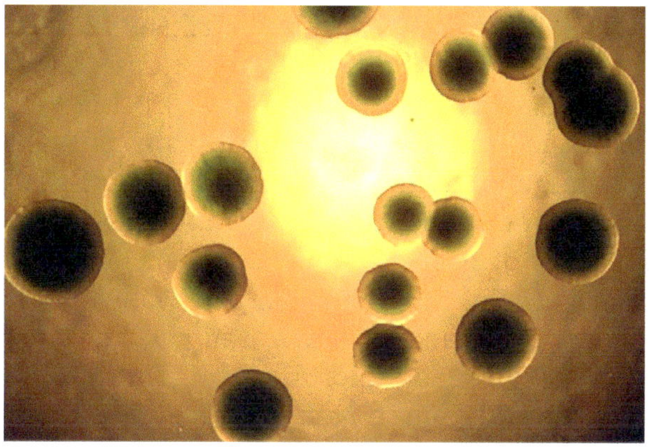

Figure 9.7. Vibrio parahaemolyticus colony morphology on TCBS agar.

Source: https://www.researchgate.net/publication/368978824/figure/fig1/AS:11431281124359783@1677933681884/brio-parahaemolyticus-colony-morphology-on-TCBS-agar.png.

The pathogenicity of Vibrio species is particularly pronounced in environments that favor their growth, , such as increased water temperature and high salinity rates. *Vibrio cholerae*, for instance, is predominantly associated with contaminated water and food substances and constitutes grave public health problem in most parts of the world (Figure 9.6). In marine ecosystems, the interaction between Vibrio species and marine animals might be particularly complex, even like the fact that certain isolates were seen to co-exist with Lactobacillus species inside fish, as uncovered in tests where Lacto*Bacillus* demonstrated antagonistic action towards Vibrio pathogens (Dhanasekaran et al., 2010). This suggests not only the ecological importance of such bacteria but also the potential for exploiting beneficial associations to improve fish health and aquaculture. Control of Vibrio-caused infections is a multifaceted strategy combining public health interventions with developments in the microbiological sciences. Vaccine manufacture and implementation of strict water quality standards are necessary in preventing hazards from Vibrio infection. In addition, studies investigating the interactions of Vibrio species with probiotics like Lactobacillus hold potential for improving fish health in aquaculture. Unraveling the dynamics of such interactions can yield novel means of controlling both bacterial pathogenicity and facilitating beneficial microbial communities. As a result, the implications of Vibrio species spread beyond human health and have profound ecological and economic implications in aquatic environments (Figure 9.7).

Test Your Knowledge

1. What are the defining characteristics of the Enterobacteriaceae family?
2. What distinguishes Pseudomonas aeruginosa from members of the Enterobacteriaceae family in terms of metabolism, pigment production, and growth conditions?
3. What are the key biochemical and morphological features used to identify Vibrio cholerae?

9.3. Pathogenicity and Disease Associations

Learning Outcome

1. Explain common infections caused by Gram-negative bacilli
2. Understand mechanisms of virulence employed by Gram-negative bacilli
3. Antibiotic resistance issues concerning Gram-negative bacilli

One of the key elements of pathogenicity in Gram-negative bacilli is their ability to grow in different environments, particularly clinical environments. The diverse mechanisms through which the bacteria cause disease have increasingly been described, particularly in vulnerable populations , such as very low birth weight infants. For instance, it has been shown through research that the fecal microbiomes of these infants have a high increase in Gammaproteobacteria, which can contribute to a high percentage of their gut microflora. This is due to various reasons , such as the mode of delivery and the administration of antenatal steroids. These correlations highlight the complexity of gut microbiome development and its implications for health outcomes, triggering a need to keep studying the dysbiotic state that may expose preterm neonates to lethal infection as well as other pathogenicity-linked complications in Gram-negative bacilli (Gilbert et al., 2018). Biofilm formation by Gram-negative bacteria is another critical feature that enhances their pathogenicity, notably in persistent infections. Biofilms are defensive structures that allow bacteria to adhere to the surface and become resistant to antimicrobial therapy. It has been noted that the majority of multidrug-resistant organisms (MDROs) produce high levels of biofilm, which complicates treatment. Certain strains like *Pseudomonas aeruginosa* and methicillin-resistant *Staphylococcus aureus* (MRSA) are famous for their capacity to produce biofilms, and hence treatment failure in chronic wound infection. In fact, presence of biofilm-forming Gram-negative bacilli in polymicrobial environments not only ensures their survival but also prevents the efficacy of antibiotics, depicting a direct correlation between biofilm formation and virulence in such pathogens (Bordignon et al., 2017). Understanding of the correlation between the pathogenicity mechanism of Gram-negative bacilli and caused diseases is crucial in order to develop effective treatment interventions. Their proclivity to form biofilms in chronic infections and the dynamic changes in their microbial communities in susceptible populations remind us of the intricacy of infection to treat. Their ability to make predictions concerning outcomes from clinical determinants, , such as mode of delivery and structure of microbial communities in infants, sheds light on the intricate interactions these bacteria have with their hosts. Such observations are of importance to both researchers and practitioners, paving the way to improved therapeutic and diagnostic paradigms in the treatment of Gram-negative bacillary infections. Last but not least, knowledge of such pathogenicity and disease associations remains a sustained overarching objective in the fight against Gram-negative bacterial infection and its effect on public health.

9.3.1. Common Infections Caused by Gram-negative Bacilli

Infection with Gram-negative bacilli is a significant public health challenge, particularly their pattern of antibiotic resistance. One of the most common infections from such bacteria is bacteremia or septicemia, which is typically lethal and is commonly seen among immunocompromised patients, e.g., those undergoing chemotherapy for cancer. A sample of this issue is a study conducted at Khartoum Oncology Hospital; in a febrile neutropenic group of patients, 63.8% of bloodstream infections were caused by Gram-negative bacilli, with *Escherichia coli* being the predominant isolate at 30.4% (Abdelaziz et al., 2022). These findings show that Gram-negative infections should be addressed in hospitals as soon as possible because high rates of multidrug resistance have a trend that complicates conventional treatment methods. Continuous monitoring of infection trends is crucial in designing effective antibiotic stewardship programs. The respiratory tract, another critical infection site caused by Gram-negative bacilli, also comes into the picture, with Klebsiella pneumoniae commonly being the implicated pathogen in healthcare-associated pneumonia. Infection is particularly stealthy in the event of underlying pulmonary disease or in hospitalized and mechanically ventilated patients. The isolation of Gram-negative bacilli from respiratory infections can lead to severe morbidity because of the inherent resistance mechanisms of the bacteria, most frequently being extended-spectrum beta-lactamases (ESBLs) responsible for resistance to numerous cephalosporins and penicillins. For instance, there have been studies that have reported high rates of resistance of Gram-negative bacilli with a significant proportion of the isolates having ESBL production (Abdelaziz et al., 2022). These findings require the clinicians to exercise care in the choice of empiric antibiotic treatment for respiratory infections and encourage an improved infection control practice within the health setting. Cervico-facial infections also yield similar proof of the existence of Gram-negative bacilli but, regretfully, diagnostic yield using cultures is not always congruent with the preliminary Gram stain results. A research at Tygerberg Academic Hospital shows that while Gram staining usually demonstrates Gram-negative bacteria in pus material, actual culture findings confirm Gram-negative bacilli less frequently, and this indicates variation in microbiological laboratory diagnosis. Such underrecognition may lead to suboptimal management strategies if antibiotic treatment is designed only on the basis of Gram staining and later confirmed by follow-up cultures. Thus, clinicians must think of cervico-facial sepsis with the expectation of both Gram-negative and Gram-positive bacterial pathogens in mind so as not to overlook broad-spectrum coverage in empirical therapy until culture sensitivities are firm enough to direct therapy definitively. These recommendations are essential to optimizing patient outcomes in such complex infection scenarios (Figure 9.8).

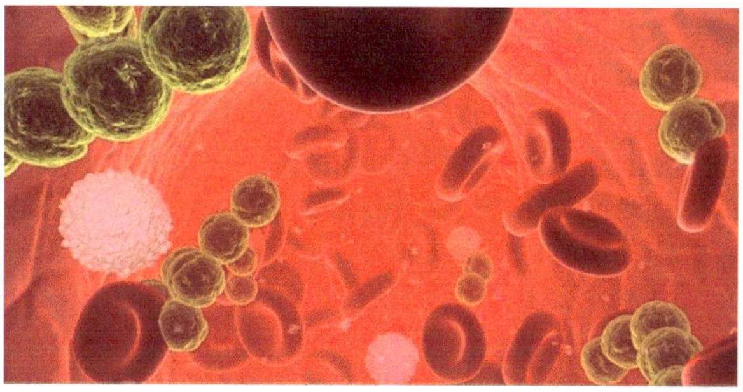

Figure 9.8. Bloodstream infection.

Source: https://clpmag.com/wp-content/uploads/2018/06/DNA-Electronics-Sepsis_highres-1280x640.jpeg.

9.3.2. Mechanisms of Virulence

The mechanisms of virulence employed by Gram-negative bacilli are complex and multifaceted, rendering them extremely pathogenic. One of their most important features is the ability to produce biofilms, which are cohesive groups of bacteria embedded in an extracellular matrix that they produce. In addition to allowing them to thrive in all types of environments, including hospitals, it also makes them resistant to antimicrobials. Studies have shown that a great majority of clinical isolates, especially multidrug-resistant strains (MDROs), are biofilm-producers. Interestingly, 80% of the tested strains were biofilm producers, and the occurrence of the biofilm-producing bacteria was especially high in chronic infections. Thus, the biofilm formation becomes a key virulence determinant accountable for the chronicity and persistence of infection irrespective of the MDRO phenotype (Bordignon et al., 2017).

Furthermore, Gram-negative bacilli have evolved sophisticated mechanisms to evade host immunity, also enhancing their virulence. The ability of uropathogenic *Escherichia coli* (UPEC), for instance, to modulate the host's inflammatory response is of particular interest. UPEC can acquire intracellular access to niches within the urinary tract, thereby escaping immune cell killing by neutrophils and macrophages. Intracellular persistence is associated with the bacterium's capacity for secretion of factors capable of inhibiting neutrophil migration and controlling the local inflammatory environment. By suppressing the host's immune response, UPEC aids in establishing infection and prolonging its life cycle, making treatment more challenging and amplifying overall pathogenicity. This specific mechanism is proof that distinguishes between pathogenic and nonpathogenic *E. coli* and the significance of continued research into their mechanisms of immune evasion (Cavalieri et al., 2016). Other than biofilm formation and immune evasion, the ability to acquire and utilize nutrient supplies is another major virulence factor in Gram-negative bacilli. The pathogens use various systems for the capture of essential nutrients, for example, siderophores that capture iron, which in most cases is not available in host environments. This capacity of the nutrient uptake facilitates not only the survival of Gram-negative bacilli during infection but also their resistance to host defense responses , such as starvation and oxidative stress. Moreover, studies have indicated that certain Gram-negative bacilli can modify their metabolic pathways to enhance growth under adverse conditions, further proving themselves to be effective pathogens. By utilizing these survival mechanisms with optimal efficiency, such bacteria not only infect but also acclimatize to the changing situations in host environments, ultimately developing an enhanced virulence portfolio and complicating their treatment modalities.

9.3.3. Antibiotic Resistance Issues

Resistance to antibiotics, particularly among Gram-negative bacilli, poses a burgeoning risk to public health. These bacteria, which include such pathogens as *Escherichia coli* and Klebsiella pneumoniae, have demonstrated an astonishing ability to acquire resistance mechanisms through horizontal gene transfer. Antibiotic misuse and abuse, especially of the broad-spectrum varieties, have accelerated the process. In light of historical context, the popularity of antibiotics initiated in the early 20th century with the discovery of penicillin has arguably led to a misconception of their limitless efficacy. As highlighted, these therapeutic agents, once hailed as cure-alls, have contributed to the rise of resistant strains that complicate treatment protocols and increase morbidity and mortality rates (Lillestolen et al., 2018). This situation highlights the need for stringent stewardship and new methods to fight antibiotic abuse and the resulting resistance patterns seen in Gram-negative bacilli. Environmental factors contributing to antibiotic resistance also need ample attention. A number of studies have established that farm practices, specifically antibiotic use in livestock, directly affect the emergence of resistant bacterial populations. Antibiotics are commonly applied to promote growth rather than treat infection, thereby selecting strains that are resistant and may then be transmitted to humans through the food chain. For instance, outbreaks caused by resistant strain-related cases have been found to be caused by imported cattle, as in the case of evidence from *Listeria monocytogenes* in red-legged partridges. Close genetic connections between the farm isolates and the imported chicks, which had identical patterns of resistance to antibiotics, demonstrate the interconnection of human and animal health systems (HJ et al., 2015). Tackling antibiotic resistance requires an integrative approach incorporating one health strategies with emphasis on the interdependence of interactions among environmental, animal, and human health. Countermeasures for antibiotic resistance must also be aimed at the production and utilization of new antibiotics and other therapeutic strategies. Research into novel agents that can bypass already established mechanisms of resistance is necessary, particularly against Gram-negative bacilli, which possess incredibly intricate mechanisms of defense. Existing antibiotics are prone to failure because they can harbor resistance genes, and the classical treatments become ineffectual. Therefore, new approaches , such as phage therapy with bacteriophages targeting certain bacteria are a promising path to overcoming resistance. Additionally, preventive vaccines against infection by resistant strains can significantly minimize the reliance on antibiotics and decrease selection pressure for resistance development. As the crisis of antibiotic resistance continues to deepen, it will become increasingly important to have a clear understanding and proactive approach in addressing such issues so that the effectiveness of present therapy is ensured and public health is safeguarded (Lillestolen et al., 2018).

Test Your Knowledge

1. What types of infections are commonly caused by Gram-negative bacilli?
2. How do Gram-negative bacilli use pili, capsules, and secretion systems?

9.4. Laboratory Identification Techniques

Learning Outcome

1. Explain culture methods and media
2. Describe biochemical tests for identification
3. Understand molecular techniques for detection

The identification of Gram-negative bacilli in the laboratory is an essential component of infectious disease diagnosis. Due to the diversity of the group of bacteria, and the presence of some of the more dangerous pathogens like *Escherichia coli* and *Salmonella* species, there is a need for accurate identification procedures. Traditionally, phenotypic methods , such as Gram staining, biochemical tests, and properties of culture have been employed to identify species. These conventional approaches, while critical, are typically time and skill-exhaustive. Thus, there has been a shift towards the utilization of high molecular methods that are more precise and faster. The use of polymerase chain reaction (PCR) and sequencing technologies provides accurate detection of bacterial species by their genetic material, revealing greater information about their potential for pathogenicity and mechanisms of resistance that are critical for clinical management and epidemiological studies. Higher developments in laboratory identification techniques have introduced machine learning algorithms to aid the identification of Gram-negative bacilli with greater diagnostic precision. Machine learning models leverage enormous amounts of microbial property data to predict organism identity based on their phenotypes or gene sequences. One area that has been in the limelight is the integration of structured methodologies that employ hierarchical information about microbial relationships to improve the accuracy of identification systems. Scientists have proven such machine learning methodology to be helpful, especially when it is a case of closely related species to which traditional methods cannot differentiate. However, studies have shown that while machine learning methodologies prove to perform better than traditional methodologies in some situations, they have not yet proven consistently that they enhance identification accuracy under all situations because traditional methods themselves already offer dramatic performance with some species (Vervier et al., 2015). Laboratory techniques for identifying Gram-negative bacilli are not only important to study but play a vital role in finding their potential applications, such as in the field of probiotics. Some recent studies have cultured spore-forming bacteria, such as *Bacillus* strains having positive attributes in animal nutrition. Through analysis of their surface properties, biosurfactant production, and pathogenic bacteria inhibition, researchers are learning about the relevant characteristics that may make them potential probiotics to be administered to animals. For instance, some *Bacillus* subtilis strains were found to inhibit Gram-positive pathogens well and displayed favorable biochemical traits in laboratory tests (Maldonado et al., 2015). These findings underscore the importance of high-level laboratory detection techniques that are highly versatile for clinical and industrial microbiology and potentially also open up new application areas in health and nutrition.

9.4.1. Culture Methods and Media

Gram-negative bacilli research is highly reliant on the utilisation of some culture methods and media that are specifically tailored to meet the unique growth requirements of such bacteria. The process begins with the selection of a good-quality medium that is suitable to provide the required nutrients without inhibiting the unwanted organisms. For instance, MacConkey agar is widely employed as it is robust enough to differentiate lactose fermenters as pink and non-fermenters, reflecting its application for the isolation of enteric Gram-negative bacilli. Other than that, other selective media , such as XLD or Hektoen Enteric agar also enhance recovery rates as they allow clinicians to isolate pathogenic strains effectively. These specialized media not only facilitate the identification of bacterial species but also allow for identification of biochemical characteristics significant in accurate diagnosis and treatment plans. In addition to solid media, liquid culture procedures are essential in the identification of Gram-negative bacilli. Broth cultures , such as tryptic soy broth or nutrient broth, support the growth of bacteria and are very handy in isolating isolates from complex samples, , such as blood or environmental samples. Successful culture methods, such as blood culture systems, are of extreme importance, as noted in studies on the incidence of bacterial contamination of blood donations. In such studies, various media and techniques are employed to isolate contaminants, with major reports indicating coagulase-negative staphylococci and Gram-positive rods can find their entry into circulation due to procedural failures in the process of blood taking (Malimu, 2012). This indicates how culture procedures are crucial not only to identify sources of infection but also to realize how bacterial presence within clinical specimens interacts. The advent of advanced molecular techniques has also transformed traditional culture methods, with improved and accelerated diagnostics for Gram-negative bacilli. Rapid molecular assays and polymerase chain reaction (PCR) enable identification of single bacterial DNA with significantly shorter turnaround times compared to traditional culture methods. Nevertheless, even in the light of these advances, culture remains a foundation for microbiological diagnosis, particularly for antimicrobial susceptibility evaluation. For example, the Kirby-Bauer disk diffusion test is utilized to identify antibiotic resistance patterns of Gram-negative bacilli, presenting concrete facts for the successful treatment of infection (Marchioro et al., 1964). As the science of microbiology advances, the union of traditional culture techniques with new technologies will further improve the knowledge base and management of infections due to Gram-negative bacilli (Figure 9.9).

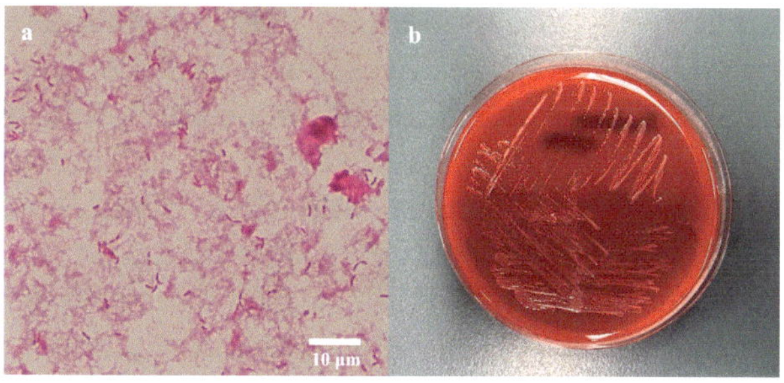

Figure 9.9. Blood culture media revealing small Gram-negative bacilli staining, Gram staining, 1000 × (a). White colonies of *Pandoraea apista* after 24 h on sheep blood agar plate (b).

Source: https://www.researchgate.net/publication/361142525/figure/fig2/AS:1164526208712727@1654656092918/Blood-culture-media-revealing-small-Gram-negative-bacilli-staining-Gram-staining.jpg.

9.4.2. Biochemical Tests for Identification

Identification of Gram-negative bacilli consists of a series of biochemical tests that are necessary to understand the pathogenic profile of such an organism. Biochemical tests exploit the metabolic properties of bacteria to differentiate species based on their ability to utilize or produce certain substrates and products. For instance, some tests , such as fermentation of sugars, citrate test, or hydrogen sulfide production can be very significant in identifying the bacteria present in a given sample. Such tests are initial, mainly due to the fact that Gram-negative bacilli can contain numerous varied species with varied pathogenic features, and therefore correct identification becomes very crucial for the development of efficient treatment strategies. Having these biochemical characteristics makes it easier for microbiologists to shortlist probable isolates, thus elucidating the presumptive pathogens causing infections, particularly in at-risk groups , such as intensive care unit patients. On clinical specimens, data from biochemical testing can be the key to the diagnosis of bloodstream infections, which are conventionally associated with Gram-negative bacilli. In a study that underscored the importance of early detection, 48.22% of blood culture specimens were positive and yielded Gram-negative bacilli as the most frequent isolates. By utilization of standard biochemical tests in the process of identification, there was critical information uncovered; e.g., Klebsiella pneumoniae and *Acinetobacter baumannii* were the most frequent organisms isolated. This brings to light an important trend where biochemical testing is at the center of pathogen identification causing multi-drug resistant infection.

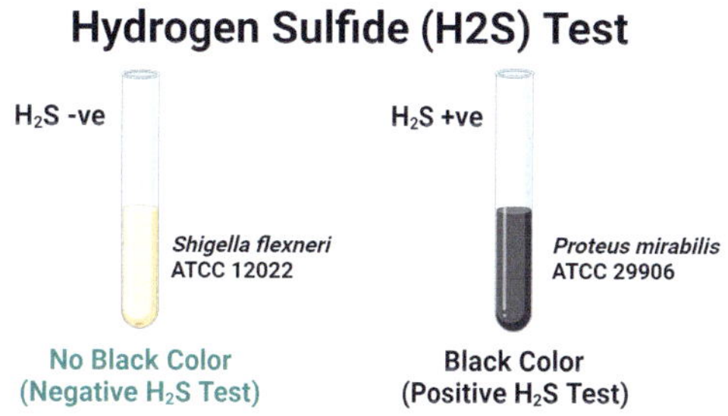

Figure 9.10. Hydrogen sulfide (H_2S) test.

Source: https://microbenotes.com/wp-content/uploads/2023/04/Hydrogen-Sulfide-H2S-Test.jpg.

The findings reveal the significance of rapid, accurate diagnosis tests that can only be obtained by employing biochemical tests strategically (Nagendra et al., 2023). Advances in biochemical testing improve the effectiveness and efficiency of identification of pathogens, and this plays a critical role in the timely application of treatment. For instance, direct testing methods with the use of automated systems , such as the VITEK are able to reduce identification and susceptibility outcome time by a considerable margin when compared to the conventional methods. Studies indicated that almost 69% of the identifications were reported to clinicians within six hours, a far cry from conventional methods. Moreover, such early reporting can trigger immediate and efficient therapeutic measures, most importantly in emergency conditions where there is an urgent need for treatment that can affect the course of patient management negatively. This integration of early screening methods into clinical microbiology testifies to the dynamic character of bacterial identification and the ongoing applicability of biochemical tests to the treatment of Gram-negative bacillary infections (Bruun et al., 2002) (Figure 9.10).

9.4.3. Molecular Techniques for Detection

Molecular detection techniques have revolutionized the art of microbiology, particularly Gram-negative bacilli, which are highly recognized for their pathogenicity and antibiotic resistance. Techniques , such as real-time PCR allow fast and targeted detection of bacterial DNA, a crucial advantage in clinical diagnosis. For instance, real-time PCR has been valuable in the detection of Mycobacterium bovis from environmental isolations, , such as soil and faeces of infected wildlife, further augmenting transmission dynamics to animals. These molecular methods not only accelerate the diagnostic rate but also enhance species specificity over traditional culture methods and thus are a critical component of infectious diseases surveillance due to Gram-negative bacilli as well as their environmental reservoirs (Sweeney et al., 1999). In addition to PCR, other molecular techniques, including DNA sequencing and multiplex tests, are significant in the determination of Gram-negative bacilli resistance profiles. With the emergence of multidrug-resistant organisms (MDROs), identifying mechanisms of resistance is crucial for effective therapeutic management. An example is the genomic sequencing, which can detect mutations involved in antibiotic resistance in bacteria like *Escherichia coli* and Klebsiella pneumoniae. Furthermore, the integration through bioinformatics tools enables sophisticated analysis of genetic information to give insight into the epidemiology of infections from Gram-negative bacilli. Improved breakdown and interpretation of complicated data enhance public health outcomes as it directs infection control practices and therapeutics in particular resistance patterns of bacteria in a clinical setting (Bordignon et al., 2017). Moreover, the detection of biofilm-producing Gram-negative bacilli by molecular techniques presents an extremely significant characteristic of their virulence. The production of biofilm is a critical factor that has been associated with chronic infection, particularly where there is wound delayed healing. Evidence supports high biofilm production levels in clinically isolated Gram-negative bacilli, which implies its virulence determinant characteristic. Quantitative characterization of biofilm formations based on molecular methods validates the identification of their persistence in chronic infections. For instance, while a significant proportion of drug-resistant strains exhibits strong biofilm production, the molecular analysis employed allows scientists and clinical doctors to develop targeted therapies that address not just the bacterial load but also biofilm-specific issues. Through targeting these characteristics, molecular techniques are valuable tools in the management of complex infections produced by Gram-negative bacilli, enhancing patient care and public health activities at large.

Test Your Knowledge

1. What selective and differential media are commonly used to isolate Gram-negative bacilli from clinical specimens?
2. Which key biochemical tests are used to identify members of the Enterobacteriaceae family?

9.5. Treatment and Management of Infections

Learning Outcome

1. Describe antibiotic options and challenges
2. Understand role of vaccines in prevention in preventing infections caused by Gram-negative bacilli
3. Discuss the importance of infection control measures

Effective treatment and management of infections caused by Gram-negative bacilli requires a multi-modal approach considering both the pathogens' antibiotic resistance pattern as well as the clinical presentation of the infection. Gram-negative bacilli are known for having intrinsic resistance to various antibiotics and thus are challenging to treat. In a study of bloodstream infections, there was an implication that a significant percentage of Gram-negative bacilli were revealed to be multidrug resistant, namely against commonly used medications like piperacillin and amikacin, projecting the dilemma faced by practitioners in choosing effective treatments (Kante et al., 2017). Resistance has the potential to lead to therapeutic failure and elevated morbidity and mortality. Therefore, early detection through blood cultures and sensitivity is crucial to guide proper antibiotic therapy and maximize patient outcomes. In therapy for Gram-negative bacillary infections, not only does the selection of antibiotics matter, but so does the need for continued surveillance of resistance patterns within specific clinical settings. The dynamic nature of bacterial populations, especially in the clinical environment, implies that there must be an adaptive response in developing resistance patterns. For instance, a study conducted at Tygerberg Academic Hospital revealed an apparent discrepancy between Gram staining findings and the actual culture yield of Gram-negative pathogens. Whereas high numbers of pus swabs were Gram-negative positive according to Gram staining, cultures yielded only a minority of these organisms, reflecting a potential loop in diagnostic effectiveness (Barnard, 2019). This emphasizes the importance of correlating laboratory findings with clinical acumen to properly manage. Preventive strategies, like infection control procedures and immunoprophylaxis procedures, need to be implemented to avoid the development of Gram-negative *Bacillus* caused infections. Hand washing procedures, safe use of personal protective equipment, and maintenance of aseptic procedures for interventions must be emphasized at hospitals and healthcare facilities to prevent transmission risk. Moreover, manufacturing and deployment of vaccine programs against pathogens that cause Gram-negative infections can be a type of prophylaxis that reduces the overall burden of disease. To complement such preventive measures by prudent application of antibiotics through good stewardship programs will not only maximize cure rates but also stem the looming landslide of antimicrobial resistance among Gram-negative bacilli, thereby supporting public health quality.

9.5.1. Antibiotic Options and Challenges

The increasing prevalence of Gram-negative bacilli renders it very difficult in the world of antibiotic therapy, and therefore there is a compelling need for effective therapeutic options. The bacteria are characterized by the presence of highly developed outer membranes, which are a hindrance to most traditional efficacious antibiotics. Therefore, therapeutic options are limited in many cases, particularly with the introduction of multidrug-resistant bacteria. The complexity involved in overcoming these resistance mechanisms involves ongoing research and development of already developed antibiotics, as well as research on new types of therapy. Antibiotic stewardship programs and the development of guidelines by organizations like the Surgical Infection Society bring into focus the need for evidence-based intervention that is aimed at both the antimicrobial selection and timing of therapy in the presence of the complexity of Gram-negative bacillus-induced intra-abdominal infections (Chang et al., 2017). Apart from the problem of resistance to antibiotics, the cost burden of unsuccessful therapy of Gram-negative infection is especially serious. Costs associated with increased morbidity and mortality due to resistant infection can reach beyond individual healthcare systems into broader public health frameworks. Unwarranted levels of antimicrobial resistance not only place a strain on hospital budgets but also complicate patient treatment. Optimizing interventions on prescribing behavior for antibiotics is thus required in order to avert the emergence of resistance and improve patient outcomes. In nations with exceedingly high levels of resistance, , such as Malta, collaboration among stakeholders is essential in order to maximize implementation of potent interventions towards the curtailment of transmission of multi-resistant organisms. This necessitates that healthcare practitioners become actively involved in promoting compliance with guidelines and optimal practice (Borg, 2009). Also, the challenge of discovering new antibiotic drugs and new treatments is continuous. Current treatment strategies must keep pace with the constantly evolving environment of bacterial resistance. The development pipeline for new antibiotics lags behind the development pace at which resistance is occurring, producing an ever-widening therapeutic gap. New approaches, such as bacteriophage therapy, immunotherapeutics, and promising vaccines are being developed as adjuncts to traditional antibiotics. Combination therapy is also becoming popular, which has the potential to enhance efficacy against resistant bacteria. While the medical community is challenged to confront Gram-negative bacilli infections and antibiotic resistance alike, the common bond of a commitment to novel, state-of-the-art approaches will be central to preserving the effectiveness of antibiotic therapy and upholding public health (Figure 9.11).

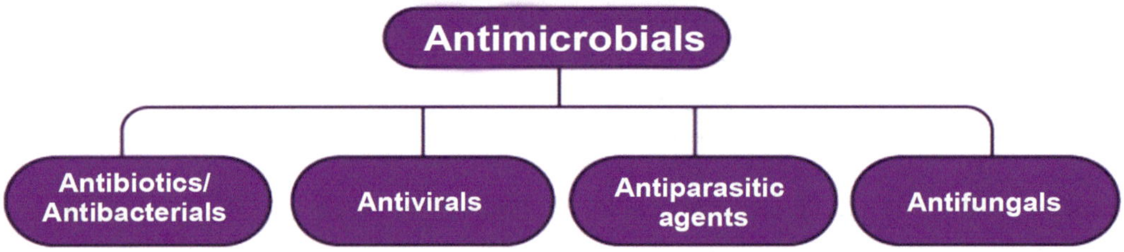

Figure 9.11. Antimicrobials.

Source: https://cdn1.byjus.com/wp-content/uploads/2018/07/Antimicrobial-Agents-700x224.png.

9.5.2. Role of Vaccines in Prevention

Vaccines play a crucial role in the prevention of Gram-negative bacillary infections, which are a polyphyletic collection of bacteria that comprise notorious pathogens, such as *Escherichia coli* and Klebsiella pneumoniae. The emerging increase in antibiotic resistance among these pathogens necessitates effective prevention. Vaccination offers a critical approach to boost immunity against specific Gram-negative infections, thus reducing disease incidence. For example, vaccines that are formulated to tackle bacterial components, , such as polysaccharide capsules, have been found to be effective in the induction of protective antibody responses, which prevent serious infection.

Thus, promotion of large-scale vaccination can contribute to the restriction of the spread of these bacteria, ultimately contributing to public health in the reduction of the danger caused by antibiotic-resistant infections that have become an emerging global problem. The development and implementation of vaccines against Gram-negative bacilli require careful consideration of the unique pathogenic strategies employed by these bacteria. Research has revealed that many of these pathogens can evade host defenses, complicating vaccine efficacy. For example, the variability in surface antigens necessitates the formulation of vaccines that can elicit broad-spectrum immune responses. Additionally, the immunocompromised status of patients, , such as liver transplant recipients, presents a unique challenge where the immune response to vaccinations may be impaired (2011 Group AST et al., 2013).

This particularly highlights the importance of targeted vaccination strategies that not only consider the general population but also the risk populations. Therefore, an individualized approach in vaccine production and delivery can achieve a maximum protective benefit, granting vulnerable segments adequate protection from these powerful pathogens. Researcher-public health provider partnerships have to unite to ensure the maximum effect of Gram-negative *Bacillus* vaccination campaigns.

Regular tracking of infection patterns and antibiotic resistance development is crucial (Lillestolen et al., 2018). This data can inform immunization policies, with an eye towards making them congruent with existing epidemiological trends. Educational and sensitization campaigns can also facilitate increased immunization acceptance, bypassing reluctance that can hinder public health progress. The integration of vaccines into routine medical practices also points to the potential for prevention of Gram-negative *Bacillus* infection complications. By prioritizing vaccination as an approach to prevention, the healthcare industry can help minimize the impacts of these bacteria and eventually see improved health results at the individual and population levels (Figure 9.12).

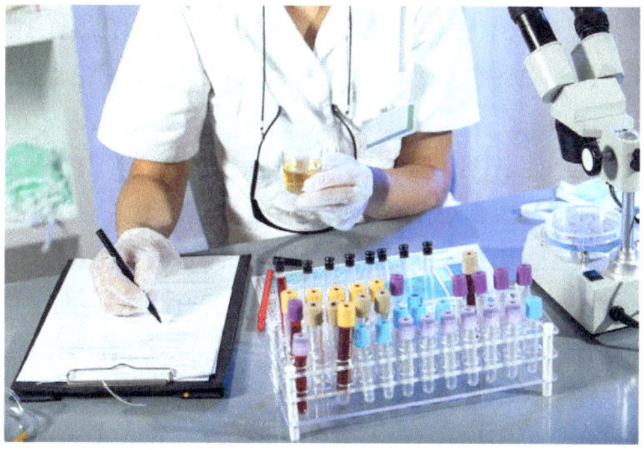

Figure 9.12. Role of vaccines in prevention.

Source: https://www.cidrap.umn.edu/sites/default/files/lab_tech_urinalysis_0.jpg.

9.5.3. Importance of Infection Control Measures

Infection control measures are crucial in avoiding the spread of Gram-negative bacilli, a significant threat to public health. The bacteria are often resistant to antibiotics and are known to cause severe infections, particularly in at-risk populations , such as immunocompromised patients and those with hospital admission. Strict infection control measures, including hand hygiene, proper utilization of personal protective equipment (PPE), and environmental cleaning, are critical within health institutions. For instance, there was a study that noted the rate of bacterial contamination in blood transfusion, where 2.8% of the blood bags were contaminated and skin-associated organisms predominated (Malimu, 2012). The above findings indicate the requirement of effective infection control protocols for ensuring patient safety and reducing the risk of nosocomial infections. Effective infection control extends beyond the healthcare environment into community centers, where education and sensitization are major determinants. Public education campaigns that make individuals aware of the importance of hygiene, immunization, and food preparation safety can considerably lower incidences of infection caused by Gram-negative bacilli. With their potential to cause outbreaks, , such as in the case of enteric pathogens in contaminated food or water sources, prevention has to be done actively. Furthermore, the heterogenic skin microbiota of the human being, including Gram-negative bacteria, necessitates the need for sustained observation and intervention activities (Gall & Riely, 1965). Via the cultivation of a culture of responsibility and awareness of infection control, communities can effectively prevent the transmission of such pathogens. Lastly, the role of research to what is known about Gram-negative bacilli cannot be overlooked. Studies that examine the antimicrobial resistance pattern and points of contamination play an imperative part in enhancing infection control policy. A good example is delineating the process through which such bacteria develop resistance to treatment as a premise for enhancing antibiotic stewardship practice and the creation of new therapeutic strategies. As evidenced by blood transfusion centers, countering contamination risks entails a multi-pronged approach based on research information and practical adjustments to ensure patients' health. In summary, the importance of infection control precautions in the handling of Gram-negative bacilli cannot be overstated because they are an important factor in preventing both individual patients and the general public from serious health dangers.

Test Your Knowledge

1. What classes of antibiotics are commonly used to treat infections caused by Gram-negative bacilli?
2. Are there any effective vaccines available for preventing infections caused by Gram-negative bacilli?

9.6. Current Research and Developments

Learning Outcome

1. Focus on advances in understanding Gram-negative Bacilli
2. Discuss new therapeutic approaches in the prevalence of antibiotic-resistant Gram-negative bacilli
3. Understand emerging strains and public health implications

Recent research has greatly assisted in enhancing our understanding of the ecological dynamics of Gram-negative bacilli, particularly in the constrained environment of the International Space Station (ISS). ISS is a unique environment in which both microbial interactions and behavior are influenced by parameters , such as microgravity and constrained spatial capacity. The environment offers means for researchers to observe the potential health impacts and functions that Gram-negative bacilli can take, both beneficial and disease-causing, on crew members. Rodgers (1986) identifies the necessity to track microbial populations, calling into focus ecological studies capable of leading to beneficial environmental control measures. This research not only has implications for the health of astronauts but to our overall knowledge base about microbial ecology in extreme environments, with possibilities of new strategies to manage microbial threats in multi-environments. In clinical settings, Gram-negative bacilli have emerged as the foremost pathogens, particularly with ventilator-associated pneumonia (VAP). The rising incidence of multidrug-resistant Gram-negative bacilli (MDR-GNB) has prompted an immediate re-evaluation of empiric guideline recommendations on the basis of the association between related morbidity and mortality. Recent evidence suggests that inappropriately administered antimicrobials are linked with higher mortality, making the need for targeted intervention critical. Recent investigations, including the MagicBullet trial, seek to equate the efficacy of colistin with that of traditional antibiotics like meropenem in treating late-onset VAP caused by MDR-GNB. This research is invaluable with the emerging antibiotic resistance patterns given its promise in establishing more specific standards for effective treatment protocols during shifting microbial resistance patterns. (Rosso et al., 2015) also identifies the trial's potential of recasting therapeutic paradigms for the treatment of life-threatening infections due to resistant pathogens. Additionally, the convergence of state-of-the-art research and microbiology offers positive directions towards fighting Gram-negative bacteria. One of such areas of investigation is the creation of new antimicrobial drugs and other therapeutic options to increase the effectiveness of treatment. New technologies, like bacteriophage therapy application, are attracting attention as possible solutions against chronic Gram-negative bacilli infections. These options have the potential to augment currently available antibiotics and offer a strategic advantage in resistance prevention. Investigators are encouraging the combined strategy that involves both the older and newer therapy modalities, stressing the importance of judicious use of antibiotics. Continued interdisciplinary collaboration between scientific disciplines and clinical practice will be important in advancing our understanding of Gram-negative bacilli and in offering effective management strategies in the future.

9.6.1. Advances in Understanding Gram-negative Bacilli

Recent advances in the science of Gram-negative bacilli have fostered a sophisticated understanding of their biology and significance to human health. The double membrane structure of these bacteria contributes to their antibiotic resistance and host immune defense evasion. Research has elucidated the intricate mechanism of their outer membranes' permeability, with the selective transfer of molecules behind an impenetrable barrier against harmful agents. Among the striking dangers of Gram-negative bacilli is that they can easily mutate and horizontally transfer genes, thereby becoming more flexible and virulent in varied environments. This evolving awareness underscores the urgency of focused research to unravel the genetic and biochemical processes responsible for antibiotic resistance, particularly against the background of the rise of infections worldwide. The increase in antibiotic resistance in Gram-negative bacilli represents a significant public health concern. Misuse and overuse of broad-spectrum antibiotics, as documented in the healthcare setting, have led to a staggering rise in resistant strains. It is reported by (Lillestolen et al., 2018) that the virulence and survival potential of some Gram-negative bacilli are extremely responsible due to their ability to transfer and acquire resistance genes. Besides, the impact of such resistant strains extends beyond individuals' health to healthcare systems and economies. For instance, infection treatment caused by drug-resistant bacteria typically requires more expensive and intensive care, extending hospitalization and increasing morbidity and mortality risks. This situation highlights the requirement for novel solutions , such as the development of new antibiotics and other therapeutic strategies aimed at the atypical biology of Gram-negative bacilli. Clinical significance of Gram-negative bacilli has increasingly become more keenly appreciated as these microbes are increasingly being identified as etiologies of severe infections, most of which afflict the pulmonary system. Current research indicates an increase in prevalence of respiratory infections due to these pathogens, documenting a disconcerting trend that needs to be addressed immediately by the medical fraternity (leo et al., 2015). The biofilm production capacity and the intrinsic virulence determinants of Gram-negative bacilli render them pathogenic, turning them into potent nosocomial infection agents. To overcome these issues, interdisciplinary solutions have to integrate microbiology, pharmacology, and clinical practice. Sophisticated surveillance and scrupulous examination of the interactions of Gram-negative bacilli are crucial to the design of effective prevention and treatment strategies. With the scientific community grappling with these new threats, the search for innovative solutions continues to be imperative in safeguarding public health and mitigating the global infectious disease burden (Figure 9.13).

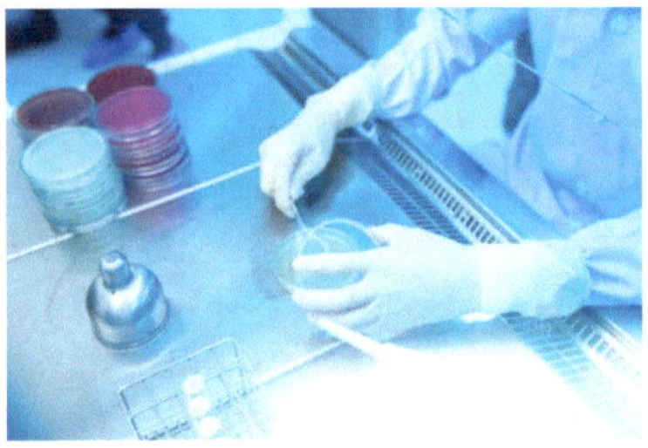

Figure 9.13. Advances in understanding Gram-negative bacilli.

Source: https://www.shutterstock.com/image-photo/hands-scientists-working-on-researchbacteria-260nw-1607717497.jpg.

9.6.2. New Therapeutic Approaches

The increased incidence of antibiotic-resistant Gram-negative bacilli necessitated the quest for new therapeutic approaches. Traditional antibiotics are incapable of treating infections with multiresistant microbes, which has resulted in the demand for new approaches that can effectively combat such microbes. Some of the strategies involve the use of new antimicrobial agents, including the utilization of bacteriophage therapy, where viruses that invade and kill bacterial cells exclusively are used. This activity not only reduces the prevalence of pathogenic bacteria but also reduces the collateral damage to good microbiota, maintaining a healthier equilibrium in the host. Furthermore, application of phage therapy along with routine antibiotics would amplify the therapeutic effect and make it easier to overcome mechanisms of resistance, a significant step ahead in the management of Gram-negative bacterial infections, particularly those with dismal clinical features, because the aforementioned high infection rates among renal transplant patients under immunosuppressive therapy fully attest (Marchioro et al., 1964). Aside from bacteriophage treatment, another possible avenue for the therapy of Gram-negative bacillary chronic infections is through the design of biofilm inhibitors. Biofilms constitute a matrix community of bacteria on a surface and are a significant problem in therapeutic control of infection because of their resistance to elimination, delayed healing, and persistent pathogenicity. With a substantial percentage of multidrug-resistant organisms that are capable of forming biofilms, as seen through clinical isolates, preventing biofilm-associated pathways can reduce infection complications (Bordignon et al., 2017). Various compounds, including targeted enzymes and surfactants, have been seen in recent research to interfere with the biofilm structures, thereby enhancing the penetration of antimicrobial agents. These advances have a dual advantage: not only do they increase the efficacy of current antibiotics, but they also offer a new measure against the virulence of Gram-negative bacilli, which is essential in clinical practice. Another innovative method being investigated in the case of infection caused by Gram-negative bacilli is immunotherapy. This method aims to build the immune response of the hosts against infections caused by bacteria, basically equipping the body to combat infections that may not be treated well by conventional therapies. By using monoclonal antibodies that specifically bind to virulence factors in Gram-negative bacteria, like lipopolysaccharides on their cell wall, researchers aim to render these microorganisms susceptible to the normal protective mechanisms of the immune system. In addition, vaccines specifically produced against each strain would guarantee the prevention of infection before it even happens, particularly among susceptible populations , such as immunocompromised patients undergoing renal transplants. The combination of immunotherapeutic methods with existing treatments not only guarantees the fight against existing infections but also assures the containment of the development of antibiotic resistance, hence ensuring an all-around strategy in treating Gram-negative bacilli infection.

9.6.3. Emerging Strains and Public Health Implications

The emergence of new Gram-negative bacilli strains has important public health consequences, particularly in terms of heightened antibiotic resistance. Gram-negative bacteria , such as *Escherichia coli* and Klebsiella pneumoniae have acquired resistance to common antibiotics, thereby complicating their treatment for health professionals. In addition to causing more morbidity and mortality, the resistance heightens hospital stay and healthcare cost. In the context of a rapidly aging population and rising incidence of chronic disease, the impact of these new strains is enhanced, with most at risk being high-risk patient populations. Generation of new therapeutic strategies and implementation of effective infection control measures are therefore most needed to manage these multidrug-resistant bacteria. Among the most dramatic examples of newly emerging strains' scale is the solid organ transplant transmission of *Francisella tularensis*, which exemplifies the interconnectedness of infectious disease and public health. Organ donors themselves infected but undiagnosed have been shown to unknowingly transfer fatal pathogens onto their recipients, with a variety of severe outcomes, including mortality. In July 2017, a donor organ transplant from a hospitalized patient who was subsequently diagnosed with tularemia resulted in fever and sepsis in some of the recipients, calling for effective donor screening protocols to be applied as quickly as possible. Involvement of these strains necessitates joint action by clinicians and public health authorities to ensure that donors are rigorously screened to prevent repetition of such events, thus protecting recipients against life-threatening infections (Annambhotla et al., 2019). Future studies on the role of the gut microbiota in contributing to pathogenesis in Gram-negative bacilli infection are needed in order to achieve the universal implications for public health. Specifically, changes in the bile microbiota were determined to have an effect on patient outcomes in patients with biliary tract and pancreatic diseases. Importantly, certain bacteria like K. pneumoniae and *E. coli* were linked with survival in malignancies of these regions. As these organisms have been found to be highly resistant to more than one class of drugs, their prevalence also underscores the utmost importance of effective surveillance and high-speed detection methods. Targeting the bile microbiota can provide a gateway to new preventive therapies that specifically target future-emerging infections, thereby enhancing outcomes for at-risk populations (Di Carlo et al., 2019).

Test Your Knowledge

1. What recent discoveries have enhanced our understanding of the mechanisms by which Gram-negative bacilli evade host immune responses?
2. What novel antimicrobial agents or combination therapies are currently being developed to combat multidrug-resistant Gram-negative bacilli?

SUMMARY

The pathogenesis of Gram-negative bacilli has a significant clinical and public health impact. Proper identification and acquaintance with these bacteria are essential in diagnosing various infections, particularly in high-risk populations , such as hospitals. Notably, the study on cervico-facial sepsis showed inconsistency in results between Gram stain and culture, challenging the efficacy of traditional diagnostic methods. The findings indicated that while a high percentage of specimens might reveal Gram-negative staining, it does not necessarily indicate the existence of viable Gram-negative organisms upon culture (Barnard, 2019). Such a discrepancy highlights that more research and better diagnostic techniques are needed to further enhance the reliability of clinical diagnosis. In addition, such implications extend beyond immediate clinical settings. Identification of Gram-negative bacilli and their activity is necessary in developing treatment options as well as infection control procedures. In the study population, the low recovery rate of Gram-negative bacteria from cultures despite having high Gram-negative staining rates suggests that anaerobic conditions may play an important role in the pathogenicity of the bacteria (Barnard, 2019). This necessitates a closer look at the conditions under which Gram-negative bacilli are capable of survival and propagation in clinical environments, requiring a rethinking of existing diagnosis methods that will disregard these concerns. Ultimately, findings from such an investigation of Gram-negative bacilli highlight the necessity of interdisciplinarity in the treatment of multifaceted infections. Scientists, microbiologists, and clinicians must come together and exchange information and forge comprehensive guidelines in an effort to recognize and combat these pathogens. Against the backdrop of unrelenting antibiotic resistance that has been observed in the majority of Gram-negative bacteria, the importance of new treatment and preventive strategies cannot be overstated. Future studies will aim to integrate emerging technologies, , such as molecular diagnostics, to increase detection rates and results, consequently resulting in better patient care and public health programs. As the epidemiology of infectious diseases continues evolving, collaboration is essential to tackle challenges posed by Gram-negative bacilli. The study of Gram-negative bacilli reveals critical details of their impact on various industries, especially food safety and medicine. Specifically, the bacteria are the major spoilers for meat, and the issue poses meat industries with challenges that results in economic loss as well as decreased consumer confidence. *Pseudomonas* species are the major refrigeration and aerobic spoilers, which encourages researchers to study their gene expression profiles. Understanding the differential expression of genes in *Pseudomonas* putida according to varied temperatures and glucose concentrations uncovers the complexity of how it survives and adapts, which indicates a strong ability to survive even in adverse conditions and complicates meat preservation. Hence, Gram-negative bacilli analysis not only illustrates how they spoilage but also demands innovative measures to encourage food safety within the meat market (Aarts et al., 2015). In clinical practice, the importance of Gram-negative bacilli is again emphasized in the management of wounds, namely under negative pressure wound therapy (NPWT). It has been discovered in studies that NPWT has an impact on the bacterial load in the wound environment, but findings present a multifaceted picture. Certain studies have demonstrated that NPWT is bacteriostatic, but there exists species selectivity, which may suppress the growth of non-fermentive Gram-negative bacilli, like *Pseudomonas* spp. The suppression may, however, allow for the growth of Gram-positive cocci, possibly leading to wound healing complications. The knowledge of NPWTs selective action emphasizes the importance of why bacterial kinetics in wound healing must be comprehended and raises doubt regarding the therapy duration and dressing regimens in the face of highly virulent bacteria (Glass et al., 2017).

The convergence of food safety and healthcare constitutes a long-standing challenge in combating Gram-negative bacilli proliferation. As researchers continue to investigate the ecological and genetic niches of these bacteria in food production and clinical settings, there may eventually emerge an integrated picture that will guide future interventions. The implications of the research suggest a need to continue investigating the ways that environmental conditions, , such as packaging and storage in food or treatment modalities for wounds, impact bacterial behavior and resistance. From research on Gram-negative *Bacillis* resilience and responses to various treatments, it is increasingly clear that effective control measures need to incorporate knowledge from the meat industry and medical practice to combat the dangers presented by these robust organisms.

KEY TERMS FROM THIS CHAPTER

Antibiotic susceptibility
Bacterial species
Biofilm formations
Cervico-facial sepsis
Food systems
Gram-negative bacilli
Health institutions
Horizontal gene transfer
Immunosuppressive therapy
Infection scenarios
Bacterial persistence
Bacteriophage therapy
Broad-spectrum antibiotics
Drug-resistant
Foodborne disease
Gram-negative organisms
Healthcare-associated infections
Host immune responses
Immunotherapeutics
Laboratory identification techniques

CRITICAL THINKING QUESTIONS

1. **Which of the following is a characteristic feature of Gram-negative bacilli?**
   a. Thick peptidoglycan layer
   b. Teichoic acids in the cell wall
   c. Outer membrane containing lipopolysaccharide (LPS)
   d. Absence of periplasmic space
2. **Which of the following organisms is a non-lactose fermenting Gram-negative bacillus?**
   a. *Escherichia coli*
   b. *Salmonella* enterica
   c. Klebsiella pneumoniae
   d. Enterobacter cloacae
3. **What is the primary virulence factor of *Escherichia coli* in causing urinary tract infections (UTIs)?**
   a. Capsule production
   b. Endotoxin production
   c. P fimbriae (adhesins)
   d. Beta-lactamase enzyme
4. **Which laboratory test is most useful in differentiating between lactose-fermenting and non-lactose-fermenting Gram-negative bacilli?**
   a. MacConkey agar culture
   b. Catalase test
   c. Oxidase test
   d. Coagulase test
5. **Which of the following antibiotics is commonly used to treat infections caused by extended-spectrum beta-lactamase (ESBL) producing Gram-negative bacilli?**
   a. Amoxicillin
   b. Ceftriaxone
   c. Erythromycin
   d. Meropenem

Short Answer Questions

1. What are the key structural characteristics that distinguish Gram-negative bacilli from Gram-positive bacteria?
2. What are the major families and genera of Gram-negative bacilli, and how are they classified based on oxygen requirements and metabolic activity?
3. How does the lipopolysaccharide (LPS) component of Gram-negative bacilli contribute to their pathogenicity and clinical manifestations , such as sepsis?
4. Compare the pathogenic mechanisms and typical diseases caused by *Escherichia coli*, Klebsiella pneumoniae, *Salmonella* spp., and *Pseudomonas aeruginosa*.
5. What are the primary laboratory techniques used to identify Gram-negative bacilli in clinical specimens?
6. How do extended-spectrum beta-lactamases (ESBLs) and carbapenemases affect the treatment of infections caused by Gram-negative bacilli?

Answers to Critical Thinking Questions

1. (c) 2. (b) 3. (c) 4. (a) 5. (d)

REFERENCES

1. Aarts, H., Cauchi, M., Doulgeraki, A. I., et al. (2015). Identification of meat spoilage gene biomarkers in *Pseudomonas putida* using gene profiling. https://core.ac.uk/download/74410385.pdf (accessed on 13th June 2025).
2. Abdelaziz, M., Bashir, T., Hamadalnil, Y., Abdelkhalig, M., et al. (2022). Bloodstream infection in cancer patients; susceptibility profiles of the isolated pathogens, at Khartoum Oncology Hospital, Sudan. https://core.ac.uk/download/552647155.pdf (accessed on 13th June 2025).
3. Di Carlo, P., Serra, N., D'Arpa, F., Agrusa, A., Gulotta, G., Fasciana, T., Rodolico, V., Giammanco, A., & Sergi, C. (2019). The microbiota of the bilio-pancreatic system: a cohort, STROBE-compliant study. *Infection and drug resistance*, *12*, 1513–1527. https://doi.org/10.2147/IDR.S200378 (accessed on 13th June 2025).
4. Akça, E., Claus, H., Debaerdemaeker, T., et al. (2005). Molecular organization of selected prokaryotic S-layer proteins. http://orbi.ulg.ac.be/bitstream/2268/57472/1/Claus05-CanJMicrobiolPP.pdf (accessed on 13th June 2025).
5. Annambhotla, P., Asad, S., Aslam, S., Basavaraju, et al. (2019). *Francisella tularensis* transmission by solid organ transplantation, 2017. https://core.ac.uk/download/323070878.pdf (accessed on 13th June 2025).
6. Ariza Cardenal, J., Bahamonde, A., Baraia Etxaburu, J., Benito Hernández, et al. (2019). The different microbial etiology of prosthetic joint infections according to route of acquisition and time after prosthesis implantation, including the role of multidrug-resistant organisms. https://core.ac.uk/download/344893862.pdf (accessed on 13th June 2025).
7. Barnard, N. (2019). Prevalence of gram-negativeGram-negative infections in cervical-facial sepsis. A mini-thesis submitted for fulfilling the requirements for the Degree of Magister Chirurgiae Dentium in the discipline of Maxillo-Facial and Oral Surgery, . A mini-thesis submitted for fulfilling the requirements for the Degree of Magister Chirurgiae Dentium in the discipline of Maxillo-Facial and Oral Surgery, Faculty of Dentistry, University of the Western Cape. Supervisor: Dr A.J. van der Westhuijzen June 2019. https://core.ac.uk/download/289120726.pdf (accessed on 13th June 2025).
8. Barnes, H. J., Basher, H. A., Fonnesbech Vogel, B., Gitter, M., Ivanics, E., Lucas, A., McDiarmid, A., et al. (2015). Outbreak of encephalitic listeriosis in red-legged partridges (*Alectoris rufa*). https://core.ac.uk/download/36778157.pdf (accessed on 13th June 2025).
9. Bordignon, V., Cavallo, I., Cilli, L., et al. (2017). Biofilm is a major virulence determinant in bacterial colonization of chronic skin ulcers independently from the multidrug resistant phenotype. https://core.ac.uk/download/188832167.pdf (accessed on 13th June 2025).
10. Borg, M. A. (2009). Addressing the challenge of antibiotic resistance in Maltese healthcare settings. Malta Medical Journal Volume 21 Issue 02 June 2009 https://core.ac.uk/download/46602217.pdf (accessed on 13th June 2025).
11. Bruun, B., Hansen, D. S., Jensen, A. G., et al. (2002). Direct identification and susceptibility testing of enteric bacilli from positive blood cultures using VITEK (GNI+/GNS-GA). https://core.ac.uk/download/pdf/81114168.pdf (accessed on 13th June 2025).
12. Burnham, C. A. D., Marshall, C., Mathias, E., et al. (2016). Culture of urine specimens by use of chromID CPS Elite medium can expedite *Escherichia coli* identification and reduce hands-

on time in the clinical laboratory. https://core.ac.uk/download/70385855.pdf (accessed on 13th June 2025).

13. Camargo, A. F., da Silva, F. O., & Treichel, H. (2024). Thermotolerant coliform bacteria present in water bodies. https://core.ac.uk/download/611862109.pdf (accessed on 13th June 2025).
14. Cavalieri, D., Godaly, G., Hagberg, L., Hedges, S., Schappert, T., & Shahin, R. (2016). Subversion of host innate immunity by uropathogenic *Escherichia coli*. https://core.ac.uk/download/80494906.pdf (accessed on 13th June 2025).
15. Chang, P. K., Diaz, J. J., Jr., Huston, J. M., et al. (2017). The Surgical Infection Society revised guidelines on the management of intra-abdominal infection. https://core.ac.uk/download/74358329.pdf (accessed on 13th June 2025).
16. Decicco, B. T. (2025). Effects of mutation and some environmental factors on the physiology and pathogenicity of selected bacteria. https://core.ac.uk/download/pdf/42895589.pdf (accessed on 13th June 2025).
17. Dhanasekaran, D., Panneerselvam, A., Rajalakshmi, M., et al. (2010). Probiotic effect of *Lactobacillus* isolates against bacterial pathogens in freshwater fish. https://media.neliti.com/media/publications/92454-EN-probiotic-effect-of-lactobacillus-isolat.pdf (accessed on 13th June 2025).
18. Drzewiecka, D., Kwil, I., Maszewska, A., Moryl, M., Ostrowska, K., et al. (2013). *Proteus* sp.–An opportunistic bacterial pathogen–classification, swarming growth, clinical significance and virulence factors. https://core.ac.uk/download/71976791.pdf (accessed on 13th June 2025).
19. Elmanama, A. A. (2007). *Diagnostic Medical Microbiology*. https://core.ac.uk/download/385924572.pdf (accessed on 13th June 2025).
20. Gall, L. S., & Riely, P. E. (2025). *Effect of Diet and Atmosphere on Intestinal and Skin Flora. Volume II–Literature Survey*. https://core.ac.uk/download/pdf/85249155.pdf (accessed on 13th June 2025).
21. Gilbert, J. A., Groer, M. W., Ho, T. T. B., et al. (2018). Dichotomous development of the gut microbiome in preterm infants. https://core.ac.uk/download/323064612.pdf (accessed on 13th June 2025).
22. Glass, G., Murphy, G. R. F., & Nanchahal, J. (2017). Does negative pressure wound therapy influence subjacent bacterial growth? A systematic review. https://core.ac.uk/download/346541612.pdf (accessed on 13th June 2025).
23. Kante, M., Muni Lakshmi, P., & Sreenivasulu Reddy, P. (2017). Bacterial profile of bloodstream infections and their antibiograms. https://core.ac.uk/download/539910262.pdf (accessed on 13th June 2025).
24. Leo, B. F., López-Heras, M., Porter, A. E., et al. (2015). Towards understanding the antibacterial activity of Ag nanoparticles: Electron microscopy in the analysis of the materials-biology interface in the lung. https://core.ac.uk/download/77002723.pdf (accessed on 13th June 2025).
25. Lillestolen, D. (2018). *Infections Not Fought: Antibiotic Resistance in Underserved Communities*. https://core.ac.uk/download/158970352.pdf (accessed on 13th June 2025).
26. Vervier, K., et al. (2015). Benchmark of structured machine learning methods for microbial identification from mass-spectrometry data. http://arxiv.org/abs/1506.07251 (accessed on 13th June 2025).

27. Maldonado, N. C., Nader, M. E. F., & Silva de Ruíz, C. (2015). *"In vitro"* evaluation of some properties in spore former bacteria isolated from calves' faces. https://core.ac.uk/download/159301332.pdf (accessed on 13th June 2025).

28. Malimu, E. Z. (2012). The prevalence of bacterial contamination in donated blood in Dar es Salaam, Tanzania. https://core.ac.uk/download/pdf/16666702.pdf (accessed on 13th June 2025).

29. Marchioro, T. L., Rifkind, D., Starzl, T. E., et al. (1964). Infectious diseases associated with renal homotransplantation: I. Incidence, types, and predisposing factors. https://core.ac.uk/download/12203488.pdf (accessed on 13th June 2025).

30. Mthembu, Wendy & Penduka, Dambudzo & Mosa, Rebamang & Shoba, Bonginkosi & Zobolo, A & Opoku, A. (2017). The bacteria profiles of wounds in diabetic patients hospitalized in northern Kwazulu-Natal, South Africa. African Journal of Clinical and Experimental Microbiology. 18. 186. 10.4314/ajcem.v18i4.2. (accessed on 13th June 2025).

31. Nagendra, M., & Trivedi, M. S. (2023). Characteristics of blood infections and phenotypic detection of extended-spectrum β-lactamases in ICU patients in Central India posing a challenge. https://core.ac.uk/download/560706615.pdf (accessed on 13th June 2025).

32. Rodgers, E. B. (1986). *The Ecology of Microorganisms in A Small Closed System: Potential Benefits and Problems for Space Station.* Document ID

33. 19870003733, Acquisition Source, Legacy CDMS, Document Type

34. Technical Memorandum (TM)

35. https://core.ac.uk/download/pdf/42839143.pdf (accessed on 13th June 2025).

36. Rosso, C., Fernández, D. E., De Blasi, R. A., Dimopoulos, G., Garnacho, J., et al. (2015). Safety and efficacy of colistin versus meropenem in the empirical treatment of ventilator-associated pneumonia as part of a macro-project funded by the Seventh Framework Program of the European Commission studying off-patent antibiotics: Study protocol for a randomized controlled trial. https://core.ac.uk/download/74318469.pdf (accessed on 13th June 2025).

37. Stabler, R. A., Larsson, J. T., Al-Jaberi, S., Nielsen, E. M., Kay, E., Tam, C. C., Higgins, C. D., Rodrigues, L. C., Richardson, J. F., O'Brien, S. J., & Wren, B. W. (2013). Characterization of water and wildlife strains as a subgroup of *Campylobacter jejuni* using DNA microarrays. *Environmental Microbiology, 15*(8), 2371–2383. https://doi.org/10.1111/1462-2920.12111 (accessed on 13th June 2025).

38. Sweeney, F. P., Courtenay, O., Hibberd, V., et al. (1999). Environmental monitoring of *Mycobacterium bovis* in badger feces and badger sett soil by real-time PCR, as confirmed by immunofluorescence, immunocapture, and cultivation. https://core.ac.uk/download/pdf/44292.pdf (accessed on 13th June 2025).

39. Toro López, M. D. del. (2019). The different microbial etiology of prosthetic joint infections according to route of acquisition and time after prosthesis implantation, including the role of multidrug-resistant organisms. https://core.ac.uk/download/231995576.pdf (accessed on 13th June 2025).

ACID-FAST BACTERIA

10

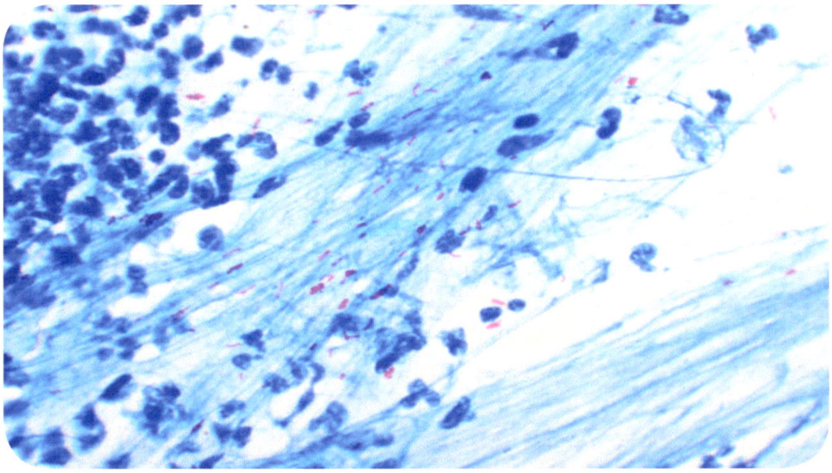

Introduction

The discussion of the topic of acid-fast bacteria paves the way to understanding their significance in microbiology and medicine. Acid-fast bacteria, particularly the genus Mycobacterium, are defined by their cell wall composition rich in lipid content, i.e., mycolic acids. In addition to affecting staining, the composition also confers resistance to environmental pressures and drugs. The determination of the distinctive structural features of acid-fast bacteria is critical in the design of appropriate diagnosis methods and treatment programs, primarily for conditions , such as tuberculosis (TB). Understanding these fundamental principles gives the foundation to discuss a comprehensive examination of their pathological and ecological roles and detection methods employed for their identification, which are critical for public health programs in disease control of TB and other mycobacterial infections. The most important principle of the detection and identification of acid-fast bacteria is the use of definite staining techniques. The traditional Ziehl-Neelsen staining technique highlights the unique features of

LEARNING OBJECTIVES

After studying this chapter, you will be able to:

1. Explain the characteristics of acid-fast bacteria
2. Describe major types of acid-fast bacteria
3. Deal with pathogenicity and disease association
4. Understand the diagnosis of acid-fast bacterial infections
5. Discuss about effective treatment and management of diseases caused by acid-fast bacteria
6. Focus on public health implications associated with acid-fast bacteria

the bacteria, enabling them to be distinguished from other microbial cells. The technique utilizes the waxy composition of the cell wall of mycobacteria, which retains the stain even through decolorization processes. Acid-fastness is thus an essential characteristic for clinical use, with clinicians being able to rapidly test for the presence of *Mycobacterium tuberculosis* in patients' samples. Further, advancements in molecular techniques and mass spectrometry, as reported in recent literature, hold promise for enhancing the diagnostic value above conventional methods (Szewczyk et al., 2013). This synergy of microbiological staining and advanced technology identifies the new face of TB diagnosis and reemphasizes the demand for ongoing investigation into acid-fast properties. The environmental and clinical implications of acid-fast bacteria extend well beyond the therapeutic consequences to involve issues of treatment resistance and infection control. Higher prevalence of multidrug-resistant *Mycobacterium tuberculosis* strains poses a significant risk to international health programs, indicative of the extreme need for new treatment and prevention programs. It has been established through research that the unique metabolic patterns and defense mechanisms employed by such bacteria facilitate their survival under stressful conditions, and hence they are challenging to eliminate (Bilcke et al., 2019). Understanding of these mechanisms not only informs the development of new therapeutic strategies but also public health policy and planning for TB control. The elegance of acid-fast organisms, therefore, is a crucial area of investigation in the grand picture of infectious diseases, requiring meticulous scrutiny in scientific as well as clinical settings.

Definition of Acid-Fast Bacteria

Acid-fast bacteria are a special group of microbes that are characterized by the specific cell structure and ability to stain. Acid-fast bacteria include such major pathogens as *Mycobacterium tuberculosis*, which causes tuberculosis. Acid-fast refers to the ability of the bacteria to retain dye upon treatment with acid-alcohol reagents after staining. This is due to their thickness and waxy cell wall that has mycolic acids. The traditional staining techniques, , such as the Gram stain, are not effective due to the rigidity of this cell wall, necessitating special staining techniques like the Ziehl-Neelsen stain. This method allows viewing acid-fast bacilli on microscopic analysis, hence it becomes feasible to determine these organisms from clinical samples. The unique structural characteristics of acid-fast bacteria reflect their ruggedness and their virulence, thus their significance in microbiological studies. The taxonomic assignment of acid-fast bacteria is largely under the genus Mycobacterium, including both pathogenic and non-pathogenic organisms. *Mycobacterium tuberculosis* remains the most clinically relevant member of this genus due to its prevalent health consequence to the general populace. In addition, leprosy is brought about by other species , such as *Mycobacterium leprae*, further relating to the public health importance of acid-fast bacteria. Importantly, *Mycobacterium avium* complex comprises non-tuberculous mycobacteria that can cause opportunistic infections, particularly among immunocompromised individuals. The diverse pathogenicity profiles of these bacteria require sophisticated knowledge about their mechanisms of infection. Later research also emphasizes the expanding roles of various mycobacteria in environmental contexts, and it has been suggested that these microorganisms may serve as indicators of the integrity of ecosystems primarily due to their varied metabolic capabilities and ability to interact with other organisms (Jones et al., 2012). The understanding of the definition and significance of acid-fast bacteria extends beyond their biological features to encompass their ecological and clinical roles. Their drug resistance poses both a challenge and a challenge area for microbiology and the prevention of infectious disease. For instance, the development of drug resistance in *Mycobacterium tuberculosis* necessitates ongoing research into new drugs and public health practices. Further, effective zoonotic acid-fast species management in animal populations highlights the importance of environmental reservoir infection surveillance, as evidenced by recent studies on Rhodococcus equi. Though associated mostly with equine infection, this bacterium calls for comprehensive strategies that integrate animal health, human health, and the environment (Jensen et al., 2012). Ultimately, studying the definition and relevance of acid-fast bacteria can reveal significant intersections between microbiology, medicine, and environmental health (Figure 10.1).

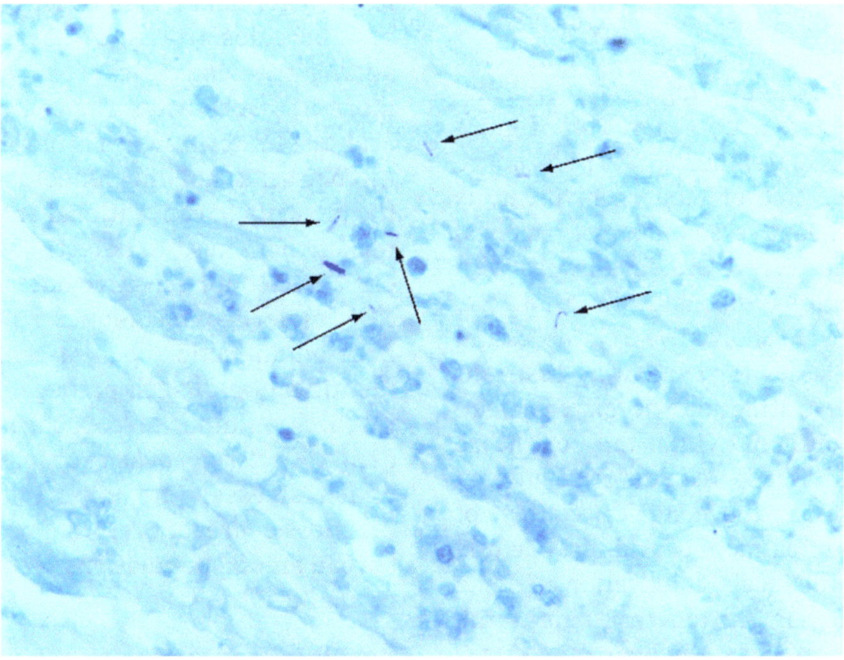

Figure 10.1. Red acid-fast bacteria (*Mycobacterium tuberculosis*) within the necrotic center of a granuloma.

Source: https://www.researchgate.net/profile/Krisada-Jongsakul/publication/49847442/figure/fig3/AS:667172879757330@1536077818728/Red-acid-fast-bacteria-Mycobacterium-tuberculosis-within-the-necrotic-center-of-a.png.

Historical Context and Discovery

Acid-fast bacteria identification, factoring in the detection of *Mycobacterium tuberculosis*, was a turning point in the history of microbiology as well as public health. Robert Koch isolated the TB-causing bacterium for the first time in 1882, which opened doors to modern bacteriology. His groundbreaking research not only provided a definitive etiological link between the disease and bacterium but also verified the germ theory of disease, revolutionizing the concept and treatment of infectious diseases. Koch's discoveries had tremendous implications in that they dictated specific public health interventions, ultimately leading in due course to guiding policies for the control of TB epidemics. Despite this revolutionary discovery over 120 years ago, TB continues to be a major health issue across the globe today, further validating the enduring relevance of Koch's work to microbial pathology and public health procedures (Seral et al., 2023).

Following Koch's initial discovery, understanding of acid-fast bacteria expanded exponentially in the 20th century, particularly through the introduction of antibiotic therapy. The emergence of the antibiotic streptomycin in the 1940s provided a novel treatment for TB, promising relief to those who had suffered from this killer disease for many years. Subsequent development of drug-resistant *Mycobacterium tuberculosis* strains eventually caused a dramatic turnaround on the clinical stage, and increasing mortality necessitated the generation of more complex regimens of treatment. This persistence of TB during the time of modern medicine is evidence of the adaptive character of bacterial resistance and healthcare systems' issues with managing infectious diseases. In response, researchers turned to alternative treatments and new antibiotic classes for combating resistant bacteria, demonstrating the persistent need for innovative solutions within the healthcare sector (Seral et al., 2023). In addition to guiding therapeutic progress, the historical context of the discovery and treatment of acid-fast bacteria also reflects broader social implications. Stigma surrounding TB has shifted throughout the course of its history based on economic status and cultural attitudes toward disease. In the early 20th century, TB was often associated with low economic status and urban living, therefore contributing to the social exclusion of patients and misconceptions regarding contagion. By contrast, the latter half of the century was marked by increasing awareness and action in favor of patients, following the advances in treatment. Public health publicity for education of communities regarding prevention and treatment once more underlined the necessity to understand both the scientific and the social facets of TB. Thus, the history of *Mycobacterium tuberculosis* is a case study of how scientific evidence comes together with public opinion and health policy, emphasizing the need for an interdisciplinary approach to health issues (Sarhan et al., 2004).

Importance in Microbiology and Medicine

The significance of acid-fast bacteria in medicine and microbiology cannot be overemphasized, particularly with their application in the diagnosis and treatment of various infectious diseases. One of the most highlighted acid-fast bacteria is *Mycobacterium tuberculosis*, the causative agent of tuberculosis (TB), a disease that remains among the leading causes of morbidity and mortality worldwide. The cell wall structure of acid-fast bacteria, which is novel and made up of mycolic acids, not only renders them resistant to the majority of conventional antibiotics but also makes them hard to detect. This highlights the critical need for sensitive detection techniques. New molecular techniques , such as PCR and DNA amplification, play a critical role in the identification of such pathogens, as evident by research on other mycobacterial species , such as *Mycobacterium avium* subsp. Paratuberculosis which stresses the importance of accurate diagnostic procedures in preventing disease spread among populations of animals (Englund et al., 2002).

Acid-fast contribution to public and veterinary health is evident in that they produce outbreaks that may impact broader ecological and economic systems. In particular, *Mycobacterium avium* subsp. Paratuberculosis is implicated in Johne's disease of cattle, a disease that results in significant economic loss through decreased milk production and reproductive potential in infected herds. The complexity in the diagnosis of *M. paratuberculosis* necessitates the development of sensitive detection systems, which remain a challenge in veterinary practice. This also raises questions concerning zoonotic transmission, highlighting the link between animal health and human health. The implications of effective management of such infections extend beyond case-by-case; they extend to industry-level procedures and demonstrate the imperative for continued research and development of diagnostic methods to more effectively counter acid-fast bacteria risks (Englund et al., 2002). Further, academic investigation of acid-fast bacteria sheds light on ecological consequences and relationships within various environments, e.g., mycobacterial infection in fish populations, such as striped bass. Mycobacteriosis has been identified as a significant disease in these species, indicative of broader environmental and health issues in aquatic communities. These outbreaks remind researchers and public health professionals of the interconnectedness of species and the need to monitor and track health issues in one species that may have implications for other species or an ecosystem. The rising instances of mycobacterial infections in fish further underscore the importance of robust surveillance systems that detect and respond to outstanding infectious diseases. These are important initiatives, not just for maintaining biodiversity but also for informing clinical and ecological management to regulate acid-fast bacterial infections effectively.

10.1. Characteristics of Acid-Fast Bacteria

Learning Outcome

1. Describe cell wall structure and composition
2. Explain staining techniques
3. Understand the growth conditions of acid-fast bacteria

Acid-fast bacteria are characterized by their unique cell wall structure, which contributes significantly to their ability to withstand numerous environmental stresses, including drying, chemicals, and even phagocytosis. Mycolic acid is the primary cell wall component, a long-chain fatty acid that renders the bacteria resistant to Gram staining as well as to most antibiotics. Instead of the traditional Gram-positive or Gram-negative classification, these bacteria are identified by applying acid-fast staining techniques, i.e., the Ziehl-Neelsen stain. This distinctive characteristic brings forward the requirement of employing specialized detection strategies for the identification of such microbes in clinical and environmental isolates. An awareness of the structural properties of acid-fast bacteria not only aids in their recognition but also highlights their role in disease, most notably tuberculosis infection caused by *Mycobacterium tuberculosis*, the responsible bacterium. In addition to their structural resistance, acid-fast bacteria have a range of physiological characteristics that enhance virulence and survival. For instance, *Mycobacterium tuberculosis* and *Mycobacterium leprae*, belonging to the genus Mycobacterium, have adapted to survive within the hostile conditions of human host tissue. They are obligate aerobes, requiring oxygen for growth, indicative of the energy requirements of these organisms. Their rate of growth, although commonly cited to take weeks to months for replication, also makes treatment more difficult, since most antibiotics require actively growing cells to be effective. This disease necessitates a chronic course of treatment with specific drugs intended to counter the characteristic properties of acid-fast microbes, e.g., the ones that act by inhibiting cell wall synthesis or metabolic processes essential to their survival and virulence (Brady, 2023). Even the taxonomic intricacy of acid-fast bacteria is an area of special concern given its implications on identification, classification, and treatment. While Mycobacterium species are the most well-characterized members, the extended group also includes other genera , such as Nocardia and Rhodococcus, which are also acid-fast in nature. The genetic affinities within such groups of bacteria have been explained through newer studies using molecular phylogeny. For example, the analysis of Rhodococcus equi revealed its distinct phyletic clade that highlights the complex affinities among acid-fast bacteria (Jones et al., 2012). This taxonomic complexity lends emphasis to the need for more advanced microbial identification methods since they depend on a good understanding of genetic and phenotypic characteristics. Research thus persists in the area not just to enhance our comprehension of acid-fast bacteria but also to inform the development of improved diagnostic tools as well as therapy.

10.1.1. Cell Wall Structure and Composition

The cell wall structure of acid-fast bacteria, particularly those within the genus Mycobacterium, has a peculiar makeup that sets them apart from other bacteria. The unusual structure is largely characterized by the existence of mycolic acids; long fatty acids that are held accountable for cell wall hydrophobicity.

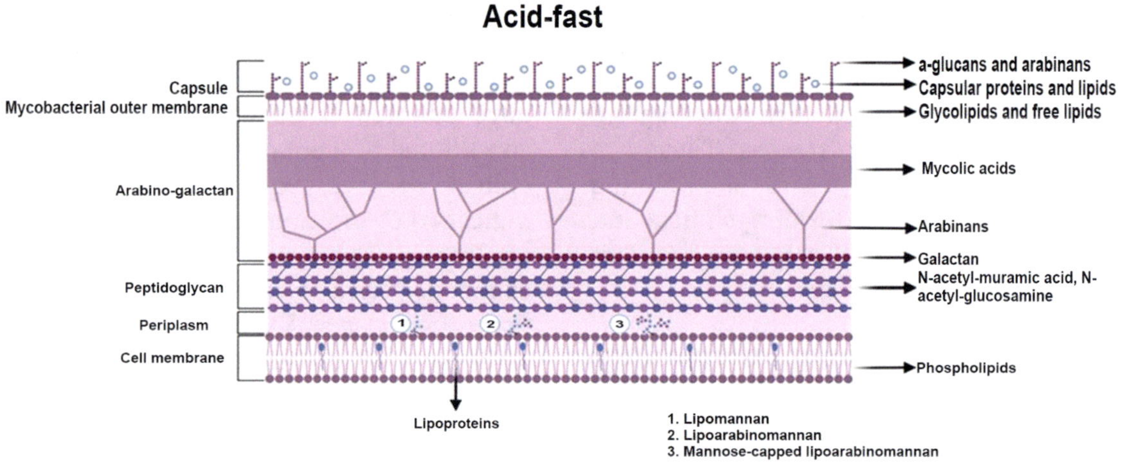

Figure 10.2. The cell wall of acid-fast bacteria.

Source: https://www.researchgate.net/publication/373812685/figure/fig2/AS:11431281209911504@1701919400151/The-cell-wall-of-acid-fast-bacteria-Created-with-BioRendercom-2023-3.png.

Such a make-up significantly enhances the resistance of acid-fast bacteria to external stress, including desiccation and antibiotic penetration. The intricate structure of these mycolic acids with peptidoglycan and other glycolipids plays a part in the formation of a waxy protective coating that is not only protective in nature but also efficient in playing a part in the virulence of these pathogens. The awareness of the specific structural details of the cell wall is hence required not just for understanding the acid-fast bacteria's biology but also for developing an effective therapeutic strategy. Further, the role of mycolic acids in the cell wall architecture is significant since they play a part in the virulence factors present in *Mycobacterium tuberculosis*, the etiologic agent of tuberculosis (TB). It has been observed from recent research that the unique patterns of mycolic acids can be accurately identified with advanced techniques , such as electrospray ionization tandem mass spectrometry. This method allows for the identification of various mycobacterial species accurately based on their unique fatty acid profiles. Profiling these molecules has provided a means for researchers to discriminate between *M. tuberculosis* and other mycobacterial species that are non-tuberculous, thereby allowing for early diagnosis. The ability to quickly and accurately identify mycobacterial species is significant in clinical practice, where intervention timing impacts patient outcome (Szewczyk et al., 2013). Furthermore, the architecture of the cell wall not only gives mechanical strength but also influences the diagnostic methods utilized for the detection of acid-fast bacteria. The presence of specific lipid structures in the cell wall can be utilized to design specific tests for the diagnosis of tuberculosis. For example, mycolic acid patterns have been found to enhance the sensitivity and specificity of tests for tuberculosis beyond the reach of routine practices, as demonstrated in studies. By refining these techniques, practitioners can achieve more rapid and uniform results and thereby improve patient management. As investigation advances further, focus on cell wall structure and composition will remain integral to the realization of the acid-fast bacteria pathogenicity and to the development of novel diagnostic approaches (Bai et al., 2013) (Figure 10.2).

10.1.2. Staining Techniques (e.g., Ziehl-Neelsen Stain)

In microbiology, staining processes are an important method of identifying and seeing bacteria, particularly those that are acid-fast. The Ziehl-Neelsen stain is one of the more widely known methods developed to specifically detect acid-fast bacilli, with *Mycobacterium tuberculosis* being the primary target. The method relies on the inherent property of the bacteria: that they resist acid decolorization when stained using a specific dye, usually carbol fuchsin. The process begins with application of the primary stain and permitting it to penetrate the waxy cell wall of the cell, followed by applying the heat to promote dye absorption. After proper staining, the specimen is treated with an acid-alcohol solution, which will dissolve the dye from the non-acid-fast organisms and leave behind only the acid-fast bacilli stained and visible. Such detail of the techniques is necessary for tuberculosis diagnosis, as this disease continues to be a significant public health problem. Closer observation of the Ziehl-Neelsen stain reveals that it can be differentiated in not just pulmonary tuberculosis but also extrapulmonary tuberculosis (EPTB), and demonstration of acid-fast bacilli is more challenging considering the smaller numbers found in various biopsy specimens. One paper emphasized the stain's utility, with a 26.1% positivity rate demonstrated in granulomatous inflammatory tissue biopsies, with variations depending on the anatomical site involved.

Pleural specimens, for instance, had an impressively high positivity rate of 35.2%, which indicates that while the sensitivity of the procedure may be limited, the utility of the stain in practice is still preserved, particularly in areas where sophisticated diagnostic techniques may not be readily available. Thus, the efficacy of Ziehl-Neelsen staining proves a key input towards confirming tuberculosis, specifically in a patient with a history of pulmonary infection, emphasizing the importance of prior medical history to the interpretation of results (Azarhoush et al., 2014). Also, beyond its routine diagnostic utility is the significance of the Ziehl-Neelsen stain in the policy of public health, where early and accurate detection of acid-fast bacilli can significantly influence interventions for disease control. Along with patient history, as encountered in the study outlined above, clinicians are better able to stratify risk appropriately and tailor treatment to those presenting with symptoms compatible with tuberculosis. In addition, developments in alternative staining techniques and rapid molecular diagnostic tests could augment, but not replace, the Ziehl-Neelsen stain, thereby equipping medical professionals with effective tools for on-site diagnosis. Constant investment in training on these staining techniques enhances diagnostic sensitivity and thereby ultimately contributes to efforts against tuberculosis and other acid-fast bacterial infections worldwide (Howell, 1966) (Figure 10.3).

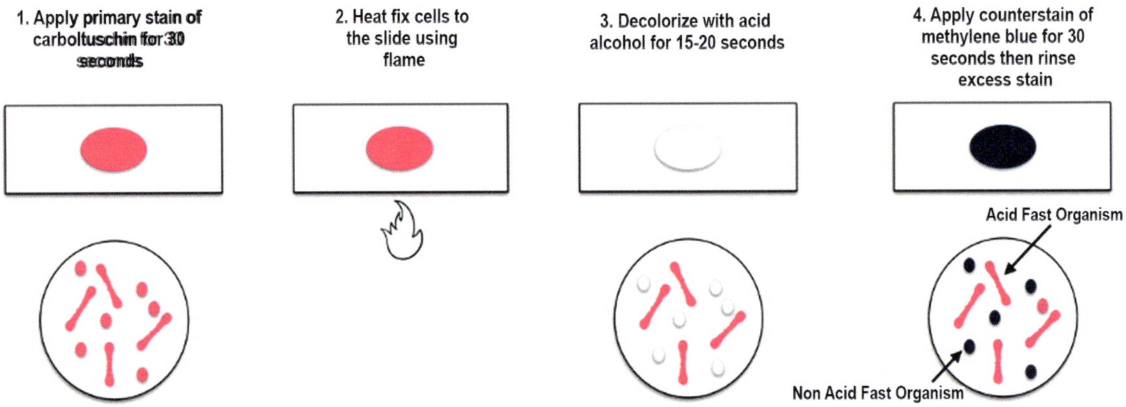

Figure 10.3. Basic steps of the Ziehl-Neelsen staining procedure.

Source: https://upload.wikimedia.org/wikipedia/commons/thumb/c/c9/Basic_steps_of_acid_fast_staining_procedure.svg/1280px-Basic_steps_of_acid_fast_staining_procedure.svg.png.

10.1.3. Growth Conditions and Metabolic Properties

The ecological conditions supporting the growth of acid-fast bacteria, particularly those in the Mycobacterium species, are highly influenced by temperature, pH, and nutrient level. The bacteria tend to acquire the capacity to thrive under nutrient-poor conditions, which necessitates a high metabolic requirement. Unlike other rapidly evolving bacteria, acid-fast bacteria exhibit low growth rates largely due to the unique cell wall structure made of mycolic acids that render them resistant to chemicals and drying. This implies that such organisms' metabolic properties are tailored to efficiently utilize available resources in a bid to survive under conditions that other microorganisms would find prohibitive. It is necessary to know these growth needs and metabolic adaptations, as this informs the pathogenesis and the chronicity of tuberculosis and leprosy due to these bacteria. Acid-fast bacteria's metabolism reveals their remarkable ability to survive in hostile surroundings while maintaining cellular functions. Aerobic respiration and fatty acid metabolism are the means by which these bacteria acquire energy primarily from a diversified set of substrates. The biochemical mechanisms of their metabolic processes are not only reflective of their ecological niche but also of their evolutionary approaches. A good example would be *Mycobacterium tuberculosis*' ability in energy metabolism with fatty acids as energy sources, the significance of which is both site-specific infection when it encounters immune responses and nutritional deprivation in host tissues. In addition, research has indicated that the metabolic properties of such bacteria can be controlled by external conditions of stress, , such as oxidative stress and salinity of the environment, which will affect growth and cell survival. All these observations for metabolic adaptability reinforce the complex equilibrium such organisms have in responding to the environment. Furthermore, acid-fast bacteria's survival is also contributed to by their chemical and physical surroundings, where temperature and osmotic pressure play central roles in controlling their growth patterns. Bacteria's growth rates, as controlled by temperature, as outlined in protein folding and metabolic stability research, provide a model explaining acid-fast bacteria's adaptation under various thermal environments. Similarly, osmotic stress through salt concentrations can inhibit growth, demonstrating just how sensitive these bacteria are to the environment. Through metabolic flexibility, bacteria that are acid-fast can survive conditions that would otherwise repress the development of other microbes and thereby solidify their position in ecological systems. This understanding of their growth conditions enhances current information and points towards lines of potential therapeutic intervention that seek to impact their respective metabolic pathways, which may further result in enhanced control of the disease of such virulent pathogens (Figure 10.4).

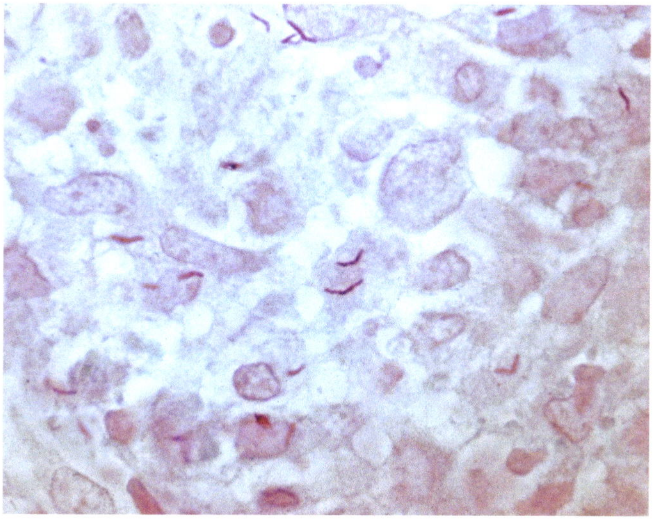

Figure 10.4. Characteristic rod-shaped acid-fast bacilli measuring 2-4 μm in length and 0.2 to 0.5 μm in width in a 34-year-old woman dying from fulminant pulmonary TB after childbirth (Zeihl-Neelson stain × 440).

Source: https://www.researchgate.net/publication/335504004/figure/fig1/AS:962703455711235@1606537798056/Characteristic-rod-shaped-acid-fast-bacilli-measuring-2-4mm-in-length-and-02-to-05mm-in.jpg.

Test Your Knowledge

1. What unique component is in the cell wall of acid-fast bacteria?
2. Which staining technique is primarily used to identify acid-fast bacteria, and what are the key steps involved?

10.2. Major Types of Acid-Fast Bacteria

Learning Outcome

1. Understand Mycobacterium tuberculosis
2. Define Mycobacterium leprae
3. Describe Non-tuberculous mycobacteria (NTM)

Acid-fast bacteria constitute a unique group in the microbial world, distinguished primarily by their very high resistance to acid decolorization in the laboratory staining process. The most well-known members are found within the genus Mycobacterium, e.g., the disease-causing members *Mycobacterium tuberculosis*, responsible for causing tuberculosis, and *Mycobacterium leprae*, responsible for causing leprosy. These microbes possess a complex lipidized cell wall composed of a majority of mycolic acids that is key to their acid-fast character. This morphological abnormality not only protects them from environmental stress but also dictates their pathogenicity and virulence determinants, making them a priority target of medical microbiology. An understanding of the specific features of Mycobacterium and their acid-fast nature not only goes to the diagnostic process but also makes us understand the challenge in the development of useful drugs and vaccines against such resilient pathogens. Another significant group of acid-fast bacteria is represented by the species of the genus Nocardia, with filamentous form and soil habit. Nocardia species have the ability to cause opportunistic infections, particularly in immunocompromised patients, with varied presentations ranging from pulmonary nocardiosis to cutaneous infection. Nocardia, like Mycobacterium, also has mycolic acid in its cell wall, which gives it acid-fastness, although with varying complexities in its pathogenic processes in comparison to Mycobacterium. Emergent literature has indicated the Nocardia genus' heterogeneity, with species defined by varying degrees of virulence and antibiotic resistance. Most notably, though, is the evolving taxonomy of these bacteria that is being determined by ongoing genomic and phenotypic investigations, continually rewriting their classifications and affiliations with other Actinomycetales members, to whom they belong. Rhodococcus species are another vital subset of acid-fast bacteria, which demonstrate an extensive ecological range and substantial ability to degrade a variety of environmental toxins. First described from horse infection and soil, Rhodococcus equi has now found interest because it is a pathogen within both horse and human hosts. Current taxonomic studies show that the majority of strains within this genus could be distinct species or even new genera as they have such unique biochemical and genetic features (Jones et al., 2012). In addition to their clinical application, Rhodococcus species are also utilized in bioremediation methods due to their enzymatic capacity to break down complex hydrocarbons and other synthetic chemicals and thus demonstrating the twofold characteristic of the organisms as opportunistic pathogens and beneficial environmental assets. The present research on the ecological role and pathogenicity of Rhodococcus is a reflection of the intricacies involved in acid-fast bacteria and indicates their relevance to public as well as environmental health programs.

10.2.1. Mycobacterium tuberculosis

The distinctive features of *Mycobacterium tuberculosis* are responsible for its pathogenicity and drug resistance. Being a member of the acid-fast bacteria, the organism has a complex cell wall composition rich in mycolic acids, which not only bestows certain resistances to antibiotics but also allows it to survive varied environmental stresses. This is particularly significant given that nonreplicating tubercle bacilli may be resistant to the cidal action of antibiotics, and hence treatment becomes more complex. A persister population of the bacilli has been isolated in sputum samples by researchers that presents New avenues for scientific investigation into response to chemotherapy and tuberculosis transmission dynamics among various populations (Alvarez et al., 2008). This unusual resilience suggests that the understanding and targeting of these persister cells could be an enhancement of current treatment protocols and, ultimately, reduce the disease burden globally as a result of tuberculosis. Compounded with the challenge of tuberculosis control is the emergence of multi-drug resistant *Mycobacterium tuberculosis* strains. These are caused by antibiotic treatment-related selective pressure, which further calls for an exploration of alternative treatment modalities and stringent diagnosis. The susceptibility of *M. tuberculosis* for developing resistance is due to its slow rate of replication, which provides for mutations of its genetic material with the passage of time. This has consequently made conventional antibiotic therapies less effective, and there is a need to design new pharmacological approaches that can either increase the efficiency of current drugs or discover new agents against metabolic pathways that are specific to M. tuberculosis. In addition, public health interventions stress the importance of early diagnosis and integrated care of high-risk groups, as they are the focal point towards curbing the transmission of resistant strains and the overall weakening of the disease's effects. Research contributes to enhancing knowledge of *Mycobacterium tuberculosis* and its host immune interactions. Studies have revealed that the bacterium has evolved sophisticated mechanisms to survive in macrophages and thus evade the host's immune attack. This ability to usurp the immune system is vitally important to facilitate active infection and disease progression. Recent reports highlight an increased imperative to determine diagnostic methodologies and therapeutic agents targeted at these interactions. For instance, more sensitive detection methods are necessary to identify latent tuberculosis infections that constitute a large reservoir for potential reactivation. Newer molecular biological techniques show potential, as they give scientists the tools to probe the intricacies of *M. tuberculosis* pathogenesis (Englund et al., 2002). With optimal technique, there is the potential to enhance diagnosis accuracy and guide treatment modalities that counter the unique challenges presented by this recalcitrant pathogen (Figure 10.5).

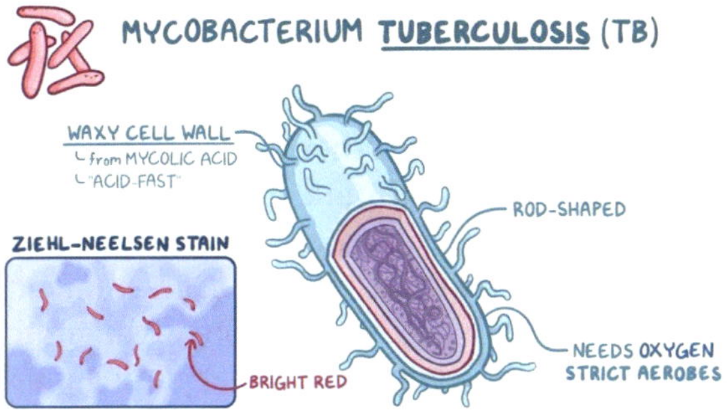

Figure 10.5. *Mycobacterium tuberculosis* (TB).

Source: https://www.osmosis.org/_next/image?url=https%3A%2F%2Fd16qt3wv6xm098.cloudfront.net%2FR_dOLeCOSt_lAlQmuaW4yztDRVmws6Ou%2F_.jpg&w=3840&q=75.

10.2.2. Mycobacterium leprae

Mycobacterium leprae, the causative organism of leprosy, is a valuable model of acid-fast bacteria because of its unique cell wall chemistry and pathogenicity. The distinctive cell wall of the organism, rich in mycolic acid, besides imparting resistance to desiccation and antimicrobial therapy, enables the organism to evade the immune system effectively. *M. leprae* as an intracellular pathogen, proliferates in the macrophages and Schwann cells of the host with subsequent clinical manifestations. Its dissemination, primarily through respiratory droplets from intimate contact, is governed by sociocultural factors and demographic determinants. Understanding these means of transmission is essential to establishing preventive measures and educating people about the disease, which is fraught with stigma and fear. In immunological language, *Mycobacterium leprae* interactions with the host immune system are complex and generally culminate in nerve injury in the periphery, resulting in crippling disabilities. The bacteria's tendency to aggregate on Schwann cells is particularly vexing because these cells have a crucial function in the maintenance of the neurons' structure and function. Experiments have demonstrated that if *M. leprae* infects Schwann cells, it alters the physiological function of these cells and therefore their output of myelin and interconnection of the neurons. Leprosy pathology can result both from the direct action of the bacterium and from amplified immune reactions against the infection. This overlap of microbial pathogenesis and immunopathology highlights the need for additional research to know more about the manner in which immune reactions can lead to the expression of the disease, , such as irreversible peripheral nerve damage (Hagge et al., 2001). Additionally, additional diagnostic techniques, , such as serological assays for the phenolic-glycolipid-1 (Phen-Gl-1) antigen, have improved the diagnosis and treatment of *Mycobacterium leprae* infection. Armadillo research, as a natural reservoir, indicates that the animals will yield detectable antibody responses to *M. leprae*, and this explains the serological picture of leprosy. A correlation of IgM antibodies against Phen-Gl-1 is found with bacterial tissue load and is a potential predictive marker for disease onset (Truman et al., 1985). However, it should be observed that antibody responses may not always correlate with clinical status in human patients due to their disparity in immune responses between different individuals. These findings suggest the need for further investigation of immunological mechanisms of leprosy and into therapeutic regimes to combat this historic but ongoing health challenge (Figure 10.6).

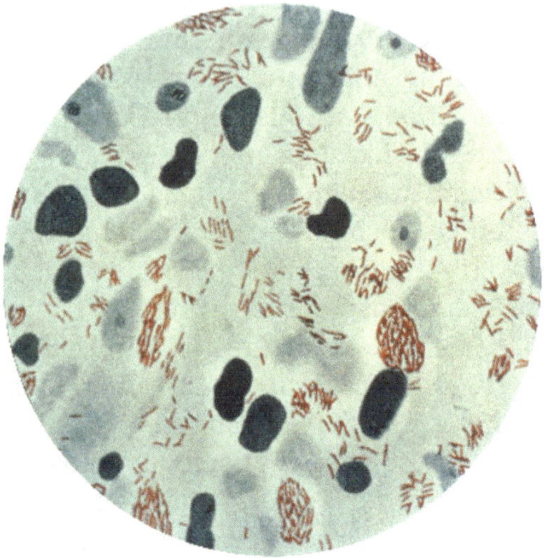

Figure 10.6. *Mycobacterium leprae.*

Source: https://upload.wikimedia.org/wikipedia/commons/d/da/Mycobacterium_leprae.jpeg.

10.2.3. Non-Tuberculous Mycobacteria (NTM)

The importance of Non-tuberculous mycobacteria (NTM) has increased in the fields of public health due to their increased identification in clinical specimens, particularly in patients with a compromised immune status. NTM have environmental reservoirs in soil and water sources, which are a public health issue as they result in opportunistic infections. Unlike their infamous cousin, *Mycobacterium tuberculosis*, NTM are not transmissible from person to person, rendering epidemiological tracking challenging. The pathogenicity of NTM is capable of producing severe morbidity, particularly in pulmonary diseases that clinically resemble tuberculosis, the reason for careful discrimination between the aforementioned mycobacterial infections. Recent evidence indicates heterogeneity of the epidemiology of NTM species by geographical region, further emphasizing the requirement for comprehensive local epidemiologic data to guide clinical practice (Cogneau et al., 2021). An awareness of NTM clinical presentations should entail a critical evaluation of their epidemiology, particularly in resource-limited settings. One example is an NTM prevalence study in The Gambia where 39.8% of sputum specimens contained NTM, and *Mycobacterium avium* complex was the most isolated species (Okoi et al., 2018). NTM diagnostic presentation varies from that of tuberculosis and can lead to misdiagnosis, consequently making treatment regimens complicated. Interestingly, the reliance on smear microscopy for the diagnosis of tuberculosis can compromise the disregard of NTM infections, particularly since certain of the species present similar clinical manifestations. Such a challenge emphasizes the critical urgency for improved diagnostic methods and clinical attentiveness toward NTM, particularly in high-prevalence areas where tuberculosis occurs equally. Secondarily, the clinical treatment of NTM infections must consider the differential antibiotic responses among species. NTM exhibit intrinsic resistance to many commonly used antibiotics, complicating treatment regimens and highlighting the need for tailored therapeutic strategies. Current guidelines often lack specific protocols for managing NTM-related pulmonary diseases, reflecting a gap in clinical standards. Enhanced understanding of molecular epidemiology can elucidate the pathogenic mechanisms of various NTM species, providing insights into potential therapeutic targets. For successful management of such problems, continuous monitoring and studies on NTM prevalence and their interaction with the host immune system are a must. With the rising prevalence of NTM infection, particularly among risk groups, it is important to have a holistic approach with education, improved diagnostics, and targeted treatment (Okoi et al., 2018) (Figure 10.7).

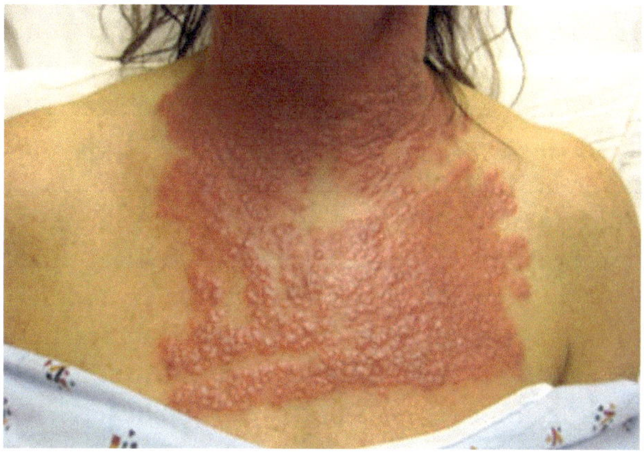

Figure 10.7. Neck and chest of a 53-year-old woman, 14 days after fractionated CO_2 laser resurfacing, showing nontuberculous mycobacterial infection.

Source: https://upload.wikimedia.org/wikipedia/commons/7/7c/Nontuberculous_Mycobacterial_Infection_on_neck_and_chest.jpg.

Test Your Knowledge

1. What disease is primarily caused by Mycobacterium tuberculosis and how is it typically transmitted?
2. Describe the characteristic clinical manifestations of Mycobacterium leprae infection.

10.3. Pathogenicity and Disease Association

Learning Outcome

1. Understand mechanisms of infection associated with acid-fast bacteria
2. Discuss about clinical manifestations of diseases caused by acid-fast bacteria
3. Explain Epidemiology and transmission routes

The relationship between pathogenicity and disease association in acid-fast bacteria, with particular focus on the genus Mycobacterium, is an interesting field of study. *Mycobacterium tuberculosis*, the bacterium causing tuberculosis, is a prime example of how bacteria manage to survive and cause disease within host environments. Pathogenicity is often considered to be caused by specific virulence factors that allow the bacteria to evade being eliminated by the host immune system, grow within host tissue, and progress disease. An understanding of such mechanisms is crucial for the creation of targeted therapeutic strategies to combat infections. The role of the microbiome in the modulation of acid-fast bacterial pathogenicity is another untapped field, and interspecies interactions could make disease relationships and outcomes more complicated. A factor highly relevant in the discussion of pathogenicity is the ability of acid-fast bacteria to form biofilms and result in chronic infection. These adaptations also render them much more resistant to antibiotic therapy and are a component of long-term disease like chronic pulmonary disease. Antibiotic resistance is also possible in cystic fibrosis, for example, as a consequence of complex microbial interactions within the lung microbiota, where pathogenic bacteria are found together with ostensibly commensal bacteria. This ecological community can influence the efficacy of antibiotics and determine the course of associated diseases. Investigation of such dynamics is crucial for understanding the broader implications of early pathogenicity and subsequent disease associations since environmental factors and composition of microbial communities are able to modulate the virulence of acid-fast bacteria. Moreover, ongoing research on acid-fast bacterial pathogen-host interaction secretion systems and gene determinants can elucidate information on mechanisms of acid-fast bacterial pathogenicity. For instance, comparative genomic studies have isolated proteins that have been implicated in modulating host immune responses or mediating the process of nutrient acquisition, demonstrating how these kinds of organisms have co-evolved to flourish in their niches. Research in these areas not only advances our understanding of Mycobacterium but also offers opportunities for novel therapeutic interventions. As reminded in recent research, the study of phytopathogenic bacteria within the Xanthomonadaceae family with common pathogenic attributes suggests that it is necessary to know common mechanisms among different bacterial families, eventually to enhance our knowledge of acid-fast bacteria pathogenicity and disease association (Assis et al., 2017; Coenye et al., 2019).

10.3.1. Mechanisms of Infection

Understanding the infection mechanisms of acid-fast bacteria, *Mycobacterium tuberculosis* in particular, is crucial in terms of preventing and treating infection. Infection typically takes place through inhalation of aerosolized droplets containing the pathogen. The bacteria, once in the host lungs, employ their unique cell wall chemistry rich in mycolic acids to manipulate the host immune system. This defense mechanism renders them capable of living and multiplying within macrophages, a family of immune cells that engulf and destroy pathogens. Additionally, inhibition of phagosome-lysosome fusion prevents the effective destruction of the bacteria by the host immune system and supports further colonization and establishment of chronic infection. Such resiliency highlights the need for stronger diagnostic tests and treatment regimens that target their unique physiological mechanisms directly, thereby augmenting patient outcomes. As the infection progresses, acid-fast organisms can cause a variety of pathophysiological reactions within the host. This can include the formation of granulomas, which are organized assemblies of immune cells that attempt to contain the infection. While this immune response appears to be protective initially, it can result in tissue damage and pulmonary dysfunction due to necrosis and fibrosis.

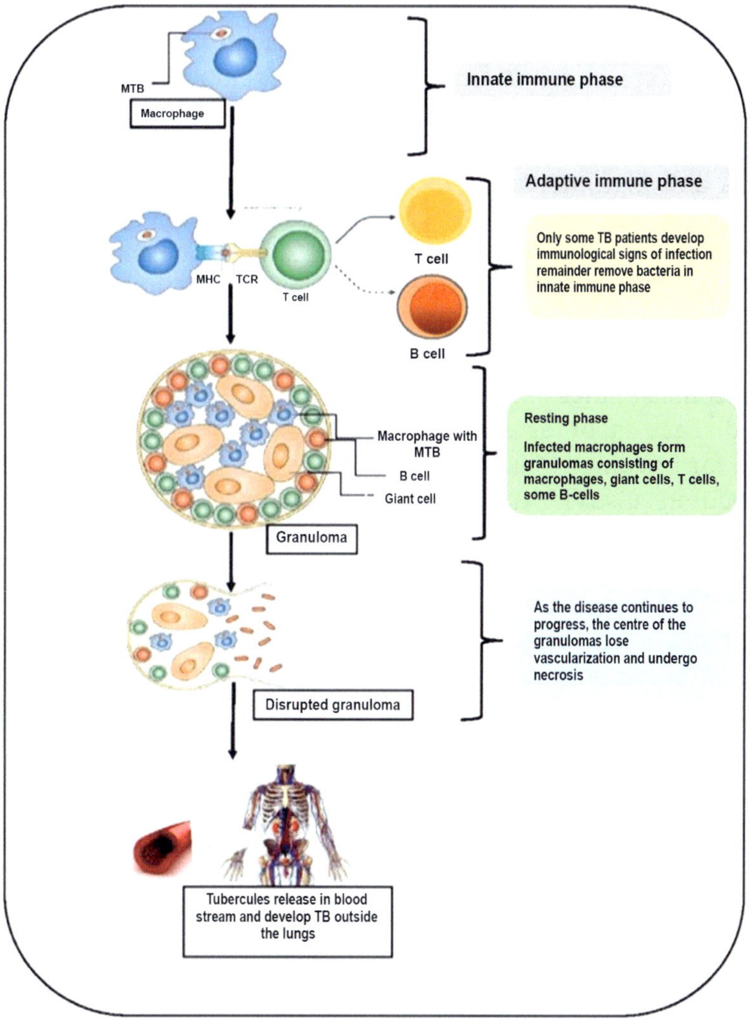

Figure 10.8. Basic mechanism of infection of *Mycobacterium tuberculosis.*

Source: https://www.researchgate.net/profile/Ajai-Singh-6/publication/291952234/figure/fig1/AS:322853292527618@1453985631436/Basic-mechanism-of-infection-of-Mycobacterium-tuberculosis.png.

Moreover, the resultant chronic inflammation after granuloma development may exert systemic manifestations with the emergence of symptoms , such as fever, anorexia, and night sweats. More significantly, some types of acid-fast bacteria are associated with the production of virulence factors that facilitate tissue damage as well as transmission. Particularly noteworthy, understanding these routes sheds light on both potential therapeutic interventions and public health measures used to control bacterial spread, particularly in risk groups. Acid-fast bacterial diseases are not confined to the lung, illustrating the diverse clinical presentation that can be caused by their pathogenicity. *Mycobacterium avium* complex, for example, may cause disseminated infection especially in immunocompromised individuals, with serious complications and high mortality. The interaction with the host immune response is multifaceted; they can evade detection and eradication by mechanisms that involve modulation of the immune response or residing in areas that are immune-privileged. The evidence of lethal outcomes of these infections, e.g., mycobacterial disease in other animals, emphasizes the need for ongoing vigilance and investigation in infectious disease. Improved understanding of infection processes, with new detection and therapy technologies, point to the need to combat the infections caused by these resilient microorganisms, a call amplified by the recent advances in biosensing technology (González-Aguilar et al., 2013) (Figure 10.8).

10.3.2. Clinical Manifestations of Diseases

The clinical presentations of acid-fast bacterium infections, particularly *Mycobacterium tuberculosis*, illustrate the complexity of diagnosis and treatment of infections. Tuberculosis (TB) can present in different ways, particularly pulmonary and extrapulmonary, with distinct clinical presentations. Pulmonary TB is presented with chronic cough, hemoptysis, night sweats, and massive weight loss, with proof of systemic disease. Conversely, extrapulmonary TB presents in many different ways based on the specific organ or area affected, e.g., lymph nodes, bones, or pleural spaces. These variations make it hard for health workers to be highly suspicious, particularly in high-prevalence contexts where TB may occur alongside other infectious illnesses, thus complicating diagnosis. Moreover, the clinical presentation of EPTB is also difficult to diagnose since the typically low bacillary load of the specimen is likely to lead to misdiagnosis or treatment delay. According to a study for the utility of acid-fast bacilli (AFB) staining in biopsy specimens for patients with EPTB, overall AFB positivity was merely 26.1%, whereas greater positivity was observed in pleural TB. This lends support to the importance of proper histopathological evaluation, especially in cases where patients present with characteristic granulomatous inflammation; the presence of such pathology can prove highly useful in establishing a diagnosis of EPTB. Clinicians therefore need to be skilled at interpreting AFB staining, particularly against the background of patients past histories of pulmonary TB since this was highly correlated with increased rates of AFB positivity.

The management of disease caused by acid-fast bacteria needs to have an understanding of the complete implications of their clinical presentation. For instance, Shiga toxins in certain species of bacteria have been discovered to exacerbate acute clinical presentation in infections (González-Aguilar et al., 2013). Although not necessarily concerning acid-fast bacteria, insight into how various bacterial infections can complicate symptoms is important towards providing proper care. Where TB and other bacterial diseases coincide, for example, in foodborne pathogens, successful treatment and diagnostic strategies are crucial. The application of biosensor technology to the rapid detection of pathogens will increase health outcomes, especially in rural or resource-poor settings. Therefore, the clinical response to acid-fast bacterial infections is to add new diagnostic strategies to traditional methods to ensure comprehensive patient care (Figure 10.9).

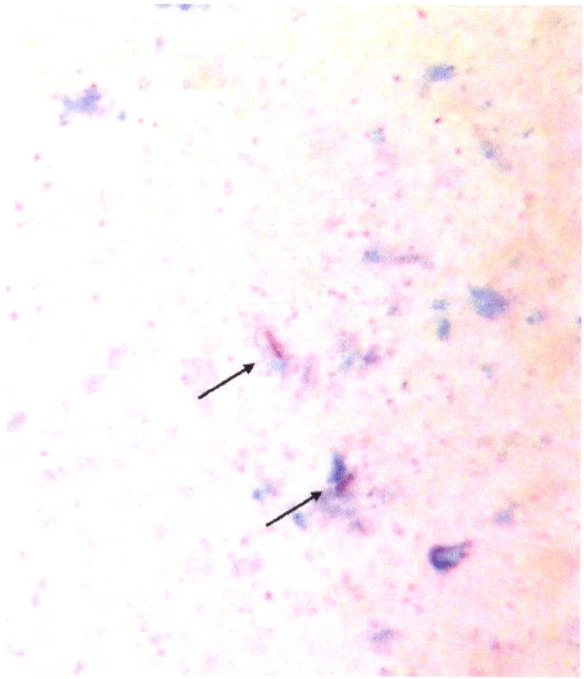

Figure 10.9. Acid-fast bacilli (black arrows) in an Ehrlich-Ziehl-Neelsen-stained smear from the patient's urine sample.

Source: https://www.researchgate.net/publication/216621759/figure/fig1/AS:276503754493958@1442935040261/Acid-fast-bacilli-black-arrows-in-an-Ehrlich-Ziehl-Neelsen-stained-smear-from-the.png.

10.3.3. Epidemiology and Transmission Routes

The study of epidemiology and transmission routes is essential to understand the mode of spread of acid-fast bacteria, particularly *Mycobacterium tuberculosis* and related pathogens, within populations. The bacteria prefer alternate modes of transmission from other pathogens due to the nature of their cellular arrangement and low rates of replication. Transmission is primarily through airborne particles discharged from the respiratory tract of infected individuals and remaining suspended in the air to be absorbed by susceptible hosts. These bacteria's epidemiologic patterns are complex, varying with socio-economics, prevalence of immune-compromising illness, and public health interventions. Effective surveillance of these patterns allows for risk groups to be defined and for targeted prevention strategies. Understanding the nuances in transmission routes is essential for effective control of acid-fast bacterium infections. Recent advances in next-generation sequencing (NGS) have revolutionized research in these pathogens for epidemiologists, enriching the understanding of their patterns of transmission. For instance, NGS technology offers high-resolution data on genetic variation and strain relationships, enabling successful outbreak investigation and effective source tracing. By demystifying the genotypic characteristics of bacteria, researchers can construct improved epidemiological models that inform public health interventions. Furthermore, integrating genomic data with epidemiological outcomes allows for the identification of transmission determinants and thus, more precise interventions that may limit disease transmission among populations

(Boon et al., 2019). Additionally, the presence of antibiotic-resistant acid-fast bacterial strains is a grave concern to public health. It is often compounded by suboptimal treatment regimens and non-compliance with prescribed treatments. Antimicrobial resistance not only complicates individual patient management but also increases epidemiological threats at a broader level, in that resistant organisms can be transmitted silently through populations. Effective monitoring and surveillance mechanisms must be available to tackle this issue, requiring an active epidemiological system consisting of traditional surveillance systems and high-tech genomic methods. With proper execution, such systems have the potential to enhance early detection of resistance patterns, transmission routes understanding, and guide treatment protocols development that target patient safety and public health preservation (Jacobs et al., 2006).

Test Your Knowledge

1. What are the primary clinical manifestations of tuberculosis, and how do they relate to the progression of infection?
2. Which populations are most at risk for developing active tuberculosis, and why?
3. How is Mycobacterium tuberculosis transmitted, and what factors influence the likelihood of transmission?

10.4. Diagnosis of Acid-Fast Bacterial Infections

Learning Outcome

1. Describe laboratory techniques for the identification of acid-fast bacteria
2. Explain the role of imaging in diagnosis
3. Focus on challenges in diagnosis

The identification of acid-fast bacterial infections, particularly mycobacterial infections related to *Mycobacterium tuberculosis*, has greatly advanced in the past few decades. Traditional methods , such as smear microscopy, have been used extensively in which the identification of acid-fast bacilli (AFB) in sputum specimens is an initial marker of infection. However, it is not without drawbacks, , such as suboptimal sensitivity in paucibacillary tuberculosis and reliance on high-quality specimens. New laboratory techniques , such as nucleic acid amplification tests, have become accessible, leading to earlier and more precise detection of Mycobacterium species. These advances in diagnostic accuracy contribute not only to enhanced treatment decisions but also to the realization of better patient outcomes in the long term. The transfer of molecular methodology to routine diagnostic laboratories is a valuable advance toward addressing the worldwide threat of tuberculosis and other acid-fast diseases. Other than conventional techniques, cerebrospinal fluid (CSF) testing is significant in the diagnosis of infections of the central nervous system due to acid-fast bacteria. Whenever fever, headache, and neurological impairment evolve, CSF testing is essential. In a study evaluating viral meningitis, HSV-1 was cultured in a few percent of CSF samples, and viral cultures and bacterial assessments are therefore considered significant (Azadfar et al., 2014). Whereas these viral infections differ from Mycobacterium infections, the principles of diagnosis remain the same. Prolonged white blood cell and protein content with normal glucose content in CSF is suggestive of mycobacterial infection. Rigorous analysis can help clinicians differentiate between infectious etiologies and tailor the treatment to suit, emphasizing the need for precise laboratory methodology in diagnosing these complex scenarios. Secondly, the increased prevalence of co-infection among vulnerable populations necessitates extensive diagnosis and treatment. For instance, respiratory syncytial virus (RSV) has emerged as a significant problem among individuals with pre-existing airway disease and older adults, with diagnostic challenges comparable to those of acid-fast bacterial infections (Fraser et al., 2016). The lack of distinctive symptoms necessitates extensive testing, particularly among vulnerable groups. Therefore, advancements in molecular diagnostic equipment capable of detecting a number of pathogens simultaneously are a potential line of development for clinical microbiology. By enhancing the diagnostic arsenal against acid-fast bacilli and other respiratory pathogens, healthcare providers can better tailor patient management regimens. Subsequently, successful diagnosis is instrumental in managing acid-fast bacterial infections, offering prompt intervention and reducing the morbidity of such life-threatening infections.

10.4.1. Laboratory Techniques for Identification

Microbiological diagnosis, including laboratory procedures for diagnosing acid-fast bacteria, particularly mycobacteria, is an integral component of diagnosing them. One such classic procedure employed is the Ziehl-Neelsen staining, which detects the presence of acid-fast bacilli visually by employing specific color differentiation with the help of a microscope. This staining process is helpful in preliminary identification but is often insensitive to produce proper species-level analysis. Owing to the diversity and complexity of pathogens that belong to the group of acid-fast organisms , such as *Mycobacterium tuberculosis* and nontuberculous mycobacteria Nocardia brasiliensis, reliance on staining alone may lead to misdiagnosis or Omission of the most significant infections requires further confirmation through culturing on selective media , such as Löwenstein–Jensen, which specifically encourage the growth of these microorganisms (Christofidou et al., 2023). Molecular techniques have increasingly become the mainstay in laboratory isolation of acid-fast bacteria with ever-better genetic and proteomic techniques. Techniques , such as the polymerase chain reaction (PCR) and DNA sequencing enable identification of the bacterial species by detecting specific genetic sequences characteristic of the pathogens. For instance, MALDI-TOF MS use has now revolutionized rapid mycobacterial species identification by their protein profiling with significantly reduced turnaround times for results. Conversely, as demonstrated by recent literature, the inclusion of these molecular tests enhances sensitivity and specificity in disease diagnosis, like tuberculosis, enhancing clinical outcomes, most significantly in immunocompromised subjects where misidentification results in severe complications (Szewczyk et al., 2013). This combined approach of routine culturing and advanced molecular diagnostics represents a paradigm shift towards more effective identification of acid-fast pathogens. Apart from the above techniques, lipid analysis has emerged as an integral part of mycobacterial detection. Mycolic acid analysis within the bacterial cell wall, facilitated by advanced techniques like electrospray ionization tandem mass spectrometry, facilitates distinctive profiling of various mycobacterial species. This technique not only aids in the diagnosis of tuberculosis but also discriminates between pathogenic and non-pathogenic species more correctly than standard biochemical screens. This highly effective tool has high potential for accelerating the diagnosis without the weeks of culturing time usually required. By involving lipid analysis, the clinical hodaminegyy is able to optimize diagnostic strategies, particularly in regions where rapid and specific identification of acid-fast bacteria is vital in ensuring timely treatment (Szewczyk et al., 2013) (Figure 10.10).

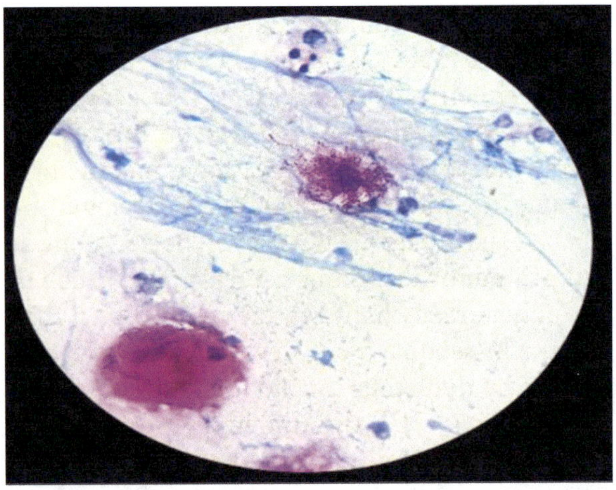

Figure 10.10. 1% acid-fast staining showing weakly acid-fast slender and filamentous bacilli conforming Nocardia.

Source: https://www.researchgate.net/publication/336200859/figure/fig3/AS:1086056258641942@1635947398119/1-acid-fast-staining-showing-weakly-acid-fast-slender-and-filamentous-bacilli-conforming.jpg.

10.4.2. Role of Imaging in Diagnosis

Imaging plays an important role in the diagnosis of acid-fast bacterial infections, particularly in tuberculosis (TB) infection. Conventional methods, , such as acid-fast bacilli (AFB) staining, have limitations, particularly with extrapulmonary infections when bacilli are present in small numbers or randomly scattered in tissues. Under such circumstances, advanced imaging techniques, including computed tomography (CT) and magnetic resonance imaging (MRI), may provide essential information about extrapulmonary tuberculosis pathology. By visualizing involved tissue, these techniques can help detect lesions that are not accessible through the traditional sampling methods, resulting in early and accurate diagnosis. Moreover, imaging can help define the extent of disease, which will guide the clinician in formulating treatment protocols for infected patients, something that is valuable given the quirks posed by various sites of infection. The use of imaging in the diagnostic process is most applicable in cases where AFB positivity is lower, such as bone and joint tuberculosis, with the positivity rate reported very low at 4.8% (Azarhoush et al., 2014). With the use of imaging modalities, clinicians can identify the presence of abscesses, osteolytic lesions, or other pathological features suggestive of active disease.

This is especially important in those patients with a history of pulmonary tuberculosis, for whom there is already a good correlation between history of past infection and AFB positivity based on multivariate models. In such a situation, imaging not only supplements the traditional diagnostic approaches but also enhances the overall understanding of the disease process and potential complications, thus offering early intervention as well as improved outcomes for patients.

Apart from aiding diagnosis, imaging can also be extremely useful in facilitating the monitoring of response to treatment in individuals suffering from tuberculosis. Traditional sputum-based measures of treatment efficacy may be compromised by the inherent heterogeneity of *Mycobacterium tuberculosis* populations, which are usually variable in drug susceptibility and immune response (Bruyn et al., 2016). Imaging, therefore, may become a helpful adjunct for assessing therapeutic efficacy, especially in extrapulmonary or drug-resistant TB. For example, a decrease in the size of lesions or the vanishing of aberrant signals on imaging techniques may provide tangible proof of the therapeutic efficacy to support clinical decision-making. With evolutions in imaging technology, the development of some biomarkers and models tailored to track treatment response will be pivotal to addressing the specific difficulties posed by acid-fast bacterial infection (Figure 10.11).

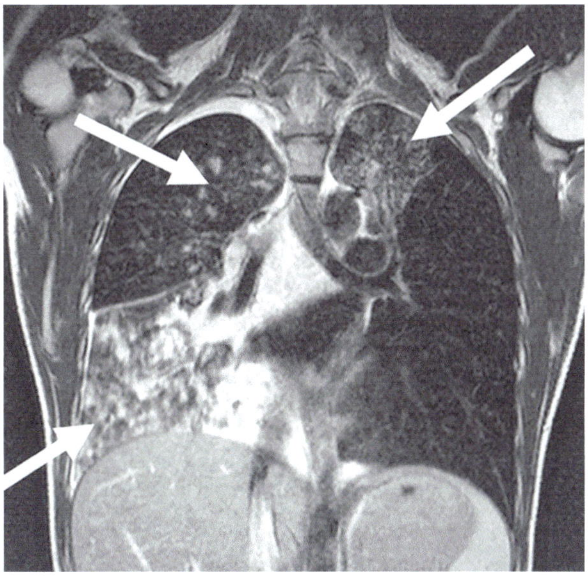

Figure 10.11. MRI of tuberculosis in a 12-year-old girl.

Source: https://www.researchgate.net/publication/338900537/figure/fig4/AS:852729840820226@1580318045656/MRI-of-tuberculosis-in-a-12-year-old-girl-Coronal-T2-weighted-turbo-spin-echo-image-MR.ppm.

10.4.3. Challenges in Diagnosis

Diagnosis of acid-fast bacterial infections, particularly *Mycobacterium tuberculosis*, poses difficulty for clinicians due to several technical and biological reasons. The cell structure with mycolic acids in acid-fast bacteria is the reason behind resistance to standard staining procedures and disinfectants. Traditional diagnosis methods, such as sputum smear microscopy are often hindered by poor sensitivity, especially under low bacillary load conditions. Moreover, the long time for culture-based methods still has to continue causing delayed diagnosis, a cornerstone in effective tuberculosis epidemic control. Research has indicated other methods, , such as mass spectrometry focused, which may have greater sensitivity and specificity, but the technologies have not yet been incorporated into routine use in mainstream diagnosis for acid-fast bacterial infections (Szewczyk et al., 2013). Other than technical limitations, the extreme variation in clinical presentation of tuberculosis further complicates the diagnostic process. Clinical presentations of tuberculosis have been discovered to mimic certain of the respiratory diseases, leading to delay in diagnosis or misdiagnosis. This is especially critical in populations with co-morbid conditions , such as HIV, where patients could be presenting atypically due to immune suppression. Moreover, non-tuberculous mycobacteria infections complicate the situation since their detection and clinical significance may be doubtful. New molecular techniques , such as real-time polymerase chain reaction (RT-PCR), have been proposed to clarify the discrepancies. However, the efficiency of RT-PCR is also affected by the stability of the bacterial membrane, making it difficult to extract genomic DNA (Bhatti et al., 2012). Accordingly, the complexity of clinical presentations requires a broad-based diagnostic strategy. Integration of advanced technologies is crucial to counter the technical limitations inherent in acid-fast bacilli detection. Advances in the technology of more recent times, , such as the use of rTDMH in combination with RT-PCR, have been encouraging to enhance the sensitivity and speed of diagnosis of tuberculosis. These advances signal the direction for a potential shift in diagnostic modalities towards the potential for amplifying mycobacterial DNA even from low bacillary burdens. The ability to diagnose tuberculosis in a more realistic timeframe not only aids patients but also addresses public health concerns regarding disease transmission. With tuberculosis still affecting millions of people worldwide, the creation and application of effective diagnostic methods are crucial in curbing transmission levels and eventually managing this infectious disease (Bhatti et al., 2012).

Test Your Knowledge

1. What are the most commonly used laboratory techniques for the identification of acid-fast bacteria in clinical samples?
2. What role does molecular testing (e.g., PCR) play in the diagnosis of Mycobacterium tuberculosis compared to traditional culture methods?

10.5. Treatment and Management

Learning Outcome

1. Describe antibiotic resistance issues
2. Focus on standard treatment regimens
3. Understand new therapies and research focused on acid-fast bacteria

Effective therapy and disease control with acid-fast organisms, particularly *Mycobacterium tuberculosis*, require an integrated approach that includes a combination of pharmacological treatments and public health practices. The traditional therapies usually constitute a regimen of first-line antimycobacterial agents , such as isoniazid, rifampicin, ethambutol, and pyrazinamide administered for a long period. This prolonged treatment is needed to attain complete annihilation of the pathogen and also to prevent the establishment of multidrug-resistant strains. However, the emerging antibiotic resistance in these bacteria necessitates the search for new therapeutic approaches. As through current research, virulence inhibition and biofilm inhibition approaches are emerging as a different option compared to conventional antibiotics (Puigdomenech et al., 2018). Inclusion of these new methods in treatment protocols can enhance efficacy and compliance and reduce the risk of treatment failure. In addition to pharmacotherapy, proper control of acid-fast bacterial infection relies significantly on public health activities aimed at prevention and early detection. Screening at-risk populations and initiation of vaccination programs are essential elements in preventing tuberculosis transmission, particularly in areas of high prevalence. Interventions at the community level, including enhancing access of care to services and transmission mechanism awareness, are crucial to the encouragement of timely treatment and diagnosis. Apart from that, the development of antimicrobial engineered materials is also another groundbreaking way of combating acid-fast bacteria infections. Researches have confirmed that hydrogels and nanoparticles are potent delivery systems for antimycobacterial drugs, and they can surpass existing limitations in the delivery of antibiotics (Puigdomenech et al., 2018). The developments would significantly transform hospital infection control practices. Lastly, therapy and care of acid-fast bacteria also have to address the widespread social determinants that can negate gains made in combating such infections. Socioeconomic determinants of poverty, hunger, and poor access to clean water and healthcare contribute significantly to the burden of tuberculosis and other acid-fast caused infections. Therefore, concerted effort among healthcare professionals, policymakers, and community agencies across professions is essential in developing sustainable interventions. Interventions targeting the stigma of tuberculosis can strengthen treatment adherence as well as community support, which are essential for successful outcome. Through the marriage of pharmacological advancements with socio-economic interventions and public health strategies, the fight against acid-fast bacteria would become more effective and thus decrease morbidity and death caused by such infections.

10.5.1. Antibiotic Resistance Issues

The development of antibiotic resistance is a major challenge in disease treatment caused by acid-fast bacteria, *Mycobacterium tuberculosis* in particular. The bacterium causes tuberculosis (TB), which has become one of the most fatal infectious diseases worldwide, with millions infected every year. Its treatment is made more difficult by the development of resistance to available antibiotics, which has led to the emergence of multi-drug-resistant (MDR) strains. The alarming statistics indicate an imperative demand for new therapeutic approaches as the current antibiotics are often ineffective in fighting the resistant pathogens (Agerberth et al., 2016). Scientists are, therefore, developing new approaches entailing the design of new drug classes to fight MDR mycobacterial disease. The challenge lies in balancing the rate of drug development with the urgent healthcare needs emanating from a changing microbial landscape. As a counter-response against the crisis of antibiotic resistance, particularly among acid-fast bacteria, research is shifting into alternative treatments that could trigger host immune responses. One such strategy involves the utilization of agents that could enhance the processes by which host cells eliminate these recalcitrant pathogens. Resistance is not just because of mutational changes in the bacteria but also because of non-replicating, latent phenotypes that are notoriously recalcitrant to therapy with standard antibiotic treatments. The quest for new drugs, like the hodamine drug D157070, has been encouraging in enhancing the intracellular killing activity of host cells against mycobacteria (Bull et al., 2009).

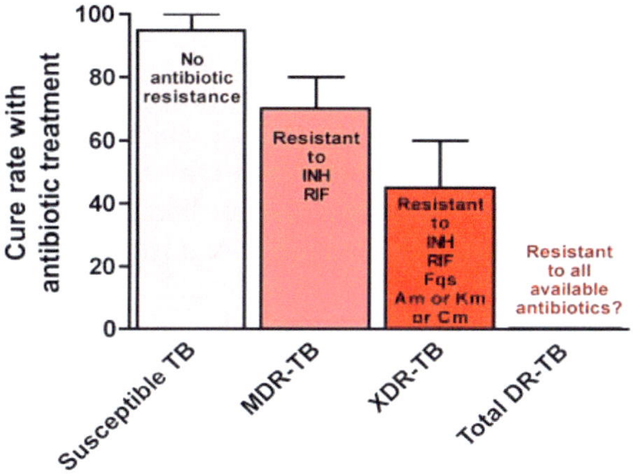

Figure 10.12. Antibiotic cure rates of TB based on drug resistance patterns.

Source: https://www.mdpi.com/pharmaceuticals/pharmaceuticals-03-02268/article_deploy/html/images/pharmaceuticals-03-02268-g001-1024.png.

Such advances would introduce a new paradigm to treatment, bypassing the limitations of existing antibiotics and eradicating the burden of drug-resistant pathogens. Additionally, the issues of acid-fast bacterial infection treatment highlight the need for novel diagnostic tools and assays capable of quantifying bacterial viability without recourse to culture techniques. Classical methods fail to account for the complexity of non-replicating strains responsible for chronic infections. New viability tests, such as the pre16S ribosomal gene RNA/DNA ratio, may provide insight into the actual state of living of mycobacterial populations and thus guide treatment regimens (Bull et al., 2009). The integration of such advanced techniques with emerging therapies can further facilitate control of acid-fast bacterial infections. Overall, the fight against antibiotic resistance requires more than a one-dimensional approach comprising not only new drugs but also new diagnostic tools to gain a better understanding of and fight common mycobacterial infections (Figure 10.12).

10.5.2. Standard Treatment Regimens

Therapy of acid-fast bacterial infections, particularly *Mycobacterium tuberculosis*, is challenging due to the special characteristics of the pathogens and the requirement of a long duration of treatment. Conventional therapy regimens typically include a regimen of first-line medications , such as isoniazid, rifampicin, ethambutol, and pyrazinamide, administered for at least six months. Such a long duration is not only imperative to the final clearance of the bacteria but also to preventing the development of drug-resistant pathogens. However, the intricate dynamics between the host's immune response and variations in bacterial sub-populations should be taken into account when controlling the infection. Consequently, the efficacy of such regimens can be very much patient-to-patient variable and thus calls for individualized approaches that consider each patient's therapeutic response (Bruyn et al., 2016).

Treatment monitoring and evaluation are critical components of tuberculosis treatment, a reflection of ongoing research in this field. Multidrug-resistant tuberculosis (MDR-TB) represents a strong challenge to conventional drug treatment regimens for acid-fast bacteria. While routine treatments are effective against drug-susceptible bacteria, the application of resistance necessitates alternative and, at times, more aggressive treatment regimens. The treatment for MDR-TB may involve second-line medications , such as fluoroquinolones and aminoglycosides, typically extending the length of the therapy to 18-24 months and beyond (Bruyn et al., 2016). This alteration, in addition to enhancing the level of complexity in handling, also enhances the likelihood of complications and side effects. Moreover, there is a critical need for identifying new pharmacotherapeutic drugs that possess the capability to act against resistant strains while not compromising patient safety. Hence, the character of bacterial strains and the sensitivity of the strains toward treatment must be properly experimented upon to ascertain the outcome of the treatment so that the treatment is maximized without subjecting the patient to further resistance generation. In the scenario of standard regimens of acid-fast bacteria treatment, monitoring and evaluation are essential. Traditional methods, , such as sputum smear microscopy, can be limited in their capacity to detect treatment failure or relapse, particularly when the population of mycobacteria is heterogeneous (Bruyn et al., 2016). The use of new biomarkers and advanced molecular techniques thus becomes increasingly critical in individualizing treatment regimens. These strategies play a critical role in the detection of active infections and tracking of host responses during treatment, which provides more accurate information concerning the effectiveness of treatment. Also, understanding the dynamics of bacterial populations in biofilms can guide improved chemotherapeutic approaches, particularly in restricting the formation of resistant strains. Thus, continuous advancements in monitoring techniques are absolutely important to optimize the effectiveness of routine treatment regimens and ensure enhanced outcomes in the management of tuberculosis (Figure 10.13).

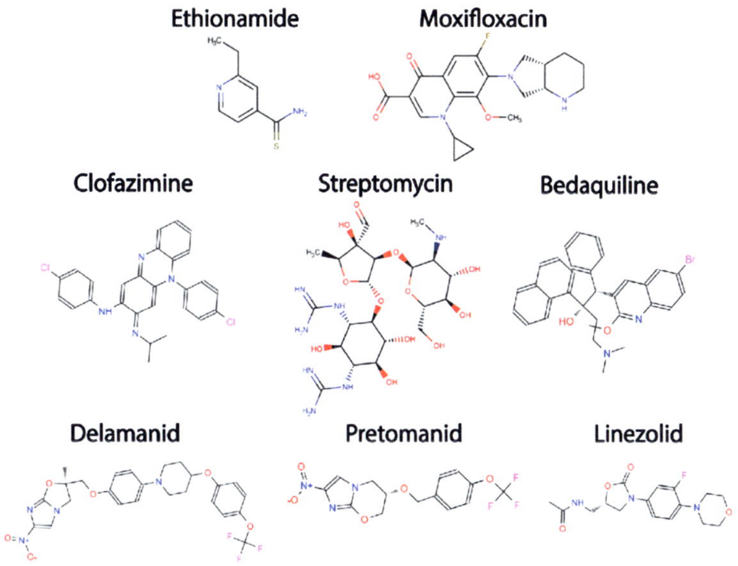

Figure 10.13. Second-line drugs used in tuberculosis treatment.

Source: https://www.researchgate.net/publication/367482615/figure/fig2/AS:1143128111535 7577@1674866312908/Second-line-drugs-used-in-tuberculosis-treatment-Structures-for-some-second-line-drugs.png.

10.5.3. Emerging Therapies and Research

The new advances in therapies and research on acid-fast bacteria, including *Mycobacterium tuberculosis* (M. tuberculosis), have also been largely in the spotlight with the growing issue of antibiotic resistance. With *M. tuberculosis* strains becoming more resistant to traditional therapy, new methods are being sought to enhance therapeutic effectiveness. The new breakthroughs in biotechnology, including the production of novel antibiotics as well as other therapies, are promising to address such issues. In addition, researchers develop innovative drug delivery methods and combination therapies that improve existing drugs against resistant bacteria. These alternatives not only attempt to counteract resistance but also seek to improve patient care where tuberculosis affects regions with poor access to healthcare, , such as Cambodia, where access to healthcare is still limited due to systemic faults (DeHart et al., 2020). Research into antimicrobial peptides and bacteriophage treatment is another promising area of defense against infection from acid-fast organisms. Antimicrobial peptides, naturally occurring immunocomponents, are capable of being specifically active on bacterial membranes and disrupting their function and are promising candidates as adjunct treatments. Bacteriophage treatment, a process that uses viruses that preferentially infect and kill bacteria, has been found to be promising for targeting antibiotic-resistant *M. tuberculosis* strains. These new therapies might be particularly useful in areas where traditional antibiotics lose effectiveness due to extensive drug-resistant strains (Panwar et al., 2024). As research is ongoing, understanding how these therapies function will be crucial to effective deployment into treatment regimens. Furthermore, acceptance of an interdisciplinary approach to research and clinical practice appears to be essential when dealing with the rising threat of antimicrobial resistance associated with acid-fast bacteria. Interdisciplinary co-operation among microbiologists, clinicians, biotechnologists, and public health experts can lead to collaborative strategies that are responsive to the complexities of drug development and resistance management. For instance, the use of biosensors in the quick identification of resistant strains of disease can significantly alter the treatment protocol, allowing interventions for curbing disease transmission. Efforts in public health should also be directed toward improving healthcare access and education in rural areas, , such as those in Cambodia, to combat the socio-economic determinants that contribute to the issue of tuberculosis (DeHart et al., 2020). The combined synergisms of research-driven innovation and social-based solutions represent a positive direction towards slowing the problematic progress of acid-fast bacteria.

Test Your Knowledge

1. What is the standard first-line antibiotic treatment regimen for Mycobacterium tuberculosis infection, and how long is the typical course?
2. What are the main treatment challenges when managing infections caused by Mycobacterium leprae?

10.6. Public Health Implications

Learning Outcome

1. Understand the global burden of acid-fast bacterial diseases
2. Describe prevention strategies and vaccination efforts
3. Explain the role of healthcare systems in managing outbreaks

In its perception of the public health implications associated with acid-fast bacteria, particularly *Mycobacterium tuberculosis*, it is imperative to appreciate the shortcomings inherent in the traditional methods of diagnosis. The continued spread of the tuberculosis epidemic emphasizes the need for sensitive and rapid diagnosis because the traditional approaches are characteristically slow and not specific enough to effectively identify infections. Traditional diagnosis tends to result in delayed treatment, thus the disease progresses unchecked. Novel technologies, , such as the integration of Real-time Polymerase Chain Reaction (RT-PCR) and targeted lysis using TDM-specific hydrolase, have the potential to raise diagnostic sensitivity significantly. The new technology may allow for accelerated diagnosis of tuberculosis, in turn making public health interventions timely and more effective and therefore reducing disease transmission rates and mortality, especially among high-risk groups like HIV doubly infected individuals (Bhatti et al., 2012).

Furthermore, the persistence of tubercle bacilli complicates treatment, emphasizing the need to monitor and limit the spread of disease. Nonreplicating persister-like *M. tuberculosis* subpopulations are resistant to multiple antibiotics, complicating final pathogen elimination. The presence of such subpopulations with dormant states complicates eradication by standard treatments. Understanding these processes is important to interventions in public health aimed at curtailing tuberculosis spread. More research into the activity and detection of such bacteria can lead to the development of certain treatment regimens that deal specifically with both latent and active bacterial populations. Consequently, such measures may curb transmission levels and lower overall disease burden in communities devastated by tuberculosis (Alvarez et al., 2008).

The economic impact of tuberculosis is not just reflected in individual health conditions but also affects public health systems and economies globally. Although tuberculosis still infects an estimated 9 million annually and kills approximately 3 million, the economic impact is massive. The expenditures appear in the form of increased medical treatment, lost productivity, and necessitating the use of public health money to stem outbreaks. Improved diagnosis, , such as that using rTDMH in combination with RT-PCR, may not only allow for early treatment but also limit the cost to the healthcare system. By limiting the occurrence and spread of tuberculosis, communities are free to direct resources towards prevention, treatment, and education and build healthier populations. Eventually, the public health impact of acid-fast bacteria like *M. tuberculosis* is key to advancing world health gains and sustaining long-term economic development.

10.6.1. Global Burden of Acid-Fast Bacterial Diseases

The global disease burden of acid-fast bacterial diseases, particularly *Mycobacterium tuberculosis* and the other mycobacteria, is a global public health issue. Tuberculosis (TB) is a severe health issue in that it has approximately 9 million new cases annually, with a staggering mortality rate, causing approximately 3 million deaths per year. The epidemic disease disproportionately affects the vulnerable groups, i.e., those who have weakened immune systems, for instance, HIV-positive individuals. The World Health Organization (WHO) continues to highlight the importance of good diagnostics, effective treatment strategies, and broad public health action to combat the threat of TB. Moreover, the synergy of increasing antibiotic resistance in mycobacteria contributes to the crisis, necessitating urgent intervention from healthcare systems and policymakers across the globe (Bristow et al., 2019). As the world struggles with this multifaceted challenge, determining the significance of acid-fast bacterial diseases remains a matter of ultimate concern to public health. In considering the epidemiology of acid-fast bacterial diseases, the profound effects of undiagnosed and misdiagnosed disease must be considered. Existing diagnostics for tuberculosis tend not to provide the rapidity and sensitivity needed to effectively face the current epidemic. Conventional techniques like acid-fast bacilli smear microscopy are generally insufficient, leading to a delay in disease detection and treatment. Novel technologies like Real-time Polymerase Chain Reaction (RT-PCR) have the potential to significantly enhance diagnostic accuracy. However, there are challenges raised by the dense *Mycobacterium tuberculosis* membrane, making it complicated to obtain DNA for amplification. Application of new strategies, , such as the application of recombinant TDM-specific hydrolase to enable lysis of mycobacterial cells, would significantly improve diagnostic sensitivity. These developments would be capable of detecting low bacterial loads in clinical specimens, ultimately reducing transmission rates and enhancing patient outcomes (Bhatti et al., 2012).

Control of acid-fast bacterial diseases calls for collective action involving various sectors, viz., research, policy, and healthcare service delivery. The stakeholders must concentrate on introducing new technologies and treatment modalities into existing health care frameworks to fill the gap in practice. New vaccines and antibiotics must be created, particularly to counteract antimicrobial resistance, which undermines the efficacy of treatment and raises the burden of acid-fast bacterial diseases. There is also a need for increased funding of research programs and international surveillance systems to identify emerging trends and challenges. Public health programs must include enhancing community education, screening practices, and the availability of treatment, particularly in high-prevalence zones. With combined efforts from academia, the public sector, and industry players, the global world can effectively combat the pervasive threat of acid-fast bacterial infections and, in the end, minimize their impact on global health.

10.6.2. Prevention Strategies and Vaccination Efforts

Control and prevention of the acid-fast bacterium-caused diseases, primarily *Mycobacterium tuberculosis*, require strategic and large-scale vaccination efforts. Current vaccination programs are primarily based on the BCG vaccine's administration, which has proven effective particularly in children but shows inconsistent effectiveness in adolescents and adults. Consequently, a growing call has been put forth to produce more efficient vaccines that will better protect against tuberculosis (TB) across all ages. Science debate, , such as the recent workshop conducted by Aeras and the Max Planck Institute, highlights the potential of employing whole mycobacterial cells as vaccine candidates, which may elicit stronger immune responses than the traditional BCG approach, thus an improved overall TB prevention measure. Other than vaccine research, preventive measures include the uptake of effective public health measures targeting early detection and intervention. High-risk groups latent TB infection screening as well as adherence to treatment are central elements of combined prevention strategies. Also, health education creating awareness about TB symptoms and transmission helps communities seek medical care in a timely fashion. Efforts must also highlight the social determinants of health, which influence the ability of individuals to use and access healthcare services. Incorporation of these educational programs into immunization activities is an integrated approach to the prevention of TB incidence, addressing both the medical and the social determinants of prevention of disease (Pinedo et al., 2018). Moreover, exploring the immunogenic potential of various strains of *Mycobacterium avium* subsp. paratuberculosis underscores the importance of vaccine development against certain acid-fast bacteria. Low-virulence strains have been identified in recent studies to hold potential as vaccine candidates for paratuberculosis that can be used as potential alternatives to further enhance immunity in livestock and possibly human populations.

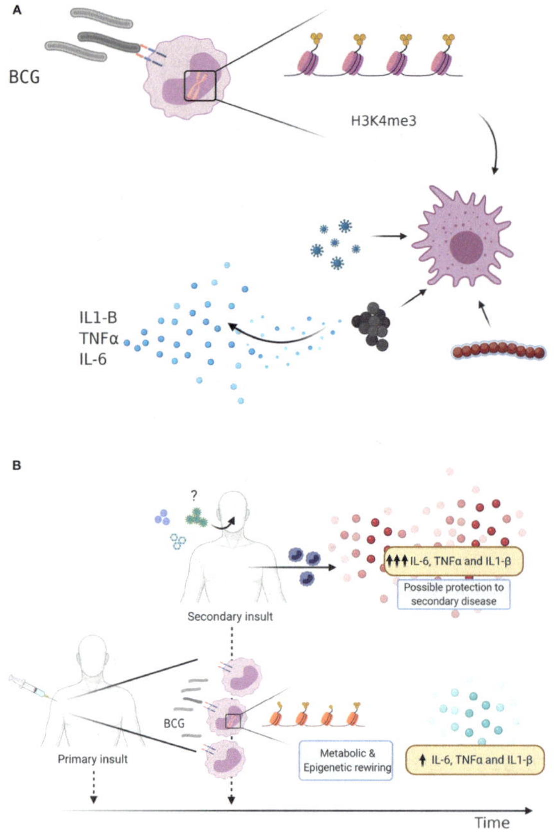

Figure 10.14. (A) BCG vaccination and trained immunity. *Bacillus Calmette-Guérin* (BCG) vaccination induces trained immunity through metabolic changes and epigenetic rewiring. (B) Trained immunity as defense mechanism against respiratory infections.

Source: https://www.researchgate.net/publication/349886215/figure/fig1/AS:11431281251020997@1718119701600/A-BCG-vaccination-and-Trained-immunity-Bacillus-Calmette-Guerin-BCG-vaccination.tif.

Research on the virulence and immunological characteristics of these strains underlines the necessity of constant assessment and innovation of vaccine candidates for ensuring more effective immunization. The findings, particularly with regard to the protective effect of live and inactivated vaccines, point to the potential of future vaccination drives and towards integrated preventive interventions against acid-fast bacteria-caused diseases (Pinedo et al., 2018) (Figure 10.14).

10.6.3. Role of Healthcare Systems in Managing Outbreaks

Healthcare systems play a critical role in the management of outbreaks, particularly for those caused by acid-fast pathogens , such as *Mycobacterium tuberculosis*, the bacterium that causes tuberculosis (TB). Effective outbreak management relies heavily on surveillance and early warning systems inherent in healthcare facilities. These systems are directed towards monitoring the prevalence and distribution of infections and providing timely information essential in public health responses. Furthermore, there should be resources, such as laboratory units for rapid detection of pathogens, raising the capacity for implementing proper regimens of treatment and isolation of infected patients. By enhancing integrated responses between various healthcare facilities, the system decreases disease transmission, thus maintaining public health while, at the same time, boosting readiness for subsequent acid-fast bacteria outbreaks (Groot et al., 2011).

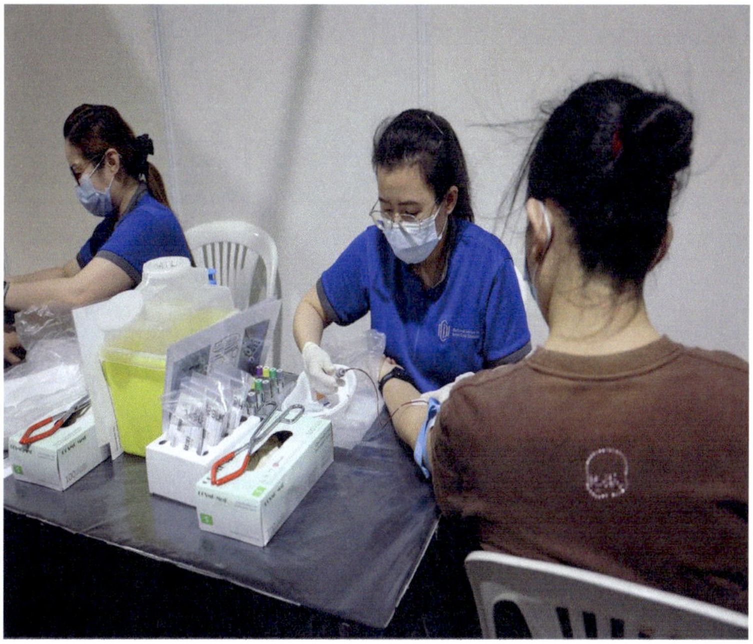

Figure 10.15. Role of healthcare systems in managing outbreaks.

Source: https://cassette.sphdigital.com.sg/image/straitstimes/a5652a1565716f 24d72f5c07d6d713adb7dfe379 70b565da0b10112a92c87a71.

Prevention is also crucial and is at times integrated into healthcare practices for outbreak control. Vaccination campaigns, sensitization programs, and rigorous enforcement of strict hygiene standards are some of the measures undertaken by healthcare systems to reduce transmission rates. These measures are particularly crucial in acid-fast bacterial disease control, which has a propensity to infect certain communities with limited access to healthcare services. Furthermore, the health systems should also focus on community involvement through collaboration with local stakeholders and leaders in responding to the sociocultural determinants of disease transmission. This joint effort not only educates about routes and prevention of transmission but also promotes trust and compliance among the affected communities, ultimately opening up avenues for better outbreak control measures (Hidalgo et al., 2016). Lastly, the ability of the healthcare system to respond to outbreaks is dependent on how robust its financing and mobilization of resources are. Adequate budgetary investment in outbreak preparedness and response activities is essential in ensuring that healthcare facilities are capable of handling the surge of cases due to acid-fast bacteria. Health workforce training, availability of essential drugs, and improvement of infrastructure are also the critical aspects that improve the resilience of a system to an outbreak. The governments and health institutions must further focus on building partnerships and networks that enhance the ability of the health systems to share information, thereby improving the coordination of responses to outbreaks. Through dedicated resources and interagency collaboration, healthcare systems can effectively manage outbreaks and contribute towards the general objective of mitigating the impact of acid-fast bacteria on public health (Groot et al., 2011) (Figure 10.15).

Test Your Knowledge

1. What is the current global burden of diseases caused by acid-fast bacteria , such as Mycobacterium tuberculosis and Mycobacterium leprae?
2. What are the key prevention strategies implemented to control the spread of tuberculosis worldwide?

SUMMARY

Acid-fast microorganisms, particularly *Mycobacterium tuberculosis*, play profound roles both in public health and the clinical practice of medicine. Advances in advanced analytical instrumentation , such as electrospray ionization tandem mass spectrometry, have revolutionized the ability to examine such microorganisms. Using mycolic acid profiling, the structural components of the bacterial cell wall integral to the rod-shaped cell, researchers have taken milestone steps toward the rapid identification of mycobacterial isolates. These novel technologies can potentially enhance diagnostic procedures for tuberculosis and outcompete the sensitivity and specificity of conventional methods. The use of modern technology in microbial diagnostics, thus, not only accelerates the identification process but can also lead to more effective treatment regimens for patients suffering from active TB (Szewczyk et al., 2013). Additionally, the survival of nonreplicating tubercle bacilli in the host is a significant challenge in the war against tuberculosis. These bacteria possess very good tolerance to antibiotic therapy and environmental stresses, which makes it difficult to manage clinically. The dynamics of this persister-like population become significant as they may inform the design of therapeutic approaches that are able to maximize treatment outcomes. To uncover the mechanisms through which these microorganisms survive chemotherapy and continue to persist throughout infection, researchers can advance to target the pathways for developing new treatment paradigms. Identification of these stable bacterial subpopulations in sputum samples presents new lines of investigation to studying transmission dynamics and holds out areas of investigation for future TB work (Alvarez et al., 2008). Overall, the role of acid-fast bateria is more than identification and classification. The evolving landscape of microbiological research highlights the necessity of continuous innovation in diagnostic technology and therapeutic strategies.

Even as science continues to unravel the mysteries of these pathogens, it is essential to have a complete picture of their biology. Efforts towards enhanced diagnostic accuracy and effective control of recalcitrant infections must be at the forefront of public health policy. With the continuous evolution of global health issues, it is essential that we remain equipped with the information and techniques necessary to combat acid-fast bacteria illnesses so that our future will be one of tuberculosis as a controllable and reduced threat. Acid-fast bacteria, of which members of the genus Mycobacterium are most significant, are significant for the study of numerous infectious diseases, particularly tuberculosis (TB) and leprosy. They are characterized by the unique cell wall chemistry composed of mycolic acids that are resistant to acid decolorization in staining methods in the lab. This acid-fastness is a paramount feature distinguishing them from other bacterial species, and their identification and following diagnosis are paramount in clinical microbiology. As Black et al. (2011) stresses, the study of microbial characteristics also extends beyond the clinical environment into other disciplines like environmental science, where soil quality indicators can play a paramount role in the understanding of microbial communities and their functions. Acid-fast bacterial pathogenicity, particularly *Mycobacterium tuberculosis*, is a public health issue. Tuberculosis remains one of the world's leading killers and continues to warrant research on its transmission dynamics, drug resistance, and treatment. Understanding the interaction of these bacteria with the host immune system is important in the development of a successful vaccine and treatment strategy. Moreover, a literary review of microbial effects in various environments, as argued in (Humphreys et al., 2010), can also illuminate the activity of acid-fast bacteria regarding waste management and containment strategies, which are crucial in guaranteeing public health safety. Besides that, the application of molecular techniques, , such as polymerase chain reaction

(PCR) and next-generation sequencing, has enhanced the research on acid-fast bacteria so that they can be understood well for their genetic diversity and antibiotic resistance. The applications allow for the rapid and precise detection of Mycobacterium species, thereby facilitating effective therapeutic intervention in time. Moreover, information on the environmental microbiology of acid-fast bacteria can inform policy to contain their spread, particularly in health institutions. The integration of microbial studies into larger-scale public and environmental health uses, noted in earlier research reports, has underscored the significance of dealing with the complete meaning of acid-fast bacteria in both clinical and environmental contexts.

KEY TERMS FROM THIS CHAPTER

Acid-fast bacteria
Acid-fast bacterial pathogenicity
Acid-fast organisms
Antibiotic therapy
Bacteria's growth rates
Bacterial infections
Cerebrospinal fluid (CSF) testing
Chronic infection
Computed tomography (CT)
DNA amplification
Drug-resistant TB
Environmental health
Extrapulmonary tuberculosis (EPTB)
Genus Mycobacterium
Health workforce training
Healthcare facilities
Healthcare systems
Leprosy pathology
Metabolic adaptability
Metabolic capabilities

CRITICAL THINKING QUESTIONS

1. Which of the following is a defining characteristic of acid-fast bacteria?
   a. They stain purple with Gram stain
   b. They have a thick peptidoglycan layer but no mycolic acid
   c. They retain carbol fuchsin dye even after acid-alcohol decolorization
   d. They are obligate anaerobes

2. Which genus is the most well-known acid-fast bacterium responsible for tuberculosis?
   a. *Staphylococcus*
   b. Mycobacterium
   c. *Clostridium*
   d. *Pseudomonas*

3. Which disease is primarily caused by *Mycobacterium leprae*, an acid-fast bacterium?
   a. Leprosy
   b. Tuberculosis
   c. Cholera
   d. Syphilis

4. Which diagnostic test is commonly used to detect acid-fast bacilli in clinical specimens?
   a. Gram stain
   b. Ziehl-Neelsen stain
   c. India ink stain
   d. Catalase test

5. Which of the following is a standard first-line treatment for tuberculosis caused by acid-fast bacteria?
   a. Penicillin
   b. Ciprofloxacin
   c. Amphotericin B
   d. Isoniazid and Rifampicin

Short Answer Questions

1. What are the key characteristics that define acid-fast bacteria and differentiate them from other bacterial groups?
2. What are the major types (genera or species) of acid-fast bacteria commonly encountered in clinical microbiology?
3. Which diseases are primarily caused by acid-fast bacteria, and what is the pathogenic mechanism of these bacteria?
4. How is the diagnosis of acid-fast bacterial infections typically performed in the laboratory?
5. What staining technique is used for the identification of acid-fast bacteria, and how does it work?
6. What are the current effective treatment options and management strategies for infections caused by acid-fast bacteria?

Answers to Critical Thinking Questions

1. (c) 2. (b) 3. (a) 4. (b) 5. (d)

REFERENCES

1. Agerberth, A., Ahsan, A., Andersson, M., Andersson, J., Andries, K., Aoki, M., Asaduzzaman, M., et al. (2016). Antimicrobial peptides as novel anti-tuberculosis therapeutics. https://core.ac.uk/download/55642138.pdf (accessed on 13th June 2025).
2. Ahmad Sarhan, M. A. (2004). *Development of Salmonella Typhi Ty21a as a Potential Oral Vaccine Against Tuberculosis: Surface Display and DNA Vaccine Carrier of a Synthetic Multi-Epitope Mycobacterial Gene* [RC311.4. A135 2004 f rb][Microfiche 7750]. https://core.ac.uk/download/11927241.pdf (accessed on 13th June 2025).
3. Akin, H., Altschul, S., Andersen, M., Andreasen, P., Aurilia, J., Barnum, R., Bartolomé, C., et al. (2010). The interplay of descriptor-based computational analysis with pharmacophore modeling builds the basis for a novel classification scheme for feruloyl esterases. https://core.ac.uk/download/pdf/289307.pdf (accessed on 13th June 2025).
4. Assis, R. A. B., Polloni, L. C., Patané, J. S. L., Thakur, S., Felestrino, É. B., Diaz-Caballero, J., Digiampietri, L. A., Goulart, L. R., Almeida, N. F., Nascimento, R., Dandekar, A. M., Zaini, P. A., Setubal, J. C., Guttman, D. S., & Moreira, L. M. (2017). Identification and analysis of seven effector protein families with different adaptive and evolutionary histories in plant-associated members of the Xanthomonadaceae. *Scientific reports*, *7*(1), 16133. https://doi.org/10.1038/s41598-017-16325-1 (accessed on 13th June 2025).
5. Alvarado Pinedo, M. F., Colombatti Olivieri, M. A., Delgado, F. O., Gravisaco, G., et al. (2018). Protection efficacy of Argentinian isolates of *Mycobacterium avium* subsp. *paratuberculosis* with different genotypes and virulence in a murine model. https://core.ac.uk/download/287883333.pdf (accessed on 13th June 2025).
6. Alvarez, A. L., Sherratt, A., Bacon, J., Beste, D., Betts, J., Canetti, G., Senner, C., et al. (2008). Cytological and transcript analyses reveal fat and lazy persister-like bacilli in tuberculous sputum. https://core.ac.uk/download/2710284.pdf (accessed on 13th June 2025).
7. Axe, A. S., Bradshaw, D. J., Lappin, G., Millhouse, E., et al. (2016). Viable compositional analysis of an eleven-species oral polymicrobial biofilm. https://core.ac.uk/download/42371960.pdf (accessed on 13th June 2025).
8. Azadfar, S., Cheraghali, F., Javid, N., Moradi, M., et al. (2014). *Herpes Simplex* virus meningitis in children in South East of Caspian Sea, Iran. https://core.ac.uk/download/52204516.pdf (accessed on 13th June 2025).
9. Azarhoush, R., Ghorbani, R., Kavian, F., Nassaji, M., et al. (2014). Acid-fast staining in formalin-fixed tissue specimen of patients with extrapulmonary tuberculosis. https://core.ac.uk/download/52205444.pdf (accessed on 13th June 2025).
10. Bai, Z., Bodé, S., Boeckx, P., Huygens, D., et al. (2013). Kinetics of amino sugar formation from organic residues of different quality. https://core.ac.uk/download/55843729.pdf (accessed on 13th June 2025).
11. Bassegoda Puigdomenech, A., Ivanova, K. D., Portés, E. R., Tzanov, T., et al. (2018). Strategies to prevent the occurrence of resistance against antibiotics by using advanced materials. https://core.ac.uk/download/157810784.pdf (accessed on 13th June 2025).
12. Basso, L. C., Basso, T. O., Walker, G. M., Walker, M. E., et al. (2019). The future of bioethanol. https://core.ac.uk/download/196581185.pdf (accessed on 13th June 2025).

13. Bhatti, A. (2012). Optimization of rTDMH as a reagent toward improving the sensitivity of the RT-PCR-based diagnosis for *Mycobacterium tuberculosis*. https://core.ac.uk/download/12210342.pdf (accessed on 13th June 2025).

14. Bilcke, G., Cirri, E., De Decker, S., De Veylder, J., et al. (2019). Associated bacteria affect sexual reproduction by altering gene expression and metabolic processes in a biofilm-inhabiting diatom. https://core.ac.uk/download/225020116.pdf (accessed on 13th June 2025).

15. Scoping biological indicators of soil quality Phase II. Defra Final Contract Report SP0534

16. (accessed on 13th June 2025).

17. Boon, N. A. M., Descamps, T., Devleesschauwer, B., Robert, A., et al. (2019). Status and potential of bacterial genomics for public health practice: A scoping review. https://core.ac.uk/download/227041617.pdf (accessed on 13th June 2025).

18. Brady, M. (2023). *Microbial Identification*. https://core.ac.uk/download/591701357.pdf (accessed on 13th June 2025).

19. Bristow, C. C., Cristillo, A. D., Dillon, J. A., Dong, W., et al. (2019). Antimicrobial resistance in *Neisseria gonorrhoeae*: Proceedings of the STAR Sexually Transmitted Infection-Clinical Trial Group Programmatic Meeting. https://core.ac.uk/download/294625789.pdf (accessed on 13th June 2025).

20. Bull, T. J., Hermon-Taylor, J., Hinds, J., Linedale, R., et al. (2009). A rhodamine agent active against non-replicating intracellular *Mycobacterium avium* subspecies *paratuberculosis*. https://core.ac.uk/download/9535330.pdf (accessed on 13th June 2025).

21. Calvet Seral, J., Asensio, G., Montañés, J. Á. M., & Carlos, M. (2023). Fighting antimicrobial resistance in mycobacteria: Development of an antivirulence screening platform and a genetic methodology to confirm drug resistance phenotypes. https://core.ac.uk/download/582230243.pdf (accessed on 13th June 2025).

22. Christofidou, M., Georgiou, S., Kolonitsiou, F., Kyriakou, D., et al. (2023). Acid-fast bacteria as causative agents of skin and soft tissue infections: Case presentations and literature review. https://core.ac.uk/download/568067010.pdf (accessed on 13th June 2025).

23. Coenye, T., Crabbé, A., Tavernier, S., Vandeplassche, E., et al. (2019). Influence of the lung microbiome on antibiotic susceptibility of cystic fibrosis pathogens. https://core.ac.uk/download/227040537.pdf (accessed on 13th June 2025).

24. Cogneau, S., & Rigouts, L. (2021). Chapter 33: *The Genus Mycobacterium*. https://core.ac.uk/download/480381998.pdf (accessed on 13th June 2025).

25. de Graff, A. M. R., Dill, K. A., Ghosh, K., Sawle, L., et al. (2016). Role of proteome physical chemistry in cell behavior. https://core.ac.uk/download/323074663.pdf (accessed on 13th June 2025).

26. DeHart, C. (2020). *Health Concerns in Cambodia Compounded by Historical and Rural Setbacks*. https://core.ac.uk/download/322850889.pdf (accessed on 13th June 2025).

27. Du Bruyn, E., Morris, T., Rockwood, N., Wilkinson, R., et al. (2016). Assessment of treatment response in tuberculosis. https://core.ac.uk/download/77015882.pdf (accessed on 13th June 2025).

28. Englund, S. (2002). *Molecular Biology Techniques as A Tool for Detection and Characterization of Mycobacterium avium subsp. paratuberculosis*. https://core.ac.uk/download/11694594.pdf (accessed on 13th June 2025).

29. Fraser, C., Jarvis, H., Jha, A., Openshaw, P., et al. (2016). *Respiratory Syncytial Virus*. https://core.ac.uk/download/77013434.pdf (accessed on 13th June 2025).

30. González-Aguilar, G., & Guerrero, Y. C. (2013). *Shiga Toxin Detection Methods: A Short Review*. http://arxiv.org/abs/1312.4748 (accessed on 13th June 2025).

31. Jones, A. L., Sutcliffe, I. C., & Goodfellow, M. (2013). Prescottia equi gen. nov., comb. nov.: a new home for an old pathogen. *Antonie van Leeuwenhoek, 103*(3), 655–671. https://doi.org/10.1007/s10482-012-9850-8 (accessed on 13th June 2025).

32. Groot, M., Kleijer-Ligtenberg, G., & Van Asseldonk, T. (2011). *Natural Swine Health*. https://core.ac.uk/download/10932084.pdf (accessed on 13th June 2025).

33. Howell, D. G. (1966). *Selected Studies of The Fluorescent Staining of Acid-Fast Bacilli in Bovine Tissues with Auramine O*. https://core.ac.uk/download/212846477.pdf (accessed on 13th June 2025).

34. Humphreys, Paul, West, J. M. and Metcalfe, R. (2010) *Microbial Effects on Repository Performance*. Technical Report. UK NDA, UK. (accessed on 13th June 2025).

35. Jacobs, J. M., & Ottinger, C. A. (2006). *USGS/NOAA Workshop on Mycobacteria in Striped Bass, May 7–10, 2006, Annapolis, Maryland*. https://core.ac.uk/download/11017969.pdf (accessed on 13th June 2025).

36. Szewczyk, R., Kowalski, K., Janiszewska-Drobinska, B., & Druszczyńska, M. (2013). Rapid method for Mycobacterium tuberculosis identification using electrospray ionization tandem mass spectrometry analysis of mycolic acids. *Diagnostic microbiology and infectious disease, 76*(3), 298–305. https://doi.org/10.1016/j.diagmicrobio.2013.03.025 (accessed on 13th June 2025).

37. Jensen, R. L. (2012). *Feed Interventions and Skatole Deposition*. https://core.ac.uk/download/10932999.pdf (accessed on 13th June 2025).

38. Miles Hidalgo, V. (2016). Optimization of an *Escherichia coli* biosensor for a rapid and *in situ* detection in water. https://core.ac.uk/download/81572434.pdf (accessed on 13th June 2025).

39. Okoi, C. B. Y. (2018). *Non-Tuberculous Mycobacteria in The Gambia: Prevalent Species, Carriage and Disease*. https://core.ac.uk/download/151394052.pdf (accessed on 13th June 2025).

40. Panwar, D. (2024). *Role of Biotechnology in Combating Antibiotic Resistance*. https://core.ac.uk/download/636456668.pdf (accessed on 13th June 2025).

41. Truman, R. W. (1985). *Host Responses to The Phenolic-Glycolipid-1 Antigen of Mycobacterium leprae (ELISA, Leprosy, Epidemiology, Armadillo, Human)*. https://core.ac.uk/download/217387118.pdf (accessed on 13th June 2025).

BASIC CONCEPTS OF IMMUNOLOGY

11

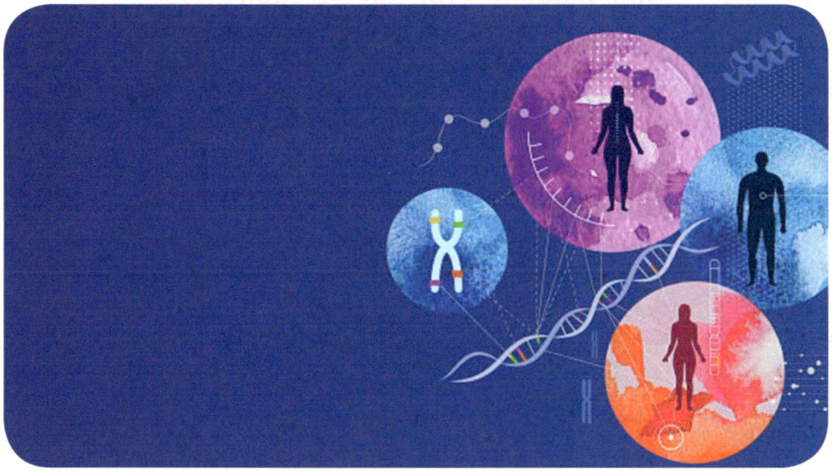

LEARNING OBJECTIVES

After studying this chapter, you will be able to:

1. Understand the basics of immune system
2. Describe innate immunity
3. Explain adaptive immunity
4. Define the terms antigens and antibodies
5. Discuss immune response mechanisms
6. Deal with immunological disorders

Introduction

The immune system is a network of complex cells, tissues, and organs necessary to safeguard the body against harmful organisms, consisting of numerous cells, tissues, and organs. Central to immunology is investigating how the body recognizes and responds to foreign bodies, known as antigens. The body tends to identify these foreigners primarily through white blood cells, which form the core of distinguishing between self and non-self bodies. Right in the middle of immunity are two fundamental branches: innate and adaptive immunity. Innate immunity is the first line of defense, producing a quick but non-specific response to infection, and adaptive immunity produces a specific response, resulting in memory to a particular infection. The exploration of these two pathways is vital in uncovering how vaccines function and how the body may be made to develop long-term immunity, and this thus confirms the importance of immunology to contemporary medicine and public health. The specificity and memory capabilities of the adaptive immune system can be attributed primarily to lymphocytes like B cells and T cells. B cells are responsible for the production of antibodies, which mark antigens for destruction, while T cells perform numerous roles, including direct cell killing and regulation of the immune system. The intricate interaction between the various elements of the immune system is a pointer to the critical need for fine coordination in the immune system. For example, the process of clonal selection allows for amplification of B cells that recognize a particular pathogen, so the response is substantial and effective when they are exposed again. Knowledge of such cellular mechanisms encourages more improved development of novel therapy regimens and vaccines to combat the impact of infectious diseases. In addition, the interaction among different immune cells highlights the importance of immunology in the clinical context and its potential to guide future research directions. Additionally, the investigation of immunology is not limited to an understanding of the body's defenses against infectious agents; it includes the implications of immune reactions on a range of health conditions. Autoimmunity, for instance, occurs when the immune system misdirects its defenses against the body's own tissues, resulting in such diseases as rheumatoid arthritis and multiple sclerosis. Immunodeficiency diseases, on the other hand, whether congenital or acquired, weaken the immune system's ability to combat infections, the best examples of which are HIV/AIDS. These examples serve to highlight the double-edged sword nature of the immune system, that of a protector and, in some cases, a participant in pathological conditions. Moreover, the ongoing research in immunotherapy is a promising area, whereby the body's immune system is used to fight cancer and other ailments. As immunology advances further, the interdisciplinary nature of the discipline and how it applies to a wide range of fields in medicine and biology are even more apparent, rendering it a significant area of study within the biological sciences.

Definition of Immunology

Immunology, as a biomedical discipline, investigates the complex interplay between the immune system and various pathogens, describing how organisms gain immunity against infection. Essentially, immunology is concerned with discovering the mechanisms of immune response, with both innate and adaptive components. The innate immune response is the initial defense, relying on physical barriers and immune cells that respond rapidly to resist or destroy potential pathogens. The adaptive immune response, however, is more sophisticated, with lymphocytes recognizing specific antigens and developing a specific response. This two-part response not only protects rapidly but also enables immunological memory, where the host can respond more efficiently upon subsequent encounters with the same disease-causing agent. Thus, the realm of immunology is greater than disease resistance; it is a dynamic interaction of biological processes that are necessary for the sustenance of life and health. Additionally, immunology is not merely limited to understanding disease resistance; it encompasses an understanding of how the immune system recognizes self and non-self, which is importantly in the context of autoimmune diseases, allergy, and cancer. Mechanisms of self-recognition are imperative to homeostasis since they prevent the immune system from attacking the body tissues in error. In autoimmune conditions, this delicate balance is disrupted, resulting in pathologies whereby the immune system mounts an attack on normal cells. The scale of immunological investigations also exists in applied sciences in the context of vaccine and therapeutic drug development to augment the immune response. Recognizing the fundamental concepts of immunology, including structures like antibodies, antigens, and cytokines, enables scientists and physicians to create efficient treatments that enhance immune function or dampen unwanted immune reactions. This encompassing awareness underlies the very paradigm according to which disease and health are presently conceived within modern medicine. The integration of practical applications into the curriculum for immunology is essential for taking theoretical constructs and turning them into applied knowledge. Having students participate in laboratory classes facilitates the comprehension of complex biological processes traditionally perceived as abstract in nature. For instance, laboratory activities enhance hands-on proficiency with techniques that illustrate fundamental immunological principles, focusing on the cultivation of critical thinking and analytical skills. Descriptive qualitative epistemic practices in such sessions, i.e., forecasting outcomes, drawing conclusions from observations, and evaluating data—highlight the importance of a dynamic learning environment. It is through this kind of experiential learning that the students can grasp the intricate interactions in the immune system and appreciate the importance of addressing public health challenges. With the encouragement of a firm foundation of immunology grounded on theoretical as well as practical foundations, the seeds are sown for innovation in medical research and clinical practice in the future, culminating in health sciences development (Bergman et al., 2010; Trivelato et al., 2016) (Figure 11.1).

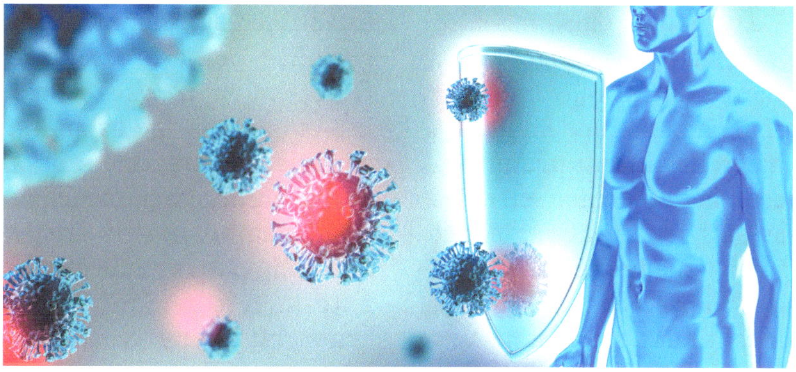

Figure 11.1. Definition of immunology.

Source: https://www.the-rheumatologist.org/wp-content/uploads/2023/11/AdobeStock_336670696.png.

Historical Background and Key Discoveries

Immunology has progressed far since centuries ago, from ancient traditions to complex molecular ideas. From the very experiences of ancient societies, witnessing that those afflicted with infectious illnesses never came down with those diseases a second time when they recovered, this phenomenon of immunity can be traced throughout history. This once triggered early inoculation methods, albeit primitive, but setting the stage for all the progress that has been made since. One of the key findings was the development of the smallpox vaccine by Edward Jenners in the late 18th century, which began the shift from empirical to a more scientific method in immunology. Jenners achievement brought with it the concept of employing attenuated pathogens for inducing immune responses and laid down the very bedrock of vaccination on which rests the cornerstone of all public health measures today. The 19th century saw revolutionary insight with the works of renowned names, such as Louis Pasteur and Emil von Behring, who advanced the field by defining the roles of antibodies and antigens in immunity. Pasteur's germ theory of disease changed prevailing notions and emphasized the significance of microbes in initiating diseases, leading to the development of anthrax and rabies vaccines. This period witnessed the birth of an understanding of the immune system as a complex web protecting the body from pathogens. In addition, von Behring's advent of serotherapy that utilized antibodies in the treatment of diphtheria laid the foundations for immunotherapeutic exploits that continue to unravel, emphasizing the vital synergy between microbes and host immunity. Later decades have seen the exploration of immunology significantly advanced by technological breakthroughs, such as monoclonal antibodies and CRISPR gene editing, which opened new fields of investigation and intervention. Debate between conventional scientific approaches and other medical paradigms, e.g., homeopathy, has also been raised, as exemplified by the collaborative research into how these systems may intersect within the realms of inflammation and immunity. Current studies have indicated promising avenues that are deserving of further scientific exploration, even as early suppositions about immunology rely largely on empirical evidence that prioritizes analytical precision and clinical trials. As the science continues, the past history combined with current information will result in new therapies and increased understanding of the complex nature of the immune system (Bellavite et al., 2005; Pace, 2012).

Importance of Immunology in Health and Disease

The importance of immunology for understanding health and disease is emphasized by its central contribution to the diagnosis of allergic illness, , such as canine atopic dermatitis (CAD). The latter, an allergic skin condition, serves to exemplify the complexity of immunity in animals as well as humans. Immunology illuminates the myriad ways through which IgE-dependent reactions to environmental allergens result in pathophysiology. In recent times, investigators have identified patterns related to CAD occurrence, which are more common in urban settings and certain breeds. Such findings support that environmental and genetic factors play a significant role in the immune response and serve to confirm that immunological concepts are absolutely essential to comprehend the multifactorial pathogenesis of allergies. Therefore, understanding of these mechanisms can lead to targeted interventions and prevention with enhanced pet health and analogues in human allergic diseases , such as eczema (Nødtvedt, 2007). The other role is seen in its ability to intervene in acute allergic reactions, for instance, the protocols for managing anaphylaxis. Anaphylaxis is a dangerous and severe hypersensitivity reaction requiring prompt treatment. Guidelines established by different allergy and immunology societies point in the direction of the key treatment approaches with an emphasis on the use of epinephrine as an initial response. This alignment in treatment approach is indicative of the underlying principles of immunology in managing health crises. The guidelines, including patient education about epinephrine auto-injectors and individual emergency action plans, are crucial in patient education and preparedness of individuals at risk and in averting anaphylactic episodes. Thus, bridging immunological knowledge and clinical practice is necessary for patient safety as well as best control of allergic disorders (Alvarez-Twose et al., 2014). Immunology does not only focus on a single disease but has implications for public health policy development and planning. Health practitioners can design successful immunization programs that are pivotal in disease prevention through the understanding of immunological mechanisms behind various diseases. Vaccines, based on the principles of immunology, have significantly cut the incidence of infectious diseases among populations. Further, ongoing research into immunological determinants of disease risk underlies the prospect of personalized medicine in the form of interventions specific to individuals' immune profiles. Such progress towards precision immunology is a prime illustration of the discipline's revolutionary potential in healthcare and reinforces its central role in improving population health outcomes. Therefore, immunology research is not just important in disease understanding but also important in the progress of medical science and public health planning in general (Figure 11.2).

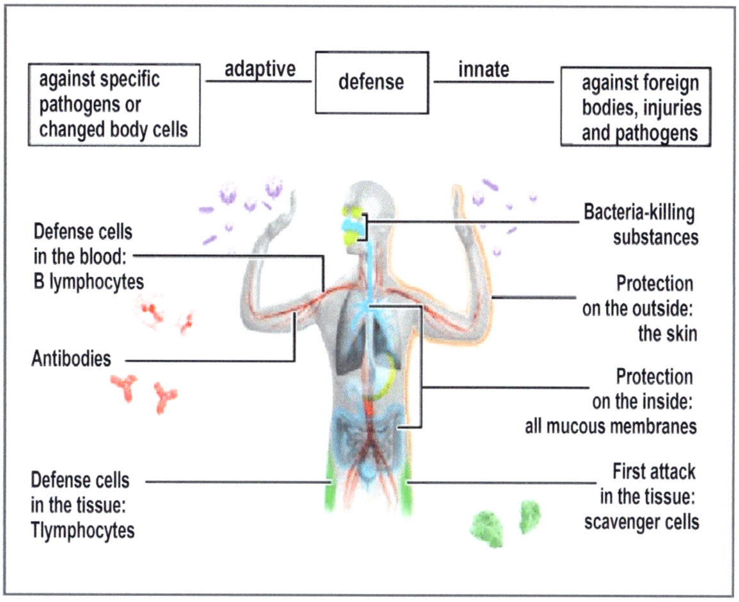

Figure 11.2. Importance of the immune system in health and disease.

Source: https://www.researchgate.net/profile/Priyanka-Namdeo-2/publication/352028771/figure/fig2/AS:1049509463326721@1627233963377/mportance-of-the-immune-system-in-health-and-disease-16.png.

11.1. The Immune System Overview

Learning Outcome

1. Understand the components of the immune system
2. Explain the types of immunity
3. Discuss the role of the immune system in homeostasis

The immune system is a multifaceted and dynamic body defense mechanism that guards the body against an array of invading organisms, such as bacteria, viruses, and parasites. This complex system consists of two major parts: the innate immune system and the adaptive immune system. The innate immune system provides immediate, non-specific responses to pathogens, depending on physical barriers, such as skin, mucosal membranes, and various types of immune cells , such as macrophages and neutrophils. The adaptive immune system, by contrast, produces specific responses later, tailored to individual pathogens through the activation of lymphocytes, such as T cells and B cells. This distinction between innate and adaptive immunity is critical to understanding the ways that the body is capable of responding to disparate immunological insults, as well as having an impact on future biomedical therapies.

The recent advances within the science of immunology have significantly enhanced our knowledge of immune processes, particularly in aquatic animals. The invertebrate immunology, for instance, has details on vertebrate-like protostome innate immune system, revealing unique pathways and pathogen receptor proteins which differ from of vertebrates. The studies have shown that there are intricate immune responses in crustaceans, involving recognition of certain effector molecules as well as regulatory pathways. These results not only expand our understanding of immune responses in non-vertebrates but also highlight the ecological significance of these interactions within aquatic environments (Adachi et al., 2012). These results can enhance disease management strategies in aquaculture, where host-pathogen dynamics are key to sustainability and biodiversity. Besides, the manufacture of biotherapeutic products also emphasizes the role of the immune system in the present medical treatments, particularly in cancer and autoimmune diseases. Genetic engineering has provided techniques for the production of pure biological products that have the ability to modulate immune responses effectively. The therapy brings its impact by improving the immune system's capacity to identify and eliminate cancer cells or to restore equilibrium to autoimmune disease. Understanding the organization and operation of the immune system is critical to its construction and offers new hope for the control of conditions that have long been aggressive clinical problems. As research into the complexity of immune reactions and their molecular mechanisms is increasingly pursued, the importance to therapeutic advances and public health is enormous (Gallucci et al., 1995).

11.1.1. Components of the Immune System

The immune system is a sophisticated system consisting of various components that work together in an effort to protect the body against infection. At the core are the innate and adaptive immune reactions, which have distinct roles in the prevention of infection. The innate immune system offers the first line of defense with barriers, such as the skin, mucous membranes, and other immune cells , such as macrophages and neutrophils, that respond immediately to any invading pathogen. This is in contrast to the adaptive immune system, which develops slowly but provides a specific response to specific pathogens. This process entails lymphocytes, T cells and B cells, discerning specific antigens, allowing for greater and longer-lasting immunity. Understanding how the immune system is designed to have a successful defense against numerous infectious diseases requires these simple distinctions. In addition, the complexity of the immune system is also evidenced by the broad array of molecules that are involved with immune signaling and recognition. Cytokines, for example, are crucial for facilitating and regulating immune response. These cell-signaling molecules, secreted by most immune cells, enable the cells to talk to each other and control the scale and time of immune responses. The function of B-cell antibodies is also crucial in identifying and disabling foreign pathogens. The antigen-presenting cell and lymphocyte interaction ensures the adaptive immune response is effective and precise. Since learning immunology is concerned with grasping these interactions is fundamental for students to put into perspective how the various immune elements function toward overall functionality. This level of understanding also aligns with educational studies research that utilizes hands-on materials to inform the students about these intricate issues, as presented in Gregory & Clarke (2009)). Finally, the theoretical model under which immune identity resides, , such as the self/non-self model, offers a useful framework for the study of immune components. First developed by F.M. Burnet, the model predicts that the immune system is capable of distinguishing between the host cell itself and alien material, which is at the core of protective immunity. More contemporary controversies, however, put forward the argument that this model needs refinement. Experiments have indicated that immune responses should also depend on the principle of continuity and not an all-or-nothing self-non-self distinction, which would better account for established immunological phenomena (Freitas et al., 2005). This fluid paradigm calls for ongoing inquiry into the mechanisms of the immune system, as it highlights the demand to revise teaching procedures and curriculum materials to reflect new knowledge. Ultimately, both the components of the immune system and the conceptual models that we use to describe them need to be questioned continuously in order to foster our comprehension of immunological principles (Figure 11.3).

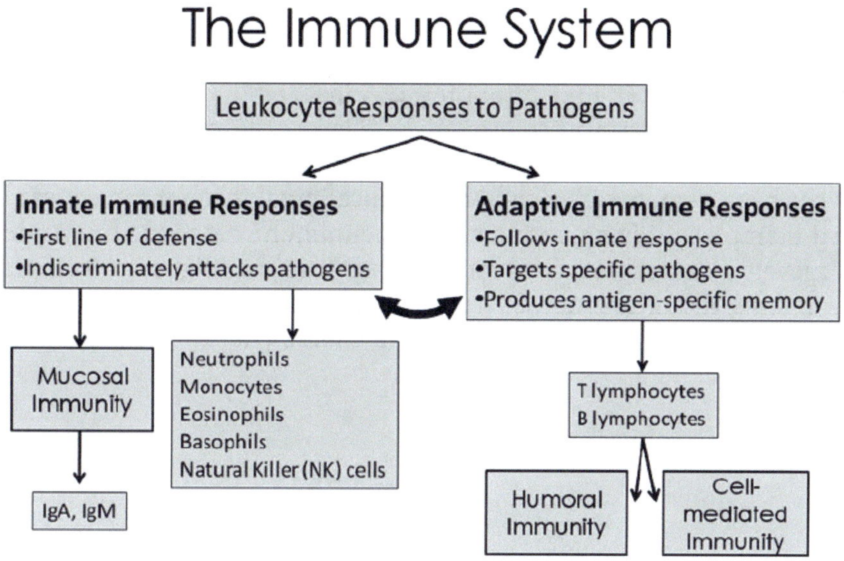

Figure 11.3. Schematic overview of the basic components of the immune system (IgA = immunoglobulin A; IgM = immunoglobulin M).

Source: https://www.researchgate.net/profile/Anthony-Hackney/publication/236091540/figure/fig1/AS:299531305537536@1448425236338/Schematic-overview-of-the-basic-components-of-the-immune-system-IgA-im-munoglobulin.png.

11.1.2. Types of Immunity: Innate vs. Adaptive

Immunity has two primary categories: innate and adaptive, which have various mechanisms and functions in the immune system. The innate immune response is the first line of defense of the body, which provides immediate, yet non-specific, protection against pathogens. This system comprises physical barriers , such as skin and mucous membranes, and cellular components , such as phagocytes and natural killer cells. These elements react quickly to identify and destroy intruders through non-specific inflammatory processes. Efficient though it is, the innate response has no memory capabilities, i.e., it is unable to recognize and recall pathogens specifically after the initial exposure. Its lack of learning is a principal deficiency of the innate system, so that if long-term protection and specific action are needed, the adaptive response must be triggered subsequently. As opposed to the natural response, adaptive immunity possesses a complicated and very specific mechanism developed over time with exposure to pathogens. Adaptive immunity is facilitated by lymphocytes, particularly T cells and B cells, that can identify specific antigens offered by pathogens. When stimulated, B cells differentiate into plasma cells that secrete antibodies, and T cells can kill infected host cells directly or assist other immune components. Another important aspect of adaptive immunity is that it can establish immunological memory, meaning that the body can react more quickly and effectively against a previously seen pathogen. This feature emphasizes the importance of vaccinations; through exposure of the immune system to a non-pathogenic form of a disease agent, vaccinations instruct the adaptive immune response to develop enduring immunity to diseases. The synergy between innate and adaptive immunity is an effective immune defense strategy, in which the speed of the innate response is supplemented by the specificity of the adaptive system. Recent advances in immunotherapy reflect the importance of understanding these two types of immunity, particularly in disease states , such as cancer and autoimmune diseases. For example, the tumor microenvironment (TME) dictates immune cell function and modulates adjustments, which need a better understanding of innate and adaptive immune capabilities to enhance therapeutic outcomes in cancer treatment. Extensive characterization of immune cells within the TME can reveal immune evasion processes and thus guide the development of new therapeutic interventions, as has been demonstrated in recent clinical breakthroughs in cancer immunotherapy, including targeted therapies utilizing both arms of the immune response to invade disease (Zhang et al., 2020). Moreover, diseases , such as multiple sclerosis highlight the complexity of immune modulation; determining the interaction between innate and adaptive immunity has the potential to reveal potential interventions that modify disease course (Reich et al., 2018) (Figure 11.4).

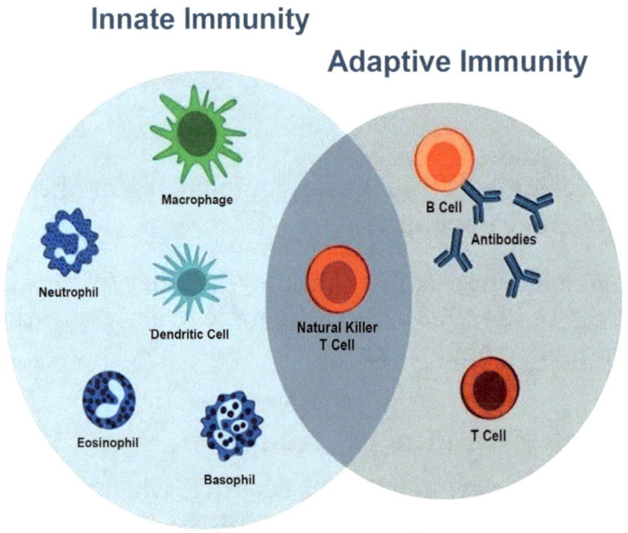

Figure 11.4. Types of immunity.

Source: https://blog.cellsignal.com/hubfs/blog/2020/19-IMO-12805%20Immunology%20SEO/Immunology_innate%20immunity%20vs%20adaptive%20immunity.jpg.

11.1.3. Role of the Immune System in Homeostasis

The immune system plays a vital role in the preservation of body homeostasis by continuously monitoring and responding to both endogenous and exogenous threats. The complexity of the systems entails cell type interaction, signaling pathways, and cytokines, all summing up to one dynamic equilibrium. For instance, ILCs have emerged as critical immune effectors with similarities in function to T helper cells but with their own unique plasticity and memory characteristics. Understanding these functions not only demonstrates the immune system's capability for plasticity but emphasizes its need to be able to function well to regulate inflammation and tissue healing. By deciphering the molecular mechanisms underlying such functions, researchers can enhance the knowledge on how the immune system retains equilibrium in response to biological and environmental stressors, thus for the maintenance of homeostasis (Sciumè et al., 2017). In addition, the function of the immune system in maintaining homeostasis also encompasses the control of allergic responses, particularly in children.

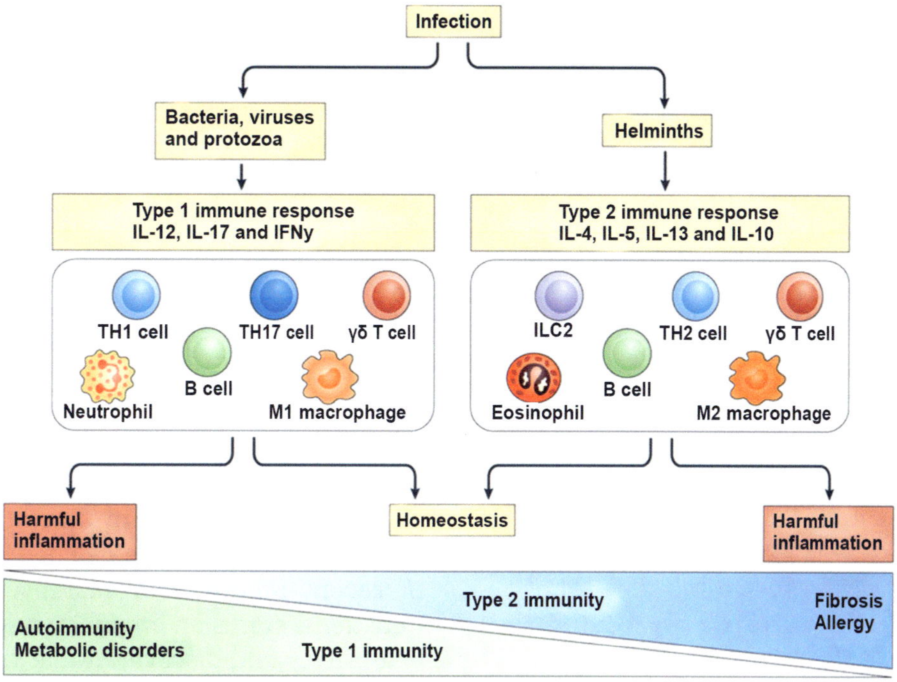

Figure 11.5. The role of the immune system in homeostasis.

Source: https://www.researchgate.net/profile/William-Gause/publication/245538135/figure/fig2/AS:279043141324831@1443540477908/The-role-of-the-immune-system-in-homeostasisHomeostasis-is-influenced-by-the-diversity.png.

Recent research has reported an increase in immune-mediated hypersensitivity among young people, and closer scrutiny of the relationship between genetic and environmental influences is called for. A combination of genetic mutation, pattern of inheritance, and environmental causes can lead to hypersensitivity reactions, making it difficult for the immune system's regulatory processes. Information gained from such studies is important, as it seeks to shed light on what is involved in such hypersensitivity reactions and on preventive measures. Such an understanding can lead to the development of specific interventions to reverse allergic responses in children, thereby highlighting the immune system's function in maintaining homeostasis and health (Burns, 2019). In general, the immune system ensures homeostasis not only through its primary function of identifying and removing pathogens but also by its homeostatic forces that suppress maladaptive reactions, , such as allergies and autoimmune disease. The dynamic nature of the immune response with regard to change in the environment highlights the importance of adaptive immunity as well as the role of memory cells. These mechanisms show the fine touch the immune system has to accomplish to attain balance within the body. As ongoing research continues to illuminate how the immune system can be influenced by a variety of factors, its relevance to medicine becomes increasingly profound, especially in the design of therapies to reassert homeostatic balance in the face of dysregulation. Overall, understanding these facets of immune function is critical toward advancing the understanding of health and disease (Sciumè et al., 2017) (Figure 11.5).

Test Your Knowledge

1. What are the primary components of the immune system, and what role does each play in defending the body?
2. How does innate immunity differ from adaptive immunity in terms of response time and specificity?

11.2. Innate Immunity

Learning Outcome

1. Understand the physical and chemical barriers of defense in the innate immune system
2. Describe cellular components: macrophages, neutrophils, and dendritic cells
3. Explain the inflammatory response

Inn Nonspecific immunity is the body's first line of defense against pathogens, as opposed to adaptive immunity in its rapid response and non-specificity. It is made up primarily of physical barriers , such as skin and mucosal membranes, and a number of cellular components , such as phagocytes , including macrophages and neutrophils. These cells have a basic function in recognizing and destroying pathogens via mechanisms , such as phagocytosis. In addition, the innate immunity has been attributed to a number of soluble molecules like cytokines and complement proteins. The rapid response of innate immunity is extremely important for regulation of the infection at the onset as well as offers a platform for the ensuing adaptive immune response by activating T and B cells. This association highlights the intrinsic significance of innate immunity as a system in itself but also as part of the entire immune system. The interaction of innate immunity with other factors within the biological system has gained much interest in recent studies. For instance, the role of nutritional status on immunity has been studied extensively and discovered that the availability of certain nutrients dictates the adequacy of innate and adaptive immune mechanisms. It is discovered through studies that the dietary constituents can enhance or suppress immune function, such that mild food deprivation leads to the augmentation of responses and severe deprivation has a negative impact. This duality suggests that effective immune responses rely not only on genetic susceptibility and pathogen exposure but also on environmental factors, including diet and environment. Such findings result in re-evaluating traditional assumptions regarding innate immunity by emphasizing the need for more comprehensive studies integrating ecological and dietary components, hence influencing human and wildlife health promotion (Strandin et al., 2018). Furthermore, advances in immunological science have underscored the need to understand the elements and function of innate immunity when seeking effective vaccines and treatments. More recent disputes among researchers, e.g., as initiated by the Global HIV Vaccine Enterprise, underscore the potential of a rational vaccine design with regard to the connection between innate immune responses and vaccine constituents. These discussions illustrated that the antigen design optimization, vector, and adjuvant need to fully grasp how innate immunity can boost a vaccine's overall efficacy. By giving more importance to building on the knowledge derived from innate immune processes, researchers are poised to enhance the efficacy of vaccines in combating infectious diseases. This holistic awareness places natural immunity at the forefront of a critical area of emphasis in immunological strategy evolution, reconciling preclinical and clinical practice (Mascola et al., 2010) (Figure 11.6).

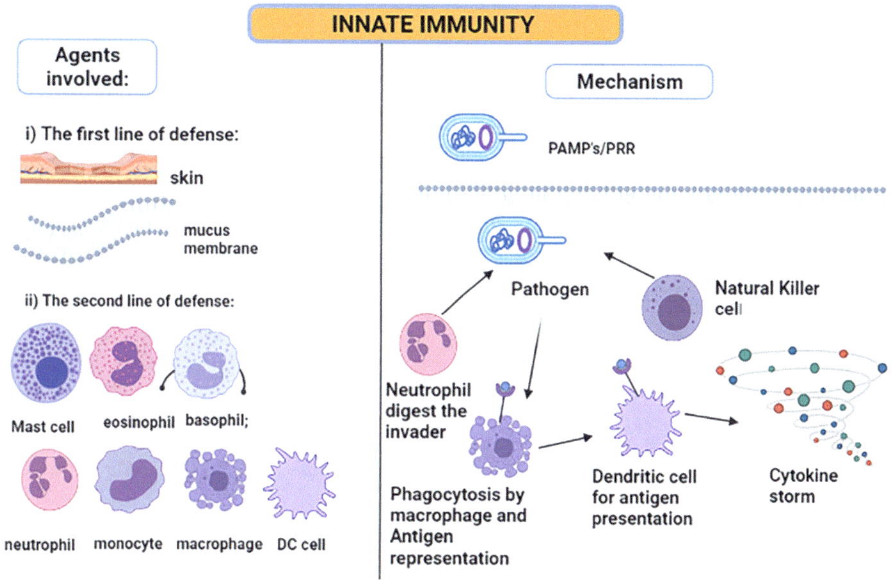

Figure 11.6. Innate immunity: pathogen-associated molecular patterns are recognized by toll-like receptors.

Source: https://www.researchgate.net/publication/359584103/figure/fig3/AS:11431281241754549@1715199575482/Innate-immunity-pathogen-associated-molecular-patterns-are-recognized-by-Toll-like.tif.

11.2.1. Physical and Chemical Barriers

Physical and chemical barriers are the innate immune system's first defense against pathogenic invasion. The skin is a prime example of such a barrier, which comes in the form of a powerful shield that has a hard outer layer which not only resists microbes but also prevents loss of water, thus maintaining homeostasis. Mucosal surfaces throughout the respiratory, gastrointestinal, and urogenital tracts also enhance defense mechanisms through secretions like mucus, which trap pathogens and permit them to be removed from the body. Finally, that cilia in the respiratory tract reveals a dynamic aspect of this barrier, sweeping dirt and microorganisms constantly. By these physical barriers, the immune system prevents infections from developing prior to an adaptive immunity being needed, illustrating how these defenses are vital for fundamental immunological principles (Gallucci et al., 1995). Chemical barriers support physical defenses by biochemical mechanisms that destroy threats. Antimicrobial peptides , such as defensins, produced by skin and epithelial cells, exhibit potent capabilities to damage microbial membranes and thereby prevent infections. In addition, secretions like lysozyme, found in salivary glands and tears, break down the cell walls of bacteria, having an initial location for invading bacterial infection. The acidic environment in the stomach is another example of a chemical barrier, being a hostile habitat for ingested microbes, effectively reducing their pathogenicity. These chemical agents indicate the sophistication of the immune system, where barriers are not just passively defensive but play an active role in biochemical warfare against a variety of pathogens. Such a confluence of physical and chemical barriers typifies an evolved pattern in our understanding of immunology (Podgórski, 2012). Physical and chemical barriers' interaction emphasizes a broad strategy towards early immune reactions, emphasizing their role in a general impression of immunological protection mechanisms. Understanding such basic principles is a foundation for the review of more evolved immune responses, , such as adaptive immunity, which are structured upon the early prevention of pathogens by these barriers. By providing a critical preventive intervention, physical and chemical barriers decrease the need for more cumbersome interventions and exhibit an extremely successful evolutionary remedy. Furthermore, with researchers seeking to develop new biotherapies that modulate immune responses, knowledge of the fundamental components of innate immunity is increasingly important. The interconnectedness of these barriers to the functioning of the immune system as a whole reveals much regarding how organisms defend their integrity from the insults of the environment (Gallucci et al., 1995) (Figure 11.7).

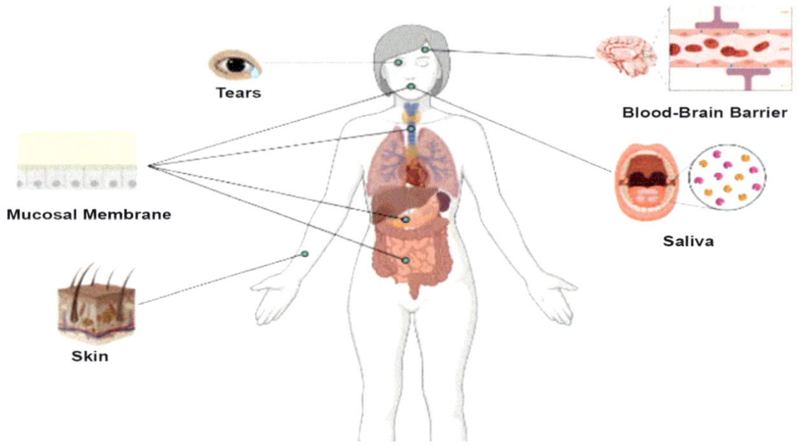

Figure 11.7. Physical barriers in innate immunity.

Source: https://i.shgcdn.com/f56874aa-3053-4f98-b47d-4439406fd243/-/format/auto/-/preview/3000x3000/-/quality/lighter/.

11.2.2. Cellular Components: Macrophages, Neutrophils, and Dendritic Cells

In immunology, macrophages are a key cellular component of immune function with a complex role. The big phagocytes are not only effective scavengers that ingest pathogens and cell debris but are also actively engaged in creating the inflammatory background by producing cytokines. Recent studies point toward the significance of autophagy in macrophages, especially for atherosclerosis, where dysfunctional autophagy has a crucial role to play in increased vascular inflammation and necrotic death of plaques. The way macrophages control such processes exhibits their key role during homeostasis as well as disease pathology (Carnuccio et al., 2013). Moreover, their ability to present antigens to T cells renders macrophages key connectors between innate and adaptive immunity, emphasizing their role within the immune hierarchy. Neutrophils, the most common leukocytes in human blood, are frontline combatants of innate immunity.

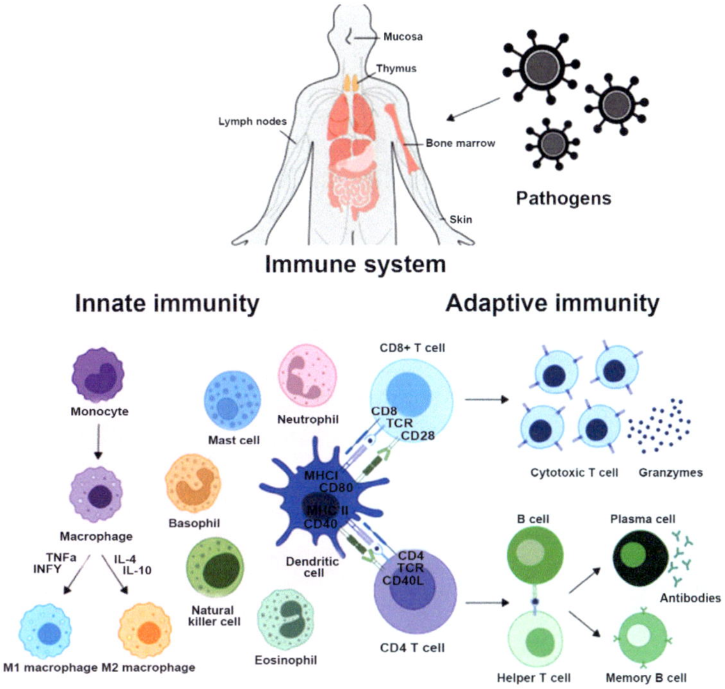

Figure 11.8. Cellular components of the immune system.

Source: https://www.researchgate.net/publication/380425653/figure/fig1/AS:11431281310460663@1739886558722/Cellular-components-of-the-immune-system-The-immune-system-comprises-various-immune.png.

These transient cells are perfectly suited to react quickly towards infections, acting rapidly on sites of inflammation through a highly coordinated interplay of chemical signals. Their recruitment is almost entirely mediated through G-protein-coupled receptors (GPCRs), which allow neutrophils to detect and react to varied chemotactic stimuli. This encompasses various forms of leukocyte movement like chemotaxis and haptotaxis, which allow for neutrophil migration through tissue efficiently (Boneschansker et al., 2019). While having the potential for rapid response, neutrophils are generally a double-edged sword, as their excessive activation leads to tissue damage and involvement in long-term inflammatory disease. Hence, familiarity with regulatory processes governing neutrophil dynamics is a must for therapeutic strategy formulation. Dendritic cells (DCs) then become the coordinators in orchestrating both innate and adaptive immunity. These antigen-presenting cells are positioned at interfaces between the body and the outside world in a strategic way and function as critical sentinels that recognize and process antigens. Once they identify pathogens, dendritic cells become mature and move to lymph nodes, where they process and present antigens to naïve T cells and stimulate adaptive immune responses. The ability of DCs to affect T cell function further underscores their significance; depending on the environment, they can drive T cell differentiation into various effector phenotypes like Th1, Th2, or Treg cells. Dendritic cells, therefore, not only have a critical role in the identification of pathogens but also in dictating the quality and degree of the adaptive immune response, thereby underscoring their significance in immunological homeostasis (Figure 11.8).

11.2.3. The Inflammatory Response

The inflammatory process is a complex biological response that is an essential part of the immune systems defense mechanism against injury and infection. Upon injury or infection of tissues by pathogens, the body mounts a cascade of signaling molecules, , such as cytokines and chemokines, that activate immune cells and induce healing.

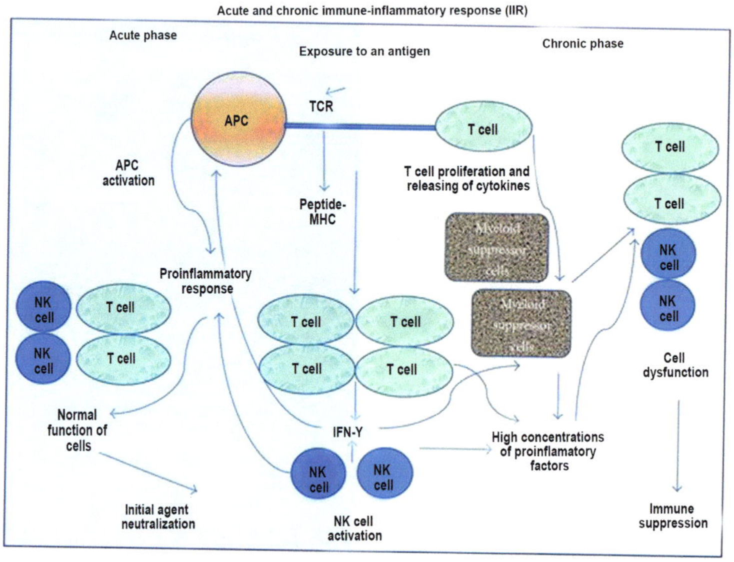

Figure 11.9. Inflammation and immune response (IIR). The primary defense mechanism of the immune system needs the activation of different cell phenotypes and intercellular signals to orchestrate all actions. Among the cytokines, the interleukins (IL) IL-1 and IL-6 and the TNFα are inducers of the IIR through the regulation of the monocytes. Immunocompetent cells are essential for an adequate immune system function, , such as the macrophages, neutrophils, fibroblasts, and endothelial cells.

Source: https://www.researchgate.net/publication/261141216/figure/fig4/AS:1088945903411244@1636636343957/Inflammation-and-immune-response-IIR-The-primary-defense-mechanism-of-the-immune.jpg.

This initial phase involves increased blood flow to the affected region, resulting in redness and swelling, as well as mobilization of immune cells like neutrophils and macrophages. These early responders are invaluable in phagocytosing pathogens and debris as well as releasing additional cytokines to perpetuate inflammation. The intricate regulation of the process makes inflammation both effective as a defense against danger and self-limiting so as not to cause unnecessary tissue damage, illustrating its double nature in disease and health. As the inflammatory process continues, there is an irrevocable turning point, from acute to chronic inflammation if the injurious stimulus is persistent. Chronic inflammation can be due to several etiologic factors, including autoimmune diseases, chronic infection, or sustained exposure to noxious substances. This is an inflammation where the immune cells remain, particularly lymphocytes and macrophages, that produce pro-inflammatory cytokines which cause sustained tissue damage rather than repair. This dysfunction can cause pathogenic processes, such as rheumatoid arthritis or inflammatory bowel disease, where the body appears to be attacking its own tissues while appearing to respond to an outside insult. Moreover, chronic inflammation has also been implicated in several other diseases, e.g., cardiovascular disease and cancer, and in this way reinforces its significance to the broader field of immunology. Inflammation-disease interface has much to tell us about the treatment of disease in modern medicine. In conditions like MS, an autoimmune disease that is chronic in nature, understanding the inflammatory cascade is crucial to devising therapeutic strategies. In MS, inflammatory demyelination is primarily due to the activation and infiltration of myelin-reactive T cells into the central nervous system, which creates a pathogenic inflammatory response leading to neurological dysfunction (Farjam et al., 2015). Current therapies for MS aim to modulate this immune response, thereby reducing relapses and tissue damage, but challenges persist in arresting disease progression (Forrester et al., 2018). Designing therapies based on specific characteristics of the inflammatory process may improve patient benefit for a wide range of inflammatory diseases, thus underscoring the merit of investigations with the goal of elucidating the pathophysiologic mechanisms of inflammation within immunology (Figure 11.9).

Test Your Knowledge

1. What are the main physical and chemical barriers that form the first line of defense in innate immunity?
2. What role do macrophages play in the innate immune response?
3. Describe the main signs and steps of the inflammatory response.

11.3. Adaptive Immunity

Learning Outcome

1. Explain the characteristics of adaptive immunity
2. Discuss the role of T cells and B cells
3. Understand the mechanisms of immunological memory

Adaptive immunity is a sophisticated arm of the immune system, developed through evolutionary processes to optimize the capacity of organisms to combat specific pathogens. It is achieved through the identification of specific antigens that occur on the surface of pathogens to elicit a specific immune response. Lymphocytes here refer to T cells and B cells and are tasked with this response and engage in a process called clonal selection and expansion. This process facilitates the development of lymphocytes that are unique to pathogen-associated antigens, ultimately resulting in effector and memory cell production. Memory cells are of critical significance because they provide long-term immunity and ensure prompt and effective response following successive exposures to the same pathogen, thereby pointing towards the efficiency and specificity that characterize adaptive immunity. The adaptive immune response can be further subdivided into two broad categories: humoral and cell-mediated immunity. Humoral immunity is primarily mediated by B cells, which produce antibodies to bind onto antigens, tagging them for destruction or neutralization. This is highly effective against extracellular pathogens. Cell-mediated immunity employs the T cells, particularly cytotoxic T cells, which kill infected cells directly. In addition, the helper T cells also play a vital role in organizing the immune response by activating the B cells and other immune cells. The coordination of these two arms of adaptive immunity is reflective of its complexity, as both of them are necessary for the overall immune defense against the entire range of pathogens.

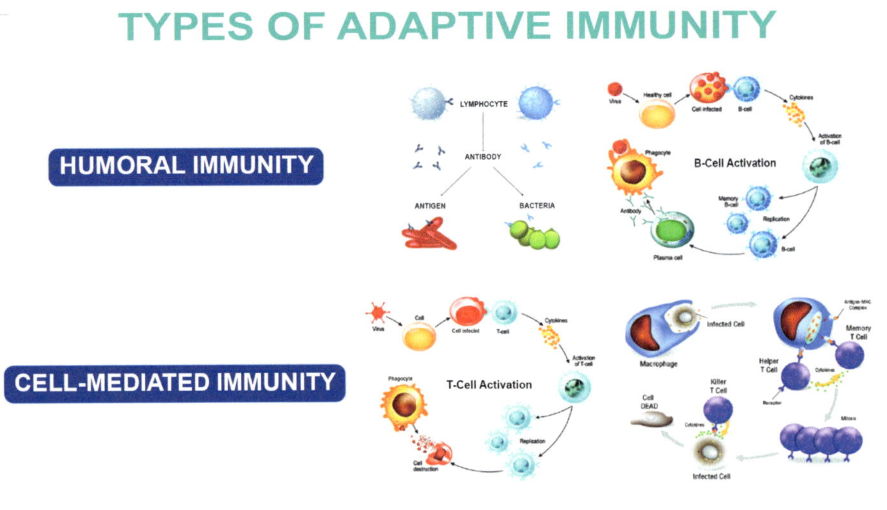

Figure 11.10. Types of adaptive immunity.

Source: https://www.biocode.org.uk/wp-content/uploads/2021/10/Blog-Thumbnail-Types-of-Adaptive-Immunity.png.

Latest findings in immunological research have unraveled the functional equivalence between innate and adaptive immune responses. For instance, studies on innate lymphoid cells (ILCs) have shown that the cells share some functions and signaling mechanisms with T cells, thus shattering traditional immune classification paradigms. Discovery of specialized cytokine profiles and T lymphocyte, as well as ILC, plasticity highlights the importance of understanding the molecular mechanisms behind adaptive immunity. A grasp of transcription factors and chromatin accessibility in these cells has opened new avenues of research in vaccine and immune therapy development, most particularly with regard to complicated diseases like HIV. As researchers continue to unveil these associations further, the emerging paradigm of adaptive immunity will more than likely shape both current and novel immunotherapeutic strategies (Mascola et al., 2010; Sciumè et al., 2017).

11.3.1. Characteristics of Adaptive Immunity

The basis of adaptive immunity is its ability to recognize and react specifically to different pathogens. Unlike innate immunity, which offers immediate nonspecific protection, adaptive immunity develops over time and is characterized by its specificity and memory. The system relies on the operation almost entirely on lymphocytes—T cells and B cells—that are able to detect distinctive antigens presented by pathogens. The lymphocytes individually proliferate and are chosen upon encountering their specific antigen so that a prompt and potent response can be mounted to subsequent encounters. Therefore, this immunological memory established by the adaptive immune system not only enhances the effectiveness against previously faced danger but also allows the system to rapidly mobilize against re-infections, demonstrating the system's good adaptability and evolutionary significance. A key characteristic of adaptive immunity is its dual response mechanism involving humoral and cellular immunity. Humoral immunity is mainly mediated by B cells, whose secreted antibodies can neutralize the pathogen or mark it for destruction by other immune cells. Cellular immunity, however, is regulated by T cells, which can directly kill infected host cells or help in other immune function by secretion of cytokines.

This balance of humoral and cellular reactions is crucial for an effective defense against an unimaginably large range of infectious pathogens, in order to tailor the response of the body to the type of pathogen encountered. Furthermore, the variety generated by somatic recombination of B and T cell receptor genes underscores the complexity of the systems, whereby a vast number of specific receptors are able to respond to an infinitude of antigenic diversities.

Recent studies highlight the contribution of natural immune cells towards shaping adaptive immunity with a complex association between the two limbs. It has been found through research that natural lymphoid cells (ILCs) have the ability to secrete cytokines analogous to those traditionally associated with T helper cells, hence bridging innate signals and adaptive responses. This mechanism highlights not only the initiating function of innate signals for priming adaptive pathways but also a degree of plasticity in immune cells responding to diverse functional demands. As ongoing research probes increasingly into the molecular underpinnings of such shared functionalities, so too does such understanding promise to illuminate the complexity of immune responses and of the potential for therapeutic intervention directed toward immune modulation in health and disease (Sciumè et al., 2017; Strandin et al., 2018) (Figure 11.11).

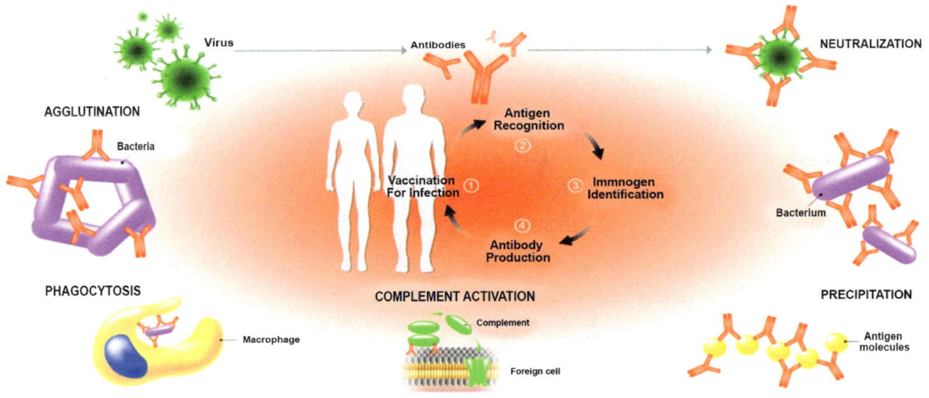

Figure 11.11. Characteristics of adaptive immunity.

Source: https://www.biocode.org.uk/wp-content/uploads/2021/11/Blog-Thumbnail-Characteristics-of-Adaptive-Immune-Response.png.

11.3.2. Role of T Cells and B Cells

The adaptive immune system is coordinated to a great extent by two central types of lymphocytes: T cells and B cells. T cells, with bone marrow origin but thymus maturation, possess the special ability to recognize specific antigens that are presented by other cells via major histocompatibility complex (MHC) molecules. T cells also subdivide into numerous subsets, including helper T cells (CD4+) and cytotoxic T cells (CD8+). Cytotoxic T cells destroy infected or tumour cells, while helper T cells are pivotal in B cell activation and the enhancement of the immune response to pathogens. The intricate interaction of T cells, their differentiation and function is governed by factors, such as cytokine milieus and transcription factor expression, which adjust their function depending on the nature of immune challenge that they encounter (Sciumè et al., 2017). B cells, however, are primarily engaged in the secretion of antibodies, which are crucial for neutralizing pathogens and marking them for phagocytic destruction. Each B cell possesses a unique membrane-bound immunoglobulin that specifically binds to a matching antigen. Activated B cells undergo clonal expansion and differentiate into plasma cells, which secrete very large quantities of antibodies. The response mediated by antibodies not only inactivates the pathogens but also makes them recognizable and susceptible to clearance. The process of affinity maturation, through which B cells refine the specificity of their antibodies, is significantly reliant upon interaction with T helper cells and is crucial to generating high-affinity antibodies (Mascola et al., 2010). This cooperation reflects synergy between B and T cells within adaptive immunity because it emphasizes their extremely crucial roles to successful immunity. A better understanding of the activities of T cells and B cells is also explained through advances in immunological technology and science. For instance, the discovery of innate lymphoid cells (ILCs) has prompted scientists to rethink functional dynamics between lymphocyte groups, finding astounding functional similarities and plasticity between ILCs and T cells. Other recent findings also feature the complexity of the immune response as an interplay of interactions instead of individual events, investigating how various cytokines and transcription factors regulate differentiation and functional outcome. An understanding of these processes not only advances our knowledge of basic immunology but also forms a platform for therapeutic strategies, , such as vaccine development and immunotherapy. Hence, the comprehensive understanding of T and B cell functions provides the background for new approaches to fight infections and cancer (Sciumè et al., 2017).

11.3.3. Mechanisms of Immunological Memory

Immunologic memory mechanisms are at the core of achieving the body's long-term immunity to infection. Upon encounter with antigen, the immune system experiences activation and differentiation, leading to the production of effector and memory lymphocytes. Effector cells perform direct action, but memory cells persist long after the first encounter, ready to respond upon subsequent contact with the same antigen.

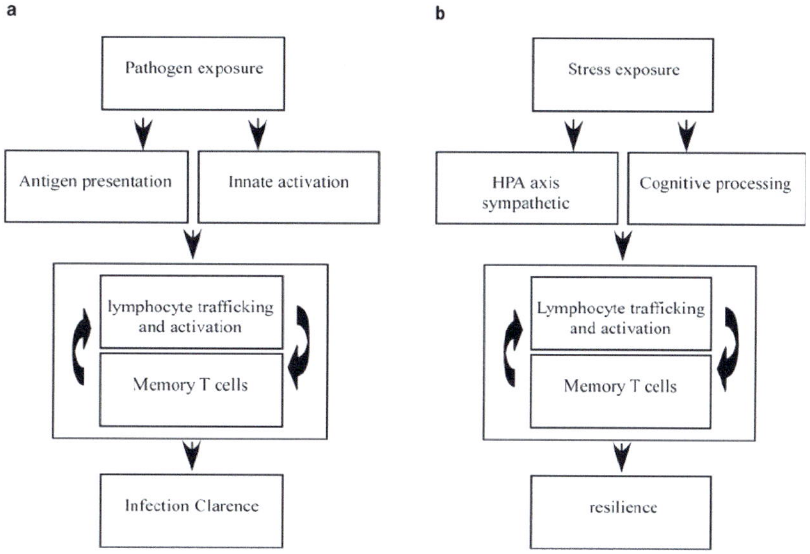

Figure 11.12. Schematic model of the induction of immunological memory. (a) Time course of induction of immunological memory following pathogen exposure and clearance of infection. (b) Time course of a protective immune response following exposure to mental stress.

Source: https://www.researchgate.net/profile/Gil-Lewitus/publication/23245592/figure/fig2/AS:277404896514059@1443149889681/Schematic-model-of-the-induction-of-immunological-memory-a-Time-course-of-induction.png.

This two-phase response not only improves more effective and quicker responses on re-exposure but also illustrates the adaptive nature of the immune system. The fine balance between these cells ensures that the body can mount an effective secondary response, highlighting the importance of memory cell populations, including memory B cells and T cells, in the general mechanism of immunity. New discoveries have clarified our understanding of the immunology of memory establishment. Investigative efforts, e.g., those spearheaded by the Global HIV Vaccine Enterprise, have emphasized rational design as a priority in vaccination strategies, particularly the optimization of factors like inserts, vectors, and adjuvants. These complexes play a central role in antigen processing and presentation, with direct implications for the generation and maintenance of immunological memory in most immune cells. Vaccine development can directly influence the competence of memory cell activation and proliferation, informing directions for boosting the immune response in at-risk populations. Consequently, successful vaccine design against challenging pathogens , such as HIV comes inevitably with memory comprehension and control, as debated in various scientific forums and workshops between distinguished immunological experts (Mascola et al., 2010). Immunological memory models and simulations have now become essential prediction technologies of immune response. By validating experimental immunological simulators, researchers can make memory theories comparable and their practical applications in a clinical setting. For instance, one model developed by authors looks at several immunological memory theories, mimicking results and comparing to in vivo readings. This allows for the chance to investigate in greater detail the heterogeneity of memory responses and its implications in immunity. These models suggest possible effect on secondary immune responses and are able to guide therapeutic treatment. While these kinds of simulations are beneficial to possess, they are more facilitatory aids than absolute evidence, supporting the nuance of immunological memory. Therefore, the integration of computational models within immunology is a significant advancement towards an improved understanding of immune system kinetics, continuing to inform vaccine research and clinical practice (Strandin et al., 2018) (Figure 11.12).

Test Your Knowledge

1. What is the primary function of B cells in the adaptive immune system?
2. How is immunological memory developed, and why is it important?

11.4. Antigens and Antibodies

Learning Outcome

1. Explain the definition and types of antigens
2. Understand the structure and function of antibodies
3. Discuss the process of antigen-antibody interaction

The immune reaction is deeply dependent on the interaction between antigens and antibodies, essentially determining the body's defense mechanisms against pathogens. Antigens, which can be described as any substance that triggers an immune reaction, encompass a wide variety of molecules, including proteins, polysaccharides, and even nucleic acids. These molecules are usually found on the surface of pathogens, thus making them recognizable by the immune system. Structural antigenic complexity is significant, as it will determine the specificity of the immune response. For instance, the presence of specific epitopes on the antigen can cause the activation of B lymphocytes and subsequent antibody production. By this process, the antigen is not only a target to the immune system but also crucial as the trigger for the whole adaptive immune response. Antibodies, or immunoglobulins, are effector molecules that are induced in response to antigens and play a vital role in the immune defense. These Y-shaped proteins have the ability to bind with specific antigens in their variable regions and facilitate various immune functions , such as neutralization, opsonization, and activation of the complement system. There are five principal classes of antibodies, IgG, IgA, IgM, IgE, and

IgD, and each has a distinct role to play in the immune system. For example, IgG plays primarily a long-term immunity role and can cross the placenta to provide passive immunity to the fetus. IgE, however, is primarily responsible for allergic responses and defense against parasitic infection. The dynamic relationship between antibodies and antigens provides the fine regulation of the immune response to allow specificity as well as a powerful resistance against thousands of pathogens. Recent research into the mechanisms of immune reactions has further elucidated the complex interrelationship between antigens and antibodies, as witnessed by seminal pieces of evidence like those of child allergies. Research into possible risk factors for hypersensitivity reactions sheds light on the importance of understanding how the immune system responds to allergens. Genetic inheritance, environmental sensitization, and immune function all play significant roles in predicting the susceptibility of individuals to allergy, particularly in children (Burns, 2019). Furthermore, efforts to develop a quantitative theoretical model for immunology can also improve our comprehension of these intricate interactions, bridging the knowledge gap between theoretical immunology and practice (Abbas et al., 2010). With research ever-progressing, the precision of our understanding of antigen-antibody interactions will be key in both the development of potent treatments and improving overall immunological health.

11.4.1. Definition and Types of Antigens

Antigens are highly significant components of the immune system and are any material capable of triggering an immune response upon contact with some lymphocytes or antibodies. They are primarily categorized into two broad categories: exogenous and endogenous antigens. Exogenous antigens originate from outside the body, typically from infectious agents , such as bacteria, viruses, and fungi, as well as from allergens and foreign tissue. Conversely, endogenous antigens are produced within the body's own cells through processes , such as normal cellular metabolism or infection by a pathogen. The immune system regards such antigens as self or foreign, and an activation process is triggered by the immune system to neutralize or destroy such perceived threats to demonstrate the fundamental role of antigens in maintaining homeostasis and health throughout the organism's life. Excavating deeper into the antigen classification, antigens can also be classified based on their characteristics, such as their immunogenicity and specificity. Immunogenic antigens are those capable of triggering a robust immune response, while non-immunogenic antigens, although identified by the immune system, do not cause robust immune activation. Of the immunogenic antigens, some are classified as hapten, small molecules that cannot elicit a response on their own but gain immunogenicity when bound to a carrier protein of larger molecular weight. Besides, antigens can differ based on origin, with native antigens highlighting the species occurring naturally in an organism and recombinant antigens generated synthetically via biotechnology processes. Each group not only signifies the complexity of antigenicity but also notes how the immune system identifies and strikes at different pathogenic threats. Finally, the application of antigens is more than mere classification; they play essential roles in vaccine manufacture and treatment determination. An understanding of the nature of antigens allows scientists to exploit their attributes in order to design vaccines that are capable of eliciting a protective immune response against specific pathogens, for instance, those of influenza or other viral infections. The production of recombinant vaccines, for instance, often means using specific antigenic components to induce a response without generating a live pathogen risk. As seen from the huge patent environment of influenza vaccine technologies, the characterization and new application of antigens reveal a pivotal engagement of science and public health programs (Barton et al., 2012), (Aickelin et al., 2010). This setting not only reflects the importance of antigen understanding to vaccine effectiveness but also reflects a global effort against emerging health issues, guaranteeing the continued relevance of immunological research and application (Figure 11.13).

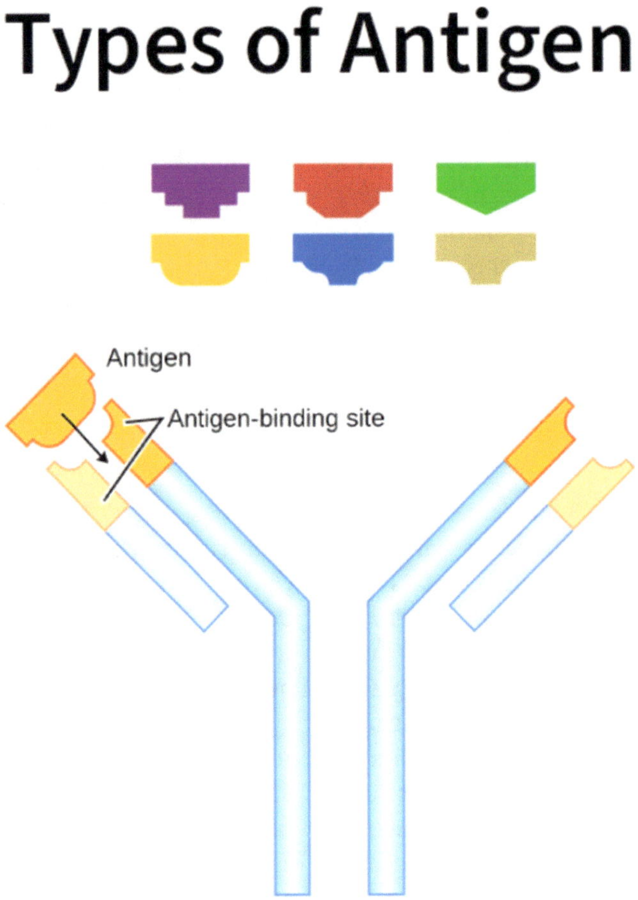

Figure 11.13. Types of antigen.

Source: https://media.geeksforgeeks.org/wp-content/uploads/20240603130902/Types-of-Antigen.png.

11.4.2. Structure and Function of Antibodies

Antibodies, or immunoglobulins, are glycoproteins derived from B cells that are the product of the body's response to antigens, and are critical components of the adaptive immune system. Their simple structure is two identical heavy chains and two identical light chains bonded together by disulfide bridges in a Y-shaped molecule. This organization is closely developed so that specific antigens can be identified, with each antibody having a different variable region capable of binding distinct antigens. The constant region is very different across different antibodies, but maintains its overall organizational pattern and functions intact. This organization is critical in enabling antibodies to perform their many roles in immune defense, including pathogen neutralization, phagocytosis activation, and complement system activation. Such knowledge of the structural characteristics of antibodies is thus critical in comprehending their diverse functions in immunological responses.

The action mechanism of antibodies is multifaceted, incorporating such processes as neutralization, opsonization, and complement pathway activation. Neutralization is the binding of antibodies to pathogens or toxins, preventing them from infecting host cells or causing harm. It is particularly crucial for viruses since it can prevent them from entering cells, preventing infection in effect. Opsonization facilitates phagocytosis by covering pathogens with antibodies, marking them for immune cell detection and destruction. Activation of the complement system again amplifies these immune reactions, which lead to augmented inflammation and the formation of membrane attack complexes that are toxic to pathogens. Incorporation of these processes demonstrates the importance of antibodies in inducing a robust defense against a broad spectrum of infectious pathogens and thereby playing an essential role in maintaining homeostasis within the immune response. Current research continues to provide insights into the complexity of the structure and function of antibodies in various situations, , such as vaccine design and immunotherapy. The understanding of how antibodies interact with antigens at the molecular level can be instrumental for making advances in disease treatment targeted to certain conditions, , such as cancer and autoimmune disorders. For instance, antibody design subtleties have been investigated via study that seeks to increase specificity and effect, for instance, in HIV vaccine development and the discovery of antigen processing routes (Mascola et al., 2010). The ability of antibodies to neutralize the targeted pathogens, for instance, through studies of bovine colostrum and its immunocomponents, suggests they can prevent gastrointestinal infections (Rokka, 2008). Together, ongoing studies in this arena not only enhance our knowledge of immune response but also guide clinical uses aimed at releasing the therapeutic utility of antibodies (Figure 11.14).

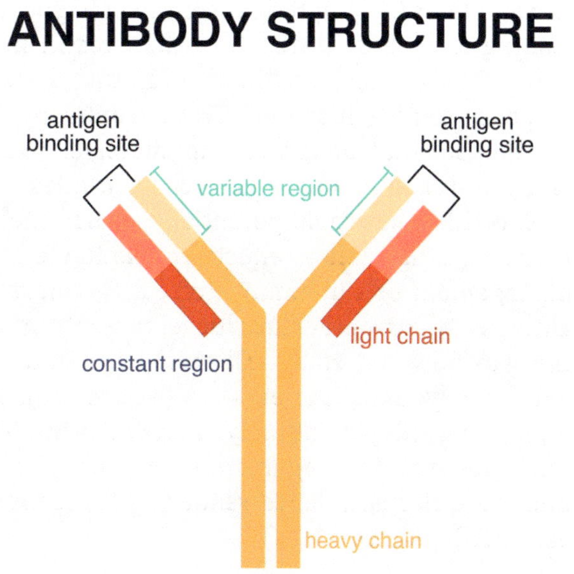

Figure 11.14. Antibody structure.

Source: https://www.news-medical.net/images/Article_Images/ImageForArticle_16427_17386091169636892.jpg.

11.4.3. The Process of Antigen-Antibody Interaction

Antigen-antibody interaction is a mechanism that assists the immune system in identifying and responding to foreign substances. The mechanism begins when an antigen, usually a protein or polysaccharide attached to the surface of disease-causing organisms, binds to a specific antibody. Antibodies, also known as immunoglobulins, are produced by B cells in response to the presence of antigens. Each antibody has a specific binding site that is designed to recognize a singular antigen, so the immune system can distinguish between a range of potential threats. The specificity of the binding is critical; it means the immune response can be highly targeted, causing minimal damage to the body's own tissues while effectively neutralizing entering organisms. When the antibody becomes bound to an antigen, it undergoes a conformational change that enhances its effectiveness in removing the antigen. Through such an interaction, various effector functions are activated, including opsonization, where the antibody is capable of tagging the antigen for phagocytic killing. Or, it can activate the complement system, leading to a chain of reactions that result in pathogen lysis. The plasticity and versatility of the antibodies are most significant, as this allows the immune system to produce a rapid, effective response to new infections. This dynamic interaction of the antigens and antibodies is the advanced mechanism that underlies immunological defense, forming the foundation for vaccine induction and natural immunity. Research continues to explore these interactions at the molecular level, with results that could potentially inform therapeutic treatments in a wide variety of diseases. For instance, drugs able to effectively modulate antigen-antibody interactions play a crucial role in the management of autoimmune diseases, where the immune response reacts against the body's own antigens by error. Further, developments in quantitative theoretical immunology seek to bridge the gap between statistical mechanics and immunological principles, hence explaining antigen-antibody dynamics in new ways (Abbas et al., 2010). The awareness of the fundamental mechanism underlying antigen-antibody interactions not only provides us with an insight into immune responses but also provides opportunities for novel pharmacological targets in disease management, like multiple sclerosis, hence rendering it a central process in contemporary immunology (Farjam et al., 2015) (Figure 11.15).

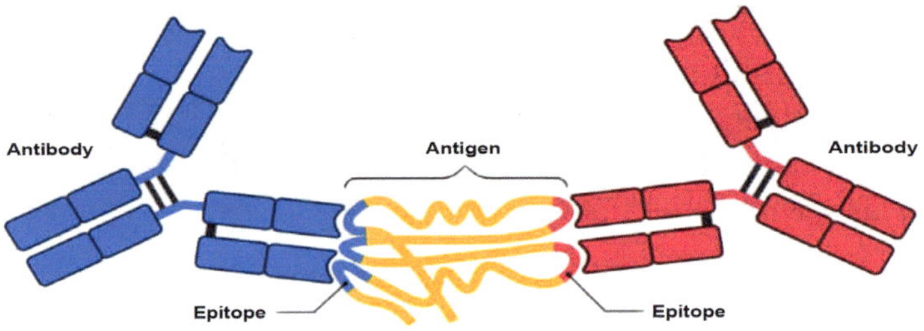

Figure 11.15. Antigen-antibody interaction.

Source: https://microbenotes.com/wp-content/uploads/2022/05/Antigen-Antibody-Ag-Ab-Interaction.jpeg.

Test Your Knowledge

1. What is an antigen, and what are the different types of antigens recognized by the immune system?
2. What are the main functions of antibodies in the immune response?

11.5. Immune Response Mechanisms

Learning Outcome

1. Understand primary and secondary immune responses
2. Describe cytokines and their role in immune signaling
3. Explain how the complement system plays a vital role in the innate immune response

Immune response mechanisms are intricate and basic in nature to guard the host organism from disease-causing agents. At the center of the response lies the recognition of foreign antigens, giving rise to a chain of immunological events. Self/non-self model, being very common among F.M. Burnet's theories, is at the heart of an explanation of how the immune system differentiates between endogenous and exogenous materials. Classically, this system takes the position that all foreign components will cause an immune response, while endogenous components will not, except for extraordinary situations. But new data indicate the limitations of this system. The low explanatory power of the self/non-self model portends the necessity of a more refined strategy that emphasizes the continuity of the biological identity, thereby broadening our description of a number of immune phenomena within the field of immunology (Freitas et al., 2005). The innate immune response is the first line of defense against infection and operates through multiple mechanisms, including physical barriers, cell-mediated recognition, and complement activation. Key players , such as macrophages, neutrophils, and dendritic cells are used for quick recognition and killing of the pathogens, mainly via phagocytosis and secretion of pro-inflammatory cytokines. This initial response sets the foundation for the adaptive immune system, which is characterized by a sluggish but differentiated response. Significant in this interaction is the role of antigen-presenting cells (APCs) since their function is to act as a link between innate and adaptive immunity. Through antigen presentation and processing to T cells, APCs initiate a targeted immune response fundamental to effective pathogen clearance and immunologic memory and thus enhance the overall function of the immune system. Besides that, psychosocial factors also influence immune responses, particularly in infectious diseases , such as tuberculosis (TB). Recent evidence suggests that adverse psychosocial determinants, , such as stress, may compromise vaccine responses and immune function overall, with positive psychosocial determinants supporting immunity. For instance, research reveals that social support may enhance the efficacy of immunity, with potential for disease like TB with the BCG vaccine (Boccia et al., 2019). With the growing insight into how psychosocial stressors intersect with immune biomarkers, this also serves to highlight the value of integrating psychological health into immunologic research and therapeutic interventions. Appreciation of these intersections has the potential to inform more integrative strategies to optimize immune responses and create public health interventions that not only address biological processes, but also the psychosocial determinants of disease and health.

11.5.1. Primary and Secondary Immune Responses

The operations of the immune system are basically classified into two types of responses: primary and secondary immune responses. The primary immune response occurs when the immune system encounters a pathogen for the first time. Naive B and T lymphocytes recognize antigens and undergo clonal selection at this time, which results in proliferation and differentiation. Typically, this is succeeded by a lag phase because it takes some time before the body can produce specific antibodies and effector cells. The produced antibodies are typically IgM isotypes, which indicate an acute response to infection. Over time, memory B cells are developed that are responsible for the immune system's recognition and defense against the same pathogen on subsequent exposures to it, thereby providing a base for an increased secondary immune response. On repeated exposure to the same antigen, the secondary immune response is initiated, resulting in a faster and more intense response. This is due to the memory B cells and T cells that have previously been generated during the primary response. Upon re-exposure of the body to the pathogen, these memory cells rapidly divide and develop into plasma cells that secrete massive quantities of antibodies, predominantly of the IgG class, that are more effective at neutralizing pathogens than IgM. The lag phase is therefore significantly reduced, and the number of antibodies produced is much higher than during the primary response. This increased and swift response serves to illustrate the importance of immunological memory, the cornerstone of vaccine policy that aims to condition the immune system against infection in the future. The complexity of immune responses is further added to by the effect of external factors like nutrition and developments in biotherapy. Experiments have shown that nutritional components may significantly affect the immune function, modulating primary and secondary responses. Certain nutrients, for instance, have been reported to enhance overall immune function, which leads to a better response against pathogens. Deficiency in certain nutrients, however, may weaken the immune effectiveness, emphasizing the relevance of nutrition to health and disease resistance. Furthermore, biotherapy is transforming immunological applications as newer innovations allow the production of purified biological compounds for the purpose of controlling the immune system. With continued advancement of biotherapy, understanding how the advancements affect existing immune response systems is essential, particularly with reference to diseases , such as cancer and autoimmune conditions, demonstrating the linkage between immunology and modern therapeutic methods (Strandin et al., 2018; Gallucci et al., 1995).

11.5.2. Cytokines and Their Role in Immune Signaling

Cytokines are a critical component of the immune system that function as signal molecules to enable communication between cells. Cytokines are small proteins secreted by various cell types like lymphocytes, macrophages, and endothelial cells. Cytokines play indispensable roles in controlling immune responses. Upon secretion, cytokines engage with particular receptors on target cells and start signaling cascades that control cellular behavior , such as proliferation, differentiation, and apoptosis. The specificity of cytokines, including interleukins, interferons, and tumor necrosis factors, is also reflected in their specialized functions in innate and adaptive immunity. Their ability to orchestrate complex immune responses highlights the decisive role played by cytokines in homeostasis and effective defense against pathogens. In addition, the abnormality in cytokine signaling has been linked with many autoimmune and inflammatory conditions, which adds even more importance to further research into their precise roles under varying physiological contexts. Among the many immune cells, innate lymphoid cells (ILCs) offer an interesting perspective on cytokine signaling because their functional properties are similar to those of T cells. Recent studies have proven that ILCs possess the ability to generate cytokines that are commonly associated with T helper subsets, rendering the traditional understanding of immune signaling questionable (Sciumè et al., 2017). The responsiveness and plasticity of ILCs reveal that they possess the ability to respond promptly to numerous stimuli and influence early as well as late phases of immune responses. Furthermore, ILCs and T cell development share in transcriptional regulation, a hint that profound mechanisms underlie cytokine production in various lymphocyte populations. It is illuminating to hear about the intricate interplay between these cell types with their respective signaling pathways and how they are implicated in understanding the intricacy of immune responses, as well as offering potential for therapeutic interventions in inhibiting cytokine-dependent pathways in disease.

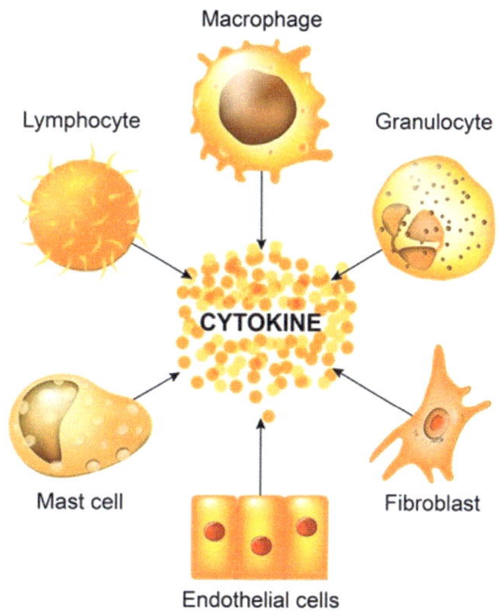

Figure 11.16. Cytokine.

Source: https://www.news-medical.net/images/Article_Images/ImageForArticle_1090_44806087938368067703.jpg.

The role of macrophages in cytokine signaling also illustrates the intricate structure of immune communication. New evidence on macrophage autophagy indicates that cellular autophagy plays a critical role in vascular inflammation, particularly in atherosclerosis (Carnuccio et al., 2013). Under early stages of disease, autophagy with normal function preserves macrophage homeostasis and is atheroprotective, while in late stages of disease, dysfunctional autophagy promotes inflammation and oxidative stress. This two-way function underlines the importance of cytokines in controlling macrophage activity and its resultant impact on adjacent tissues. Because they are resident immune cells of several tissues, macrophages release cytokines that not only recruit other immune cells but also define the local immune environment. The complex interaction between macrophage and cytokine function highlights the need for a more subtle understanding of cytokine signaling to develop targeted therapy for inflammatory diseases (Figure 11.16).

11.5.3. The Complement System

The complement system is an important part of the innate immune response and serves as the bridge between innate and adaptive immunity. It is a complex cascade of proteins found in tissues and blood, which is activated by three primary pathways: the classical, lectin, and alternative pathways.

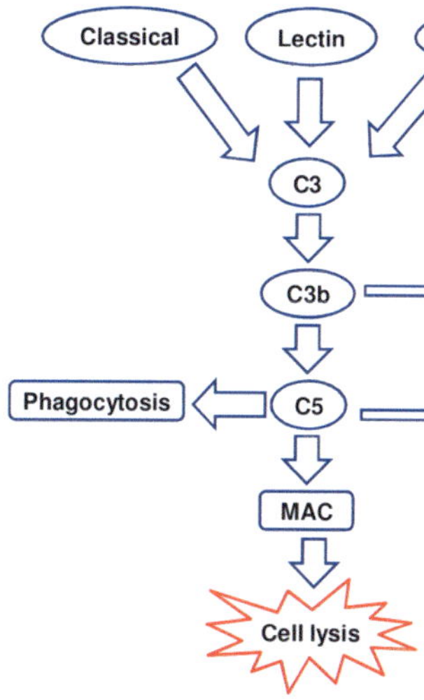

Figure 11.17. The complement system is a central component of the innate immune system and plays a pivotal role in host defense against infection.

Source: https://www.researchgate.net/profile/Praveen-Srivastava-6/publication/276288343/figure/fig1/AS:391855918338049@1470437139286/The-Complement-system-is-a-central-component-of-the-innate-immune-system-and-plays-a.png.

These are all triggered by specific stimuli, , such as antibody detection of pathogens or pathogen-associated molecular pattern detection. Activated complement proteins pass through a series of enzymatic processes to ultimately result in pathogen opsonization, inflammation, and cell lysis via membrane attack complex (MAC) assembly. This polyvalent mechanism ensures that the pathogens are efficiently targeted and eliminated, subsequently enabling the adaptive immune response to occur in addition to enhancing overall immunological memory. The complement system is also significant in regulating immune responses and in homeostasis. This is well evidenced by its action with other immune cells like macrophages and neutrophils. By enhancing opsonization, complement components enhance phagocytosis of the pathogens so that immune cells are able to clear the infection. Furthermore, complement activation initiates the release of pro-inflammatory mediators, which attract immune cells to infected sites, thus enhancing inflammatory responses. However, deregulation of the complement system results in tissue destruction or autoimmune diseases due to excessive inflammation or inappropriate targeting of self-tissues. Awareness of this fine balance is essential for grasping the role of the complement system in protective immunity as well as in possible pathologies. Beyond the direct defense against pathogens, the usefulness of the complement system extends to shaping the success of diverse therapies. The activity and efficacy of the complement system, for example, in the fight against infections, has been influenced by certain dietary factors in some studies. Of special interest are therapies and immunizations acting on the complement system, as observed to enhance the overall immunogenicity of vaccines by the interactions between selected antibodies and complement proteins. Experiments show that adding colostral immune preparations with selected probiotics can be highly effective in enhancing complement and opsonizing functions in neonatal hosts, suggesting new ways for immune response enhancement at critical development stages. Overall, the complement system is not just a cornerstone of innate immunity but also a key player in realizing the efficacy and effectiveness of adaptive immune responses, as further research unveils its overall role in immune modulation (Rokka, 2008; Strandin et al., 2018) (Figure 11.17).

Test Your Knowledge

1. What is the difference between a primary and a secondary immune response?
2. What are cytokines, and what role do they play in the immune system?
3. How does the body ensure a more rapid and effective response during a secondary immune response?

11.6. Immunological Disorders

Learning Outcome

1. Understand autoimmune diseases
2. Describe allergies and hypersensitivity reactions
3. Explain immunodeficiency disorders

Immunological diseases are a group of diverse disorders that are characterized by dysfunction of the immune system, and either inappropriate response to foreign antigens or inability to recognize and eliminate pathogens. Autoimmune illnesses , such as rheumatoid arthritis and lupus are a notable subgroup of these diseases, in which the body's own tissues are recognized and attacked by the immune system inappropriately. These diseases can cause inflammation, tissue damage, and a plethora of systemic manifestations, complicating their diagnosis and management. Furthermore, the burden of disease in autoimmune diseases extends beyond physical well-being, often impacting psychological well-being. The complex nature of such diseases necessitates an integrated approach to decipher their pathogenesis and design more effective interventions, further emphasizing the importance of immunological research in uncovering the pathogenic processes responsible for such deranged immune responses. Yet another significant aspect of immunological disorders is their overlap with infections, particularly in immunocompromised patients or in the presence of underlying conditions , such as HIV/AIDS. The ability of the immune system to respond against infectious agents may be grossly compromised so that it becomes more prone to opportunistic infections with potentially disastrous consequences. Illnesses like tuberculosis (TB) illustrate the intricate relationship between psychosocial forces and immune responses as adverse psychosocial influences can exacerbate immune impairment, which then impacts disease course. Evidence suggests that stressed individuals may have compromised vaccine efficacy and heightened immune responses to some pathogens, , such as TB, thus illuminating the importance of psychosocial context in immunologic health. Therapy of both the psychosocial and biological aspects can enhance preventive interventions for infectious disease, and additional research is necessary to ascertain the interaction of these elements and their roles in immune functions (Boccia et al., 2019). In addition to autoimmune illnesses and infectious disease complications, neuroinflammatory disease , such as multiple sclerosis (MS) also demonstrate immunological disorder complexities. MS is characterized by central nervous system inflammatory demyelination, which is triggered primarily by atypical immune reactions. Activation of myelin-reactive T cells is the crucial mechanism implicated in its pathogenesis, causing substantial neuronal damage and disruption of nervous system communication. Despite advances in disease-modifying therapy aimed at immune response modulation to reduce relapse rates, issues with the prevention of long-term disability in MS course remain. New therapeutic strategies designed to counteract the individual autoimmune mechanisms are under development, which underscores the dynamic nature of the science of immunology and the need for new ways to successfully treat these incapacitating diseases (Farjam et al., 2015). Definition of the immunopathogenesis of such illnesses not only facilitates the development of targeted therapies but also increases the general discourse within the science of immunology.

11.6.1. Autoimmune Diseases

Autoimmune diseases are one of the biggest research concerns in the field of immunology, with the immune system attacking the body's own tissues and cells by mistake. Many different disorders fall under this category, including rheumatoid arthritis, lupus, and multiple sclerosis (MS), each presenting its own complications and presentations. In autoimmune diseases, the regulatory mechanisms that should maintain self-tolerance are disrupted, leading to tissue damage and inflammation. The pathogenesis of such conditions generally consists of complex interactions between genetic predisposition and environmental provocation, the latter inducing or exacerbating the dysregulated immune process. Mechanistic explanation of the former is extremely crucial for the development of effective therapeutic regimens aimed at the restoration of normal immunity and reduction of symptoms of these disabling diseases.

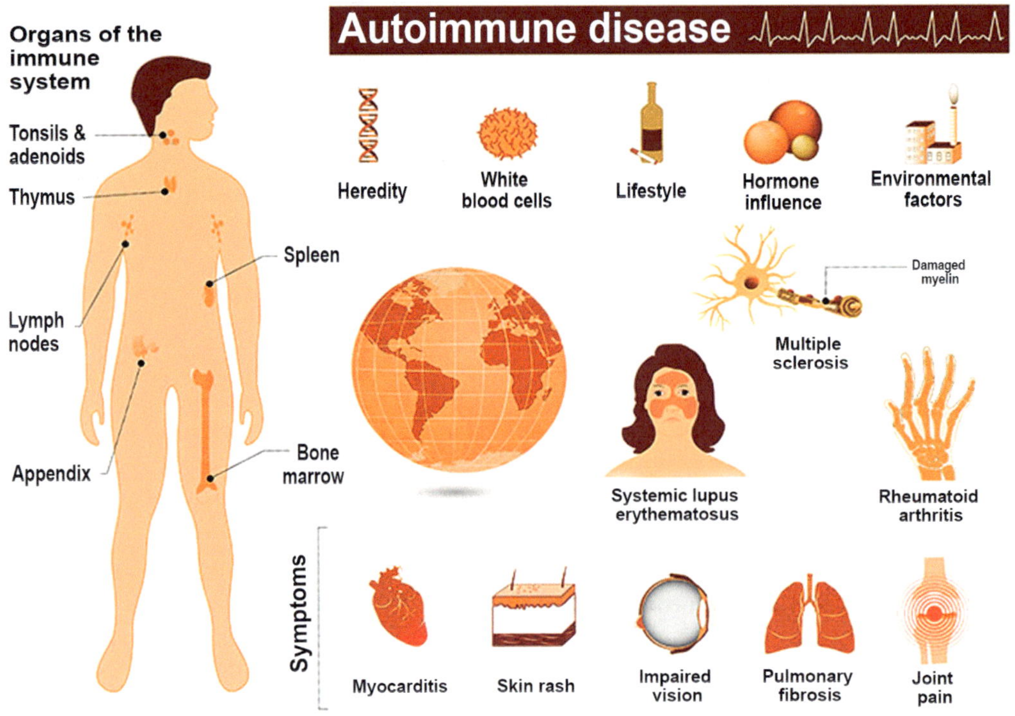

Figure 11.18. Autoimmune disease.

Source: https://www.niehs.nih.gov/sites/default/files/health/assets/images/autoimmune_disease.jpg.

Multiple sclerosis (MS) is a classic example of an autoimmune disease illustrating the complexity of immunity-mediated pathology. The characteristic feature of MS is central nervous system inflammatory demyelination, in which disease-driving myelin-reactive T cells are responsible. Research indicates that such autoreactive T cells infiltrate the CNS, precipitating an inflammatory cascade that leads to demyelination and axonal damage, significantly impacting neurological function. Current treatments primarily target immune-modulation to prevent tissue injury. Although existing disease-modifying therapies are effective in reducing relapse frequency in relapsing-remitting MS, they often do not succeed in preventing long-term disability accumulation. As improvements emerge in the area, there exists an imperative to explore new therapies that target specifically the pathogenic immunologic processes of MS, thereby enhancing treatment effectiveness without amplifying adverse effects (Farjam et al., 2015). The discovery of new pharmacological targets for autoimmune diseases like MS is a reflection of an evolving understanding of their immunopathogenesis. Through the investigation of more targeted interventions on autoreactive immune cells and their mediators, researchers are looking to improve the specificity and effectiveness of therapies. These advances are likely to reduce the global immunosuppression that occurs, which can result in increased susceptibility to infections and other comorbidities. Furthermore, the translation of complex immunological principles could provide the basis for new modalities to possibly reshape autoimmune disease treatment paradigms. Current research into the complex interaction between immune mechanisms involved in these disorders has potential for a breakthrough that optimizes patient outcomes and quality of life, emphasizing the active process of autoimmune disease regulation and the decisive role of developments in immunology in this effort (Forrester et al., 2018) (Figure 11.18).

11.6.2. Allergies and Hypersensitivity Reactions

The complex interaction between the immune response and allergy has attracted a lot of focus in immunological research, especially on the processes involved in hypersensitivity reactions. Hypersensitivity occurs when the immune system overreacts to harmless antigens with resultant detrimental effects. It is classified into four categories, of which type I hypersensitivity, or immediate hypersensitivity, is most common. In such a reaction, the sensitization by the allergen causes the synthesis of Immunoglobulin E (IgE) antibodies that bind to mast cells. Upon re-exposure to the same allergen, the mast cells release inflammatory mediators that result in symptoms, such as vasodilation, edema, and bronchoconstriction. The importance of studying these immune responses lies in the potential for the creation of targeted therapeutic strategies for allergies, particularly among pediatric populations, where the incidence of allergic illnesses continues to increase (Burns, 2019). The emergence of pediatric allergies has instigated enormous research into risk factors for hypersensitivity in younger patients. Genetic background, environmental exposures, and lifestyle variables have been identified as the main elements of this multifaceted interaction. Studies indicate that certain genetic mutations predispose children to develop specific allergies, whereas environmental factors , such as early exposure to allergens or the hygiene hypothesis can enhance sensitization risks. This multi-factorial perspective is critical to meet the escalating burden of allergic reactions, as it provides an individualized comprehension of susceptibility. By investigating these risk factors, researchers aim to find methods that will be able to prevent developing allergies in susceptible individuals (Burns, 2019). Thus, a clearer insight into , such associations could lead to effective preventive measures and treatments. Clinical signs of hypersensitivity reactions, especially in type I hypersensitivity, are extremely diverse and may exert an immense impact on the quality of life. These responses may be anything from mild allergic rhinitis to severe anaphylaxis, and therefore early diagnosis and treatment are crucial. It is to be noted that not only in humans but also in animals, allergic reactions occur, making the hypersensitivity disorders universally applicable. As seen through veterinary medicine, diseases like canine atopic dermatitis have a similar immunological basis to human allergies. The identification of the pathological processes, including the release of mediators from the mast cells, enables an expanded comprehension of the whole range of allergic disease. In addition, further research into the immunologic nature of allergy might lead to new methods of therapy to desensitize individuals to allergens and eventually reduce the public load imposed by these diseases.

11.6.3. Immunodeficiency Disorders

Immunodeficiency illnesses are a critical problem in immunological science because they constitute a class of illnesses resulting from a defective ability of the immune system to effectively combat infection and other disease. Immunodeficiency illnesses are also classified into two broad classes: primary and secondary immunodeficiencies. Primary immunodeficiencies (PIDs) are typically presentat birth and result from congenital genetic abnormalities that compromise immune function and lead to recurrent infection and complications associated with the immune system. Secondary immunodeficiencies are acquired, typically secondary to external factors , such as viral infection, malnutrition, or immunosuppressive therapy. Both their pathogenesis are of great importance to understand in order to be able to devise successful management regimens and improve outcomes. Their complexity is due to heterogeneity of PIDs and diversity of causative genetic mutations underlying them. Variable presentations on clinical grounds make diagnosis even challenging. Variable presentation, ranging from recurrent infection to autoimmune conditions, to malignancy, complicates diagnosis. Physical examination and thorough clinical history are crucial to evoking suspicion for PIDs. Laboratory tests form a major component of the diagnostic process, assessing antibody as well as cellular immunity. Techniques , such as flow cytometry and genetic testing are now widely utilized to confirm diagnoses and to identify specific genetic abnormalities. As highlighted in the literature, recent developments in genetic testing have immensely improved the identification of known and new mutations, hence knowledge on immunodeficiency disorders (Chen et al., 2019). The management of immunodeficiency disorders has significantly improved with advances in the field of immunological science and clinical practice. New therapies , such as gene therapy and monoclonal antibodies, are being researched and applied in the clinical setting to correct or circumvent the intrinsic immunodeficiency. Approaches to vaccination are also being tailored to enhance the immune response in individuals. With improved understanding of the immune system acquired in recent years, the healthcare professionals are now ready to implement targeted interventions to improve the quality of life for such patients suffering from these disorders of complicated nature. In general, sustained advances in immunologic science are of utmost significance in developing effective treatment regimens to achieve improved clinical outcomes in various immunodeficiency disorders (Chen, 2019) (Figure 11.19).

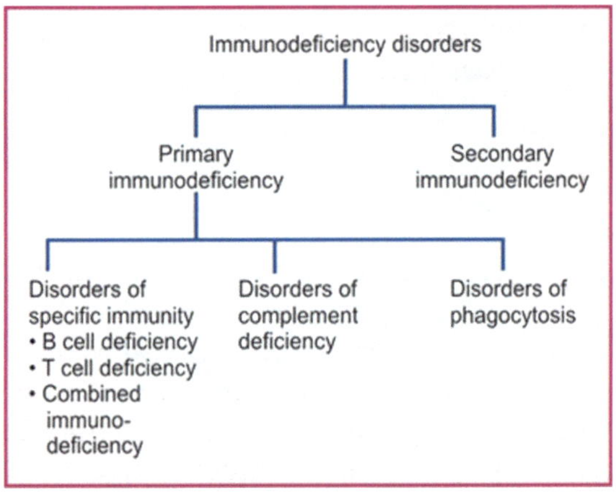

Figure 11.19. Immunodeficiency disorders.

Source: https://d45jl3w9libvn.cloudfront.net/jaypee/static/books/9788184480610/Chapters/images/142-1.jpg.

Test Your Knowledge

1. What is an autoimmune disease, and how does it affect the immune system's normal function?
2. Give two examples of autoimmune diseases and the organs or systems they primarily affect.
3. What is the difference between primary and secondary immunodeficiency disorders?

SUMMARY

In assessing the foundational concepts of immunology, it is evident that understanding the immune system's complexities is essential for advancing medical science and therapeutic interventions. The dynamic interactions between various components, particularly lymphocytes and high endothelial venules (HEV), illuminate critical processes in immune response mechanisms. These interactions can dictate how effectively the immune system can respond to pathogens and cellular damage. Specifically, lymphocyte homing to secondary lymphoid organs relies on this interaction, as illustrated by GlcNAc6ST-2's important role in forming and producing functional ligands for lymphocyte homing []. This interaction offers the potential for targeting specific molecular processes in inflammatory diseases with an inflammatory background, e.g., rheumatoid arthritis. Also, more than the simple role of immune system is the effect on public health, particularly for children. As allergic reactions and hypersensitivity become increasingly widespread among children, the underlying foundation must be understood. By means of research, the determinants of genetic inheritance, the environment, and immune system function have been proven to make up the foundation of such conditions []. Through further study of such risk factors and their interaction, immunology not only provides theoretical knowledge but also guides clinical practice in prevention and management. Thorough knowledge can lead to effective interventions that minimize the impact of allergy in susceptible groups. Ultimately, the topic of immunology is a vital and involved aspect of health sciences that unifies theoretical concepts and practical applications. The ongoing progress in our knowledge about immune responses and their uses in various diseases is of great promise for therapeutic advances. As the science evolves, targets , such as the targeting of HEV interactions in autoimmune disease and in pediatric hypersensitivities will transform treatment strategies. Worldwide, the tenets of immunology not only form the basis for scientific knowledge but also open the doors to the treatment by design philosophy of effective targeted therapies capable of dramatically enhancing patient care and disease control in heterogeneous populations.

The basic concepts of immunology involve the understanding of how the immune system functions to protect the body against harmful pathogens. Essentially, the immune system is founded on the cooperative actions of heterogeneous cell types, including lymphocytes, dendritic cells, and macrophages. Each cell possesses a unique role in the identification and destruction of foreign pathogens. For instance, lymphocytes like T cells and B cells are essential to adaptive immunity through their provision of tailored responses to specific antigens. Dendritic cells are vital in activating T cells through antigen presentation as well as acting as a bridge between the innate and adaptive immune responses. This balance of cellular engagement emphasizes the intricacy of the immune response and its ability to respond to diverse challenges imposed by pathogens. Understanding how psychosocial factors influence immune function is another new research field within immunology. It has been established from recent research that psychosocial stressors have profound impacts on the modulation of immune responses as well as the advancement of diseases, as in the case of TB. For instance, adverse psychosocial events , such as acute stress, have been proven to compromise the efficacy of vaccines, e.g., the BCG vaccine against TB, leading to weak immunity and higher susceptibility to infections. This connection stresses the importance of the holistic approach in immunology, where not only biological determinants but also social and psychological determinants are taken into account in immune response and disease susceptibility. The fine balance between psychosocial stress and immune biomarkers underlines the importance of better understanding the roles these play in infectious disease and responses to vaccination (Boccia et al., 2019). In applied immunology, artificial immune system technology applies fundamental principles in immunology to address contemporary problems, , such as cybersecurity. Through the implementation of theories like the Danger Theory, where the role of dendritic cells to detect danger messages in infected tissues is emphasized, researchers designed programs mimicking immune functions. These systems perform tasks like intrusion detection through the analysis of data analogies between biological immune systems and machine learning processes. Dendritic cell dynamics in algorithmic forms allow for the possibility of performing effective real-time analysis and anomaly detection within diverse datasets. These developments not only enhance technological frameworks but also reiterate the relevance of understanding immunological concepts in solving modern issues, bridging the gap between technology and immunology (Aickelin et al., 2006).

KEY TERMS FROM THIS CHAPTER

- Adaptive immunity
- Antigen-presenting cells (APCs)
- Autoimmune illnesses
- B-cell antibodies
- Canine atopic dermatitis (CAD)
- CRISPR gene editing
- Epithelial cells
- Helper T cells (CD4+)
- Homeostatic balance
- Immune classification paradigms
- Antigen-antibody interaction
- Antigen-presenting cells are
- Autoimmunity
- Cancer immunotherapy
- Chronic inflammation
- Cytokine profiles
- G-protein-coupled receptors (GPCRs)
- Homeostasis
- Hypersensitivity reactions
- Immune modulation

CRITICAL THINKING QUESTIONS

1. Which of the following is a component of the innate immune system?

a. B cells

b. T cells

c. Natural killer (NK) cells

d. Plasma cells

2. What is the primary function of antibodies?

a. To directly destroy pathogens

b. To produce cytokines

c. To present antigens to T cells

d. To recognize and bind specific antigens

3. Which type of immunity provides long-lasting protection after vaccination?

a. Innate immunity

b. Passive immunity

c. Artificial passive immunity

d. Adaptive immunity

4. Autoimmune diseases occur when:

a. The immune system fails to recognize foreign antigens

b. The immune system attacks the body's own cells

c. Antibodies are not produced

d. T cells are not activated

5. Which of the following best describes the difference between innate and adaptive immunity?

a. Innate immunity is antigen-specific; adaptive immunity is not

b. Innate immunity has memory; adaptive immunity does not

c. Innate immunity responds immediately; adaptive immunity takes time to develop

d. Innate immunity is only found in vertebrates; adaptive immunity is in all organisms

Short Answer Questions

1. What are the primary functions of the immune system, and what are its main components?
2. How does innate immunity differ from adaptive immunity in terms of specificity and response time?
3. What roles do B cells and T cells play in adaptive immunity?
4. What is an antigen, and how do antibodies recognize and neutralize antigens?
5. Describe the steps involved in a typical immune response from the first exposure to a pathogen to the elimination of the threat.
6. How does immunological memory contribute to the effectiveness of vaccines?
7. What is the difference between autoimmune diseases and immunodeficiency disorders? Give one example of each.
8. What is the role of inflammation in the immune response, and how can chronic inflammation be harmful?

Answers to Critical Thinking Questions

1. (c) 2. (d) 3. (d) 4. (b) 5. (c)

REFERENCES

1. Abbas, A. K., Barra, A., Agliari, E., Amit, D. J., Burnet, F. M., et al. (2010). A statistical mechanics approach to autopoietic immune networks. http://arxiv.org/abs/1001.3857 (accessed on 13th June 2025).
2. Acín Tresaco, C., Bolea Bailo, R. M., & Salord Torres, F. X. (2017). La reacción de hipersensibilidad tipo I en la especie canina: Dermatitis atópica canina y otras enfermedades alérgicas. https://core.ac.uk/download/289988574.pdf (accessed on 13th June 2025).
3. Adachi, T., Aleivar-Warren, J., Amparyup, P., Antony, S., Arts, E., Bachère, E., et al. (2012). The scope of the crustacean immune system for disease control.
4. Aickelin, U., Garrett, S., Robbins, M., Walker, J., et al. (2025). Modelling immunological memory. https://core.ac.uk/download/98245.pdf (accessed on 13th June 2025).
5. Aickelin, U., Greensmith, J., & Twycross, J. (2006). Dendritic cells for anomaly detection. https://core.ac.uk/download/328347420.pdf (accessed on 13th June 2025).
6. Aickelin, U., Greensmith, J., & Whitbrook, A. (2010). Artificial immune systems. https://core.ac.uk/download/42495389.pdf (accessed on 13th June 2025).
7. Alvarez-Twose, S., Muraro, A., Arga, M., Armstrong, R., Arroabarren, E., Sheikh, A., Barnett, C., et al. (2014). International consensus on (ICON) anaphylaxis. https://core.ac.uk/download/28978204.pdf (accessed on 13th June 2025).
8. Strandin Tomas, Babayan Simon A. and Forbes Kristian M. 2018Reviewing the effects of food provisioning on wildlife immunityPhil. Trans. R. Soc. B37320170088
9. http://doi.org/10.1098/rstb.2017.0088(accessed on 13th June 2025).
10. Barton, J., Cavicchi, J. R., Janovetz, J., Kowalski, M., et al. (2012). Patent landscape of Influenza A virus prophylactic vaccines and related technologies. https://core.ac.uk/download/72052387.pdf (accessed on 13th June 2025).
11. Bat-Erdene, A., Choijilsuren, G., Lkhagvasuren, G., & Enkhsaikhan, T. (2019). *Clinical Immunology*, Fifth edition. https://core.ac.uk/download/617921726.pdf (accessed on 13th June 2025).
12. Bellavite, P., Conforti, A., Ortolani, R., Piasere, A., et al. (2005). Immunology and homeopathy. 1. Historical background. https://core.ac.uk/download/pdf/3814031.pdf (accessed on 13th June 2025).
13. Bergman, A., Force, A., Kurakin, A., Minai, A., Seth, A., Wagner, A., Wagner, A., et al. (2010). Networked buffering: A basic mechanism for distributed robustness in complex adaptive systems. https://core.ac.uk/download/pdf/1631279.pdf (accessed on 13th June 2025).
14. Boccia, D., Dowd, J. B., Fletcher, H., Hayward, A., et al. (2019). A systematic review of the impact of psychosocial factors on immunity: Implications for enhancing BCG response against tuberculosis. https://core.ac.uk/download/286270876.pdf (accessed on 13th June 2025).
15. Boneschansker, L., Brandt, S. L., Chan, E. C., Filippo, K., Freedman, N. J., Hjorto, G. M., Hons, M., et al. (2019). Concepts of GPCR-controlled navigation in the immune system.
16. Burns, H. (2019). *The Development of Hypersensitivity Reactions in The Pediatric Population: A Review*. https://core.ac.uk/download/213464303.pdf (accessed on 13th June 2025).
17. Carnuccio, R., Grassia, G., Ialenti, A., Maffia, P., et al. (2013). Macrophage autophagy in atherosclerosis. https://core.ac.uk/download/9652208.pdf (accessed on 13th June 2025).

18. Chen, R. (2019). *Primary Immunodeficiency*. https://core.ac.uk/download/322444930.pdf (accessed on 13th June 2025).

19. SJ Gregory, F Clarke - Proceedings of The Australian Conference on Science ..., 2009https://core.ac.uk/download/229413587.pdf (accessed on 13th June 2025).

20. Forrester, J. V., Kuffova, L., & Dick, A. D. (2018). Autoimmunity, Autoinflammation, and Infection in Uveitis. *American journal of ophthalmology, 189*, 77–85. https://doi.org/10.1016/j.ajo.2018.02.019 (accessed on 13th June 2025).

21. Frateschi Trivelato, S., Manzoni-De-Almeida, D., & Marzin-Janvier, P. (2016). Analysis of epistemic practices in reports of higher education student groups in carrying out the inquiry-based activity of immunology. https://core.ac.uk/download/47344847.pdf (accessed on 13th June 2025).

22. Freitas, A. A., Tauber, A. I., Silverstein, A. M., Buscaglia, C. A., et al. (2005). The self-model and the conception of biological identity in immunology. https://core.ac.uk/download/11921231.pdf (accessed on 13th June 2025).

23. Galindo, M., Pablos, J. L., Palao, G., Rosen, A., et al. (2005). A HEV-restricted sulfotransferase is expressed in rheumatoid arthritis synovium and is induced by lymphotoxin-alpha/beta and TNF-alpha in cultured endothelial cells. https://core.ac.uk/download/323073701.pdf (accessed on 13th June 2025).

24. Gallucci, B. B., & McCarthy, D. O. (1995). *The Immune System*. https://core.ac.uk/download/213081395.pdf (accessed on 13th June 2025).

25. Mascola, J., Steinman, R., King, R. C., & The Working Group convened by the Global HIV Vaccine Enterprise. (2010). Immunogens and antigen processing: Report from a Global HIV Vaccine Enterprise Working Group. https://core.ac.uk/download/pdf/289325.pdf (accessed on 13th June 2025).

26. Sciumè, G., Shih, H. Y., Mikami, Y., & O'Shea, J. J. (2017). Epigenomic Views of Innate Lymphoid Cells. *Frontiers in immunology, 8*, 1579. https://doi.org/10.3389/fimmu.2017.01579 (accessed on 13th June 2025).

27. Nødtvedt, A. (2007). *Epidemiology of Canine Atopic Dermatitis*. https://core.ac.uk/download/11695161.pdf (accessed on 13th June 2025).

28. Pace, O. (2012). *Complementary and Alternative Medicine: Facts and Figures (Part I)*. https://core.ac.uk/download/46603042.pdf (accessed on 13th June 2025).

29. Podgórski, J. S. (2012). Who is on guard for harmony? On harmony, phagocytes and immunological identity. https://core.ac.uk/download/pdf/27183808.pdf (accessed on 13th June 2025).

30. Reich, D. S., Lucchinetti, C. F., & Calabresi, P. A. (2018). Multiple sclerosis. *New England Journal of Medicine, 378*, 169–180. https://doi.org/10.1056/nejmra1401483 (accessed on 13th June 2025).

31. Rokka, S. (2008). *Bovine cloistral antibodies and selected lactobacilli as means to control gastrointestinal infections*. https://core.ac.uk/download/10928087.pdf (accessed on 13th June 2025).

32. Farjam, M., Zhang, G. X., Ciric, B., & Rostami, A. (2015). Emerging immunopharmacological targets in multiple sclerosis. *Journal of the neurological sciences, 358*(1-2), 22–30. https://doi.org/10.1016/j.jns.2015.09.346(accessed on 13th June 2025).

33. Steele, K. F. (1998). *Directory of Water Related Courses Offered at Colleges and universities in Arkansas as of November 1998.* https://core.ac.uk/download/145191276.pdf (accessed on 13th June 2025).

34. Zhang, Y., & Zhang, Z. (2020). The history and advances in cancer immunotherapy: Understanding the characteristics of tumor-infiltrating immune cells and their therapeutic implications. *Cellular and Molecular Immunology, 17,* 807–821. https://doi.org/10.1038/s41423-020-0488-6 (accessed on 13th June 2025).

CELLS AND ORGANS OF THE IMMUNE SYSTEM

12

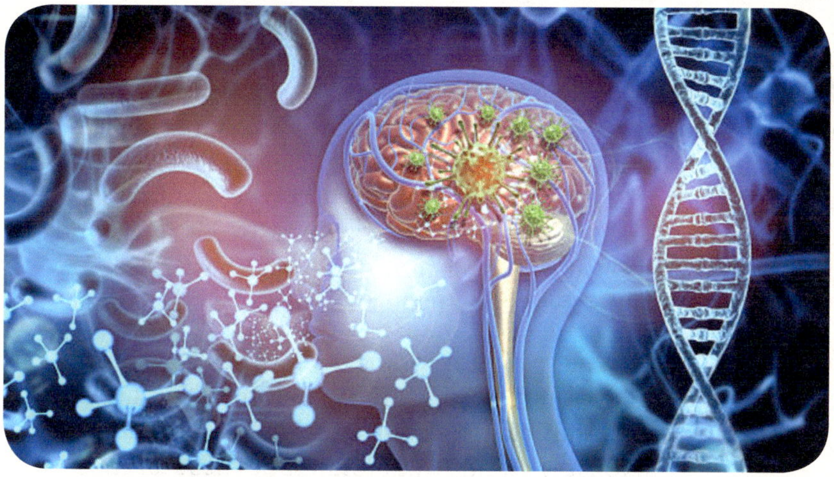

LEARNING OBJECTIVES

After studying this chapter, you will be able to:

1. Understand lymphocytes and macrophages
2. Describe antigen-presenting cells (APCs)
3. Explain the role of the thymus in adaptive immunity
4. Discuss how bone marrow serves as a crucial component of the immune system
5. Define Lymph Node

Introduction

The immune system is a complex network of organs and cells dedicated to protecting the body against cancers, foreign bodies, and infections. The foundation of the system is made up of lymphocytes, macrophages, and other antigen-presenting cells (APCs) that collaborate in order to coordinate innate and adaptive immunity. Operation by specialized organs like the thymus, bone marrow, lymph nodes, and spleen enables maturation, activation, and effective deployment of immune cells. This general understanding of types of immune cells and their particular roles is the context for an examination of the intricate relationship among these factors. This type of research emphasizes the role of the immune system in homeostasis and its responsive function towards shifting environments. Lymphocytes, including B cells, T cells, and natural killer (NK) cells, play a primary role in the immune response. B cells secrete antibodies, while T cells control the immune response and kill infected or malignant cells themselves. Present studies have stressed that NK cell interaction with

APCs, i.e., dendritic cells, is crucial for effective functional competence in human as well as in murine systems. Indeed, the activation of NK cells is reliant on their perception of signals from APCs , such as cytokines and ligands, which boost their functionality in resistance to infections and tumors. The interaction plays a significant role in the establishment of new immunotherapeutic strategies to enhance innate and adaptive immunity and hence improve disease outcomes (Chijioke et al., 2011). The path of immune cells begins in the bone marrow, where hematopoietic stem cells differentiate into varying lineages of immune cells. Upon maturation, the cells travel to the thymus, where selection is experienced by T cells prior to gaining entry to the circulation system. Lymph nodes and the spleen are major locations for lymphocyte activation and proliferation against a particular antigen. Study of the immune function of these organs reveals not only their role as a center for immune activity but also how tumors can take over such functions for growth and survival, further making it difficult for therapeutic intervention. Particularly for high-grade brain tumors, the mechanisms of the immune response are central to revealing issues with treatment and developing useful interventions. This context thus provides the background for examining the unique roles and interactions of immune cells under both health and disease conditions, with an emphasis on the necessity for new modalities in cancer therapy (Lister, 2003).

Importance of Understanding Immune Cells and Organs

The comprehension of immune organs and cells is key to comprehending how the immune system functions as an ensemble. The central participants, namely lymphocytes, macrophages, and antigen-presenting cells (APCs), cooperate in an attempt to recognize and eliminate pathogens. Lymphocytes, for instance, differentiate into T-cells and B-cells, each suited for specific tasks, such as direct killing of infected cells and antibody production. Macrophages, which are responsible for engulfing pathogens, play a central part in not only eliminating pathogens but also warning other immune cells that there is an ongoing threat. Thus, a deep understanding of such cell and organ associations provides the basis for future research within immunology, directing vaccine development and therapy for immune disorders (Arkestål, 2019). The immunological plasticity and immunological flexibility are, to a large degree, determined by the organs involved, , such as the thymus, bone marrow, lymph nodes, and spleen. Each of these organs contributes uniquely to the immune cell differentiation, maturation, and function. The thymus has a key function in T-cell maturation, where naïve T-cells undergo intense selection that determines their ability to respond effectively to antigenic stimulation.

Bone marrow is the primary site of hematopoiesis, generating the diverse repertoire of immune cells that can be required to build an effective defense system. Understanding these organs' specific functions, together with cross-talk between immigrating immune cells and local microenvironments, is essential in order to understand how systemic and local immune responses are organized (Arkestål et al., 2019). Moreover, the importance of comprehending the cellular and organ components of the immune system translates into clinical use, , such as the creation of immunotherapies and vaccines. Having a good understanding of how these cells and organs interact determines strategy in the context of modulating immune responses in numerous diseases, , such as cancer and autoimmune disease. For example, enhancement of T-cell function with checkpoint inhibitors is based on insights gained from investigations into T-cell activation and trafficking patterns. In addition, the unravelling of immune organ complexity allows researchers to create enhanced interventions at such critical moments of life as infancy or senescence, when the immune system is radically different. Lastly, knowing the intricacies of immune cells and organs is important to enhancing healthcare outcomes and tailored medical interventions (Arkestål, 2019) (Figure 12.1).

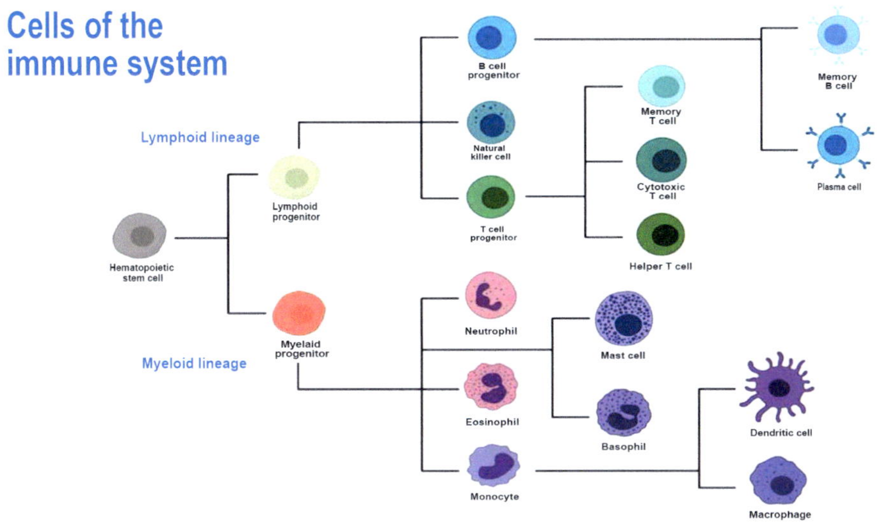

Figure 12.1. Cell of the immune system.

Source: https://www.ibiology.org/wp-content/uploads/2019/03/iBioImmunologyIntro.jpg.

12.1. Lymphocytes

Learning Outcome

1. Explain the types of lymphocytes
2. Understand the functions of lymphocytes in immune response
3. Discuss the role of lymphocytes in memory and immunity

In immunology, lymphocytes play a central role in the adaptive immune system. The white blood cells differentiate into two major groups: B cells and T cells. B cells provide humoral immunity, which releases antibodies that bind to antigenic sites, and T cells for cell-mediated immunity, enabling the recognition and elimination of infected or cancerous cells. The development of lymphocytes occurs primarily in the bone marrow and thymus, where precursor cells undergo complex processes of development. The particular ability of lymphocytes to identify an impressive array of pathogens is caused by their special antigen receptors. The enormity of this diversity is established by the mechanism of somatic recombination, allowing the immune system to react against an immense range of potential aggressors. The concerted functioning of lymphocytes depicts the intricacies of immune system vigilance. Movements and location of the lymphocytes within the body are delicately regulated by various signals, primarily chemokines and their corresponding receptors. Chemokines are small proteins that participate in leukocyte migration, including lymphocytes, to foci of infection or inflammation. As lymphocytes possess numerous G-protein-coupled receptors (GPCRs), they can effectively respond to the complex chemokine environment in order to move across tissue (Boneschansker et al., 2019). Such chemotaxis is crucial to ensure effective immune surveillance and response because lymphocytes need to transit through lymph nodes and other tissues most effectively. Chemokines also induce other migratory phenomena beyond directed locomotion, which influences lymphocyte behavior during inflammation as well as homeostasis. Understanding these intricate signaling pathways increases our knowledge of immune responses and uncovers new therapeutic targets for immunological disorders.

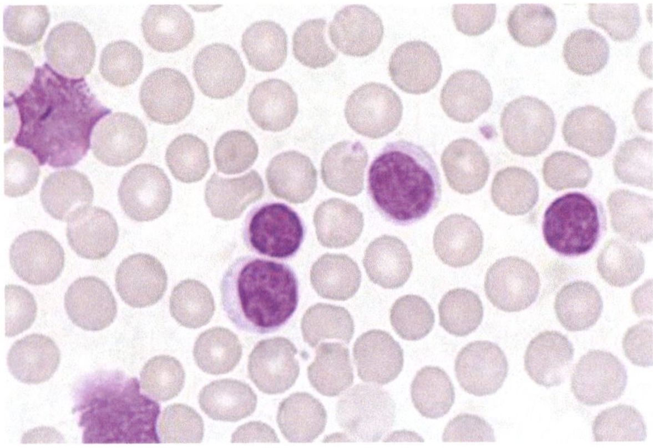

Figure 12.2. Large lymphocyte cells.

Source: https://www.researchgate.net/profile/Aiman-Al-Sabaawi/publication/337928097/figure/fig1/AS:1140869088452608@1649015795562/Large-lymphocyte-cells-in-one-image-RBCs-and-background-from-4.jpg.

The functions of lymphocytes and antigen-presenting cells (APCs) also underscore their significant role in the immune system. APCs, including dendritic cells and macrophages, are important in the capture, processing, and presentation of antigens to lymphocytes, which is essential for T cell activation. This interaction initiates a cascade of immune reactions that result in antigen-specific lymphocyte proliferation and the development of a robust adaptive immune memory. Recent studies have suggested that the effectiveness of this cooperation hinges on the dynamic expression of chemokines and adhesion molecules on the lymphocytes and the APCs (Braun et al., 2018). Lymphocytes' ability to synthesize the information from the local cellular environment, as well as their communication with APCs, is crucial in orchestrating the immune response. Through such mechanisms, lymphocytes not only contribute to eliminating the pathogens but also create durable immunologic memory that is significant for future immunity against reinfection (Figure 12.2).

12.1.1. Types of Lymphocytes: B Cells and T Cells

The immune system comprises a complex network of organs and cells that work together to detect and destroy pathogens. Among the principal players in the system are lymphocytes, more specifically B cells and T cells, with complementary but separate functions. B cells play a primary role in humoral immunity by producing antibodies that respond to particular antigens. Upon activation by contact with pathogens or antigen-presenting cells (APCs), B cells become plasma cells, which secrete antibodies, or memory B cells, which trigger lasting immunity. The process demonstrates the responsiveness of the immune response and how B cells are modified based on previous encounters with pathogens. Further, the dynamic functionality of B cells is supplemented by their functionality in conjunction with T cells, demonstrating the immuno-dependency (Arkestål, 2019).

In contrast to B cells, T cells are vital for cell-mediated immunity and bear the primary responsibility of virus-infected cells and tumor cells detection and destruction. T cells are derived in the bone marrow and develop within the thymus, where they experience a strict selection process to guarantee self-tolerance. The selection eliminates autoreactive T cells, hence avoiding autoimmune conditions. Following maturation, T cells are split into some of their subgroups, that is, they have cytotoxic

T cells, which kill infected cells directly, and helper T cells, which aid and regulate the immune response by coordinating the actions of other immune cells. This sophisticated equilibrium and differentiation allow T cells to respond effectively, allowing the immune system to appropriately respond to an enormous range of pathogens (Chijioke et al., 2011). T cell and B cell synergy is important for a successful immune response. After antigen exposure, T helper cells activate the B cells through cell-to-cell contact and cytokine production. The synergy allows for the high-affinity antibody production as well as memory cell formation, allowing for an enhanced response against the same pathogen upon re-exposure. These interactions are a prime example of the complexity of coordination of the adaptive immune response, further asserting the dual importance of the two lymphocyte types in immunological health. With new research constantly uncovering the complexity of the activities of B and T cells, the therapeutic potential, , such as the use of vaccines and immunotherapy, increases exponentially, illuminating the path toward improved disease control and prevention (Arkestål, 2019) (Figure 12.3).

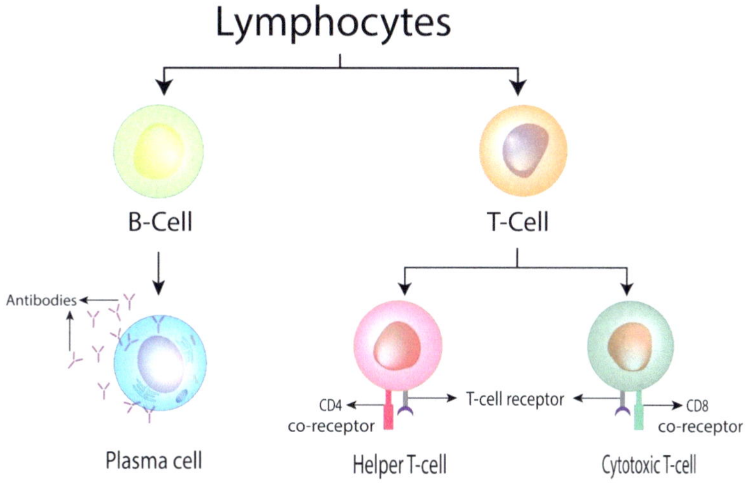

Figure 12.3. Types of lymphocytes.

Source: https://stgaccinwbsdevlrs01.blob.core.windows.net/newcorporatewbsite/blogs/october2023/Anatomy-of-Lymphocytes.jpg.

12.1.2. Functions of Lymphocytes in Immune Response

The immune response is strongly dependent on the function of lymphocytes, which are primarily classified into the T cells, B cells, and natural killer (NK) cells. T cells, which mature in the thymus, are crucial in cell-based immunity. They specialize in various subpopulations, such as helper T cells, which activate B cell proliferation and antibody production, while cytotoxic T cells destroy infected or malignant cells. This adaptability is important for the modulation of responses to numerous pathogens and maintaining immune homeostasis. In addition, lymphocytes do not operate alone; rather, their activity is enhanced by coordination with antigen-presenting cells (APCs), which enable necessary signals during lymphocyte activation and proliferation. The synergistic nature of these components provides a function to support the complex orchestration for a good immune response. B cells are not as important in the functions of humoral immunity and antibody production. After recognizing specific antigens, they are activated by undergoing clonal expansion and differentiation into plasma cells, which secrete large amounts of antibodies. The antibodies are key to the process of inactivating pathogens and marking them for destruction by other immune cells. The production of memory B cells is another important characteristic of the B cell response because it enables the immune system to mount a quick and effective response upon future exposure to the same pathogen.

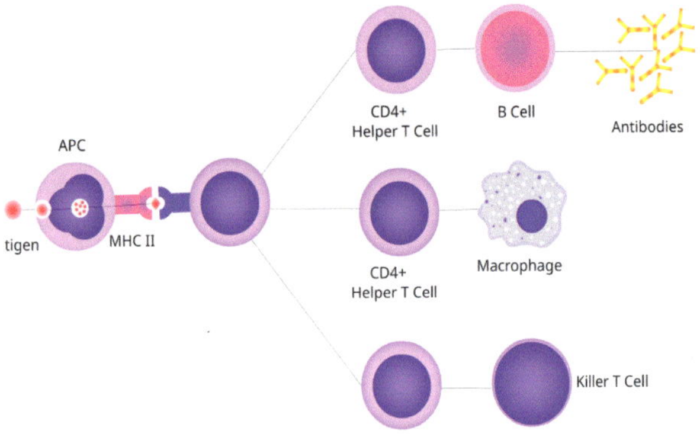

Figure 12.4. Immune response of lymphocytes.

Source: https://upload.wikimedia.org/wikipedia/commons/thumb/7/7e/Immune_response_of_Lymphocytes.svg/1200px-Immune_response_of_Lymphocytes.svg.png?20200414145504.

This aspect of lymphocyte function not only emphasizes the body's memory for infections but also the value of vaccinations, which are intended to mimic exposure and enhance immunological memory. In concert, the varied roles of B cells complete the complex immunology of the immune system. Natural killer (NK) cells are another essential member of the lymphocyte family, particularly in the field of innate immunity. Though they are born with the ability to recognize and destroy virus-infected and tumor cells, recent evidence has demonstrated that their full functional maturity is achieved via their interaction with APCs, specifically dendritic cells (DCs). This interaction primes NK cells, sensitizing and responding more strongly to pathogens, demonstrating the interface of innate and adaptive immunity. These functions of NK cells are important, especially during the initial stages of infection, before the full activation of the adaptive response. The evolving information on NK cells' functions, particularly their preactivation pathways, is a fascinating topic, particularly in the application of the cells to the development of vaccines to augment innate and adaptive immunity (Chijioke et al., 2011). The synergistic activities of lymphocytes are a display of complexity and efficiency in an immune system activity (Figure 12.4).

12.1.3. Role of Lymphocytes in Memory and Immunity

Lymphocytes are responsible for the formation of immunological memory, an essential element of the adaptive immune system. The specialized white blood cell subset consists of two prominent types: T cells and B cells. T cells, originating from the thymus, play a key role in the coordination of immune response as well as directly killing infected cells. B cells, which are produced in the bone marrow, are responsible for the production of antibodies. When the T and B cells see an antigen for the very first time, they get activated and differentiated. A few of these differentiated cells are memory cells that remain in the body even after the first infection has cleared. This memory formation process is crucial as it enables a quicker and better response by the immune system upon subsequent exposure to the same pathogen, minimizing the risk of acute disease and enhancing host survival, as supported by current research in immunology (Arkestål, 2019). Lymphocytes' functional activity is not only for the primary immune response but also for lifelong protection against a broad array of pathogens. This is particularly evident in vaccinations, which exploit the principle of acquired immunity. Vaccines expose the immune system to harmless components of pathogens and thereby condition lymphocytes to know and combat subsequent infection. In the face of the real pathogen, pre-existing memory B cells will rapidly produce specific antibodies, significantly reducing the immune response time.

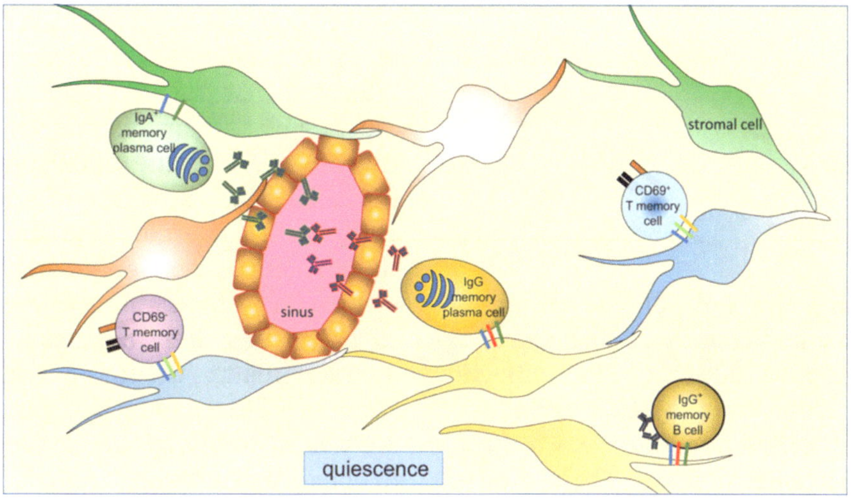

Figure 12.5. Organization of the resting memory lymphocytes in the bone marrow.

Source: https://www.researchgate.net/publication/351723062/figure/fig1/AS:1143128117430 3691@1689178735856/Organization-of-the-resting-memory-lymphocytes-in-the-bone-marrow-Following-the.png.

This is a rapid reaction similar to having an armed force waiting in readiness to attack, which can easily overwhelm the aggressor before it finds space to settle. Therefore, the function of lymphocytes in memory creation not only represents the intricacy and effectiveness of adaptive immunity but also underscores the significance of vaccination in public health (Gillen et al., 2020). In addition to their roles in immunity and memory, lymphocytes also have a complex interaction with other immune cells to enhance the overall immune response. Antigen-presenting cells , such as dendritic cells and macrophages, are instrumental in activating naive T cells; APCs engulf and present antigens to lymphocytes, bridging the innate and adaptive immune responses. This interaction is critical as it allows the lymphocytes to distinguish between self and non-self, and thus, immune activation becomes specific and accurate. Additionally, once an immune response is initiated, cytokines secreted by activated lymphocytes further tune the response, guiding the activity of other immune cells and enabling coordination across various immune components. Thus, the cooperative function of lymphocytes with the APCs highlights their very intrinsic location within the complex immune milieu, which ultimately serves to make the host's immune response effective and specific (Arkestål, 2019) (Figure 12.5).

Test Your Knowledge

1. What are the main types of lymphocytes involved in the adaptive immune response, and how do they differ?
2. What is the role of B lymphocytes in the adaptive immune response?
3. What is immunological memory, and how do lymphocytes contribute to it?

12.2. Macrophages

Learning Outcome

1. Understand the origin and development of macrophage
2. Explain the functions of macrophages in phagocytosis
3. Discuss the role of macrophages in antigen presentation

Macrophages are the hub of the immune system and serve as the movers and shakers of innate and adaptive immunity. Macrophagic cells, derived from monocytes, permeate the tissues and constitute the body's first line of defense against disease. Their multi-faceted role comprises the phagocytosis and ingestion of invaders, and the release of pro-inflammatory cytokines to facilitate the recruitment of other immune cells to sites of infection. Early responses do more than just kill invaders; they initiate a cascade of immune processes, ultimately deciding the adaptive immune response. Therefore, macrophages connect innate and adaptive immunity, which highlights their function in coordinating overall immune defense mechanisms. Macrophages are significant in activating lymphocytes, particularly T cells, as antigen-presenting cells (APCs). By phagocytosing pathogens, macrophages process antigens and present them on the cell surface along with major histocompatibility complex (MHC) molecules. This interaction is required for further activation and proliferation of naïve T cells, which are responsible for an adequate immune response. The functional interaction between macrophages and lymphocytes is also pointed out by the fact that macrophages are capable of controlling the differentiation of T cells into various functional subsets, e.g., Th1 or Th2 cells. In so doing, they help determine the nature of the immune response depending on the nature of the encountered pathogen as well as the nature of the immunological environment, thereby contributing to the adaptability and diversity of the immune response. Furthermore, the functional life of macrophages can be significantly conditioned by their environment as well as ongoing physiological adaptations, such as in pregnancy or senescence. Evidence has indicated that during pregnancy, macrophages must regulate their immune response to protect the mother and the embryonic fetus, which typically means a degree of tolerance to semi-allograft tissues. Likewise, as organisms age, the role of macrophages might decline, and this compromises their ability to respond effectively to pathogens, based on canine research on overall health throughout their life span (Arkestål, 2019). Identifying these interactions is essential in therapeutic strategy development to enhance macrophage function and, therefore, overall immune capacity in various clinical conditions, including vaccination and infection, as they play an important role in the immune system (Chijioke et al., 2011) (Figure 12.6).

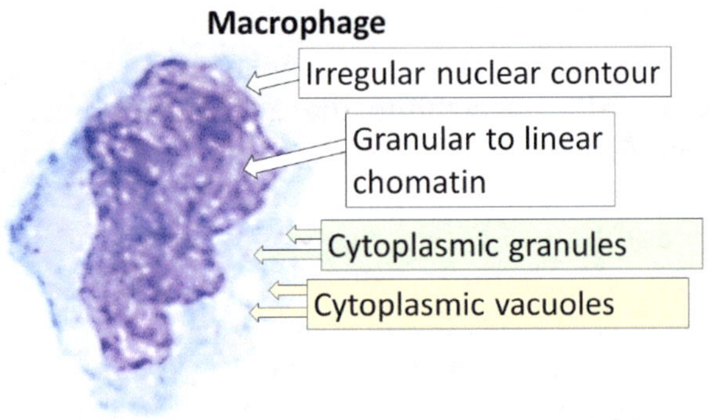

Figure 12.6. Macrophage.

Source: https://upload.wikimedia.org/wikipedia/commons/c/cc/Cytology_of_a_macrophage.png.

12.2.1. Origin and Development of Macrophages

Origin and development of macrophages are the key components in unraveling the broader context of the immune system, more particularly within the hierarchical organization of immune cells. Macrophages primarily develop from monocytes, hematopoietic precursors that are produced within the bone marrow. After being released into the bloodstream, monocytes travel through tissues and become macrophages through various signals from the environment, particularly in sites of inflammation or injury. This transformation enables them to become phagocytic cells that engulf pathogens and debris, playing a significant role in innate and adaptive immunity. Furthermore, the functional heterogeneity of macrophages is induced by their environment, allowing them to differentiate into different phenotypes that facilitate inflammation or healing.

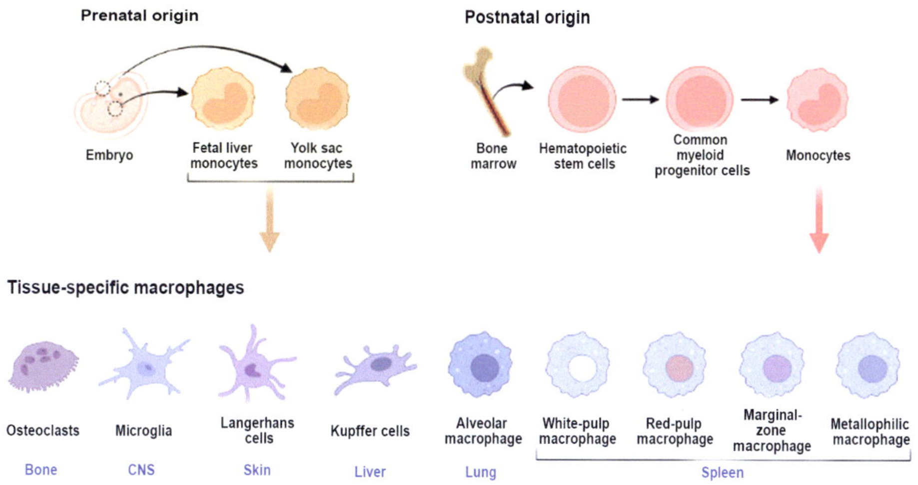

Figure 12.7. Macrophages: Origin and development.

Source: https://cdn.prod.website-files.com/621e95f9ac30687a56e4297e/64a8d7cd2dab97f77b8c64aa_V2_1675790496251_c22da989-0402-4164-8518-4b28e3cf8458.png.

The intricate development of macrophages involves numerous signaling pathways and interaction with other immune cells. As an example, G-protein-coupled receptor (GPCR) signaling has been demonstrated to be crucial in the regulation of leukocyte dynamics during immune responses through the modulation of macrophage migration towards injured or infectious sites. Cell ability to recognize and respond to chemokines enables them to migrate within various tissues efficiently and become actively involved in immune responses. Macrophages also have a close interaction with lymphocytes and dendritic cells that allow for concerted immunity. Their ability to integrate signals from various sources points to the complexity of their function within the immune system as they are able to adapt adjustments to fulfill particular functions in various microenvironments, either initiating inflammation or promoting resolution. In addition to origins and functions, the ontogenetic pathways of macrophages highlight important implications for immunological therapy. The recent publication has shown the potential for the regulation of macrophage function by targeted therapies, notably in transplantation and tolerance. For instance, the presence of donor-derived dendritic cells (DCs) in recipients of allografts was shown to induce tolerance, and this may be attributed to the regulation of macrophage functions and interactions with T cells. Understanding mechanisms of macrophage development and function is essential for designing new therapies for immune diseases and improving transplantation outcomes. Overall, macrophage research represents an essential link between innate and adaptive immunity, emphasizing their critical role in maintaining immune homeostasis and responding to various pathological conditions (Figure 12.7).

12.2.2. Functions of Macrophages in Phagocytosis

Macrophage role in phagocytosis in the immune response is pivotal to maintaining homeostasis and resisting infection. As professional phagocytic cells, macrophages possess a remarkable ability to recognize, internalize, and degrade pathogens and cellular debris. The mechanism begins with the detection of foreign material by various receptors on the macrophage surface, such as pattern recognition receptors (PRRs) that detect pathogen-associated molecular patterns (PAMPs). With the adhesion and subsequent binding, the process of phagocytosis is induced, which causes internalization of the target material into a phagosome that further merges with lysosomes to degrade the content inside by enzymatic activity.

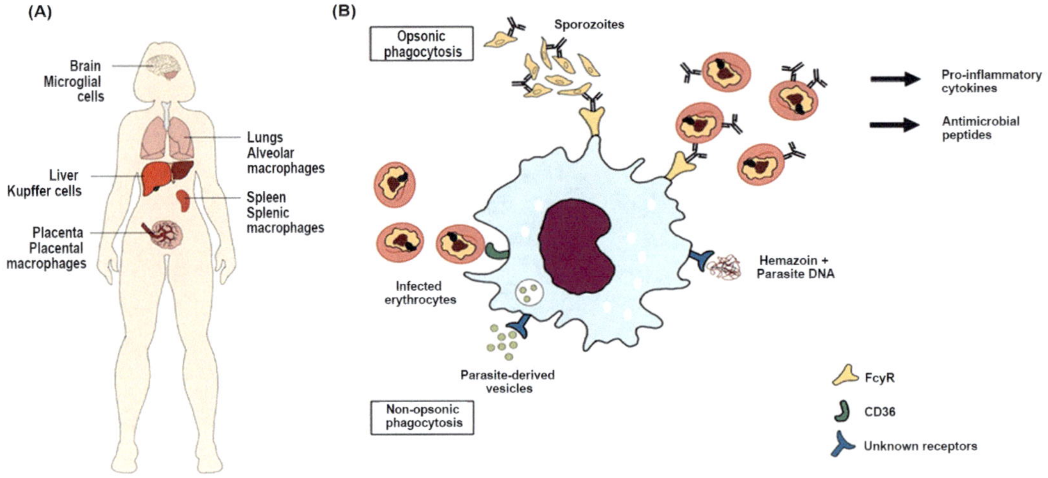

Figure 12.8. The role of macrophages in phagocytosis of *Plasmodium falciparum*. A There are different populations of macrophages that may interact with the parasites during an infection. B Macrophages can perform opsonic phagocytosis of IEs, which often results in the production of pro-inflammatory cytokines and antimicrobial peptides that play a role in inhibiting parasite growth.

Source: https://www.researchgate.net/publication/353306150/figure/fig2/AS:1046432983314433@1626500473860/The-role-of-macrophages-in-phagocytosis-of-Plasmodium-falciparum-A-There-are-different.png.

This combined process not only removes infections but also facilitates tissue remodeling and the resolution of inflammation, pointing towards the two-faced activity of macrophages in active defense as well as restorative mechanisms in the immune environment. Apart from their phagocytic activity, macrophages are also important antigen-presenting cells (APCs), bridging innate and adaptive immunity. Following phagocytosis of pathogens, macrophages digest ingested material and present peptide antigens on their surface via major histocompatibility complex (MHC) molecules. Specific MHC class II molecules present derived antigens to CD4+ T lymphocytes, thereby triggering adaptive immune responses. This activation is crucial to T cell differentiation and proliferation, which subsequently leads to the coordination of a more specialized defense mechanism that enhances the body's overall efficiency of defense mechanisms. The encounter between macrophages and T cells also leads to cytokine synthesis, which further modulates immune response and leads to a coordinated attack on the pathogens, illustrating the sophisticated interaction among the various elements of the immune system. Macrophages are also extremely plastic and have their functional functions changing based on the microenvironment and the received signals. They can polarize into subtypes under their plasticity, essentially divided into M1 and M2 macrophages. M1 macrophages are typically associated with pro-inflammatory responses, capable of eliminating infectious microbes by exuberant phagocytic activity and inflammatory cytokine production. On the other hand, M2 macrophages have a reparative function, participating in tissue repair, inflammatory resolution, and are frequently engaged in tumor microenvironments. This multifunctionality, dictated by local signaling molecules and factors, is critical for mounting the correct immune response. The attainment of insight into macrophage dual functions and plasticity not only enlarges our knowledge of immune function but also has implications for therapeutically targeting disease approaches in autoimmunity and cancer, which involve dysregulated macrophage functions (Vardakis, 1948; Iseki et al., 2019) (Figure 12.8).

12.2.3. Role of Macrophages in Antigen Presentation

The role of macrophages as antigen-presenting cells is key to the immune system. As professional APCs, macrophages phagocytose, process, and present antigens to T lymphocytes, connecting innate and adaptive immunity. Activated macrophages phagocytose pathogens and subsequently degrade them into peptide pieces. These are loaded onto major histocompatibility complex (MHC) molecules, where they are recognizable by T cells. This communication is crucial for the activation of CD4+ Th cells, which subsequently produce cytokines that also enhance the immune response. Importantly, macrophage proficiency in antigen preparation relies on their activation status, which may differ depending on environmental signals , such as cytokines or pathogen-associated molecular patterns. Hence, understanding the complex mechanisms of macrophage activity is essential for the continued advancement of therapeutic strategies that modulate immune responses in disease and infection. Additionally, the phagocytic activity of macrophages is not simply the ingestion of antigens; it has the active potential to modulate the quality of the immune response. For instance, evidence shows that macrophage signals play a role in determining whether T cells develop as helper or cytotoxic T lymphocytes, thus determining the type of immune response triggered. Frequency and context of antigen encounter are also factors of significant value. As demonstrated with the interaction of virulent microbes and macrophages, , such as *Mycobacterium tuberculosis*, mechanisms employed by such pathogens to evade phagocytic digestion could impair antigen presentation. Here, the ability of macrophages to distinguish intracellular bacteria for digestion in lysosomes plays a critical role, as evidenced in the fact that some virulence factors possess the ability to interfere with the intracellular antigen traffic, rendering the process of immune activation burdensome. This underscores the key role that macrophages play in resolving the mechanisms of host defense and pathogen evasion, thereby defining the effectiveness of the immune response (Combaluzier, 2008). Macrophages are also flexible in their functions, which can be transformed according to the tissue's microenvironment and the nature of antigens they recognize. In chronic inflammatory conditions, for example, macrophages can switch to a tissue repair and immunosuppressive-associated phenotype rather than antigen presentation. This transformation indicates that macrophages are not only sensors and effectors of the immune response but also key regulators of immune homeostasis. Therefore, the activity of macrophages is not limited to their antigen-presenting capacity; it is also their capacity to control the immune setting on responding to different immunologic challenges. Recent research has clarified the intricate molecular pathways of macrophage activation and their significance in the progression of specific immunotherapies. As researchers explore these dynamics further, the bidirectional role of macrophages in mediating and moderating immunity highlights their significance in immune system pathology and physiology (Arkestål, 2019) (Figure 12.9).

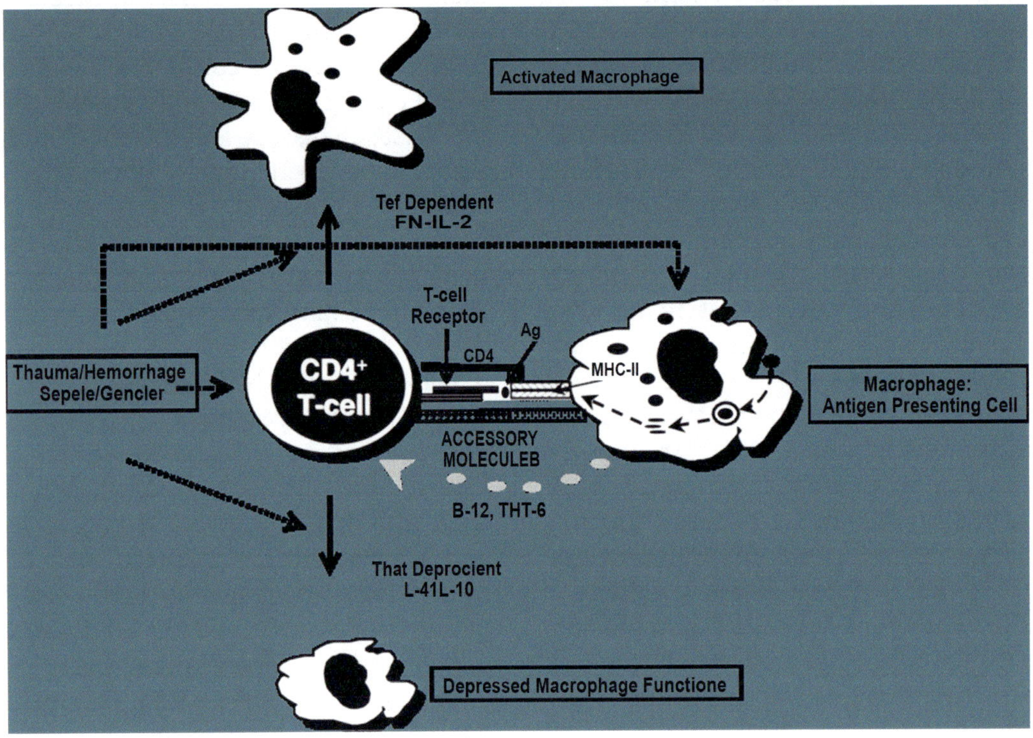

Figure 12.9. Antigen processing and presentation. Foreign antigen is phagocytized by the macrophage and undergoes lysosomal catabolism into small antigenic peptides.

Source: https://www.researchgate.net/profile/Martin-Angele/publication/7748167/figure/fig1/AS:601780190724098@1520486986984/Antigen-processing-and-presentation-Foreign-antigen-is-phagocytized-by-the-macrophage.png.

Test Your Knowledge

1. Where do macrophages originate from, and how do they develop?
2. What are the main functions of macrophages in the immune response beyond phagocytosis?

12.3. Antigen-Presenting Cells (APCs)

Learning Outcome

1. Understand the definition and types of APCs
2. Explain the mechanism of antigen processing and presentation
3. Discuss the importance of APCs in activating T cells

Antigen-Presenting Cells or APCs are the key to the mediation of the immune response by processing and presenting antigens to the lymphocytes, most importantly T cells. This is critical for activating the adaptive immunity, which demonstrates the way APCs play an intermediary role between the innate and adaptive immune response. Dendritic cells, macrophages, and B cells are the most significant APCs, each with different roles to play in immune response and surveillance. For instance, dendritic cells are uniquely designed for antigen capture in peripheral tissues, migration into lymph nodes, and presentation of processed antigens to naïve T cells. Their effective antigen presentation is central to ensuring a robust immune response against pathogens. In this complicated mechanism, APCs not only enhance the activation of T cells but also provide essential co-stimulatory signals, which play a crucial role in T cell proliferation and differentiation and consequently dictate the immune landscape. The interaction between APC and natural killer (NK) cells illustrates the complicated dynamics of immune activation. Recent studies have also stressed that NK cells are not fully matured within the bone marrow but acquire functional capability while interacting with APCs, i.e., dendritic cells, during their journey to the infectious sites.

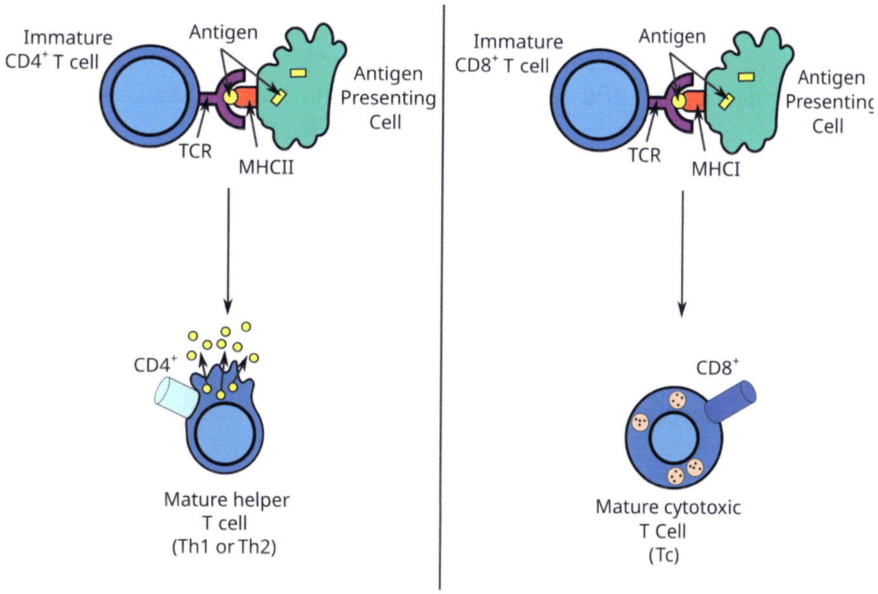

Figure 12.10. Antigen presentation stimulates immature T cells to become either mature "cytotoxic" CD8+ cells or mature "helper" CD4+ cells.

Source: https://upload.wikimedia.org/wikipedia/commons/thumb/4/4d/Antigen_presentation.svg/1280px-Antigen_presentation.svg.png.

This means APCs play a role not only in activating T cells but also in preactivating NK cells, thereby enhancing the innate immunity. Once NK cells come into contact with APCs, they are signaled to activate a response against pathogens effectively, most importantly at the onset of infection. The increasing recognition of these interactions emphasizes the pivotal function of APCs in coordination of both the innate and the adaptive immune systems and suggests that the exploitation of this collaboration may lead to novel therapeutic approaches to immune response enhancement during vaccines and disease, as evidenced in current studies. APCs also bear a crucial function in immune tolerance, which is required for homeostasis maintenance in the immune system. This balance is particularly relevant at the level of individual physiological states, i.e., pregnancy, where APCs have to promote tolerance so that the growing fetus is not rejected as being immunologically foreign to the mother. APCs' capacity to promote tolerance rather than an immune response is a multifaceted process involving the secretion of specific cytokines as well as the presentation of co-inhibitory molecules. Here, APC function modulation can determine whether an immune response in an aggressive manner is mounted against foreign antigens or tolerance is developed. This regulatory role highlights the necessity for further studies into the functional diversity of APCs, especially in those conditions where immune tolerance is critical, i.e., organ transplant and autoimmune disease, thereby shedding new light on emerging concepts of immunotherapy and vaccine strategies, as indicated by recent studies (Figure 12.10).

12.3.1. Definition and Types of APCs

Antigen-presenting cells (APCs) play a central role in the immune system by processing and presenting antigens to T lymphocytes. Immune cells that comprise mainly dendritic cells, macrophages, and B cells activate and regulate immune responses by facilitating recognition of foreign pathogens. Dendritic cells are considered the most effective APCs and are efficient at antigen capture in peripheral tissues, where they migrate into lymph nodes to present the antigens to naïve T cells. Macrophages, in addition to presenting antigens, possess intense phagocytic activity and can degrade pathogens to be presented at a later time as their antigenic components. The function of the B cells as APCs enhances their contribution beyond antibody production, thereby specifying their importance in facilitating the adaptive and innate immune response. This shows that the definition and versatile functions of the APCs is a core concept in the comprehension of the overall functioning of the immune system. The APCs are generally divided into professional and non-professional subsets. Professional APCs, including dendritic cells, macrophages, and B cells, present an array of major histocompatibility complex (MHC) molecules necessary for effective antigen presentation. These cells engage in direct contact with T cells, which activate and propagate them. Non-professional APCs, however, may be an array of tissue cells that are able to present antigens under specific circumstances but lack the characteristics of professional APCs as a default function. They expose antigens mainly upon inflammatory responses, emphasizing their role in initiating the immune system. Understanding the variety of APC types is essential since it reveals the various means through which the immune system responds to danger while remaining in balance so as not to form pathological conditions, , such as autoimmunity, where the immune system harms host tissue in error. Functionally, APCs also play a role in the modulation of the adaptive immune response through the regulation of the differentiation of T cells. Processing and presentation capacity of the APC is extremely variable, and this can be the key determinant of the success or failure of an immune response. For example, some APC-T cell interactions trigger distinct T cell subsets to induce different immunological outcomes, like the generation of effector T cells, regulatory T cells, or memory T cells. These kinds of interactions are very important in infections and in vaccination regimens. This APC-T cell interaction is further complicated by the ability of pathogens to evade recognition by the immune system; of special interest is the example of *Mycobacterium tuberculosis*, which can interfere with the function of APCs so that its own survival in host cells is enhanced (Combaluzier, 2008). As APCs remain a focus of immunological study, their multifaceted roles shed light on potential therapeutic avenues for enhancing immune responses against disease (Figure 12.11).

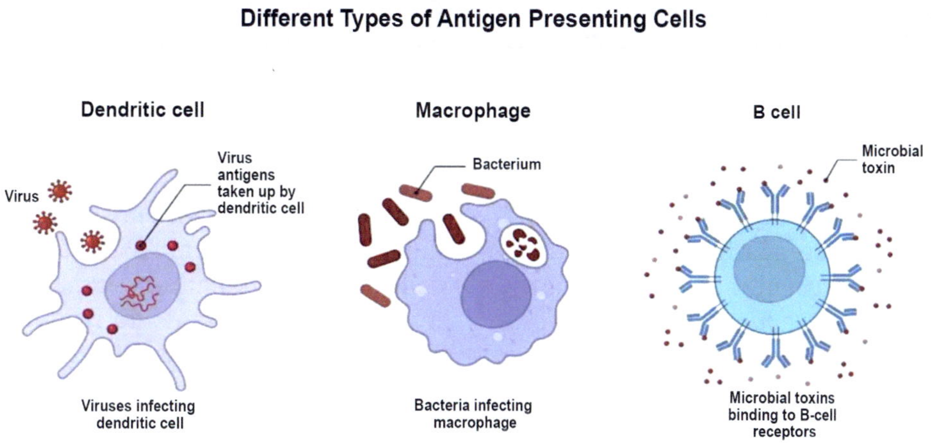

Figure 12.11. Different types of APCs.

Source: https://biologynotesonline.com/wp-content/uploads/2024/04/image-1441.png.

12.3.2. Mechanism of Antigen Processing and Presentation

Antigen processing and presentation are critical immune response mechanisms by which pathogens become recognized by lymphocytes, particularly T cells. Professional antigen-presenting cells , such as dendritic cells, macrophages, and B cells are the core of this process by capturing, processing, and presenting the antigens on their surface through the form of major histocompatibility complex (MHC) molecules. The classical and cross-presentation pathways of this process highlight the sophisticated mechanism of immune surveillance. For instance, dendritic cells phagocytose or endocytose exogenous antigens and they get broken down to peptide fragments. These fragments are displayed on MHC class II molecules to CD4+ T helper cells, initiating adaptive immune responses. Knowing the intricacies of these processes is important in developing successful vaccines and immunotherapies as they dictate the body's response against pathogens and cancer. In addition to the classical pathway, cross-presentation allows APCs to present antigens from extracellular sources on MHC class I molecules, which is the important process for activation of CD8+ cytotoxic T cells. This pathway is of great importance in immune response to viruses and tumor cells, which have a tendency to escape direct recognition by downregulating expression of MHC class I. Research shows that dendritic cells can effectively translocate such antigens to MHC class I, leading to a productive cytotoxic response. Vaccine experiments show that effective delivery of the antigen correlates with enhanced T cell activation as manifested in the observation of DNA vaccination and its impact on

T cell responses within cervical lymph nodes. Especially, dendritic cells were transfected directly in a cell population, leading to maximum T cell activation, highlighting the essential role played by dendritic cells in immune responses (Akbari et al., 1999). Furthermore, the ability of APCs to control antigen processing is also important in determining the flexibility and effectiveness of the entire immune system. Successful antigen recognition is crucial to prevent inappropriate immunity, which can result in autoimmune disease or continuous inflammation. For instance, studies have delineated the ways in which mycobacterial infection reverses macrophage function and escapes lysosomal degradation and winds up affecting aetiology presentation and immunity. Pathogens , such as *Mycobacterium tuberculosis* can avoid immune surveillance by persisting within macrophages, thereby disrupting normal pathways of processing. Despite these problems, effective antigen presentation from various sources remains vital in initiating and sustaining immune defense mechanisms. The understanding emphasizes the importance of researching capabilities of APC under different conditions, that is, how they develop as they respond to varied pathogens and how they influence lymphocyte reactions within the broader immune system (Combaluzier, 2008).

12.3.3. Importance of APCs in Activating T Cells

T cell activation plays a critical role in adaptive immune responses, and antigen presenting cells (APCs) play a vital role in this process. APCs , such as dendritic cells, macrophages, and B cells are responsible for antigen capture, processing, and presentation to T cells. This interaction also occurs by and large in secondary lymphoid organs, , such as lymph nodes, when T cells identify particular antigens presented by APCs bound to major histocompatibility complex (MHC) molecules. The significance of this interaction cannot be overstated because, apart from initiating T cell differentiation and proliferation, it also initiates the formation of memory T cells that provide long-term immunity against pathogens. The ability of APCs in this role is underscored by their ability to produce the co-stimulatory signals needed for the activation of T cells, thereby enabling the body to provide an appropriately tuned immune response. The ability of APCs to recognize and absorb antigens of various types makes them unique in comparison with other components of the immune system. This capacity is particularly important in the creation of the immune landscape, particularly under chronic infections and foreign substance exposure. For instance, professional APCs , such as dendritic cells possess a remarkable capability to migrate from peripheral tissues to lymph nodes where they present processed antigens to naïve T cells. This migration is modulated by many factors, including the expression of chemokine receptors necessary for APCs to migrate within the complex immunoevironment. Most importantly, the generation and maturation of APCs, including their transcriptional and migratory adaptations, can determine whether or not they are effective at stimulating T cells. Clarification of how these processes are regulated is important for understanding the mechanisms by which the immune system gains homeostasis and mounts productive responses to infections and disease (Arkestål, 2019). Furthermore, interaction with T cells and APCs is a precisely controlled process that not only stimulates T cells but also represents an important mechanism for limiting unproductive immune responses. For example, the crosstalk between APCs and Tregs is crucial for immune tolerance as well as autoimmunity evasion. APCs have been shown to regulate Treg differentiation by providing intrinsic signals and a supportive niche for their generation. Such coordination is particularly beneficial in the case of pathogenic infection since certain pathogens have evolved immune evading capabilities and downmodulated T cell activation. Studies on such interactions shed light on how specific pathogenic mechanisms, such as those of *Mycobacterium tuberculosis*, affect the maturation and the function of APCs, ultimately deciding the immune response and the capacity of the hosts to clear infections (Combaluzier, 2008). This dynamic again underscores the pivotal role of APCs in stimulating T cells as well as in shaping immune responses in an effective manner (Figure 12.12).

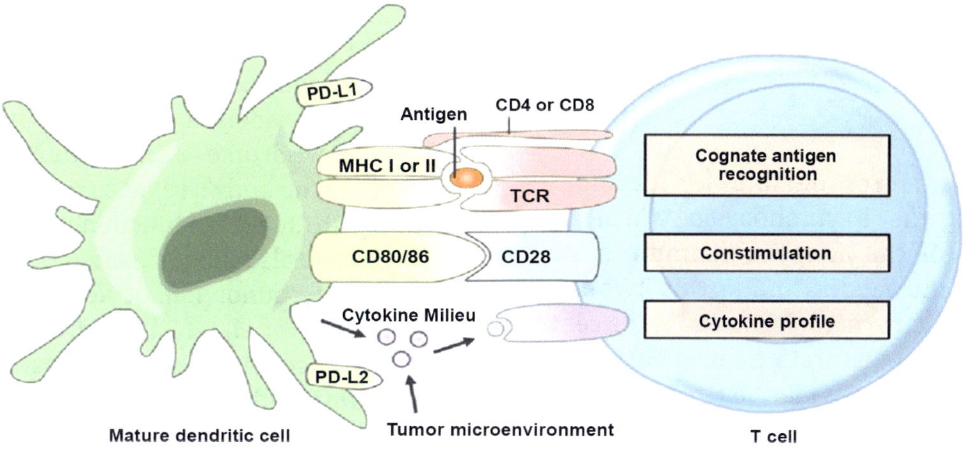

Figure 12.12. T-cell activation. T cells require three signals from an antigen-presenting cell (APC) in order to be effectively activated and primed. First, T cells must recognize their cognate antigen in the context of the correct MHC. Second, T cells require appropriate co-stimulation by an APC. Finally, the T cell receives instructive cytokines from immune cells and the tumor microenvironment, which dictate its phenotypic differentiation.

Source: https://www.researchgate.net/publication/352074154/figure/fig2/AS:1030441244917850@1622688432580/T-cell-Activation-T-cells-require-three-signals-from-an-antigen-presenting-cell-APC-in.png.

Test Your Knowledge

1. What are antigen-presenting cells (APCs), and why are they important in the immune response?
2. What are the main types of professional antigen-presenting cells in the body?

12.4. Thymus

Learning Outcome

1. Understand structure and location of the thymus
2. Explain the role of the thymus in T cell maturation
3. Discuss the importance of thymic education in immune tolerance

The thymus is responsible for developing and growing the T lymphocytes, which are a component of the adaptive immune system. Located in the mediastinum, this two-lobed organ is very active in early life and is the central site where T cell maturation takes place. In the thymus, bone marrow-derived precursor cells travel to undergo several complex processes of differentiation, including positive and negative selection. This selection permits only those T cells that have the ability to recognize self-MHC molecules and are non-reactive to self-antigens to develop, thereby promoting immune tolerance and preventing autoimmune disease. This fine tuning is achieved by virtue of the unique thymic microenvironment that is replete with dendritic cells and specialized epithelial cells, enabling a functional and tolerant T cell repertoire that can respond efficiently to pathogens. In addition to its role in T cell maturation, the thymus is also an important component in the interplay of various immune cells, particularly antigen-presenting cells (APCs), such as dendritic cells. These APCs, , such as the Langerhans cells referred to in (Flotte et al., 1980), act as a bridging entity between innate and adaptive immunity by antigen processing and T cell presentation. Thymic dendritic cells play an important role in the regulation of T cell responses and the establishment of immunocompetent conditions in the environment. Recurrent interaction between thymocytes and APCs permits the T cell response to be finely tuned so that the cells can recognize heterogeneous antigens and remain self-tolerant. Consequently, the thymus is not only involved in the maturation of T cells but also serves as a key site for the creation of a robust immune response, highlighting its position as part of the immune systems architecture. The loss or malfunction of the thymus can have significant consequences for the immune system, including susceptibility to infection and autoimmunity. Illnesses , such as thymic hypoplasia or complete agenesis typically result in extremely low T cell counts, as with DiGeorge syndrome. Such immunodeficiencies emphasize the body's reliance on the thymus for an adequate supply of functional T lymphocytes. Studies have also demonstrated the presence of multilineage donor leukocyte microchimerism in recipients of allografts, and thymic function and tolerance considerations (Demetris et al., 1995). Donor-derived dendritic cell survival and engraftment in the host further illuminated the thymus's role in immunological tolerance, illustrating how the organ is not only a T cell-producing destination, but also an immune adaptation and modification focal point under both endogenous and exogenous inputs.

12.4.1. Structure and Location of the Thymus

Strategically positioned in the upper portion of the chest, behind the sternum and between the lungs, the thymus is a key immune system organ. The bilobed organ develops greatly throughout an individual's life, with peak activity occurring during puberty. The thymus is engaged in T lymphocyte maturation, which plays a vital role in adaptive immunity. It is a specialized niche with precursor cells from the bone marrow migrating there to proliferate and differentiate. Its position in the body makes it efficient with other components of the immune system, hence playing a key role in ensuring the production of immunocompetent T cells that are effective in response to pathogens while ensuring tolerance to self-antigens. The thymus is anatomically divided into two distinct lobes, each consisting of a number of lobules that are disposed around an interconnecting network of epithelial cells. The epithelial cells play an important role in the supply of the proper microenvironment for the maturation of T cells, and they secrete hormones like thymosin and thymopoietin. Each lobule consists of a cortex and medulla, with the cortex containing predominantly immature T cells (thymocytes) and the medulla containing mature T cells.

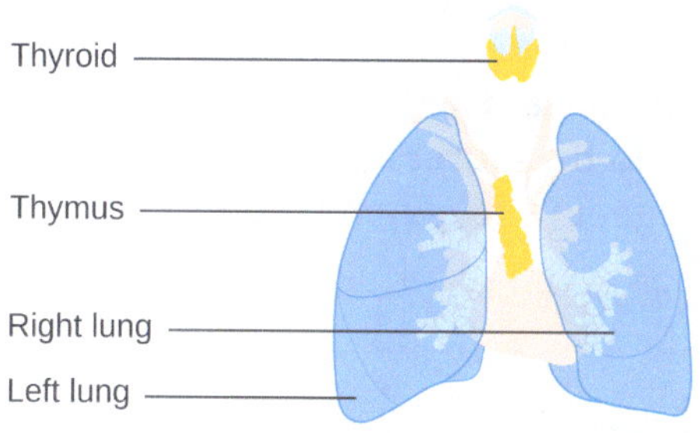

Figure 12.13. Diagram showing the position of the thymus gland.

Source: https://upload.wikimedia.org/wikipedia/commons/thumb/3/37/Diagram_showing_the_position_of_the_thymus_gland_CRUK_362.svg/1280px-Diagram_showing_the_position_of_the_thymus_gland_CRUK_362.svg.png.

Besides that, the medulla has specialized epithelial cells that are involved in the process of negative selection, whereby T cells with the potential to be autoreactive are eliminated. The thymus is consequently a well-developed organ with a complex architectural design that supports its vital role in immune competence formation. The thymus involutes, i.e., gradual reduction and shrinkage and activity decline, throughout life, particularly after puberty. This involution is linked to the reduction in the generation of new T cells, which may impact the capacity of the body to develop effective immune responses as a function of aging. Apart from this involution, nonetheless, the thymus retains its indispensable function in the preservation of immune homeostasis and tolerance. Its engagement with other immune organs, such as the spleen and lymph nodes, further determines its status in the network of the immune system. To understand more about the intricate mechanisms of the immune response, studies continue to validate how the structure and function of the thymus complements other immune cells, including dendritic cells that are involved in antigen presentation and triggering T cell responses (Flotte et al., 1980; Krishnamoorthy et al., 2010) (Figure 12.13).

12.4.2. Role of the Thymus in T Cell Maturation

The thymus has a principal function in T cell maturation, with the thymus serving as the organ where precursor cells mature into functionally competent T lymphocytes. The gland resides in the anterior mediastinum and is charged with mechanisms critical in the construction of a healthy adaptive immune response. T cells originate from bone marrow hematopoietic stem cells and migrate to the thymus, where they undergo a couple of cycles of maturation. During their stay in the thymus, these precursors experience positive and negative selection, a process designed to build self-tolerance and the ability to react to foreign antigens in the appropriate fashion. Without gradual, subtle T-cell maturation in the thymus, the immune system might become impaired, possibly leading to autoimmune diseases or an attenuated adaptive response to infections. In addition, the function of the thymus in T cell maturation is not limited to selection processes themselves, but rather actually shapes the repertoire of competent T cells capable of recognizing heterologous antigens. The specialized microenvironment of the thymic stroma plays a pivotal role in the generation of key molecules and cytokines enabling T cell development. These thymic epithelial cells play a crucial role in the expression of Major Histocompatibility Complex (MHC) molecules to display self-antigens to immature T cells. This is crucial in the selection of T cells to allow only those cells capable of recognizing MHC-peptide complexes appropriately to undergo maturation. The intricate networks of thymic signaling not only cause the development of T cells but also contribute to the induction of immunologic tolerance, underlining the gland's important role in immune well-being. Over time, the functional potential of the thymus diminishes, a process known as thymic involution. This age-related loss impacts the immune profile mainly, with fewer naive T cells being produced by the thymus, which are required to respond to new pathogens. Subsequently, infections may become more tolerable and vaccines have diminished impact, highlighting the long-term influence of thymic function on immune competence. Decreased thymic output can lead to an accumulation of memory T cells and a decrease in the naive T cell reservoir, which inhibits the adaptive immune system's capacity to mount vigorous responses to new antigens encountered later. It is vital to understand processes responsible for governing T cell development in the thymus because it provides insight into how therapeutic intervention to promote immunity in older age could be addressed, demonstrating the long-standing function for preserving immune wellness throughout life (Figure 12.14).

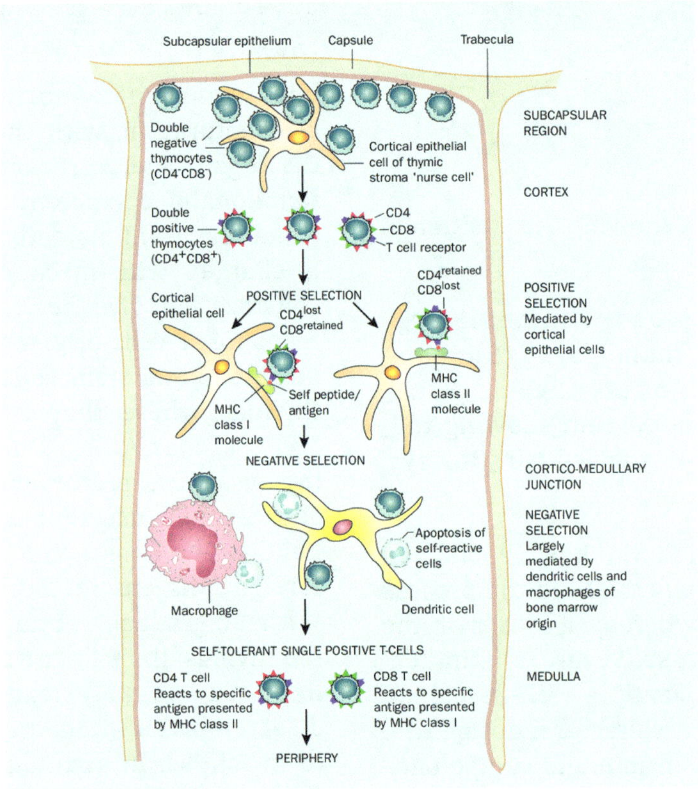

Figure 12.14. T cell development in the thymus.

Source: https://www.researchgate.net/profile/Mel-Storey/publication/23790088/figure/fig2/AS:667204605444098@1536085382222/T-cell-development-in-the-thymus-Thymocytes-enter-the-thymus-in-the-subcapsular-region.png.

12.4.3. Importance of Thymic Education in Immune Tolerance

Thymic training is essential to the development of immune tolerance, a critical process that regulates the balance between immunogenic reaction to infections and the prevention of autoimmunity. The thymus is the principal organ for the maturation of T cells, where immature thymocytes undergo a rigorous process of selection. This comprises positive selection, whereby thymocytes that can bind to self-MHC molecules are selected, and negative selection, whereby T cells that respond too vigorously to self-antigens are eliminated. These mechanisms are crucial because they prevent lymphocytes from targeting the tissues of the body and thereby lower the risk of autoimmune diseases. Apoptosis of potentially autoreactive thymocytes has been demonstrated by studies to be the major mechanism for these selection pressures, and thereby enhancing the foundation of immune tolerance in the thymic environment (Sotomayor & Rabinovich, 2000). Throughout thymic education, cytokines and specific antigens play vital roles in dictating the repertoire of T cells that can distinguish between self and non-self. There has been increased focus on the contribution of galectin-1, a protein that causes immature thymocytes to undergo apoptosis, resulting in the removal of cells that could stimulate undesirable immune reactions (Rabinovich et al., 2000). Not only is this helpful in maturing functional, self-tolerant T cells, but it also contributes to the systemic homeostasis of the immune system. In addition, the thymus has also been discovered to engage in specialized interactions with a variety of immune stimuli, , such as infections, that further impact T cell development and function. For instance, it has been discovered that the presence of mycobacterial infections has been able to modulate thymic output, which further implies that the thymus is not just an inactive organ but an active one in regulating immunity. The significance of thymic education extends beyond the immediate generation of self-tolerant populations of T cells. Properly educated pools of T cells ensure that the immune system is able to respond effectively to non-self pathogens and escape the possibility of autoimmunity. Perhaps surprisingly, thymic educational failure has the potential to lead to autoreactive T cells that can be implicated in many autoimmune diseases. Therefore, processes , such as the recruitment of mature T cells from peripheral organs with the ability to recirculate back to the thymus are indicative of a dynamic interaction between the thymus and the peripheral immune environment. This interaction highlights the necessity for continuous and efficient thymic schooling, indicating its critical role in maintaining immune tolerance and the integrity of the global immune system.

Test Your Knowledge

1. Where is the thymus located in the body, and what is its general structure?
2. What is the primary role of the thymus in the adaptive immune system?
3. How does positive selection in the thymus contribute to T cell maturation?

12.5. Bone Marrow

Learning Outcome

1. Understand the structure and function of bone marrow
2. Explain the role of bone marrow in hematopoiesis
3. Discuss the importance of bone marrow in immune cell production

Bone marrow is a crucial component of the immune system and is the principal site for hematopoiesis, the production of blood cells, including critical immune cells. It is within this specialized tissue that stem cells are differentiated into various lineages of immune cells, , such as lymphocytes and myeloid cells. The role of bone marrow is not only confined to the mere generation of blood cells but also serves as a key reservoir for B cells, which receive maturation in this environment before they migrate towards peripheral tissues. The homeostasis of hematopoiesis in the bone marrow showcases the intricate modulation of immune cell growth and function, which emphasizes its significance in immune homeostasis during an organisms lifetime. As the immune system changes with varying physiological demands, functions of the bone marrow become increasingly important. Importantly, the alteration in bone marrow functionality can be triggered by all stages of life, for example, stress, pregnancy, or ageing. Of special concern, pregnant females must deal with the complexities of immune tolerance, honoring maternal health as well as fetal security while ensuring a nurturing space for embryonic growth. In the later years of life, there is extensive loss of bone marrow integrity that can lead to reduced immune competence and make individuals susceptible to disease as well as infection. This intricate relationship places an accent on the necessity of ongoing research to comprehend bone marrows evolving role on immune dynamics over an organism's life span, particularly with respect to its involvement with agents like disease and aging.Moreover, current research has determined that bone marrow-derived natural killer (NK) cells are not yet fully functionally competent during their initial appearance. Instead, their activation and maturation are heavily determined by interaction with antigen-presenting cells (APCs), most notably dendritic cells. This complex interaction makes clear the importance of coordinated immune responses since the potential of NK cells can exert a powerful influence on innate and adaptive immunity. Ongoing research into these interactions not only makes more clear about immune cell precursors, but it also discloses significant information about potential therapeutic directions for enhancing immune responses. By the elucidation of mechanisms that regulate such interactions, we may have better control over NK cell functions, therefore resulting in more effective vaccination and enhanced overall immunity against pathogenic stimuli (Arkestål, 2019; Chijioke et al., 2011).

12.5.1. Structure and Function of Bone Marrow

The osseous framework of bone marrow is paramount to its intricate function in the immune system. Located within the cavities of the bones, bone marrow exists in two types: red marrow and yellow marrow. Red marrow is dedicated solely to hematopoiesis, the process by which blood cells like lymphocytes and macrophages are created. Red marrow contains a highly developed vascular network within this spongy tissue, which feeds the growth and maturation of these critical immune cells. Within the red marrow, hematopoietic stem cells differentiate into various lineages and therefore generate not just leukocytes but also erythrocytes and platelets. This double function indicates that the bone marrow plays a critical role in nourishing both immune response and overall body health and indicates its profound connection to other immune organs , such as the thymus and lymph nodes. Aside from its physical properties, bone marrow is also crucial in organizing immune reactions. Lymphocytes, particularly B and T cells, are generated in the bone marrow and thymus, which are central to adaptive immunity. B cells are processed in the bone marrow, where they undergo somatic hypermutation and class switch recombination, enabling them to respond with pathogen-specific antibodies. T cells, however, go to the thymus for further maturation and selection such that only functionally capable cells make it to the circulation. The interaction between the bone marrow and the thymus emphasizes the balance of the immune system with its timely and effective response to infections as well as self-antigen tolerance. The ability to generate variant immune cell populations is therefore reliant upon the structural and functional niches offered by the bone marrow.

The significance of bone marrow involvement in immune regulation is further evidenced by its role in disease, in particular within the tumor microenvironment. Current studies highlight processes by which bone marrow-derived cells, , such as myeloid-derived suppressor cells and regulatory T cells, are involved in cancer immunosuppression. The cells can modify local immune responses and promote tumor growth by inhibiting effective antitumor immunity, thus demonstrating how bone marrow-mediated production of immune cells can have complex implications for disease and health. In addition, the ability of marrow to respond to signals of inflammation marks it for its flexibility in the different physiological states necessary in maintaining homeostasis. Describing bone marrow organization and function not only enlightens its role in the immune system but also provides potential routes for therapy to manipulate this organ for greater immunotherapeutic benefit in oncology (Eroukhmanoff, 2010; Georgoudaki, 2015) (Figure 12.15).

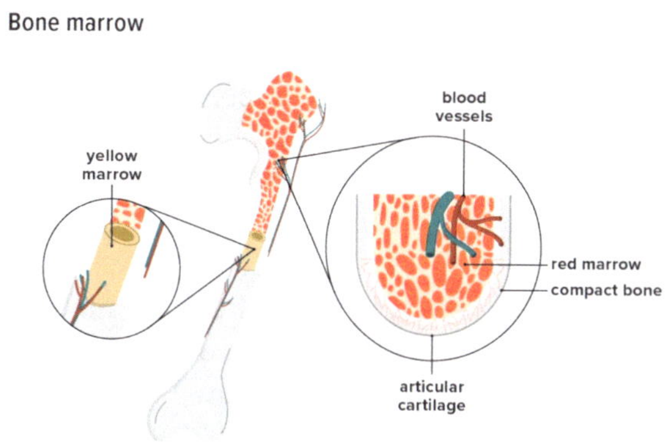

Figure 12.15. Bone marrow structure.

Source: https://i0.wp.com/post.healthline.com/wp-content/uploads/2022/01/1907952_What-Is-Bone-Marrow-and-What-Does-It-Do-01.jpg?w=1155&h=1997.

12.5.2. Role of Bone Marrow in Hematopoiesis

The bone marrow plays a vital role in hematopoiesis, the formation of all blood cells, including lymphocytes. Located inside bone cavities, the marrow is richly supplied with blood and represents a microenvironment that includes hematopoietic stem cells (HSCs). The multipotent stem cells are differentiated into a range of progenitor cells that further develop into the enormous range of blood cells that are required for immunity. This differentiation process is controlled by a number of different signaling molecules and cytokines that facilitate lineage specification. In addition, the niche formed by the bone marrow not only sustains the HSCs but also controls their development into a particular type of immune cell, such as B and T lymphocytes required for adaptive immunity. Therefore, the bone marrow is not just a production facility but a dynamic niche critical for functional coordination of the immune system. As hematopoietic stem cells divide, they go through a cascade of processes tightly regulated and responsive to physiological needs. One key aspect of this regulation is the role of the bone marrow microenvironment, made up of stromal cells and extracellular matrix elements that regulate the fate of HSCs. These interactions are necessary for the maintenance of HSC quiescence as well as the prevention of premature differentiation. Under conditions of stress, such as infection or blood loss, demand for hematopoietic output increases. In such circumstances, the bone marrow triggers signaling pathways that trigger precursor cell proliferation and lead to white blood cell creation rapidly, which is critical for initiating an immune response. This reactivity demonstrates the bone marrow's central role in rendering the body susceptible to various immunological challenges. Further, the relationship between the immune system and bone marrow extends beyond the mere production of blood cells; it also encompasses maturation and release of lymphocytes into circulation. Immature B cells that are produced in the bone marrow travel to secondary lymphoid organs , such as lymph nodes and the spleen, to undergo further maturation and selection processes. This transition is crucial to the development of B cells generating high-affinity antibodies, the mechanism that underlies humoral immunity. In much the same way, while T cells originate from precursors within the bone marrow, they develop in the thymus, indicating coordinated work between the two organs in the process of gaining a fully potent immune response. Thus, the bone marrow is not just a core reservoir of immune cells but also a core regulatory center for immune competence against infection in both localized and systemic character (Lister, 2003Combaluzier, 2008) (Figure 12.16).

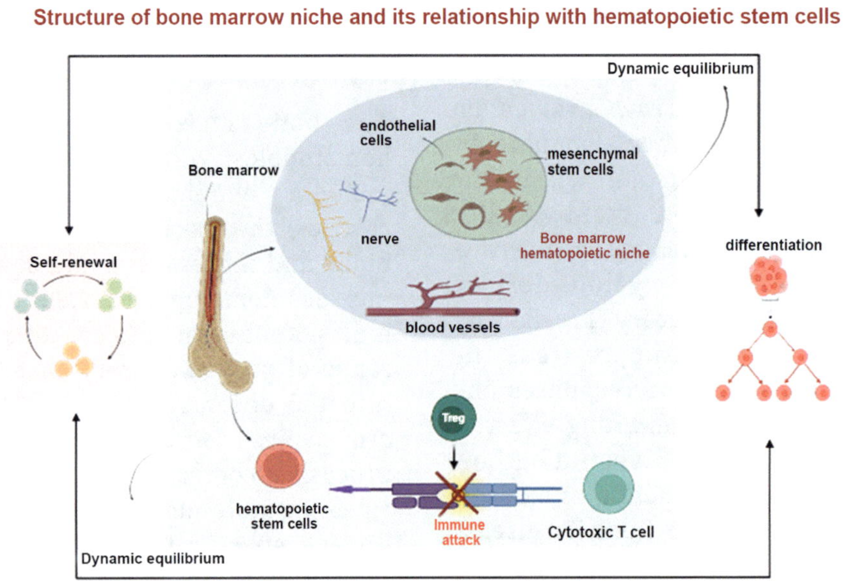

Figure 12.16. Structure and function of the bone marrow hematopoietic niche.

Source: https://www.researchgate.net/publication/369941761/figure/fig4/AS:11431281143245246@1681232440728/Structure-and-function-of-the-bone-marrow-hematopoietic-niche-The-bone-marrow.png.

12.5.3. Importance of Bone Marrow in Immune Cell Production

Bone marrow is a critical site for the production of immune cells, in essence forming the foundation of the body's defense systems. This spongy bone tissue, located in bone cavities, is, in essence, committed to hematopoiesis, that is, to producing blood cells, , such as leukocytes, which contain immune cell types like lymphocytes and macrophages. Lymphocytes, which are key players of the adaptive immune system, arise from bone marrow-derived hematopoietic stem cells. The cells undergo differentiation and selection processes necessary to mature into functional immune cells that can recognize and combat diverse pathogens. The role of the bone marrow should not be underestimated; its ability to generate a very heterogeneous repertoire of immune cells is important not only for responding to acute infections, but also for the establishment of long-term immune memory. In addition to the production of lymphocytes, bone marrow has a key function in the overall immune homeostasis. The microenvironment of bone marrow is specifically created for the support and sustenance of a range of immune progenitor cells towards survival and development. Signaling molecules and stroma cells work synergistically to enable progenitor cells to develop into fully capable immune cells. In addition, it is during this stage that crucial maturation processes take place, influencing the phenotype and the cells' function, , such as natural killer (NK) cells, which do not fully mature functionally within the bone marrow alone. They need interactions with antigen-presenting cells (APCs) to gain their full immune competence. This reliance is working to accentuate the bone marrow's role not only in the generation of immune cells, but also in generating an effective immune landscape ready for instant response to pathogens (Chijioke et al., 2011). In addition, the role of bone marrow is not only in generating immune cells but also as a reservoir for stem cells that aid in tissue repair and regeneration. The ability of bone marrow cells to migrate to the infected area and aid in healing demonstrates potential in immune function. Bone marrow structure evolves with age and has a significant impact on immune responses as well, further emphasizing its importance throughout an individual's lifetime. A case in point is that with increasing dog age, the immune system, including bone marrow function, deteriorates, rendering immune responses against pathogens and vaccines useless (Arkestål, 2019). This age-related loss not only affects the yield of leukocytes but also modulates the quality of immune memory, thus emphasizing the relevance of having an intact, healthy microenvironment of bone marrow for good immunity. In summary, the complex function of bone marrow in producing immune cells and regulating systemic immunity underscores its central role in the overall immunological system.

Test Your Knowledge

1. What is the structure of bone marrow, and where is it primarily located in the body?
2. Which immune cells are produced in the bone marrow?
3. How does the bone marrow microenvironment support immune cell development?

12.6. Lymph Nodes

Learning Outcome

1. Understand structure and organization of lymph nodes
2. Explain the role of lymph nodes in filtering lymphatic fluid
3. Discuss the importance of lymph nodes in immune surveillance

Lymph nodes play a significant role in the immune system as they offer needed sites for lymphocyte activation and growth. Lymph nodes are small, bean-shaped organs that are distributed throughout the body, filtering lymph fluid and allowing the association of immune cells with pathogens. Every lymph node consists of personalized zones, , such as the cortex, paracortex, and medulla, allowing specialized function. Upon interacting with antigens, dendritic cells transport such foreign substances from peripheral tissues to the lymph nodes for activation of T and B cells. The process calls out the lymph node role as an antigen-presenting site where immunity starts. Organizing the lymph nodes in such a way ensures efficient identification of pathogens and highlights their role in adaptive and innate immunity. In the examination of lymph node function, of note is the consideration of how the nodes have dynamic interactions with various immune cells, , such as lymphocytes and antigen-presenting cells (APCs). The communication between lymphocytes and APCs, including dendritic cells, is crucial in the stimulation of NK cells as well as their functional capacity. Studies show that NK cells mature their function in the context of such interactions, underlining the role of lymph nodes in generating robust immune responses. Interestingly, the cross-talk between immune cells in lymph nodes not only enhances the humoral response through B cell differentiation but also enhances cellular immunity through T cell activation. Such a complex mechanism maximizes the immune system's ability to recognize and respond to diverse pathogens and thereby maximizes overall immune homeostasis and surveillance. Furthermore, the role of lymph nodes extends beyond mere pathogen filtering; they are important for immune system regulation and immunity as well.

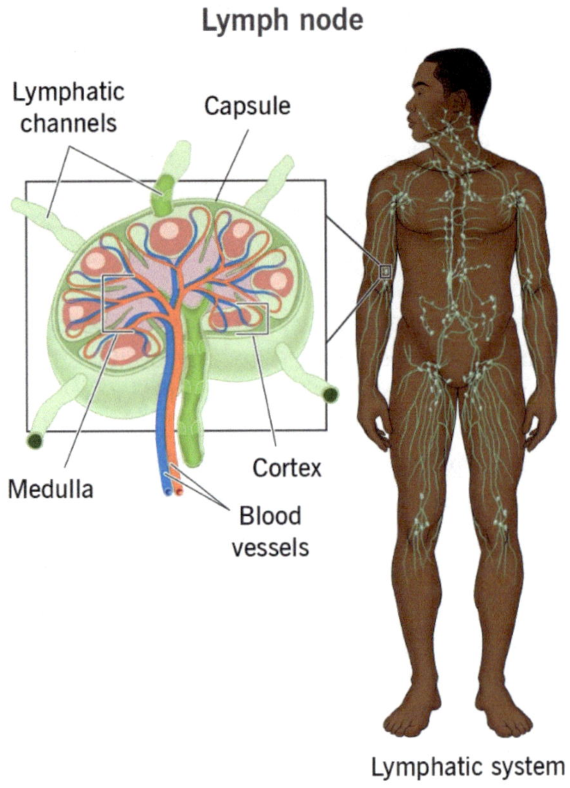

Figure 12.17. Lymph nodes.

Source: https://my.clevelandclinic.org/-/scassets/images/org/health/articles/23131-lymph-nodes.

In early infections, lymph nodes orchestrate an acute migration of immune cells that results in an intensely effective response that primes the organism for repeated contact with the same pathogens. This formation of memory is highly complemented by the clonal growth of B and T memory cells within the lymph nodes, which retain the capacity to reply more efficiently with re-infection. This property of lymph nodes is a demonstration of the dynamic nature of the immune system, particularly through different stages of life, as expressed through fluctuating immunity capabilities during pregnancy and aging (Arkestål, 2019). Valuing the roles of lymph nodes in such processes not only highlights their importance in terms of instantaneous immunity responses but also elucidates their effect on overall long-term immune health and acclimatization (Figure 12.17).

12.6.1. Structure and Organization of Lymph Nodes

Lymph nodes are an integral component of the immune system that are strategically located in the body to filter lymph and influence the immune response.

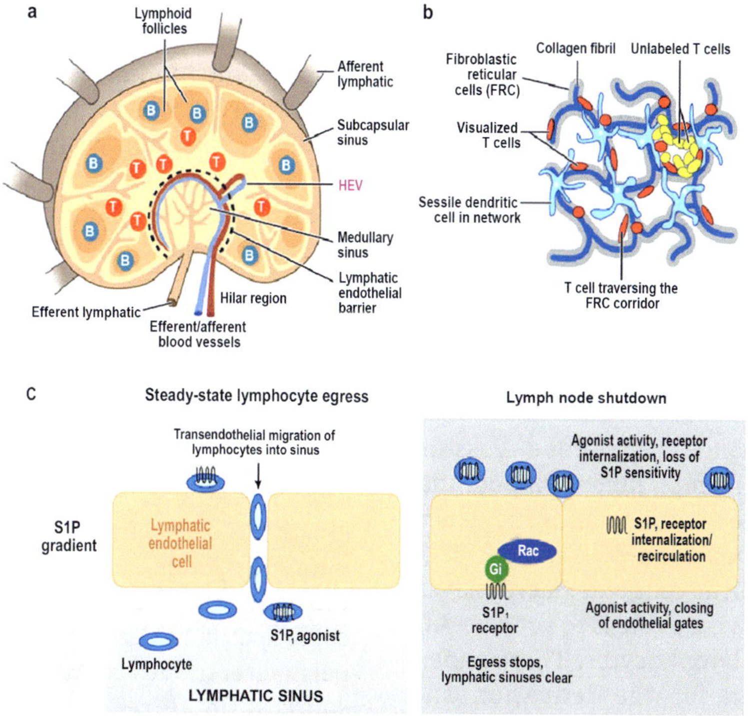

Figure 12.18. Structural and functional aspects of lymph node organization. (a) Macroscopic organization of lymph node regions, illustrating B cell follicles, T cell localization within the paracortex, and high endothelial venules (HEVs). (b) Schematic illustrating the motility of labeled T cells (orange) along and across the fibroblastic reticular scaffolding, in the presence of DC and an excess of unlabeled T cells (yellow), only a small fraction of which are shown in one region. (c) Hypothesis for regulation of lymphocyte egress by sphingosine 1-phosphate (S1P), illustrated under conditions of steady-state egress (left) and lymphopenia (right). T cells are shown with S1P 1 receptors either exposed or internalized in the presence of S1P. Junctions between the lymphatic endothelial cells close in the presence of an S1P1 agonist.

Source: https://www.researchgate.net/profile/Ian-Parker-11/publication/5677378/figure/fig2/AS:280841872789511@1443969328736/Structural-and-functional-aspects-of-lymph-node-organization-a-Macroscopic.png.

They are made up of a variety of specialized compartments, including the cortex, paracortex, and medulla, which have unique cell patterns and functions. The outer cortex is occupied mostly with follicles containing B lymphocytes that enable the quick production of antibodies upon encounter with antigens.

The paracortex, which contains T lymphocytes, is the critical location where the T cells are activated by antigens presented by dendritic cells. Such compartmentalization not only emphasizes the success of immune responses but also allows for the retention of the fine balance to avoid uncontrolled immune responses, reflective of the complex architecture unique to optimal immune function and adaptation to varied pathogens, , such as those using highly evolved evasion strategies like *Mycobacterium tuberculosis* (Arroz-Madeira et al., 2023). The lymph vessels linked with lymph nodes are also significant initiators of immune responses by transporting antigens and immune cells to peripheral locations.

The vessels, independent of blood vessels, enable the passage of lymph fluid with potential pathogens, cellular detritus, and antigens. There exist professional antigen-presenting cells (APCs) , such as dendritic cells and macrophages, within lymph nodes whose role is to process and present antigens to lymphocytes. This enables a good environment for the activation and clonal expansion of naïve lymphocytes in the generation of an adaptive immune response. Such coordinated movement of the immune cells in and across the lymph nodes is promoted by specific chemokines and adhesion molecules that lead to efficient targeting of immune resources at locations where they are most required. Generally, this coordinated cell response helps the body's ability to formulate effective defenses against infection (Arroz-Madeira et al., 2023). Additionally, the organization of lymph nodes is not just a static anatomical process but also a dynamic structure that supports physiological demands placed upon it in the context of immune threats. The compilation of various cell types, including follicular helper T cells and regulatory T cells, provides an association of complex relationships forming a network that mediates tight control over immunity activation and tolerance. Emerging discoveries of the molecular regulation of lymph node organization show that alteration of the structural elements, i.e., lymphatic vasculature, can greatly affect immune responses and disease outcomes in disease models.

This knowledge is critical for designing therapy to augment immune responses in vaccination or suppress them in autoimmunity. With studies increasingly unfolding the intricacies of lymph node biology, the potential for use in immunotherapy and regenerative medicine grows, opening up new avenues to treat a wide variety of diseases (Combaluzier, 2008) (Figure 12.18).

12.6.2. Role of Lymph Nodes in Filtering Lymphatic Fluid

The function of filtering lymphatic fluid by lymph nodes is paramount to the function of the immune system, acting as sentry structures in the body that filter out pathogens, toxins, and ill cells. Lymph nodes receive lymphatic fluid from peripheral tissues containing antigens of various sources. On entry into the lymph node, lymph fluid enables naïve lymphocytes and antigen-presenting cells (APCs), primarily dendritic cells, to come into contact and process and present antigens. Such contact is essential for activating lymphocytes and initiating adaptive immunity responses.

In filtering in this manner, lymph nodes also have specialized microenvironments that facilitate immune cell maturation and proliferation to help the body respond efficiently to infection. Thus, the filtration apparatus of the lymphatics is mechanically significant in fluid balance as well as playing a critical function in coordinating immune surveillance and subsequent immunity response (Arroz-Madeira et al., 2023). The capacity of lymph nodes to filter is particularly noteworthy, as the dynamic balance of lymphatic fluid must run continuously through the lymphatic channels. Lymph nodes also filter out not only germs but also waste products and cell detritus from tissues, contributing to the overall health of the lymphatic system. This is controlled by numerous immune cells, some of which are macrophages that reside within the nodes and are scavengers for germs and dead cells.

The interactions between these cells optimize immune reactions to infection. Besides, the lymph fluid enables a vehicle through which signaling molecules , such as cytokines, can drive immune cell behavior. These interactions spotlight the complex function not merely as filters but as active players in guaranteeing immunity and homeostasis within tissues (Tadayon et al., 2022). Additionally, their structural organization provides optimal filtration and immune modulation. Each lymph node is conditioned with differentiated regions, , such as the cortex and the medulla, which allow for specialized immune activities.

The cortex contains follicles with B cells, while the paracortex consists of T cells, which allows specialized immune interaction. This structure is necessary for the rapid activation of specialized immune pathways against known threats. Recent studies show that the capacity of lymph nodes to regulate lymphocyte trafficking and activation is even enhanced by molecules , such as Clever-1, which has been seen to regulate leukocyte migration into these organs. Understanding how lymph nodes regulate filtration of lymphatic fluid and coordination of immune response is thus vital in the design of specific therapies for some immune-related diseases (Arroz-Madeira et al., 2023).

12.6.3. Importance of Lymph Nodes in Immune Surveillance

Lymph nodes are critical nodes in the immune surveillance network, allowing for the detection and response to pathogens within the body. Located in strategic areas about the lymphatic system, lymph nodes act as filters, sifting lymph fluid for foreign invaders, , such as bacteria and viruses. This filtration process is crucial because it allows lymphocytes, i.e., B cells and T cells, to interact with antigens carried by antigen-presenting cells (APCs) in the lymph nodes. The architecture within lymph nodes, , such as differentiated zones for B cell and T cell activation, facilitates a good immune response. By concentrating immune cells within these differentiated compartments, lymph nodes enhance the likelihood of a robust adaptive immune response, thereby establishing an indispensable bridge between the innate and adaptive branches of immunity. Lymph node anatomy is more than anatomical; it is significant to immune surveillance dynamics. Dendritic cells, a subtype of APC, play the key role. These cells capture antigens in tissue and migrate to lymph nodes, where they present the antigens to naive T cells. This encounter, often accompanied by co-stimulatory signals, leads to T cell activation and expansion. Lymph nodes also offer proper training for T cells so that only the cells capable of recognizing specific antigens are amplified and distributed. This mechanism is a paradigm for the lymph node function in immune tolerance and prevention of autoimmunity, but efficient defense against pathogens. Lymph nodes are not passive structures; they are active players in orchestrating immunity. While beyond their direct function in pathogen recognition and T cell activation, lymph nodes also play a critical systemic function in coordinating immunity. They provide an avenue for communication among categories of immune cells so that the messages from the various parts of the body can be harmonized. Besides, the lymphatic system is a conduit, transporting immune cells to various tissues and allowing immune responses to be mobilized on time wherever they are needed. This transport system is particularly critical during infections or tissue injury episodes when swift immunological responses can be the determining factor in recovery or severe disease onset. Lymph nodes are vital, in fact, in coordinating the synchronized immune responses that can deal with the diverse threats, solidifying their places as critical immune system structures (Lister, 2003; Arkestål, 2019).

Test Your Knowledge

1. Explain the role of forensic pathologists.
2. Write a short note on post-mortem computed tomographic angiography (PMCTA).
3. What is exhumation?

SUMMARY

The intricate interaction among the various cells and organs of the immune system gives a clear picture of how our body's defense operates. Lymphocytes, macrophages, and antigen-presenting cells (APCs) all play pivotal roles in recognizing and responding to pathogens, thereby rendering immune responses effective and precise. The architecture of the immune system, with principal sites , such as the thymus, bone marrow, lymph nodes, and spleen, provides the stage on which this exquisite ballet of recognition and response takes place. As described, the dynamic image of charting these interactions is a demonstration of the beauty of biological complexity, wherein specially adapted cells collaborate to maintain homeostasis and combat disease (Combaluzier, 2008). Additional research verifies that the immune system's ability to adapt underlies its evolutionary significance. As pathogens have become increasingly devious at avoiding immune systems, our immune cells have adapted to create ingenious means of destroying such enemies. This type of adaptability suggests that immune cells are learning and adapting their attack methods constantly, often employing different organs to do their job most effectively. The role of macrophages and lymphocytes is of particular interest in this respect because they not only respond to immediate threats but also contribute to immunological memory. This dual role is a significant component of long-term immunity and emphasizes the imperative for ongoing investigation into these cell interactions (Georgoudaki, 2015). In addition, the understanding of these cellular dynamics is opening new avenues for therapeutic intervention, especially for conditions , such as cancer and autoimmune diseases. Immune process manipulation offers potential therapeutic avenues for immunotherapy, using the body's defense mechanisms to combat malignant cells or restore balance where the system fails. By attributing certain targets and mechanisms to the immune landscape, scientists can design better drugs that harness the strength of the immune system. Thus, knowing the roles of lymphocytes, macrophages, APCs, and the organs used provides us with the foundation knowledge necessary to advance medical science's fight against disease (Combaluzier, 2008; Georgoudaki, 2015).

In understanding immune system function, the role of the various cells and organs is most relevant. Lymphocytes, i.e., T and B cells, orchestrate adaptive immunity by identifying specific antigens presented by antigen-presenting cells (APCs). The thymus is especially crucial for T cell maturation so that only cells that are able to interact in a proper manner with self-MHC molecules survive, thereby preventing autoimmunity. Moreover, bone marrow is the site of major hematopoiesis, which forms all the immune cells, , such as lymphocytes, playing a crucial part in the immune response. Communication among these cells and organs provides a large network that accelerates immune surveillance and the ability to react against pathogens, emphasizing the complex interaction of the immune system (Eroukhmanoff, 2010). Macrophages are primary cells of the immune system that serve both as APCs and phagocytes. Macrophages capture and incorporate microbes, presenting antigens to T cells on MHC class II molecules to initiate an adaptive immune response. The spleen is a secondary lymphoid organ where macrophages and dendritic cells reside and interact with lymphocytes in order to generate an effective immune response. These interactions are critical, especially in the context of blood-borne pathogens. Recent research has established how specific conditions, , such as the absence of specific proteins, can impact these critical processes, revealing intricate processes controlling macrophage function and immune competence. Identification of these processes helps explain how pathogens like *Mycobacterium tuberculosis* can escape immune surveillance and sheds light on the planning of targeted therapies

(Combaluzier, 2008). In addition to that, lymph nodes are also important centers of immune cell activation and expansion. Lymphocytes, upon exposure to antigens, get activated and expand to facilitate a rapid immune response. The anatomy of lymph nodes is favorable for such activation, with effective interaction among the lymphocytes, APCs, and other immune cells. It is aided by the activity of dendritic cells, which phagocytize pathogens and travel to lymph nodes to induce an immune response. Lymphocyte response in such sites depends heavily on their previous maturation and the presence of necessary co-stimulatory signals from other immune cells. Hence, the very concerted interactions between lymphocytes, macrophages, and immune system organs highlight the complexity level of immune response, justifying ongoing research into mechanisms to address immunological challenges efficiently (Eroukhmanoff, 2010).

KEY TERMS FROM THIS CHAPTER

- Antigen-presenting cells (APCs)
- Blood cells
- Cancer therapy
- Chemokines
- Cytotoxic T cells
- Dendritic cells (DCs)
- G-protein-coupled receptor (GPCR) signaling
- Humoral immunity
- Immune function
- Immune response
- Autoimmunity evasion
- Bone marrow
- CD8+ cytotoxic T cells
- Co-inhibitory molecules
- Cytotoxic T lymphocytes
- DNA vaccination
- Hematopoietic stem cells (HSCs)
- Immune cells
- Immune organs
- Immune system pathology

CRITICAL THINKING QUESTIONS

1. **Which of the following cells are primarily responsible for the adaptive immune response?**
   a. Neutrophils
   b. Erythrocytes
   c. Lymphocytes
   d. Platelets
2. **What is the main function of macrophages in the immune system?**
   a. Produce antibodies
   b. Engulf and digest pathogens
   c. Activate cytotoxic T cells
   d. Regulate blood pressure
3. **Which of the following are considered professional antigen-presenting cells (APCs)?**
   a. B cells, dendritic cells, and macrophages
   b. T cells
   c. Neutrophils and basophils
   d. Natural killer cells and erythrocytes
4. **What is the primary role of the thymus in adaptive immunity?**
   a. Producing antibodies
   b. Filtering lymph
   c. Maturation of T lymphocytes
   d. Engulfing foreign particles
5. **Which of the following best describes the role of bone marrow in the immune system?**
   a. It filters lymph and traps pathogens
   b. It is the site of T cell maturation
   c. It is where antigen-antibody complexes are destroyed
   d. It produces all blood cells, including immune cells

Short Answer Questions

1. What are the primary functions of lymphocytes in the immune system?
2. How do macrophages contribute to the innate and adaptive immune responses?
3. What is the role of antigen-presenting cells (APCs) in adaptive immunity?
4. Describe the function of the thymus in T cell development.
5. What are the structural components of a lymph node, and how do they function in immune surveillance?
6. How does the bone marrow serve as a critical organ in the immune system?
7. Differentiate between central and peripheral lymphoid organs. Provide examples.
8. Explain how lymphocytes circulate between the blood, lymph, and lymphoid tissues.

Answers to Critical Thinking Questions

1. (c) 2. (b) 3. (a) 4. (c) 5. (d)

REFERENCES

1. Akbari, O. (1999). *Analysis of the Basis for Induction and Maintenance of T Cell Responses in DNA Vaccination*. https://core.ac.uk/download/376910702.pdf (accessed on 13th June 2025).
2. Arkestål, Kurt (2019). Immunological aspects of migration and tolerance. Karolinska Institutet. Thesis. https://hdl.handle.net/10616/46589(accessed on 13th June 2025).
3. Arroz-Madeira, S., Bekkhus, T., Petrova, T. V., Ulvmar, M. H., et al. (2023). Lessons of vascular specialization from secondary lymphoid organ lymphatic endothelial cells. https://core.ac.uk/download/590305668.pdf (accessed on 13th June 2025).
4. Boneschansker, L., Brandt, S. L., Chan, E. C., Filippo, K., Freedman, N. J., Hjorto, G. M., Hons, M., et al. (2019). Concepts of GPCR-controlled navigation in the immune system.
5. Braun, A., Dyer, D. P., Garton, K. J., Gupta, S. K., Hundelshausen, P., Janssens, R., Murphy, P. M., et al. (2018). A guide to chemokines and their receptors. https://core.ac.uk/download/155789735.pdf (accessed on 13th June 2025).
6. Brekelmans, P. J. M., Jacobs, R., van Ewijk, W., Wisse, E., et al. (1988). Lymphoid microenvironments in the thymus and lymph node. https://core.ac.uk/download/424960015.pdf (accessed on 13th June 2025).
7. Chijioke, O., & Münz, C. (2011). Interactions of human myeloid cells with natural killer cell subsets *in vitro* and *in vivo*. https://core.ac.uk/download/pdf/8558792.pdf (accessed on 13th June 2025).
8. Combaluzier, B. M. (2008). *Studies on The Relation Between Antigen Presentation and Mycobacterial Trafficking and On the Importance of Coronin 1 in Mycobacterial Pathogenesis, Neutrophil- and B Lymphocyte Functions*. https://core.ac.uk/download/18234246.pdf (accessed on 13th June 2025).
9. Demetris, A. J., Lu, L., Murase, N., Rao, A., et al. (1995). Micro chimerism, dendritic cell progenitors and transplantation tolerance. https://core.ac.uk/download/12205240.pdf (accessed on 13th June 2025).
10. Eroukhmanoff, L. (2010). *Tolerance and Immunity: Opposite Outcomes of Microbial Antigen Stimulation*. https://core.ac.uk/download/83747716.pdf (accessed on 13th June 2025).
11. Flotte, T. J., Silberberg-Sinakin, I., & Thorbecke, G. J. (1980). Langerhans cells as macrophages in skin and lymphoid organs. https://core.ac.uk/download/pdf/82473634.pdf (accessed on 13th June 2025).
12. Georgoudaki, A. M. (2015). *Exploring Immunotherapeutic Targets in The Tumor Microenvironment*. https://core.ac.uk/download/70343749.pdf (accessed on 13th June 2025).
13. Gillen, A. L., & Keoprommony, H. (2020). *Wise Blood: The Principle of Overcoming in Disease and Immunity (Part 1)*. https://core.ac.uk/download/286570787.pdf (accessed on 13th June 2025).
14. Iseki, M., Ishihara, K., Kashihara, N., Kawahara, H., et al. (2019). *Sh3bp2* gain-of-function mutation ameliorates lupus phenotypes in B6.MRL-*Faslpr* mice. https://core.ac.uk/download/228066095.pdf (accessed on 13th June 2025).
15. Krishnamoorthy, S. (2010). *In Vivo Labeling of Immune Cells for Tracking Using Magnetic Resonance Imaging*. https://core.ac.uk/download/614714874.pdf (accessed on 13th June 2025).

16. Lister, A. M. (2003). *Mechanisms Underlying Protection Against RT-2 Glioma Genesis in Rat Brain Utilizing Primary and Secondary Vaccination.* https://core.ac.uk/download/215482202.pdf (accessed on 13th June 2025).

17. Sotomayor, C. E., & Rabinovich, G. A. (2000). "Galectin-1 induces central and peripheral cell death: implications in T-cell physiopathology". *Developmental immunology*, *7*(2-4), 117–129. https://doi.org/10.1155/2000/36321 (accessed on 13th June 2025).

18. Rodrigues, B. M. C. (2011). *Caracterização Da Resposta Imune No Timo Em Resposta a Infecções Micobacterianas.* https://core.ac.uk/download/534410340.pdf (accessed on 13th June 2025).

19. Saraiva-Marques, C., da Fonseca, I. P., Graça Maria, & Alexandre-Pires, G., et al. (2019). From *in utero* to elderly. https://core.ac.uk/download/427721780.pdf (accessed on 13th June 2025).

20. Tadayon, S. (2022). *Role of Clever-1 in Leukocyte Trafficking and Inflammation.* https://core.ac.uk/download/535017333.pdf (accessed on 13th June 2025).

21. Vardakis, J. (1948). *Lymphoid Tissue and Resistance to Infection.* https://open.bu.edu/bitstream/2144/21494/1/lymphoidtissuere00vard.pdf (accessed on 13th June 2025).

HYPERSENSITIVITY AND AUTOIMMUNITY

13

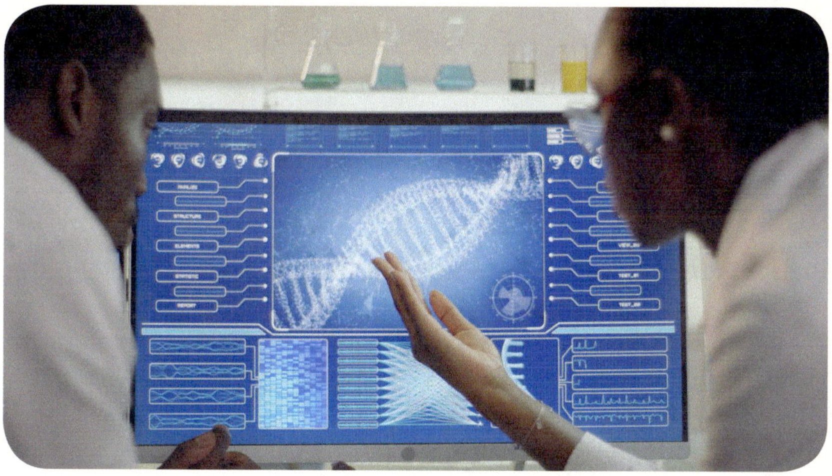

LEARNING OBJECTIVES

After studying this chapter, you will be able to:

1. Explain the types of hypersensitivity reactions
2. Understand the mechanisms of autoimmunity
3. Describe common autoimmune diseases
4. Deal with the diagnosis of hypersensitivity and autoimmunity
5. Discuss the treatment options for hypersensitivity and autoimmunity

Introduction

Both hypersensitivity and autoimmunity are immune disorders, but the targets are different. Hypersensitivity is an exaggerated immune reaction to nonactive substances, while autoimmunity is an inappropriate response of the immune system targeting the body's own tissue. Both are linked with inflammation and tissue injury, but the causes and mechanisms are distinct.

Definition of Hypersensitivity

Hypersensitivity is a pathological increase in the immune response to a foreign substance, which normally causes tissue damage and clinical manifestations ranging from mild to dangerous. It is caused by a number of factors, including allergens, autoimmunity, and other drugs. The immune system of the body tends to distinguish between nonhazardous and hazardous substances; however, in hypersensitivity, the immune response gets erroneous, resulting in deleterious effects on the body. This disease is not merely a bother but can lead to potentially life-threatening conditions , such as anaphylaxis. Understanding mechanisms of hypersensitivity is critical in accurate diagnosis and treatment because inappropriate immune responses can threaten overall health and welfare. The complexity of these reactions underlines the need for a broad definition that will capture their diversity and implications for affected individuals. There are four main types of hypersensitivity reactions: Type I (immediate), Type II (cytotoxic), Type III (immune complex-mediated), and Type IV (delayed-type). Each demonstrates various immunological mechanisms and processes, which illustrate the multi-aspect nature of hypersensitivity. For instance, Type I reactions, which are typically seen in the context of allergies, are caused by IgE antibodies binding to allergens, leading to the histamine and other mediator release by mast cells, creating symptoms like itchiness, swelling, and anaphylaxis. Type II reactions consist of the destruction of host cells via the binding of IgG or IgM antibodies with antigens present on cell surfaces, commonly giving rise to diseases like hemolytic anemia. Understanding these classifications assists doctors in identifying certain hypersensitivity conditions and administering effective therapeutic measures, thus requiring further study and education in this area. Clinical significance of hypersensitivity involves immediate reactions as well as long-term plans for patients. In allergic rhinitis or asthma, recognition of hypersensitivity as a chronic state of disorder can cause healthcare professionals to enforce preventive measures, lifestyle modifications, and pharmacological interventions. Furthermore, the integration of a multidisciplinary model is imperative in facilitating the advanced complexity of hypersensitivity, as can be witnessed in diagnosing idiopathic pulmonary fibrosis (IPF) within a collaborative healthcare environment. Existing guidelines are directing attention to the necessity of multidisciplinary discourse among specialists in order to increase diagnostic quality and treatment outcome, since such discourse allows for demarcation of the role of autoimmune manifestations in lung disease and adds sophistication to the concept of hypersensitivity as a broader health concern (Brown et al., 2017). Therefore, general awareness of hypersensitivity definitions and classifications leads to improved patient outcomes by facilitating the delivery of evidence-based, targeted, and patient-specific therapeutic interventions across various medical specialties (Carnevale et al., 2019) (Figure 13.1).

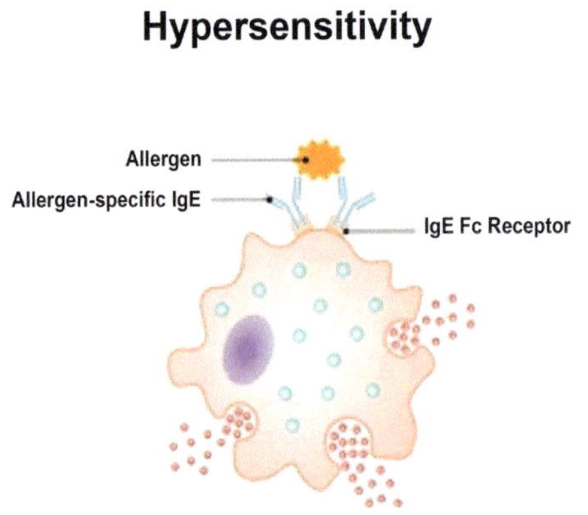

Figure 13.1. Hypersensitivity.

Source: https://www.shutterstock.com/image-vector/hypersensitivity-reaction-scientific-design-vector-260nw-2381436389.jpg.

Definition of Autoimmunity

Autoimmunity is a multifaceted and significant branch of immunological research, in which the defense system of the body begins to attack its own tissues in an uncontrolled immune response. The crux of autoimmunity lies in the failure of self-tolerance, the process that would otherwise prevent immune cells from responding to the antigens of the host as harmful. Such decomposition may lead to various autoimmune conditions, , such as rheumatoid arthritis, lupus, and multiple sclerosis, each with varied presentations and etiopathogenesis. The intricate dance among genetic susceptibility, environment, and microbial forces is at the core of the development of autoimmunity. It has been found that various exogenous factors are capable of inducing this dysregulated immune reaction, corroborating the complexity of how autoimmunity can be both a child of host genetics and external triggers, therefore making management and treatment processes complicated. Also entering the picture through increased research of autoimmunity are the levels of T cell involvement, in that these cells are key to facilitating immune reactions. Single T cell subsets, particularly those which become ineffective through mechanisms of exhaustion, can contribute to the chronic inflammatory state found in the majority of autoimmune diseases. The presence of effector memory T cells, on the other hand, can increase tissue damage and exacerbate disease. The difference between these types of T cells illustrates the delicate balance in the immune milieu and suggests the sophistication of autoimmune disease. Understanding this balance is important to the creation of new therapeutic strategies since an improved knowledge of T cell dynamics may lay the foundation for more efficient therapy aimed at the recovery of normal immune function and pathogenesis arrest. Additionally, mechanisms of autoimmunity extend into the realm of chronic infection-induced disease. The post-acute sequelae of SARS-CoV-2 (PASC), or Long Covid, are an example of this interaction between infectious agents and autoimmune mechanisms.

There is growing evidence that individuals who recover from COVID-19 can suffer ongoing symptoms due to autoimmune effects, which means the virus may accidentally reactivate dormant autoimmune pathways. This phenomenon illustrates the multifactorial character of autoimmunity, where inaugural exposure to pathogens can potentially lead to multifactorial chronic inflammatory and immune dysregulatory patterns, thus rendering clinical outcomes more complicated. With increased understanding of infections like PASC, it increasingly becomes evident that investigation of interfaces among autoimmunity, infection, and systemic inflammation responses is critical to designing practical prevention as well as treatment strategies in modern medicine (Canter et al., 2020; Bussolati et al., 2022) (Figure 13.2).

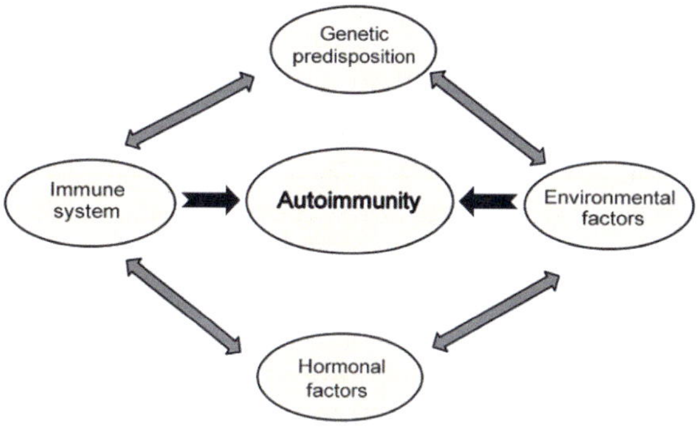

Figure 13.2. Autoimmunity.

Source: https://carolinatotalwellness.com/blog/wp-content/uploads/2023/01/autoimmunity--768x506.jpg.

Importance of Understanding These Conditions

Understanding the varied conditions that shape co-housing schemes is essential to successful urban planning and community development. The complexity of these factors accounts for how various stakeholders—ranging from planning authorities to community activists—interact in complex ways to construct innovative housing options. Given that social need tends to be fluid, such understanding allows planners to address the hazards that are an integral part of co-housing. As studies indicate, adaptive navigation of processes by such projects mirrors overall shifts in society. By recognizing the role of actor networks and self-organization, planners can better navigate different aspirations of communities and enhance the co-housing environment. Apart from that, this knowledge facilitates more cooperative collaborations between different stakeholders, ultimately leading to enhanced life quality in cities, coupled with higher satisfaction among residents involved in such initiatives (Boonstra et al., 2016). Moreover, the effects of recognizing these conditions reach public health and welfare. The connection between housing and well-being is gaining importance as a substantial element for residents and communities. Inadequate housing conditions have the potential to exacerbate a wide variety of health conditions that impact not just the body but also the mental wellbeing and social stability. Understanding the complexity of co-housing conditions, therefore, can unlock paths towards sustainable lifestyles that support the wellbeing of residents.

It is evident that urban planners are increasingly supporting design principles that encourage community connection and wellbeing. By encouraging settings within which physical activity, social connections, and mental health can thrive, the importance of such knowledge cannot be overstated, particularly with respect to urban regeneration and public health policy (Appelbaum et al., 2019).

Finally, transforming needs in society requires the integration of the circumstances under which co-housing exists. With more and more dense and diverse city environments, affordable and acceptable housing is more essential than ever. Neglecting such conditions can lead to ill-planned communities that do not meet the diverse needs of the population.

By adopting an integrative planning process that includes the perspectives of diverse stakeholders, the process can lead to sustainable co-housing developments that are also sensitive to potential challenges in the future. By embracing these conditions, the co-housing and urban development principles underlying them are reinforced to enable the creation of spaces that are responsive to current and potential future community needs. As the nature of urban life becomes increasingly complex, this knowledge is critical to developing creative and sustainable housing alternatives (Boonstra et al., 2016).

13.1. Types of Hypersensitivity Reactions

Learning Outcome

1. Describe Type I: immediate hypersensitivity
2. Explain Type II: Antibody-mediated hypersensitivity
3. Understand Type III: Immune complex-mediated hypersensitivity
4. Discuss Type IV hypersensitivity

Immune reaction is classified into four broad categories of hypersensitivity reactions: Type I, Type II, Type III, and Type IV. Type I hypersensitivity, or immediate hypersensitivity, is mediated by IgE antibodies. During the first encounter with an allergen, such as pollen or pet dander, the immune system releases IgE, which attaches to basophils and mast cells. After repeated exposure, these cells secrete histamine and other mediators of inflammation, which bring about symptoms , such as anaphylaxis, allergic rhinitis, and asthma. All this is significant to understand since it demonstrates how minimal environmental stimuli could generate huge physiological responses, and these need to be managed well if severe reactions are to be prevented. In contrast, Type II hypersensitivity occurs when IgG or IgM antibodies bind to cellular surface antigens and lead to cell lysis through mechanisms , such as complement fixation or phagocytosis. Hemolytic anemia and drug reactions are such reactions in which the defense mechanism of the body attacks its own cells by mistake. The clinical presentation of Type II reactions tends to be severe because normal cell destruction is very harmful to the patient in morbidity. The understanding of the mechanism of this type of hypersensitivity not only serves to emphasize the complexity of autoimmune reactions but also to highlight the relevance of further research on targeted interventions aimed at preventing such adverse effects on health. Type III hypersensitivity or immune-complex-mediated hypersensitivity is the deposition of antigen-antibody complexes in tissues, leading to inflammation and tissue injury. This can occur in systemic lupus erythematosus and rheumatoid arthritis. In contrast to the above, Type III reactions may take hours to weeks to manifest after exposure to an antigen and thus are more difficult to treat. The research reveals that many different factors, such as genetic predisposition and environmental triggers, contribute to the pathogenesis of these immune-mediated hypersensitivity reactions, particularly in children. Understanding the mechanisms of pathophysiologic processes becomes important in initiating therapeutic interventions that are effective, particularly for vulnerable populations, , such as those mentioned in the scenario of pediatric allergies and their increasing incidence in younger populations (Burns, 2019). Knowledge growth in this field is important for improved clinical outcomes and quality of life in those affected.

13.1.1. Type I: Immediate Hypersensitivity

Type I hypersensitivity, or immediate hypersensitivity, is an acute reaction to a few specific allergens by immunoglobulin E (IgE). Upon initial exposure to an allergen, the immune system develops IgE antibodies that bind to mast cells and basophils. With future exposure to the same allergen, these cells are activated to release histamines and other inflammatory mediators, leading to symptoms of itching, swelling, and bronchoconstriction. The hypersensitive reaction occurs within minutes and is thus distinct from other types of allergic reactions, which may be of a delayed nature. The clinical significance of Type I hypersensitivity is most alarming in cases involving repeated allergens , such as pollen, pet dander, and certain food items, where appropriate control measures have to be adopted in order to prevent acute episodes. Genetic susceptibility studies for Type I hypersensitivity, particularly in relation to ß-lactam antibiotics, offer crucial information on the pathogenic processes of this condition. A good example was a study that showed a significant correlation between the HLA-DRB1*10:01 allele and penicillin-induced immediate hypersensitivity reactions in patients with such a proven reaction. The findings suggested that this hereditary factor could predispose an individual towards catastrophic allergic reactions, and the significance of genetic screening for risk stratification in patients with established allergies was emphasized.

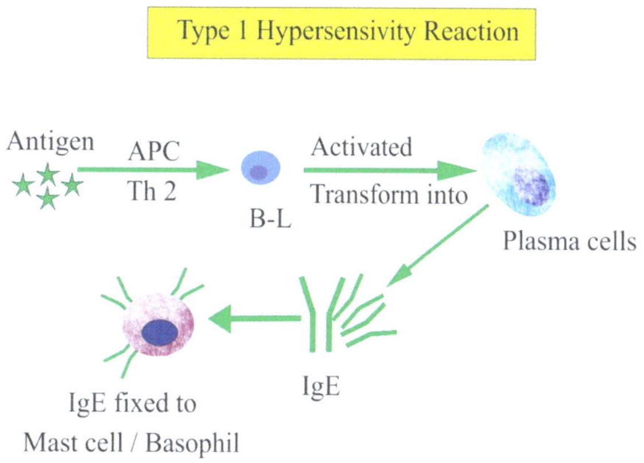

Figure 13.3. Type-1-hypersensitivity reaction.

Source: https://www.labpedia.net/wp-content/uploads/2020/04/Type-1-hypersensitivity-reaction-2.jpg.

The awareness of such genetic markers enables medical practitioners to personalize antibiotic prescriptions during the treatment process, minimizing the threat of life-threatening reactions and improving patient outcomes overall (Barrett et al., 2020). In children, drug hypersensitivity reactions, particularly those caused by antibiotics, are of utmost importance in diagnosis and treatment. The Italian Pediatric Society for Allergy and Immunology has made recommendations with the aim of maximizing the accuracy of the diagnosis of such reactions through the employment of the drug provocation test (DPT). The drug provocation test is central to the determination of a definitive etiology of allergic reactions because routine laboratory tests are found to be inaccurate. The DPT protocol takes into account the duration and degree of the reaction, thereby increasing the diagnosis of immediate hypersensitivity to commonly prescribed drugs. These combined measures in pediatric units are geared towards decreasing the risks caused by prescriptions of antibiotics while making sure that children are given necessary therapeutic interventions without undue exposure to possibly dangerous allergens (Arasi et al., 2018) (Figure 13.3).

13.1.2. Type II: Antibody-Mediated Hypersensitivity

Antibody-mediated hypersensitivity, which is of the Type II hypersensitivity form, is a significant aberration in immunity involving the production of antibodies against self-antigens or foreign antigens bound to cell surfaces. This process has unwanted implications where antibodies , such as IgG and IgM bind to target antigens, activating the complement system or immobilizing immune cells that lead to cell lysis or phagocytosis. Common manifestations of such hypersensitivity are autoimmune hemolytic anemia, purpura thrombocytopenia, and certain drug reactions. Pathologic mechanisms underlying show how the defense mechanism of the body, designed to protect it, can misinterpret its own components as threats. Therefore, effects of Type II hypersensitivity have both acute and chronic implications and pose a serious challenge to the individuals involved and need proper clinical handling. It is important to understand the mechanisms that underlie the induction of Type II hypersensitivity in order to design useful therapeutic interventions. Current research suggests that genetic susceptibility, environmental factors, and interaction with the microbiome can play a role in susceptibility to developing these hypersensitivity responses. The hygiene hypothesis, for instance, proposes that decreased exposure to microbes during development may bias immune function towards hypersensitivity disease, including Type II responses. Specifically, it implies that an inability of microbial diversity will impact the immune system's development in a way that predisposes one to the production of autoantibodies or antibodies to host tissues inappropriately.

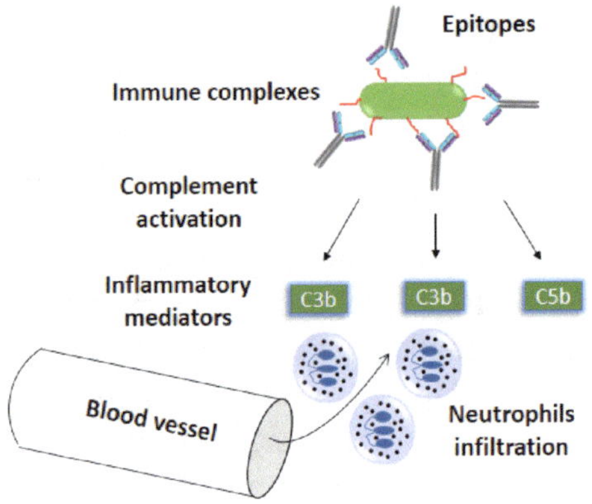

Figure 13.4. Mechanism of type II hypersensitivity reactions. IgM or IgG binding to either cell membrane or extracellular matrix induces lysis firstly through the formation of the membrane attack complex, secondly by antibody-dependent cell-mediated cytotoxicity. Type II sensitivity reactions could also enhance phagocytosis by opsonization.

Source: https://www.researchgate.net/profile/Faisal-Anjum/publication/342105656/figure/fig57/AS:11431281179698001@1691355242063/Mechanism-of-Type-II-hypersensitivity-reactions-IgM-or-IgG-binding-to-either-cell.png.

This indicates the subtle interactions between the immune system and environmental factors and requires additional effort to delineate the subtle dynamics underlying the onset and development of Type II hypersensitivity (Apostol et al., 2020). Furthermore, the role of dietetic factors in the formulation of immunological responses has gained increasing attention, most prominently their functions in hypersensitivity diseases. There is evidence to suggest that there are foods proven to modulate innate and acquired immunity and thus offer therapeutic possibilities for vulnerable people to Type II hypersensitivity. Some foods have been known to be useful in enhancing immune function, and the immune system can, thereby, modulate allergic reactions. For instance, probiotic or omega-3 fatty acid treatment has been reported to improve immune parameters in hypersensitivity patients. The investigation of the interaction between immunity and diet is therefore significant as it may provide insight into prevention and therapy of Type II hypersensitivity control. Emphasizing the importance of this interaction underscores the complexity of immune regulation and the degree to which alterations in diet can influence clinical expression (Kaminogawa & Nanno, 2004) (Figure 13.4).

13.1.3. Type III: Immune Complex-Mediated Hypersensitivity

Type III hypersensitivity reaction, which is otherwise called immune complex-mediated hypersensitivity, occurs when antigen-antibody complexes accumulate in particular tissues, leading to inflammation localized or generalized. These immune complexes, formed by the interaction of certain antigens with antibodies, get lodged in tissues , such as the kidneys, skin, and joints and activate the complement system and an inflammatory reaction.

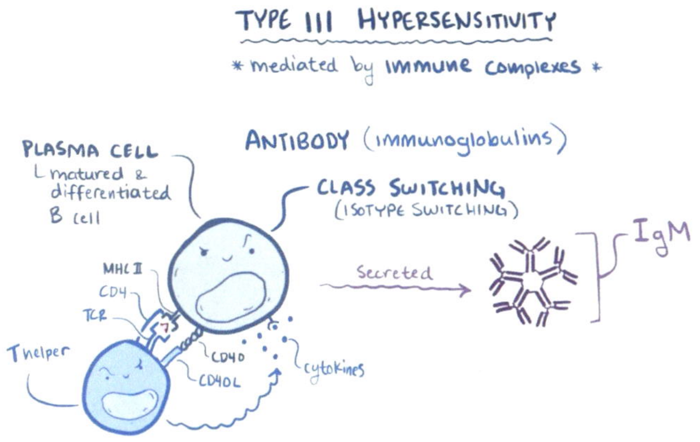

Figure 13.5. Type III hypersensitivity.

Source: https://d16qt3wv6xm098.cloudfront.net/Nlun7xJeTMeB7us_Np_CdYuvQlKEx2Jm/_.jpg.

This reaction is fundamentally a double-edged sword; while it is central to the elimination of pathogens, wrongful deposition or formation of such complexes is injurious and causes an assortment of diseases , such as systemic lupus erythematosus and rheumatoid arthritis. The characterization of mechanisms that are accountable for Type III reactions is critical in coming up with therapeutic interventions that might potentially inhibit tissue damage in conjunction with guaranteeing effective immunity against invading pathogens. The immune complex formation and deposition processes have several important factors, , such as the size, charge, and solubility of the complexes and the specific tissues involved. Larger complexes become trapped in tissue, while smaller ones might be circulating until eliminated by the kidneys. Dysfunctional immune responses increase these processes, increasing tissue damage and inflammatory responses. In pregnancy, for instance, more recent research has taken into account the fact that maternal food allergies are able to affect the immune development of the fetus, suggesting a potential link between maternal health and immune complex-mediated responses in offspring. The interface between maternal immune status and fetal immunity points to the intricacy of Type III hypersensitivity to both maternal and infant health outcomes, and research into how maternal immune status can impact perinatal health is required (Seita et al., 2013). The impact of Type III hypersensitivity extends beyond the immediate allergic reaction, as it is also significant in chronic inflammatory disease and autoimmune disease. New evidence shows that improper microbial exposure at windows of increased development has the capacity to influence immune maturation and amplify hypersensitivity responses. This is particularly relevant when taking the hygiene hypothesis into account, where diminished microbial exposure creates an immune imbalance of regulation, which has the capacity to activate the immune response towards hypersensitivity-type features (Apostol et al., 2020). With a deeper appreciation of Type III mechanisms and how they influence maternal-fetal health and the advancement of chronic disease, researchers hope to be able to identify effective strategies for prevention and treatment, introducing opportunities for improved health in impacted groups (Figure 13.5).

13.1.4. Type IV Hypersensitivity

Type IV hypersensitivity, in the Gell and Coombs division of hypersensitivity responses, or delayed-type hypersensitivity, is one of the hypersensitivity reactions that may take a day or more to develop. It is the only one not humoral (not antibody-mediated) but rather a cell-mediated response. The reaction is an interaction among T cells, monocytes, and macrophages. This reaction is because of the identification of foreign antigen in combination with the MHC class II on the surface of antigen-presenting cells by CD4+ Th1 cells. These can be macrophages that secrete IL-12, which induces further growth of CD4+ Th1 cells. CD4+ T cells secrete IL-2 and interferon gamma (IFNγ), which induces the further secretion of other Th1 cytokines, thus resulting in the immune response. Activated CD8+ T cells kill target cells upon contact, whereas activated macrophages release hydrolytic enzymes and, upon antigen presentation with certain intracellular pathogens, transform into multinucleated giant cells (Figure 13.6).

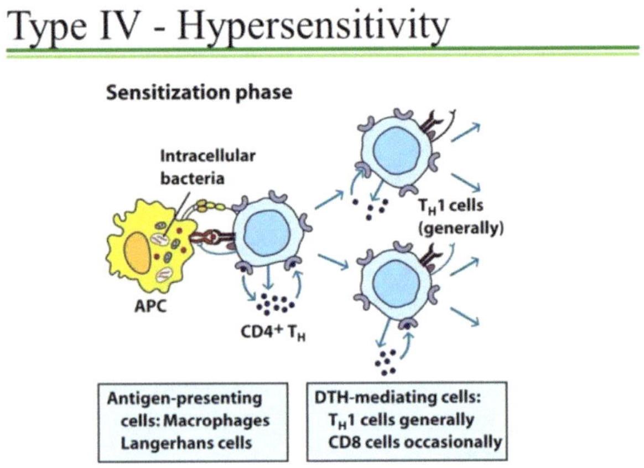

Figure 13.6. Type IV hypersensitivity.

Source: https://i0.wp.com/microbeonline.com/wp-content/uploads/2022/10/Hypersensitivity-type-IV.jpg?w=678&ssl=1.

Test Your Knowledge

1. What are the four types of hypersensitivity reactions?
2. Which type of hypersensitivity reaction is responsible for anaphylaxis and what is the primary immune mediator involved?
3. What distinguishes Type II from Type III hypersensitivity reactions in terms of antigen location?

13.2. Mechanisms of Autoimmunity

Learning Outcome

1. Explain the term genetic predisposition
2. Understand environmental triggers affecting autoimmunity
3. Focus on immune system dysregulation

The mechanisms of autoimmunity are intricate and include a broad understanding of the immune system complexities. One such critical aspect is the breakdown of immune tolerance, which normally safeguards the organism against its own antigens. Autoimmune diseases predominantly arise when the immune system incorrectly identifies self-tissues as foreign and launches an immune response against them. Such dysregulation may be influenced by genetic vulnerabilities, environmental etiologies, and hormonal effects. For instance, individuals with specific genetic markers may be susceptible to autoimmune disease, and environmental exposures , such as infections or chemicals trigger or exacerbate the disease process. Systemic review of these determinants points towards the intricate interplay between genetics and environment and hints at potential preventative and therapeutic maneuvers to prevent autoimmunity-related illness. Another important mechanism is the role of autoantibodies, which are antibodies created by the immune system that target the body's own cells. In many autoimmune disorders, the presence of such autoantibodies leads to inflammation and tissue damage. For example, systemic lupus erythematosus and rheumatoid arthritis are characterized by the presence of particular autoantibodies, not only beneficial as diagnostic biomarkers but also central to the pathophysiology of the conditions. Chronic production of autoantibodies can suppress cellular function and induce chronic inflammation, which goes on to feed back into the cycle of immune deregulation.

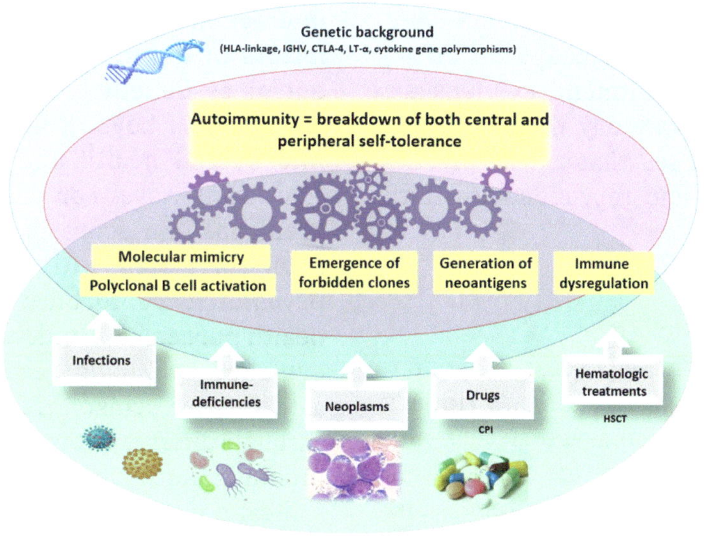

Figure 13.7. Mechanisms of autoimmunity.

Source: https://www.researchgate.net/publication/350419075/figure/fig1/AS:11431281210401626@1702051858741/Mechanisms-of-autoimmunity-The-pathogenic-mechanisms-of-autoimmunity-involve-a-genetic.tif.

Understanding the mechanisms of autoantibody production and their pathogenic effects is crucial to the discovery of targeted therapies that restore immune balance as well as improve patient outcomes. Considering the broader applications of autoimmune mechanisms, an understanding of how they intersect with problems of fertility, particularly in females, is critical. More recent studies have indicated that endocrine autoimmunity has a significant impact on reproductive function, and as such, diseases like infertility become more complicated conditions to treat. As an example, autoimmune disorders of the hypothalamus, thyroid, or ovaries can disrupt normal hormonal control necessary for ovulation and conception. Thus, a multidisciplinary approach to managing infertility must include careful evaluation for potential autoimmune contributions. For the patient, determination of such factors is important for the purpose of making intelligent decisions regarding reproductive health. Greater insight into autoimmunity processes can lead to improved diagnostic and therapeutic interventions, hence enabling women to achieve their reproductive aspirations in spite of autoimmune challenges (Josephine et al., 2023). Such integrated treatment regimens are becoming the norm of the day in overcoming difficult health challenges that cut across the fields of immunology and reproductive health (Figure 13.7).

13.2.1. Genetic Predisposition

Genetic susceptibility is an important component to look into in understanding an individual's susceptibility to many characteristics and disorders. There is no question that certain genetic characteristics predispose one towards cognitive capacity, health condition, personality characteristics, and even physical looks, which can significantly influence an individual's academic and economic success. The combination of genetic components and environmental components determines an individual's capability and potential for economic and social mobility. For instance, Kronstadt (2008) indicates the contribution of contextual factors that can enhance or diminish the advantage that they gain from genetic predispositions. This requires realization of the necessity of incorporating both genetic tendencies and environmental circumstances in complete understanding of success trajectories among individuals. Additionally, the intricate relationships between genetic predispositions and some psychiatric conditions reveal insight into the shared etiological pathways they have on mental health. Recent studies have demonstrated robust genetic correlations between illnesses , such as schizophrenia and eating disorders and the way that multiple genetic risk factors overlap to produce risk for multiple psychiatric disorders. As an example, Zhang (2022) offers a family study of eating disorder-schizophrenia co-occurrence and finds that eating disorder patients have a highly increased risk of developing schizophrenia. These findings not only enlarge our understanding of genetic predispositions but also illuminate the complexities of the interaction between genetic and environmental factors in the manifestation of various health outcomes. Genetic predisposition has extended implications beyond mental illness, reaching into overall health and clinical outcomes in significant ways. For example, higher genetic predisposition scores for schizophrenia have been correlated with higher risks for other psychiatric comorbidities as well as other health burdens. As underscored in the research evidence by Zhang (2022), individuals with a history of schizophrenia in their family go through different somatic conditions, and also mental health challenges, that constitute a critical point where genetic factors can dictate life courses. This convergent information regarding genetic factors indicates the necessity for certain interventions that account for both environmental and genetic factors in developing effective models of mental health care and disease prevention (Figure 13.8).

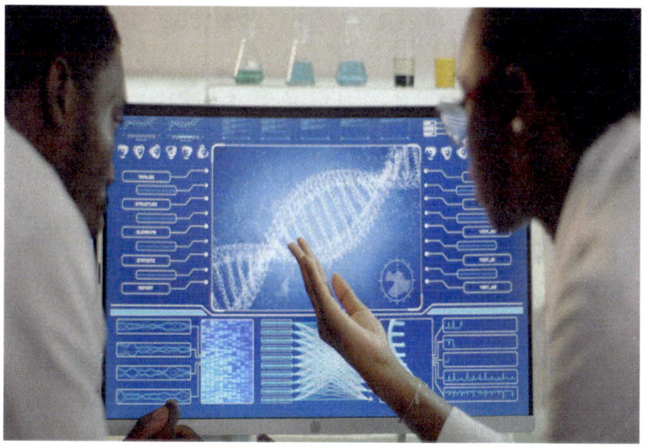

Figure 13.8. Understanding genetic predisposition.

Source: https://www.verywellhealth.com/thmb/FW2aC0KwK-L4xzBI0QxbInLm2bE=/1500x0/filters:no_upscale():max_bytes(150000):strip_icc()/VWH-GettyImages-1345098965-779be2ac96934cb998ab1ce83470318b.jpg.

13.2.2. Environmental Triggers

Environmental conditions play the most important role in initiating natural disasters, with landslides being one of their notable characteristics. They are often the result of a combination of conditions that constitute topography, ground material, and climate. Landslides, which refer to the movement of earth materials by gravity, can be as destructive as they have immense loss of human life and property. Early forecasting of the events is required in order to restrict damage. Current progress in predictive modeling, particularly with the use of convolutional neural networks, has been able to identify such environmental triggers. Through the advancement of models to support diversified spatial characteristics, researchers have developed frameworks that enhance predictability, hence improving the safety of exposed groups. This intersection of environmental science and technology highlights the importance of understanding environmental triggers within systems previously difficult to quantify, ultimately leading to innovations that can conserve resources and lives (Hajimoradlou et al., 2020). Further, the broader implications of environmental triggers must be considered beyond the immediacy of physical risk like landslides. These stimuli are not isolated; they are part of an overall ecosystem involving biological responses, urban growth, and public safety measures. The greater the extent to which the city intrudes into vulnerable areas, the greater the knowledge of ecological nuances becomes the standard. Ecological components typically interact in a way that resists simple description because complexity arises from interactions among flora, fauna, and human activity. For instance, deforestation can increase landslide susceptibility, and urban growth can alter drainage patterns. An inclusive methodology that recognizes these interactions can enhance our ability to create effective mitigation plans. This is also a pressing necessity given the increasing frequency of such climate change-related natural hazards, which accentuates the frequency of extreme weather phenomena and, by extension, the environmental stimuli occurring there (Jaffe et al., 1989). Critically, integrating holistic environmental data into software requirements is crucial to driving predictive models with an environmental trigger focus. A successful software system must portray an integrated sense of many different factors to guarantee that the software can take in and scrutinize real-time data for landslides and other environmental risks. Software that is strong, extensive, and sufficient to handle questions prompted by environmental variability must be created. Such systems must include a list of conditions, such as timing, safety, and strength, to provide credible predictive capacity. Through the development of robust methodologies for software requirement specifications, developers and researchers can be able to ascertain that predictive models not only work effectively but will also play an important role in achieving sustainable management of our environment and effective disaster preparation strategies (Jaffe et al., 1989; Hajimoradlou et al., 2020).

13.2.3. Immune System Dysregulation

Immune system dysregulation is a new area of study, particularly in light of its applicability to most autoimmune diseases and to chronic inflammatory conditions. If the immune system is unable to maintain the delicate balance between tolerance of self-antigen and recognition of non-self pathogen, it has the potential to cause hazardous hyper-inflammatory responses. For example, those with an intense inflammatory reaction may establish a deviation in systemic inflammatory mediators that can evolve to a hyper-inflammatory phenotype (HIP). This dysregulation could lead to more intense local inflammatory reactions, particularly at tissue niches that are susceptible to chronic infection or injury, making the treatment regimen for diseases associated with dysregulated immunity, , such as osteological lesions from infections by pathogens like *Porphyromonas gingivalis* or *Staphylococcus aureus* (Duncanson, 2019). Explaining these interactions is crucial in developing effective interventions for restorative immune balance. The impact of genetic predispositions on immune dysregulation has become more evident with the progress made in genomic research. Genome-wide association studies have revealed many of the genes involved in immune-mediated illnesses, and it has been observed that the majority of disease-causing variants are non-coding and tend to reside in enhancer regions. This finding underscores the importance of regulatory elements in the regulation of immune responses. To see how the common genetic differences influence enhancer function and subsequently immune dysregulation, researchers employ various statistical and experimental methods. Among these, some notable strategies are fine-mapping for the identification of causal variants and the application of massively parallel reporter assays to determine the modulation of gene expression (Lee et al., 2023). This genetic research not only sheds light on the mechanisms behind immune compromise but also offers windows into potential therapeutic interventions. In addition, the interplay between environmental exposures and gene susceptibilities in immune system dysregulation holds the key to unraveling the pathogenesis of chronic inflammatory diseases. Numerous studies have demonstrated that environmental factors, , such as infections, diet, and exposure to toxins, can initiate or exacerbate immune responses in genetically at-risk individuals. This complex interaction typically establishes a feedback loop whereby dysregulated immune activity serves further to enhance the sensitivity of an individual to environmental insult, leading to a cycle of inflammation and damage. As an illustration, the interaction between local tissue response and systemic inflammation demonstrates how environmental initiators can augment the action of predisposing genetic susceptibilities. The treatment of immune dysregulation thus necessitates a multi-dimensional approach that addresses both the environmental and genetic determinants in an attempt to optimize therapeutic interventions in these affected patients.

Test Your Knowledge

1. How can genetic predisposition contribute to the development of autoimmune diseases?
2. Name two environmental triggers that have been linked to autoimmune diseases and explain how they might contribute.
3. Describe one way in which immune system dysregulation can lead to autoimmunity.

13.3. Common Autoimmune Diseases

Learning Outcome

1. Describe rheumatoid arthritis
2. Understand systemic lupus erythematosus
3. Explain multiple sclerosis

Autoimmune illnesses, characterized by the immune system mounting an attack against the body's own cells in error, constitute a heterogeneous group of ailments that have the potential to significantly impact an individual's quality of life. Among the most prevalent autoimmune diseases are rheumatoid arthritis, lupus, multiple sclerosis, and type 1 diabetes. Each of these conditions is characterized by unique symptoms and complications, yet they share an identical underlying pathophysiology of immune dysregulation. For instance, rheumatoid arthritis initially involves the joints, leading to chronic inflammation and pain, while lupus can affect a number of organ systems, including skin, kidneys, and heart, and has a complex clinical presentation. Because these conditions are prevalent and long-lasting, they need to be understood and managed effectively, and autoimmune diseases thus represent an area of study of greatest significance in contemporary medicine. The impact of autoimmune diseases is not merely on the physical manifestations but also considerably on psychological well-being, as well as the overall well-being. The psychological burden of chronic disease puts patients in a position of increased susceptibility to depression and anxiety. Vitiligo, with its depigmentation effect on the skin, again goes to reflects the psychosocial discomfort of the patients. In fact, vitiligo patients have diminished quality of life and greater psychological distress, particularly those with darker skin tones who may be more conspicuous in its effects from the condition. The identification of a link between vitiligo and other autoimmune illnesses, as the relationship between this disease and autoimmune thyroid conditions shows, confirms that the disease is interlinked and requires comprehensive treatment that addresses both physical and psychological factors (Baldini et al., 2017). findings regarding the pathogenesis of autoimmune disorders have led to insights into potential therapeutic avenues and interventions. Genetic, environmental, and immunological factors have been identified by research to work together to cause these diseases and provide the groundwork for more effective therapy. For example, present research on the molecular mechanisms of autoimmune attacks has led to the introduction of novel biologic therapies designed against the immune system. The efficiency of these treatment methods could lead to improved treatment in patients with diseases , such as rheumatoid arthritis and systemic lupus erythematosus. Further, with continuous advances, particularly on the autoimmune aetiology of liver disease, the healthcare community must keep up with the integration of this research into practice to enhance patient outcomes and care (Alisi et al., 2015).

13.3.1. Rheumatoid Arthritis

Rheumatoid arthritis (RA) is not only a struggle for the diagnosed patient but also for the healthcare systems of the world. It is an inflammatory disease that predominantly affects joints, leading to pain, swelling, and ultimately joint destruction. The complexity of RA makes it the second most common cause of disability globally, hindering the functionality of patients to lead their day-to-day lives and participate in social activities. Interestingly, in Australia alone, there are about 3 million people who are affected, highlighting the far-reaching prevalence and persistent effects of this disease (Smedley et al., 2014). The impact of RA is not just physical limitations because it also leads to mental health concerns, such as depression and anxiety, making management strategies and interventions for individuals affected even more complex. It is vital to identify the patient preferences for rheumatoid arthritis treatment in order to maximize the outcomes of treatment. In a recent study, patients and rheumatologists have been shown to prefer different features influencing the selection of treatment, which they prioritize differently according to their perception. Patients tend to prefer the time required to achieve optimal quality of life and the route of administration of the therapies, which are critical factors in making their decisions (Comellas et al., 2020).

Furthermore, patients' desire to engage in shared decision-making highlights their desire to be autonomous and have a stake in healthcare decisions. The shift from paternalistic care models to collaborative models not only empowers patients but also is linked to increased compliance with treatment guidelines and thus improved health outcomes, which is evidence of the worth of , including patients' input in plans for management. Furthermore, with the implementation of the National Disability Insurance Scheme in Australia, an understanding of how RAs influence daily life becomes increasingly important. There is evidence that the management of the challenges of arthritis requires a multi-disciplinary approach to supporting services that addresses physical, psychological, and social components of care (Smedley et al., 2014). Proper service delivery should consider the life world of individuals struggling with RA, promoting not only medical treatments but also rehabilitative and psychological therapy related to their unique situations. To this end, increased awareness and knowledge regarding RA can encourage policymakers to create better frameworks that enable better patient outcomes and care services, ultimately improving the quality of life for millions afflicted by this debilitating condition (Figure 13.9).

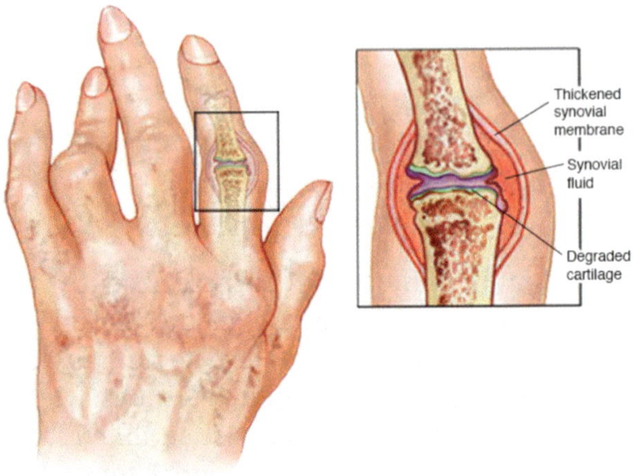

Figure 13.9. Rheumatoid arthritis.

Source: https://www.mayoclinic.org/-/media/kcms/gbs/patient-consumer/images/2013/08/26/10/47/ds00020_im02689_r7_rheumatoidarthritisthu_jpg.jpg.

13.3.2. Systemic Lupus Erythematosus

Systemic lupus erythematosus (SLE) is a systemic autoimmune disease where the body's immune system attacks its own tissues in error. It is a disease with a wide range of symptoms that can affect any or all organ systems, including the skin, joints, kidneys, and cardiovascular system. SLE's heterogeneity complicates diagnosis and treatment because symptoms are hugely variable between patients. Typical features include fatigue, arthralgias, and the classic butterfly rash across the cheeks and nose. SLE's complexity requires interdisciplinary treatment for managing both the systemic and organ-related aspects of the disease, not only testifying to its complexity but also to the ongoing need for research attempting to elucidate further its pathophysiology. Effective management of SLE, particularly lupus nephritis, a severe complication of kidney involvement, is reliant on adherence to treatment protocols formulated. Various international bodies have established comprehensive protocols for the diagnosis and treatment of lupus nephritis with a focus on systematic approaches of induction and maintenance therapy tailored to the different histological classes of renal involvement.

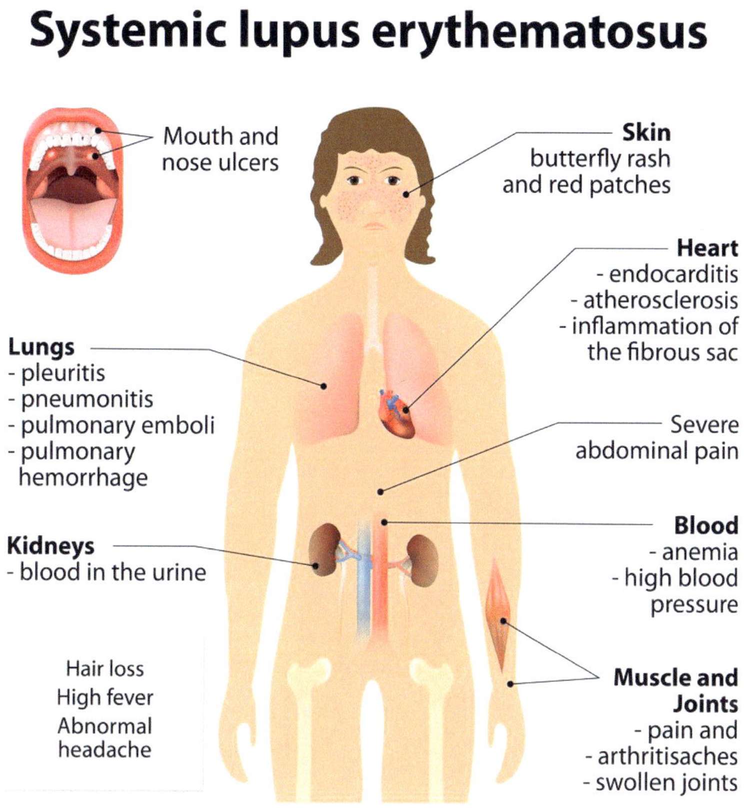

Figure 13.10. Systemic lupus erythematosus (SLE).

Source: https://s16736.pcdn.co/wp-content/uploads/sites/207/2016/12/shutterstock_302168915.jpg.optimal.jpg.

These recommendations also encompass vital considerations like patient observation, treatment response, and the requirement for repeat renal biopsies in case. A review indicates that guidelines encompass data from several randomized trials, referring to the dynamic course of lupus treatment and requirement for a holistic approach catering to the specific patient circumstances, , such as pregnancy-related complications and pediatric issues (Bajema et al., 2015). These recent developments in SLE treatment, , such as the launch of belimumab, are a paradigm in the therapeutic landscape of SLE. Belimumab, a monoclonal anti-BLyS antibody, has been shown to improve patient outcomes, particularly in individuals with specific serological patterns, e.g., antinuclear and anti-double-stranded DNA antibody-positive patients. Meta-analyses of randomized trials show that belimumab significantly enhances the SLE Responder Index at week 52, suggesting its promise in minimizing disease symptoms and improving patient quality of life (Clarke et al.,

2013). Notwithstanding, there may be differences in response based on variations in patient demographics, including ethnicity and geography, emphasizing the importance of personalized therapeutic approaches. While investigations continue, the study of new treatments in combination with existing guidelines is a prospective avenue for enhancing patient treatment in systemic lupus erythematosus (Figure 13.10).

13.3.3. Multiple Sclerosis

Multiple sclerosis (MS) is a complex neurological disease , including the abnormal attack of the immune systems on the central nervous system. This autoimmune disorder leads to demyelination of the nerve fibers, and therefore, a wide range of clinical manifestations which can differ greatly between individuals. Common symptoms include fatigue, visual defects, and loss of motor functions. The randomness of the condition makes it extremely challenging for both the patients and the clinicians.

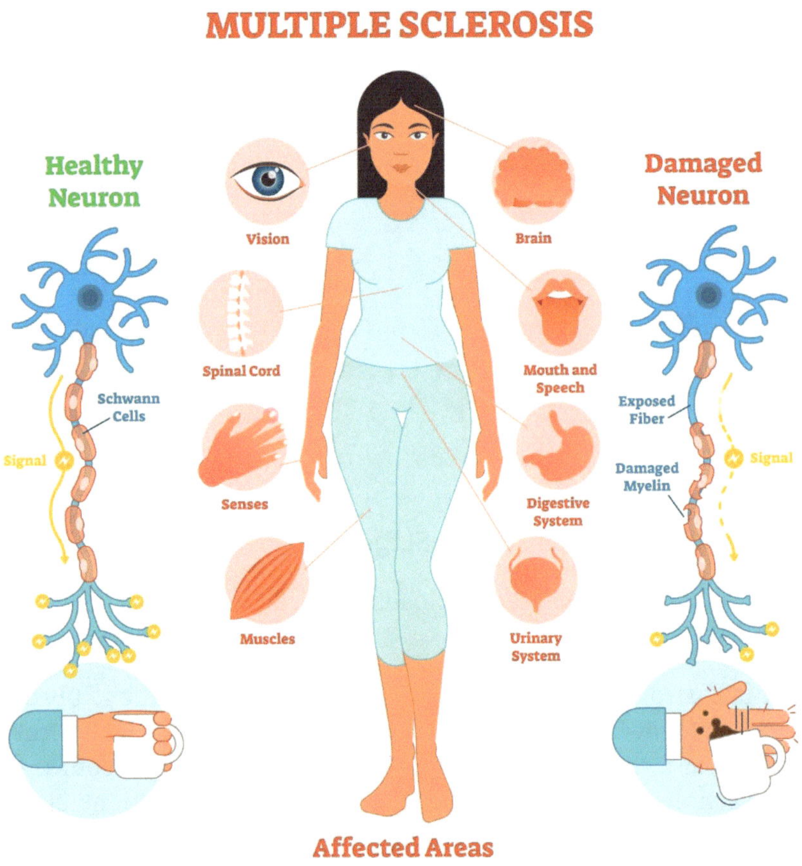

Figure 13.11. Multiple sclerosis infographic.

Source: https://shelteringarmsinstitute.com/wp-content/uploads/2023/12/Multiple-Sclerosis-Infographic.jpg.

With increasing research, unraveling the mechanisms of MS has become imperative in order to plan effective therapies. Refining immunology and neurobiology has also shed light on the significance of early intervention, which can possibly modify the disease's course as well as the severity of symptoms. The therapeutic scenario of MS has seen a significant change over the past decade, with new therapies on the horizon that take into account the multifaceted clinical features of the disease. Of these, ocrelizumab has been of particular interest because of its success in the treatment of both relapsing and primary progressive MS. In clinical trials, it has proven to significantly reduce annualized relapse rates and disability accumulation and record encouraging patient outcomes. However, integration into real-world clinical practice remains necessary to determine the long-term benefits. Initial results indicate that the effectiveness of ocrelizumab across different patient populations mirrors results from seminal clinical trials, demonstrating its potential as a go-to treatment for patients with MS (Matthews et al., 2023). Despite the rise in treatment options, multiple sclerosis remains a complicated condition needing an individualized treatment regimen. Progressive and severe patients typically experience few treatment options, which aggravate their symptoms and compromise their quality of life. New treatment paradigms, including new disease-modifying therapies and symptomatic treatments, are key in addressing the complexities of MS. Multidisciplinary care models comprising neurologists, physiotherapists, and mental health professionals are also vital in the delivery of multidisciplinary care. The patient education and engagement in the process of care decision-making cannot be overstated because it calls for patients to actively participate in self-care management. An enthusiastic approach towards MS care, whether pharmacological or non-pharmacological, is the way forward towards achieving the best possible health outcomes in patients (Shah et al., 2020) (Figure 13.11).

Test Your Knowledge

1. What is the primary immune target in Rheumatoid Arthritis, and what joints are most commonly affected?
2. Which autoantibodies are commonly associated with Systemic Lupus Erythematosus (SLE)?
3. What neurological structure is primarily affected in Multiple Sclerosis (MS), and what is the consequence?

13.4. Diagnosis of Hypersensitivity and Autoimmunity

Learning Outcome

1. Discuss about clinical evaluation and history for diagnosis of hypersensitivity and autoimmunity
2. Understand laboratory tests and biomarkers
3. Describe imaging studies and their relevance

Diagnosis of hypersensitivity and autoimmunity is a multifaceted process that involves clinical assessment, laboratory testing, and immunologic testing. Doctors normally begin with a thorough patient history and physical examination to identify evidence of hypersensitivity or autoimmune illness, , such as allergic response or systemic symptoms. Following clinical assessment, official tests like skin prick test or serological tests are employed to assess specific immune reactions. A knowledge of the aetiopathogenesis of these diseases is necessary, as both hypersensitivity diseases and autoimmunity are brought about by an immunologically malfunctioning system. In addition, diagnostic markers have a significant role to play in making presumptions, particularly in long-standing cases where there might be overlapping presentations that give rise to other illnesses. By taking into account clinical observations together with laboratory findings, clinicians can arrive at a more accurate diagnosis, which can lead to effective treatment regimes. In one specific situation, illnesses like Vernal Keratoconjunctivitis (VKC) are one instance of the diagnostic challenge presented by hypersensitivity. VKC occurs with ocular surface inflammatory responses and symptoms that can easily be misinterpreted as other allergic or autoimmune illnesses. Research lays greater emphasis on the assessment of biomarkers , such as vascular endothelial growth factor (VEGF) in both tear and blood liquids to assess the disease's severity as well as its pathophysiology. In patients presenting with an acute attack, elevated levels of VEGF in the tears would suggest enhanced inflammatory activity, and hence, this marker would be a valuable diagnostic test and monitoring tool for VKC. As more research continues to define the role of such biomarkers, they can enhance diagnostic accuracy and lead towards personalized therapeutic approaches for patients who are affected by hypersensitivity disorders like VKC (Aventaggiato et al., 2018). Besides, hypergammaglobulinemia is another dominant factor that one must consider while diagnosing autoimmune diseases in children. Analysis of clinical records shows a strong correlation between elevated immunoglobulins and the prevalence of autoimmune diseases. The finding of hypergammaglobulinemia can be the first indication of underlying immunological dysregulation, at times preceding the clinical presentation of systemic lupus erythematosus and other autoimmune disorders of the gastrointestinal tract. Notably, the diagnostic algorithm designed to assess the likelihood of autoimmunity based on the levels of immunoglobulin and ancillary laboratory findings serves to underscore the value of a multimodal diagnostic approach. Quantitative assessments of blood components, including indicators like C-reactive protein (CRP) and white blood cell count, help practitioners differentiate between autoimmune and non-autoimmune diseases efficiently. The method enhances the predictability of probable autoimmune emergence, hence promoting early intervention and improved patient outcomes (Lo et al., 2014).

13.4.1. Clinical Evaluation and History

Patient history and clinical evaluation are the foundations of diagnostic and treatment processes in healthcare. When patients visit practitioners, thorough evaluations are underway in stages, beginning with an overall patient history that involves medical, social, and psychological aspects. The detailed story allows healthcare professionals to identify pertinent health trends and issues, which ultimately guide the decision-making process. Above all, in vulnerable populations, such as adolescent refugees, subtle judgments become the focal point. For instance, one research on Syrian adolescent refugees demonstrated how the differential experiences of war and resettlement influence their constructions of harm and moral judgments, revealing complex interplays between cultural contexts and personal accounts (Teja, 2019). These reflections point out that clinical evaluation is more than a technical process; it must also be culturally responsive and sensitive to individual life context. Beyond history taking, the clinical evaluation usually includes physical examination and systemic inquiry that provides valuable information about a patient's health status. The evaluations must integrate the symptom patterns presented by the patient with the results of clinical objective measures to produce a comprehensive picture of their condition. For example, working with adolescent refugees, clinicians would have too many psychological and emotional problems to be assessed and interpreted. In one study, Syrian refugee younger adolescents based their decisions about harm on authority and societal standards, compared to older adolescents who had more mixed reasoning (Teja, 2019). This difference requires specific assessment methods that allow for differences in development and context while ensuring clinical evaluations reflect the entire range of a patient's health profile. Lastly, although clinical evaluation is necessary, it is also necessary to engage in them with an empathic and understanding eye. A close analysis of the refugee and other marginalized groups' experiences betrays the necessity for health professionals to be aware of the broader socio-political forces that shape individual health. Cultural competency in care requires that practitioners attend critically to patients' narratives in order to inform treatment approaches that are sensitive to their unique contexts. The study of Syrian adolescent refugee patients reveals that harm responses are not merely individual but are embedded within social and environmental contexts that shape judgments and actions (Teja, 2019). Bringing this information to bear in clinical practice enables practitioners to optimize effectiveness in assessment, ultimately producing improved health outcomes and patient-practitioner trust.

13.4.2. Laboratory Tests and Biomarkers

Laboratory tests and biomarkers are key components in the modern healthcare system, providing valuable information regarding patient status and disease progression. Laboratory tests are designed to measure biological markers that represent physiological or pathological alterations. A proper understanding of laboratory tests helps medical practitioners diagnose, predict disease progression, and treat accordingly based on the same.

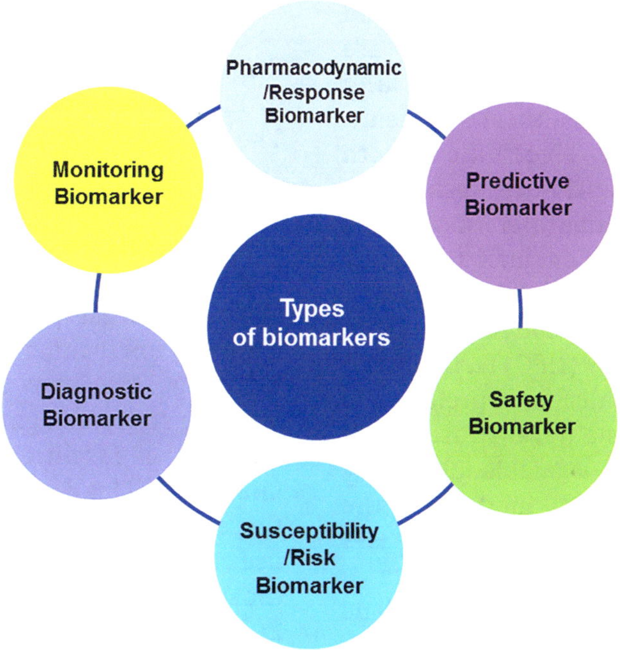

Figure 13.12. Types of biomarker.

Source: https://www.frontiersin.org/files/Articles/527209/fpsyt-11-00432-HTML/image_m/fpsyt-11-00432-g001.jpg.

For diseases , such as COVID-19, the role of some biomarkers came to the forefront. For example, a study showed that laboratory values , including the neutrophil-lymphocyte ratio and C-reactive protein, have significant correlations with patient outcomes and are therefore important in adding to medical decision-making processes (Antón et al., 2022). While valuable, the prognostic value of routine laboratory tests can sometimes be overshadowed by redundancy, as demonstrated in COVID-19 studies. There is evidence that while testing in the lab is helpful, information available through it can be restricted due to redundancy. Specifically, it was demonstrated that the majority of laboratory tests merely revealed inflammatory or organ damage processes rather than appropriately assessing immune responses ; a critical indicator of patient outcome (Antón et al., 2022). This limitation underlines the necessity of employing a comprehensive method that uses traditional laboratory tests and novel immunological biomarkers to enhance predictive value and clinical utility. Technology developments are also revolutionizing laboratory tests and biomarker utilization in healthcare systems. The standardization of electronic health records (EHR) with nomenclature, such as the Laboratory Observation Identifier Names and Codes (LOINC), allows for enhanced tracking and analysis of laboratory results. Furthermore, techniques to map LOINC-coded values to Human Phenotype Ontology (HPO) terms offer a means to interpret the clinical interpretation of laboratory results. This is a novel strategy that allows clinicians to utilize available laboratory tests in deep phenotyping, increasing the detection of biomarkers for particular diseases like asthma. As the technology continues to advance, the challenge in the future will be to adopt these advancements in technologies to enhance diagnostic precision and tailored treatment plans (Figure 13.12).

13.4.3. Imaging Studies and Their Relevance

Imaging methods have become indispensable throughout numerous industries, but particularly within medicine and education. Their significance cannot be emphasized enough, as they allow for a sophisticated comprehension of complex structures and functions that cannot easily be directly observed through conventional means. In medicine, MRI and PET scan imaging technologies provide us with details regarding the structural and functional brain abnormalities, hence improving the accuracy of diagnosis and treatment outcomes. Practitioners can detect conditions at earlier stages by the systematic application of these studies with enhanced capacity to customize patient care. This groundbreaking capability overflows into the educational environment as imaging technologies enable teachers and researchers to monitor cognitive processes in learning. As imaging studies are evolving through adoption, they increasingly serve as central tools for diagnostics and pedagogic development, leading to more sophisticated results in both sectors. The impact of artificial intelligence (AI) has significantly enhanced the usability of imaging studies and the environments where they are applied across sectors. As found through recent research, AI technologies have revolutionized the learning process, particularly within vocational training environments, by offering tailored teaching strategies that support individual learning styles. Imaging tests, when augmented with AI capabilities, provide personalized analysis of learner behavior and progress, thereby informing pedagogical planning. The use of systematic literature reviews, particularly those that view developments from 2018 to 2023, reveals how AI can enhance the efficacy of imaging studies in education by promoting student engagement as well as the overall learning process. The innovative potential of AI combined with imaging studies is a paradigm shift towards efficient educational strategies, drawing attention to the significance of adaptive approaches in contemporary models of learning. In addition to educational progress, imaging studies have an important function to fulfill in pharmacological research, particularly in assessing the effect of new therapeutics on the CNS. Guidelines drawn by many organizations, such as the International Pharmaco-EEG Society stress the implementation of standardized protocols to achieve good data collection and analysis. The use of advanced imaging techniques aids in understanding the pharmacokinetic and pharmacodynamic action of drugs, thus overcoming the imperfections caused by inconsistent methodologies in research. Standardization not only enables more credible comparisons but also enables the pooling of data necessary to validate new biomarkers and analytical algorithms. As the field matures, imaging research will be a necessity in advancing drug development innovation and enhancing therapeutic intervention safety and efficacy (Babiloni et al., 2012; Rosyadi et al., 2023).

Test Your Knowledge

1. What key elements in a patient's clinical history can help differentiate between immediate (Type I) and delayed (Type IV) hypersensitivity reactions?
2. What imaging modalities are most useful in assessing organ damage in autoimmune diseases?

13.5. Treatment Options for Hypersensitivity

Learning Outcome

1. Explain the role of antihistamines and corticosteroids in the management of allergic reactions and inflammatory disorders
2. Describe immunotherapy approaches
3. Focus on lifestyle modifications and avoidance strategies

The control of hypersensitivity involves a multifaceted treatment plan, with the initial intervention being the determination and avoidance of triggering stimuli. Most patients experience hypersensitivity reactions that are potent in their effect, so the determination of the causing stimuli is paramount to avoiding detrimental effects. Sensitizers are hugely varied, from food, pollen, and insect stings to medications and toxins. By employing diagnostic methods , such as skin prick tests and specific IgE, clinicians are able to determine the offending allergens. Following identification, effective avoidance measures are the cornerstone of treatment, whereby individuals change their lifestyle or environment to prevent exposure. Not only does this specific reduction in allergen exposure reduce the frequency and severity of hypersensitivity reactions, but it also enhances the overall patient quality of life and offers a firm foundation for future therapeutic interventions, where necessary. When avoidance measures prove insufficient to adequately manage hypersensitivity, pharmacological intervention becomes the mainstay. Antihistamines, corticosteroids, and leukotriene receptor antagonists are the typical medicines that are prescribed to counteract signs of allergic reactions. Antihistamines inhibit histamine receptors, thus preventing itching, sneezing, and hives. Corticosteroids are utilized to reduce inflammation and modulate immune response, aiding in more extreme cases. As hypersensitivity can occur in varying ways in various individuals, personalized treatments are necessary. Along with pharmacotherapy, patients may also be treated with immunotherapy, which is a process of building tolerance by slow exposure to allergens. The treatment works most effectively in allergic rhinitis and food allergy. This combination of drug and immunological therapy is a complete management approach, enabling the patient to cope more effectively with their hypersensitivity. In some instances, specific types of treatment must be administered for more advanced hypersensitivity diseases, , such as hypereosinophilic syndrome (HES) and diffuse parenchymal lung diseases (DPLD). HES involves an elevated eosinophil count resulting in multisystem pathology and necessitates individual treatment plans, which are typically corticosteroids and other immunomodulatory treatments (Brys et al., 2015). Similar to children with DPLD, there is a need for a tailored treatment program due to the heterogeneity of the condition that may involve genetic components and presentations. Systematic approaches in the form of advanced classification systems and centralized data gathering offer insights for particular therapeutic recommendations based on the individual patient profile (Clement et al., 2009). These sophisticated approaches are the reflection of the need for an interdisciplinary and personalized management strategy to hypersensitivity diseases to provide improved prognosis and functional results in the involved patients.

13.5.1. Antihistamines and Corticosteroids

Antihistamines and corticosteroids are significant pharmacological agents in the management of allergy and inflammatory disorders. Antihistamines are merely drugs that inhibit the effect of histamine, an allergic chemical released during an allergic response, and thus free the subject from itching, swelling, and inflammation.

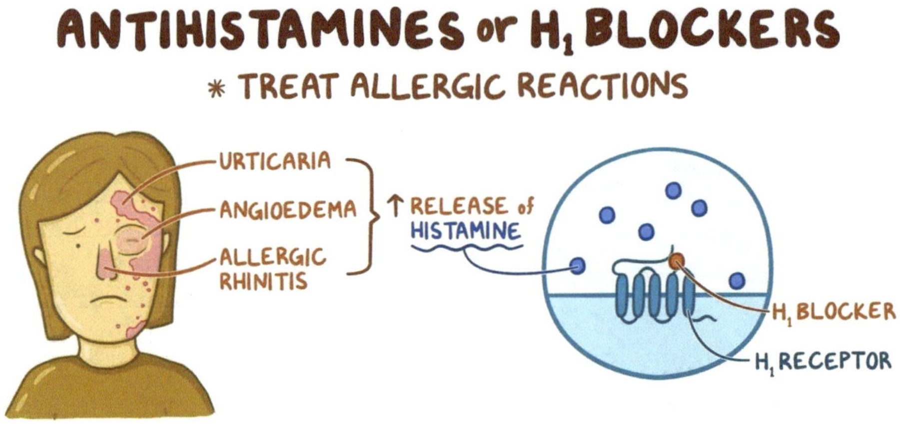

Figure 13.13. Antihistamines.

Source: https://d16qt3wv6xm098.cloudfront.net/QtD33TiHTI2K8hLzhLCY_ExlSC6qXGF0/_.jpg.

They are often prescribed to manage allergic rhinitis and urticaria. The second category, corticosteroids, has a generalized role of modulating the immune response and also inhibiting inflammation. They are of value in the treatment of more serious allergic reactions and long-term inflammatory disease , such as asthma, where rapid control of inflammation is crucial. Combined, these medications have a profound effect on patient care by improving symptoms and blocking the progression of allergic reactions. Although useful, antihistamines and corticosteroids are not without risk with their administration, particularly when administered concomitantly. Their interaction can augment their effect, and therefore physicians can consider in terms of dose adjustments based on patient profiles. For example, patients on venom immunotherapy (VIT) must be shielded with prophylactic medication with antihistamines and corticosteroids, as it has been reported in a study evaluating various factors in successful VIT. Even though the study had reported that high baseline serum tryptase level was not strongly correlated with treatment failure, anti-allergic medications were protective in this context (Aberer et al., 2013). Thus, it is imperative to learn about the interaction and timing of these drugs to maximize therapeutic interventions in allergic disorders. Besides, the therapeutic benefit of antihistamines and corticosteroids varies greatly in different patient populations and allergic conditions (Figure 13.13). Other studies indicate that age, gender, and allergy type can influence treatment efficacy, making certain strategies necessary to select medications. Clinically, data on symptom severity and patient history need to guide the inclusion of these medications. For instance, patients with a history of known honey bee venom allergy may require more aggressive management strategies, , such as using antihistamines in addition to corticosteroids during desensitization (Bosnic-Anticevich et al., 2017). By these considerations, the health providers can ensure maximum safety and effectiveness of the treatment such that the patients not only achieve immediate relief but also receive optimal long-term care of allergic diseases (Figure 13.14).

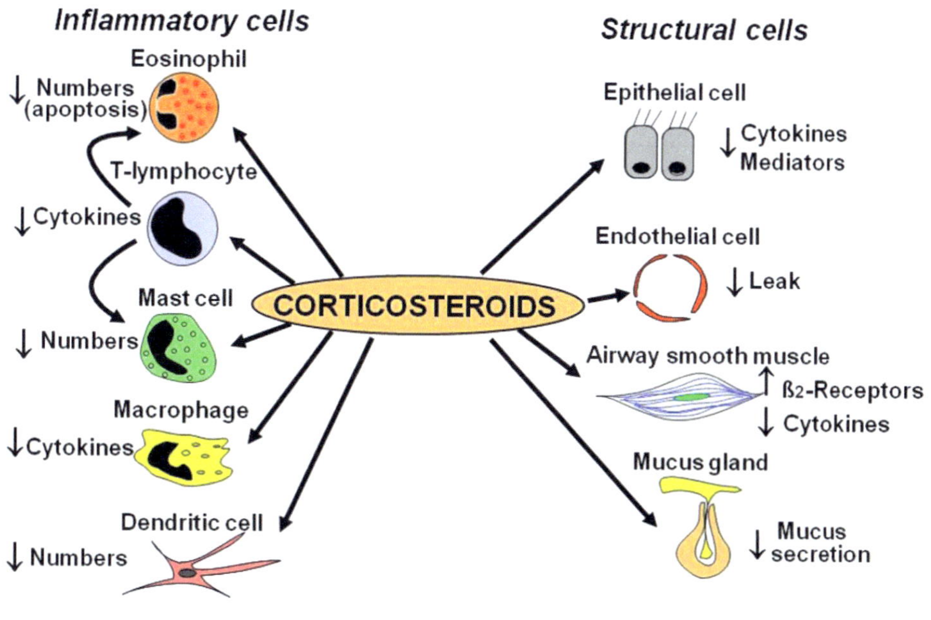

Figure 13.14. Corticosteroids.

Source: https://pub.mdpi-res.com/pharmaceuticals/pharmaceuticals-03-00514/article_deploy/html/images/pharmaceuticals-03-00514-g001.png?1401953885.

13.5.2. Immunotherapy Approaches

Immunotherapy approaches are a paradigm-shifting aspect of the treatment for a lot of cancers, employing the body's own immune mechanism as a weapon against cancers. Outstanding among these are the immune checkpoint inhibitors that block inhibitory molecules , such as PD-1 to reactivate exhausted T cells. This reactivation of immune function has led to significant clinical responses, particularly in solid tumors and hematological malignancies. However, the field is now exploring new areas beyond T cells, looking to reinvigorate other forms of immune cells. The greater focus is critical as researchers explore the less-understood field of natural killer (NK) cell exhaustion, which may be key in developing effective cancer therapies. Recognizing the personalized aspects of NK cell dysfunction can reveal new horizons for improving patient survival with increasingly innovative immunotherapy approaches as the discipline adeptly evolves to support a range of tumor niches (Canter et al., 2020). The big data and AI era has also revolutionized the discipline of immunotherapy science, with researchers now being able to study complex immunological interactions at a scale never thought possible. With the advancement of omics technologies, researchers can combine and interpret large data sets that shed light on the sophisticated dynamics of the immune system. Such analytical capability makes it possible to identify new targets for therapy and can guide individualized treatment regimens according to patient profiles. Through new hypothesis generation and new mechanisms of modulating immunity, AI plays a key role in addressing traditionally challenging fields, such as autoimmune disorders and cancer. But ethical considerations for the application of AI in immunotherapy must be considered, reflecting the need for regulation to manage these technological advancements in clinical applications (Desjardins et al., 2024). As immunotherapy continues to pick up steam, the merger of various techniques will likely offer more effective treatments. Combining checkpoint inhibitors with other treatments, such as cytokines or cancer vaccines, can optimize the overall efficacy of immunotherapeutic interventions. Identification of the distinctive mechanisms of immune cell exhaustion—namely, in T cells and NK cells—can direct adaptive strategies targeting these critical components of immune response. Blocking the pathways to T cell dysfunction, for instance, could refunction exhausted cells, yielding improved antitumor responses. With further research, the promise of combinatorial therapies or creating personalized immunotherapy regimens holds a promising future for oncology, paving the way for a new era in cancer treatment where immune modulation holds the secret to longer survival and better quality of life for the patient (Canter et al., 2020) (Figure 13.15).

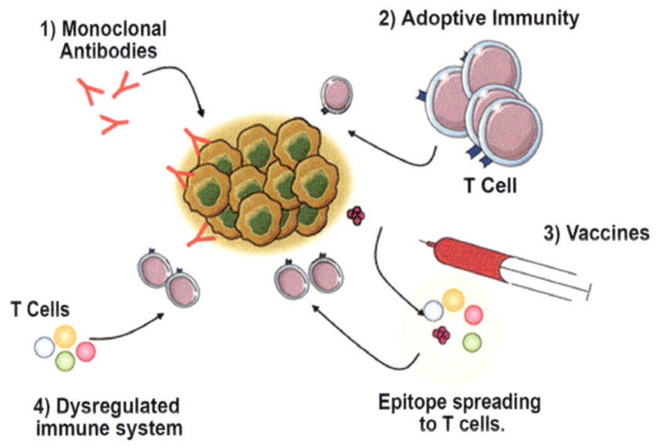

Figure 13.15. Forms of immunotherapy.

Source: https://onlinelibrary.wiley.com/cms/asset/ed2dd94f-6b4e-4bc6-97b0-0ed99b4ecc65/jo4508794-fig-0001-m.png.

13.5.3. Lifestyle Modifications and Avoidance Strategies

The past decades have seen lifestyle modification as a central theme in the management of chronic disease, including hypertension. Lifestyle modification has been touted as an initial line of action to disease management as it can profoundly influence patient outcomes. Some of the interventions that have been highlighted as part of the essential components of hypertension management include dietary modification, exercise adaptation, smoking cessation, and stress control. Interestingly, a systematic review has found that a high proportion of clinical trials for the treatment of hypertension will consistently ignore widespread use of lifestyle change, as 54% of studies did not refer to these changes whatsoever. This omission suggests significant questions regarding the effectiveness of existing therapeutic interventions and highlights the necessity for a greater focus on lifestyle change as a core preventative strategy in the treatment of hypertension (Brendin P Schievink et al., 2014). By prioritizing changes in lifestyle, health practitioners can better replicate evidence-based practice guidelines to provide more holistic care to patients. The situations of food allergies and intolerances also emphasize the advantage of lifestyle modifications and avoidance strategies. With increasing rates of these disorders in the United States, people will adopt restrictive diets as a way of avoiding such reactions. Although avoidance techniques may be lifesaving in the short term, they have the unintended consequence of causing disordered eating habits, especially in susceptible groups like college students. Studies have shown a positive correlation between the removal of some foods from the diet based on allergy and the development of poor eating habits. This connection means that the avoidance mechanisms ought to be managed cautiously and guided by wise nutritional advice since they affect not only physical health but also mental well-being (Scholma et al., 2025). It is thus critical to raise awareness of such risks while promoting balanced food consumption to guarantee general health. Last but not least, the convergence of lifestyle modifications and avoidance strategies gives rise to an intersection of behavior, health status, and quality of life. Effective lifestyle modifications demand an integrated solution that not just addresses physiological requirements but psychological and social needs as well. Tailored interventions combining behavior modification techniques with in-depth education on health habits can significantly empower individuals to manage their health actively. Moreover, the coordination of healthcare facilities and community support systems can prepare individuals to overcome the challenges posed by their health situations successfully. This wider perspective insists that lifestyle changes are not reductionally viewed as reactionary interventions but instead, at best, as preventative interventions used as part of holistic health management, which underlines the importance of continuous research and debate among the health community.

Test Your Knowledge

1. How do antihistamines and corticosteroids differ in their mechanism of action when treating hypersensitivity reactions?
2. What are the main types of immunotherapy used in managing hypersensitivity, and how effective are they in long-term symptom control?
3. In what scenarios are corticosteroids preferred over antihistamines for managing allergic reactions?

13.6. Treatment Options for Autoimmunity

Learning Outcome

1. Understand disease-modifying antirheumatic drugs (DMARDs)
2. Describe biologic therapies
3. Focus on supportive care and symptom management

The treatment setting for autoimmune disorders is a combination of modalities aimed at reversing the abnormal immune response characteristic of these conditions. Pharmacological treatments are usually first in line, and they include the use of corticosteroids, immunosuppressants, and biologic agents. Corticosteroids are commonly used due to their acute anti-inflammatory effect, which provides symptom relief along with the potential for halting disease activity. However, chronic use of corticosteroids has serious side effects, so there is a need for a fine balance between symptom control therapy and patient safety. Ultimately, treatment strategies must be individualized in consultation with medical professionals to suit the specific condition and therapy response of the patient, which can differ quite markedly from one patient with autoimmune disease to another. Additional treatment approaches for autoimmune diseases can involve lifestyle interventions and alternative modalities for overall health and disease management. Modifications in dietary habits, exercise practices, and stress management techniques can have significant functions in improving the quality of life of patients and effectively preventing flares of disease. For others, complementary therapy , such as acupuncture or supplements may even induce relief from symptoms, but these are to be utilized cautiously in view of variations in efficacy as well as the lack of regulation in the alternative medicine field. Given that treatment modalities are not standard, a multidisciplinary approach is ideal for customized management strategies for the heterogeneous expressions of autoimmune diseases. Also, new research developments highlight the importance of personalized medicine to optimize treatment modalities in autoimmune disease. With increasing knowledge on disease mechanisms, new biomarkers and targeted therapies are being discovered, which hold the promise to revolutionize traditional treatment paradigms. For instance, there is evidence that certain proteins within the immune pathways can be effective therapeutic targets, as seen in the case of research on conditions like IgA nephropathy. By combining omics information and clinical observations, it is possible to create not just effective but also personalized therapies based on the unique molecular profiles of a specific patient. These developments bring to light the necessity of ongoing research and evidence-based interventions in the dynamically changing field of efficient treatment modalities for the management of autoimmune diseases for improved patient outcomes and quality of life (Cisek et al., 2017).

13.6.1. Disease-Modifying Antirheumatic Drugs (DMARDs)

Disease-modifying antirheumatic drugs (DMARDs) also play a critical role in the management of rheumatoid arthritis (RA), a polyarticular autoimmune disorder characterized by chronic synovial inflammation and subsequent cartilage destruction. Treatment with DMARDs early on is necessary, as studies have indicated that early treatment is linked with favorable long-term outcomes, particularly in patients who have high-risk features of heightened disease activity and the presence of autoantibodies. DMARDs modulate the inflammatory mechanisms causing joint damage, to achieve remission or low disease activity. Efficacy of the treatment strategy depends on proper application of a treatment-to-target strategy, which requires regular surveillance of disease activity using composite indices to guide therapeutic alterations (Aletaha et al., 2016). Beyond their disease-modifying effects on joint integrity, rheumatoid arthritis and associated comorbidities represent a broader public health concern. DMARDs, both traditional synthetic and newer biological agents, are formulated to change the course of disease by targeting the fundamental biological pathways of the inflammatory process. Recent advances have yielded a diverse array of DMARDs with varying degrees of efficacy and safety profiles. Whereas conventional DMARDs like methotrexate have been cornerstones of the therapeutic drug armamentarium, the development of biologic agents has revolutionized managing practices. The biologics tend to act against platelets, interleukins, or other inflammatory mediators, thereby offering targeted strategies for potentially better mitigating damaging disease impacts (Chaplain et al., 2019). The ongoing evolution of DMARD therapy also mirrors the necessity of rigorous clinical appraisal and regulation. Today's research is not only exploring the pharmacokinetics and pharmacodynamics of these medications but also their cost-effectiveness in the treatment of RA. With new treatment strategies developing constantly, practicing clinicians must be vigilant in modifying therapeutic paradigms based on emerging clinical findings and patient response. Lastly, the goal of DMARD therapy is relief of symptoms as well as achieving a sustainable remission that maximizes quality of life while minimizing the long-term impact of the disease. Bridging treatment gaps, including looking for new therapeutic agents that meet the unmet needs of patients, continues to be an urgent priority for researchers and doctors (Aletaha et al., 2016) (Figure 13.16).

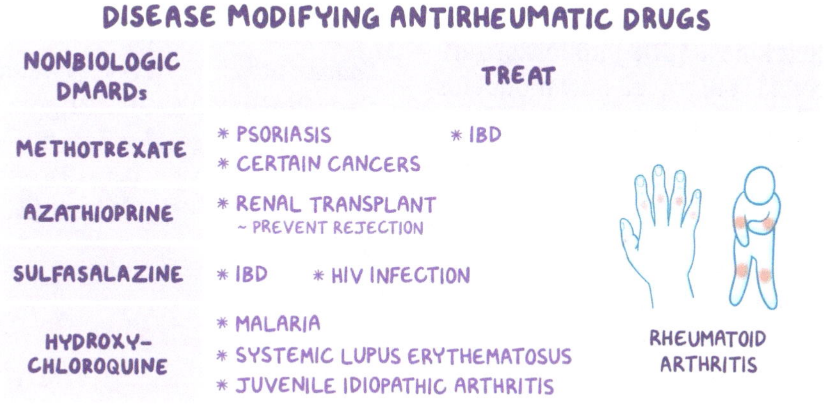

Figure 13.16. Disease-modifying antirheumatic drugs (DMARDs).

Source: https://www.osmosis.org/_next/image?url=https%3A%2F%2Fd16qt3wv6xm098.cloudfront.net%2FobpdEsfvQ0iWgxDYlQHSVdSsRb6r3z65%2F_.jpg&w=3840&q=75.

13.6.2. Biologic Therapies

Biologic therapies represent a revolutionary disease treatment approach, particularly cancers and autoimmune diseases. Biologic therapies employ advanced biological molecules, primarily proteins, to bind to the intended entities in the body and hence offer a more precise and potent drug mechanism. Biologics are typically composed of monoclonal antibodies, recombinant proteins, and vaccines, which are formed to stimulate or inhibit inflammatory mechanisms resulting in disease progression. As cancer therapies evolve, for example, biologic therapies come to be viewed more and more as having the capacity to directly modulate tumor behavior, possibly to the advantage of the patient. Cellular complexity dictates an advanced understanding of the biological underpinnings of these therapies, which emphasizes their reliance upon discrete molecular mechanisms within tumor microenvironments and immune networks. Investigation of the role played by cyclins in biologic therapy yields useful information on oncogenesis and cell proliferation regulation. Cyclins, which are central proteins in regulating the cell cycle, are overexpressed in cancer cells and lead to uncontrolled proliferation and tumor development. Cyclins D1 and E have also been found to play a role in cancer, with several research studies suggesting that cell cycling processes can be normalized by inhibiting their activity for enhanced treatment responses. Furthermore, biologic maneuvers in these pathways, in association with strategies , such as cyclin-dependent kinase (CDK) inhibition, are also being explored to construct a new model for treating cancer. The modular analysis of signaling networks, proposed in recent theoretical frameworks, also contributes to understanding how biologic therapy can effectively counteract the dysregulation of cell cycle kinetics of cancers, opening the doors to novel clinical trials that seek to restore cell cycling inhibition in metastatic cells (Baianu, 2011). In addition, the interface between biologic therapies and neurobiology highlights the promise of novel treatment modalities for both oncology and neurodevelopmental disorders. The latest studies highlight the significance of the role of cyclins in neural cell proliferation and differentiation, especially during early development of the organism. Defective differentiation associated with cyclin signaling can lead to abnormal neural cell growth, and such has implications for Alzheimers' disease. By targeting these pathways using biologic therapies, researchers hope to make inroads into the mechanistic underpinnings of cognitive impairments associated with neural development. Application of intricate systems biology modeling in these cases not only enhances our knowledge of the roles of cyclins in cancer and neurodevelopment but also encourages research into individualized therapeutic regimens that could possibly optimize outcomes with a broad range of patient populations (Baianu et al., 2004) (Figure 13.17).

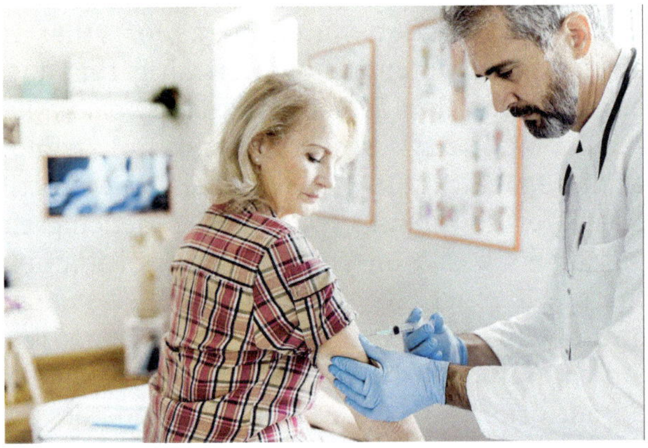

Figure 13.17. Biologic therapies.

Source: https://www.verywellhealth.com/thmb/CXdgGBGBzlFkX4GvntRKgpm9NmE=/1500x0/filters:no_upscale():max_bytes(150000):strip_icc()/making-sure-she-stays-healthy-1280865275-3e79f10ccf2042f3bef7cdb640a52861.jpg.

13.6.3. Supportive Care and Symptom Management

Supportive care and symptom control are important components of palliative care, particularly for individuals with life-shortening illnesses. This is an acknowledgment that the most important features of disease are not merely concerned with the physical symptoms but also the emotional, spiritual, and social challenges faced by the patient and their families. Effective symptom control requires a complete assessment to tailor interventions that can alleviate distressing symptoms , such as pain, nausea, and fatigue. The growing emphasis on this complex strategy points to the importance of healthcare providers having conversations with patients and families regarding their desires and values to ensure that care received is consistent with their desired outcomes and values. With regard to this, research has established that the experience of relatives, especially with regard to decreased use of a dying relative, is vital to enhance patient care and support systems (Pettifer et al., 2019). Additionally, supportive care complexities extend beyond the clinical environment to encompass psychological and emotional support for patients as well as relatives. Family caregivers feel anxious and stressed out as they witness their loved ones worsening, particularly in terms of decreased fluid intake in the dying period. The problem can be a significant psychological burden, leading to conflict and miscommunication between family members and health workers. Studies point out that open communication measures and empathetic care can ease some tension emanating from such an experience. Enhancing the awareness of healthcare professionals to the emotional framework that accompanies such situations may benefit family members in the role of carers, thereby facilitating a more empathetic and cooperative culture of care (Pettifer et al., 2021). Finally, the research determines areas of most important professional support that can be utilized in order to boost the experience for families suffering from the loss of their loved ones. The identification of effective strategies for carrying out discussions about hydration and nutrition, especially in hospital settings, is important for enhancing the quality of end-of-life care. Framing the experiences of families within a pragmatic outlook assists healthcare providers in developing complex protocols that address the family members' unique needs and concerns. This realization paves the path towards innovative supportive care to make sure that the voice of family caregivers is also heard and that their agency is maintained in decision-making. The integration of these measures of support not only benefits the families but ultimately brings honor and comfort to the patients during their final days (Pettifer et al., 2019).

Test Your Knowledge

1. What is the primary role of Disease-Modifying Antirheumatic Drugs (DMARDs) in the treatment of autoimmune diseases?
2. How do biologic therapies target specific components of the immune system?
3. What are the potential risks and benefits of long-term DMARD or biologic therapy for autoimmune disease management?

SUMMARY

In summarizing from conversations included in this chapter, there is a basic significance in emphasizing the change potential of such things as social innovation and moral phenomenology. These theories not only impact theoretical discourse but also policy practice and ethical reasoning. Social innovation development highlights the radical shift in understanding societies dynamics, from merely maximizing personal utility to creating collective processes that address structural imbalances. As highlighted in the study, this shift highlights the need to integrate holistic approaches for addressing complex social issues. The need for interdisciplinarity emerges most strongly, as an encounter with various disciplines is able to yield richer information and more effective solutions to contemporary issues, aligning exactly with adaptation and expansion required in today's policy space (Ayob et al., 2016). The dialogue between moral phenomenology and ethical issues also accounts for the intricate character of decision-making on an individual and collective level. By analyzing the experiential aspects of moral life, researchers can gain a deeper insight into how moral judgments guide behavior and shape social norms. Through a consideration of the root challenges that have been established by the study of moral phenomenology, it is evident that these subjective experiences are not only real but also extremely influential in forming the moral terrain. This overlap of experience and ethical theory demands more nuanced knowledge of moral reasoning, bridging gaps among rival philosophical stances and thus enhancing the discourse on morality and ethics. It is thus imperative to integrate these findings into more comprehensive social policies to ensure that ethical issues are placed at the forefront of societal advancement (Kriegel et al., 2020). Finally, the consequences of combining social innovation and moral phenomenology extend beyond scholarly analysis; they require practical steps that promote social justice and ethical practice. Seeing the complexities of human experiences and collective activities will unlock innovative solutions to society's biggest problems. As described in this chapter, embracing these transdisciplinary approaches makes it possible to gain a profound understanding of the interconnectedness of policy development and ethical consideration. The need for new structures highlighting cooperation, empathy, and moral responsibility is more acute than ever. Through an open climate of critical reflection and collective conversation, we can drive the effective change that produces a more equitable future, demonstrating the significance of social innovation and moral phenomenology in contemporary discourse (Ayob et al., 2016; Kriegel et al., 2020).

Complete comprehension of academic writing calls for the cultivation of various higher-order thinking abilities, most notably evaluation and synthesis. As evidenced studies show, undergraduate learners are prone to falter in applying such higher-order thinking skills. Such difficulty could be due to either underestimating the importance of such skills in written coursework or realization that such skills are exertion-demanding beyond description writing. Critical thinking workshops are front and center in bridging this gap. Research indicates that students who participate in directed sessions whose intent is to build a question that they resolve in their chapter perform better than students who do not participate in such courses. As a result, the development of an environment that encourages critical engagement and questioning is likely to greatly improve academic performance and understanding among learners (Henri et al., 2015). The role of ownership within the learning process cannot be overemphasized. By providing learners with the opportunity to choose areas of interest, teachers are in a position to encourage motivation and passion for complicated assignments, which are essential in the acquisition of critical thinking skills. The aforementioned workshops showcase the same principle, where the capability to make choices leads to higher levels of ownership in the learning material, which is directly related to higher engagement levels. The same process also transcends what is rote and encourages students to appreciate using critical thinking in the context of learning their subject matter. Interacting with content on which they are focused not only serves to facilitate memorization of content but also guarantees fuller understanding of the content. Thus, incorporating strategies that emphasize student agency is essential for academic success (Henri et al., 2015). Legal scholarship, especially in areas of judicial interpretation, also communicates the importance of sophisticated understanding and application of critical thinking. Katyals treatment of originalism is indicative of such subtlety, as he creates distinct interpretative frameworks for the judiciary and legislative courts. His treatment encompasses foundational pillars , such as history, precedent, and moral philosophy, thus indicating how they converge to direct judicial decisions. Above all, Katyal demonstrates that courts' interpretative method may be substantially different from legislative interpretation, demanding more context and application scrutiny. This separation is crucial to understanding the broader application of legal texts and how meaning can vary based on the perspective of analysis. Thus, coming at the different views enlarges not just critical analysis in a legal context but also ensures a more refined discussion about the complexities of law and governance.

KEY TERMS FROM THIS CHAPTER

- Allergic rhinitis
- Antigen-antibody complexes
- Autoimmunity
- Basophils
- Biomarkers
- Dangerous allergens
- Diffuse parenchymal lung diseases (DPLD)
- Electronic health records (EHR)
- Genetic factors
- Hemolytic anemia
- Antibody-mediated hypersensitivity
- Autoimmune reactions
- Autoimmunity-related illness
- Biologic therapies
- Corticosteroids
- Diagnostic quality
- Drug provocation test (DPT)
- Foreign substance
- Genetic predisposition
- Hypereosinophilic syndrome (HES)

CRITICAL THINKING QUESTIONS

1. Which of the following is an example of a Type II hypersensitivity reaction?

a. Allergic rhinitis caused by pollen

b. Hemolytic anemia due to autoantibodies against red blood cells

c. Contact dermatitis caused by poison ivy

d. Serum sickness caused by immune complex deposition

2. Which mechanism best explains the development of autoimmunity?

a. Excessive production of IgE antibodies

b. Breakdown of self-tolerance leading to an immune response against self-antigens

c. Overproduction of complement proteins

d. Deficiency of neutrophils leading to recurrent infections

3. Which autoimmune disease is characterized by antibodies against the thyroid peroxidase enzyme?

a. Rheumatoid arthritis

b. Systemic lupus erythematosus

c. Hashimoto's thyroiditis

d. Multiple sclerosis

4. Which diagnostic test is commonly used to detect systemic lupus erythematosus (SLE)?

a. Antinuclear antibody (ANA) test

b. Anti-cyclic citrullinated peptide (anti-CCP) antibody test

c. Rheumatoid factor (RF) test

d. Serum IgE level measurement

5. Which of the following is a common treatment option for hypersensitivity and autoimmune diseases?

a. Antibiotics targeting bacterial infections

b. Vaccination with live attenuated viruses

c. Antihistamines only

d. Immunosuppressive drugs , such as corticosteroids

Short Answer Questions

1. What are the four types of hypersensitivity reactions, and what immune mechanisms characterize each type?
2. How do Type I hypersensitivity reactions (immediate hypersensitivity) develop, and what role do IgE antibodies and mast cells play in this process?
3. Describe the mechanism behind Type II hypersensitivity reactions and provide examples of autoimmune diseases caused by this reaction.
4. What is the role of immune complexes in Type III hypersensitivity reactions, and which diseases are commonly associated with this type?
5. Explain how Type IV hypersensitivity differs from the other types in terms of immune response and timeline, and give examples of clinical conditions where it is seen.

Answers to Critical Thinking Questions

1. (b) 2. (b) 3. (c) 4. (a) 5. (d)

REFERENCES

1. Aberer, W., Biló, M. B., Bodzenta-Lukaszyk, A., Bonifazi, F., et al. (2013). Clinical effectiveness of Hymenoptera venom immunotherapy. https://core.ac.uk/download/12175772.pdf (accessed on 13th June 2025).
2. Adamusiak, A. M., Alkhatib, E. H., Bellin, M. D., Brooks, J., et al. (2023). Case report: Insulin hypersensitivity in youth with type 1 diabetes. https://core.ac.uk/download/604217912.pdf (accessed on 13th June 2025).
3. Aletaha, D., McInnes, I. B., & Smolen, J. S. (2016). *Rheumatoid Arthritis.* https://core.ac.uk/download/77600864.pdf (accessed on 13th June 2025).
4. Alisi, A., Alterio, A., Della Corte, C., Mosca, A., et al. (2015). Pediatric liver diseases: Current challenges and future perspectives. https://core.ac.uk/download/84688423.pdf (accessed on 13th June 2025).
5. Antón, A., Arrese Muñoz, I., Bas Minguet, J., Blanco Grau, A., et al. (2022). Exposing and overcoming limitations of clinical laboratory tests in COVID-19 by adding immunological parameters: A retrospective cohort analysis and pilot study. https://core.ac.uk/download/586702700.pdf (accessed on 13th June 2025).
6. Apostol, A. C., Beaudin, A. E., & Jensen, K. D. C. (2020). Training the fetal immune system through maternal inflammation–A layered hygiene hypothesis. https://core.ac.uk/download/288432714.pdf (accessed on 13th June 2025).
7. Appelbaum, B., Black, R., Bradshaw, T., Short, B., Ceri, D., Delaney, C., Darveau, R., et al. (2019). Polymicrobial oral biofilm models: Simplifying the complex. https://core.ac.uk/download/293867880.pdf (accessed on 13th June 2025).
8. Arasi, S., Barni, S., Bottau, P., Caffarelli, C., et al. (2018). SIAIP position paper: Provocation challenge to antibiotics and non-steroidal anti-inflammatory drugs in children. https://core.ac.uk/download/188829702.pdf (accessed on 13th June 2025).
9. Aventaggiato, M., Bruscolini, A., Duse, M., Iannaccone, A., et al. (2018). Vascular endothelial growth factor (VEGF) serological and lacrimal signaling in patients affected by vernal keratoconjunctivitis (VKC). https://core.ac.uk/download/188829646.pdf (accessed on 13th June 2025).
10. Ayob, N., Fagan, K., & Teasdale, S. (2016). How social innovation "came to be": Tracing the evolution of a contested concept. https://core.ac.uk/download/293880907.pdf (accessed on 13th June 2025).
11. Babiloni, C., Boeijinga, P. H., Brunovsky, M., Drinkenburg, W. H., Ffytche, D. H., Freeman, J., et al. (2012). Guidelines for the recording and evaluation of pharmaco-EEG data in man: The International Pharmaco-EEG Society (IPEG). https://core.ac.uk/download/54522901.pdf (accessed on 13th June 2025).
12. Baianu, I. C. (2011). Complex systems analysis of cell cycling models in carcinogenesis. https://core.ac.uk/download/pdf/290191.pdf (accessed on 13th June 2025).
13. Baianu, I. C., & Prisecaru, M. S. V. (2004). Complex systems analysis of arrested neural cell differentiation during development and analogous cell cycling models in carcinogenesis. https://core.ac.uk/download/pdf/85970.pdf (accessed on 13th June 2025).

14. Bajema, I. M., Bertsias, G. K., Boumpas, D. T., Gordon, C., et al. (2015). Lupus nephritis management guidelines compared. https://core.ac.uk/download/77009956.pdf (accessed on 13th June 2025).

15. Baldini, E., Carbotta, G., Catania, A., D'Armiento, M., et al. (2017). Vitiligo and autoimmune thyroid disorders. https://core.ac.uk/download/127588138.pdf (accessed on 13th June 2025).

16. Barrett, S., Blanca, M., Blanca-López, N., Carr, D. F., et al. (2020). Beta-lactam-induced immediate hypersensitivity reactions: A genome-wide association study of a deeply phenotype cohort. https://core.ac.uk/download/334954369.pdf (accessed on 13th June 2025).

17. Barry, P. D., & O'Farrell, A. G. (2014). *Geometry in the Transition from Primary to Post-Primary*. https://core.ac.uk/download/297019125.pdf (accessed on 13th June 2025).

18. Bennett, T. D., Callahan, T. J., Carmody, L., Champion, J., et al. (2019). Semantic integration of clinical laboratory tests from electronic health records for deep phenotyping and biomarker discovery. https://core.ac.uk/download/228991424.pdf (accessed on 13th June 2025).

19. Boonstra, B. (2016). *Mapping Trajectories of Becoming: Four Forms of Behavior in Co-Housing Initiatives*. https://core.ac.uk/download/55743980.pdf (accessed on 13th June 2025).

20. Bosnic-Anticevich, S. Z., Carney, A. S., Carter, V., Christian, R., et al. (2017). Seasonal patterns of oral antihistamine and intranasal corticosteroid purchases from Australian community pharmacies: A retrospective observational study. https://core.ac.uk/download/131024570.pdf (accessed on 13th June 2025).

21. Brown, K. K., Colby, T. V., Galvin, J. R., Goldin, J., et al. (2017). Diagnostic criteria for idiopathic pulmonary fibrosis: A Fleischner Society white paper. https://core.ac.uk/download/148790433.pdf (accessed on 13th June 2025).

22. Brys, A. K., Sheth, M. R., Sohn, D. D., Sweidan, R., et al. (2015). Diagnostic and therapeutic considerations in idiopathic hyper eosinophilia with warm autoimmune hemolytic anemia. https://core.ac.uk/download/323075654.pdf (accessed on 13th June 2025).

23. Burnett, C., Chen, L., Edwards, P., Norman, G., et al. (2014). TRAAC: Trust and risk aware access control. https://core.ac.uk/download/42130694.pdf (accessed on 13th June 2025).

24. Burns, H. (2019). *The Development of Hypersensitivity Reactions in The Pediatric Population: A Review*. https://core.ac.uk/download/213464303.pdf (accessed on 13th June 2025).

25. Bussolati, G., Mantovani, A., Morrone, M. C., Patrono, C., et al. (2022). Long COVID: Where we stand and challenges ahead. https://core.ac.uk/download/614026981.pdf (accessed on 13th June 2025).

26. Canter, R. J., Judge, S. J., & Murphy, W. J. (2020). Characterizing the dysfunctional NK cell: Assessing the clinical relevance of exhaustion, anergy, and senescence. https://core.ac.uk/download/323070535.pdf (accessed on 13th June 2025).

27. Carnevale, A., Casoni, G. L., Cavagna, L., Furini, F., et al. (2019). The role of the multidisciplinary evaluation of interstitial lung diseases: Systematic literature review of the current evidence and future perspectives. https://core.ac.uk/download/275692836.pdf (accessed on 13th June 2025).

28. Cebrian-de-la-Serna, M., Lemos-de-Carvalho-Júnior, G., Raposo-Rivas, M., Sarmiento-Campos, J. A., et al. (2018). Analysis of the pedagogical perspective of the MOOCs available in Portuguese. https://core.ac.uk/download/214842676.pdf (accessed on 13th June 2025).

29. Chaplain, M. A. J., Eftimie, R., & Macfarlane, F. R. (2019). Quantitative predictive modelling approaches to understanding rheumatoid arthritis: A brief review. https://core.ac.uk/download/286356117.pdf (accessed on 13th June 2025).
30. Cisek, K., Delles, C., Filip, S., Gakiopoulou, H., et al. (2017). Identification of novel molecular signatures of IgA nephropathy through an integrative-omics analysis. https://core.ac.uk/download/96883268.pdf (accessed on 13th June 2025).
31. Clarke, A., Connock, M., Court, R. A., Cummins, C., et al. (2013). *Belimumab: A Technological Advance for Systemic Lupus Erythematosus Patients? Report of a Systematic Review and Meta-Analysis.* https://core.ac.uk/download/16664132.pdf (accessed on 13th June 2025).
32. Clement, A., Laverty, A., Freihorst, A., Hartl, D., et al. (2009). Incidence and classification of pediatric diffuse parenchymal lung diseases in Germany. https://core.ac.uk/download/pdf/8364093.pdf (accessed on 13th June 2025).
33. Comellas, M., Dilla, T., Díaz Torne, C., Díaz, M., et al. (2020). What matters most to patients and rheumatologists? A discrete choice experiment in rheumatoid arthritis. https://core.ac.uk/download/304372039.pdf (accessed on 13th June 2025).
34. Croce, A., D'Aguanno, V., De Vincentiis, M., De Virgilio, A., et al. (2018). Audio-vestibular symptoms in systemic autoimmune diseases. https://core.ac.uk/download/188823057.pdf (accessed on 13th June 2025).
35. Desjardins, E., Jevnikar, A. M., & Singh, B. (2024). Artificial intelligence, big data, and regulation of immunity: Challenges and opportunities. https://core.ac.uk/download/621598864.pdf (accessed on 13th June 2025).
36. Duncanson, M. E. (2019). *Experimental Immunology and The Potential for Osteopathological Reconstructions: Pursuing an Experimental Foundation for The Skeletal Inflammatory Index.* https://core.ac.uk/download/223224095.pdf (accessed on 13th June 2025).
37. Hajimoradlou, A., Poole, D., & Roberti, G. (2020). Predicting landslides using locally aligned convolutional neural networks. Proceedings of the Twenty-Ninth International Joint Conference on Artificial Intelligence
38. Henri, D., Morrell, L., & Scott, G. (2015). Ask a clearer question, get a better answer. https://core.ac.uk/download/151157342.pdf (accessed on 13th June 2025).
39. Jaffe, M. S., & Leveson, N. G. (1989). Completeness, robustness, and safety in real-time software requirements specification. https://core.ac.uk/download/484245953.pdf (accessed on 13th June 2025).
40. Josephine, A., Renjith, K. R., Sindhu, K., Simi, N., et al. (2023). Endocrine autoimmunity in association with female infertility. https://core.ac.uk/download/591404113.pdf (accessed on 13th June 2025).
41. Rosyadi, M. I., Tetehfio, M., et al. (2023). The role of AI in vocational education: A systematic literature review. https://core.ac.uk/download/599141043.pdf (accessed on 13th June 2025).
42. Kaminogawa, S., & Nanno, M. (2004). Modulation of Immune Functions by Foods. *Evidence-based complementary and alternative medicine : eCAM, 1*(3), 241–250. https://doi.org/10.1093/ecam/neh042of immune functions by foods. https://core.ac.uk/download/pdf/3552804.pdf (accessed on 13th June 2025).

43. Katyal, N. K. (2000). Impeachment as congressional constitutional interpretation. https://core.ac.uk/download/62568827.pdf (accessed on 13th June 2025).
44. Kriegel, U. (2020). Moral experience: Its existence, describability, and significance. https://core.ac.uk/download/131213466.pdf (accessed on 13th June 2025).
45. Kronstadt, J. (2008). *Genetics and Economic Mobility.* https://core.ac.uk/download/71351453.pdf (accessed on 13th June 2025).
46. Kros, J. M., Li, J., & Zheng, P. P. (2018). Approved CAR T cell therapies. https://core.ac.uk/download/154410949.pdf (accessed on 13th June 2025).
47. Lee, J. C., & Stankey, C. T. (2023). Translating non-coding genetic associations into a better understanding of immune-mediated disease. https://core.ac.uk/download/558911414.pdf (accessed on 13th June 2025).
48. Lo, M. S., Son, M. B. F., Sundel, R. P., Zurakowski, D., et al. (2014). Hypergammaglobulinemia in the pediatric population as a marker for underlying autoimmune disease: A retrospective cohort study. https://core.ac.uk/download/28947012.pdf (accessed on 13th June 2025).
49. Matthews, P. M., Montalban, X., Petrie, J. L., Ramagopalan, S. V., et al. (2023). Real-world evaluation of ocrelizumab in multiple sclerosis: A systematic review. https://core.ac.uk/download/581114593.pdf (accessed on 13th June 2025).
50. Pettifer, A. (2021). *The Experiences of Family Members Witnessing the Diminishing Drinking of a Dying Relative in Hospital: A Narrative Inquiry.* https://core.ac.uk/download/478153186.pdf (accessed on 13th June 2025).
51. Pettifer, A., Bird, A., Froggatt, K., Kuhn, T., Meares, C. J., Neuberger, J., & Hughes, S. (2019). The experiences of family members witnessing the diminishing drinking of a dying relative: An adapted meta-narrative literature review. https://core.ac.uk/download/228158270.pdf (accessed on 13th June 2025).
52. Schievink, B. P., Wilson, D. E., Dean, E., Doak, E. B., Shane, J. S., & Van Vlack, T. (2014). Lifestyle factors in hypertension drug research: Systematic analysis of articles in a leading Cochrane report. https://core.ac.uk/download/205351283.pdf (accessed on 13th June 2025).
53. Scholma, L. M. (2025). *The Relationship Between Food Allergies and Intolerances and The Development of Disordered Eating Patterns.* https://core.ac.uk/download/651275692.pdf (accessed on 13th June 2025).
54. Seita, H. M. (2013). *Food Allergies in Pregnant Women: A Study of Prevalence in Expecting Mothers and Association with Neonatal Outcomes.* https://open.bu.edu/bitstream/2144/12219/6/Seita_Helene_2013.pdf (accessed on 13th June 2025).
55. Shah, P. L., & Slebos, D. J. (2020). Bronchoscopy interventions for severe emphysema: Where are we now? https://core.ac.uk/download/363146082.pdf (accessed on 13th June 2025).
56. Smedley, C., Fisher, K., Wong, M., Kayess, R., & Bates, S. (2014). *Arthritis and Disability.* https://core.ac.uk/download/pdf/30673486.pdf (accessed on 13th June 2025).

INDEX

B

C

H

I

S

T

U

V

W

Z